HANDBOOK OF DIAGNOSTIC IMAGING

VOLUME 1

PRINCIPLES, PHYSICS, AND TECHNOLOGIES

Dr. José Abraham Amaya Duarte

ALLIED HEALTH PRESS

Handbook of Diagnostic Imaging Volume 1

Principles, Physics, and Technologies

Author: **Dr. José Abraham Amaya Duarte**

Allied Health Press
4164 Lakeshore Road
Burlington ON L7L 1A4
Canada
www.alliedhealthpress.com
Email: orders@arclereducation.com

ISBN: 978-1-77956-865-6

ABOUT THE AUTHOR

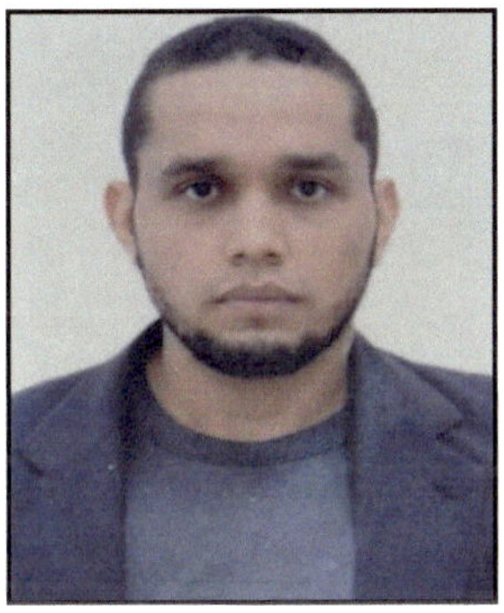

Dr. José Abraham Amaya Duarte is a radiologist with extensive clinical and academic experience in diagnostic imaging, advanced image interpretation, and image-guided procedures. His expertise includes ultrasound, computed tomography (CT), magnetic resonance imaging (MRI), and radiography across a broad range of clinical applications.

He earned his Doctor of Medicine and Surgery degree from the Universidad Nacional Autónoma de Nicaragua (UNAN-León) and completed his specialization in Diagnostic Imaging at the Universidad de Defensa de Nicaragua (UDENIC). To further enhance his expertise, Dr. Amaya pursued advanced subspecialty training in musculoskeletal, neuro, and women's imaging, and is currently completing a Master's degree in Obstetric and Gynecologic Ultrasound.

Dr. Amaya currently serves as a Radiology and Imaging Specialist at Sugar City Medical Center in Belize, where he provides comprehensive diagnostic evaluations and supports multidisciplinary clinical teams. His professional background also includes academic instruction, pediatric medicine, and international teleradiology services for hospitals and clinics worldwide.

A dedicated educator and researcher, Dr. Amaya's professional focus lies in improving diagnostic accuracy, clinical workflow, and imaging quality through continuous education and collaboration. His commitment to excellence and his contributions to clinical radiology continue to advance the field across Latin America and beyond.

Brief Table of Contents

Detailed Table of Contents

CHAPTER 5

Magnetic Resonance Imaging Fundamentals 123

CHAPTER 6

Ultrasound Physics and Instrumentation 155

CHAPTER 9

Contrast Media in Imaging: Types, Administration, and Safety 245

CHAPTER 10

Radiation Dosimetry and Patient Safety 275

CHAPTER 11

Digital Image Acquisition and Quality Control 305

CHAPTER 12

Picture Archiving and Communication Systems (PACS) in Medical Imaging 335

LIST OF FIGURES

PREFACE

Diagnostic imaging has transformed the practice of medicine by providing a glimpse into the human body without the need for invasive intervention. From the first identification of X-rays to the advanced modalities of today, imaging technologies have expanded diagnostic capabilities and influenced treatment choices across nearly every field of medical specialization. By applying principles of physics and engineering, these methods transmute biology's shape and function into observable signals so that clinicians can detect disease at an early stage, monitor the response to therapy, and plan surgical treatment more precisely. Advances in imaging have been provoked by ongoing advances in radiation physics, detector technology, and computational reconstruction, producing images with ever greater detail and diagnostic power.

The convergence of various imaging techniques—ranging from conventional radiography and computed tomography to magnetic resonance imaging and nuclear medicine—has provided a broad range of tools for evaluating anatomy and physiology. They employ various physical interactions and equipment, but all aim to present as much diagnostic information as possible while minimizing risk to patients. This image quality and safety balance invokes an understanding of principles of radiation management, detector operation, and system calibration. As medical imaging is increasingly applied to functional imaging and hybrid systems, competent practitioners well-versed with theory as much as practice have never been more needed.

Handbook of Diagnostic Imaging Volume 1 is intended as a comprehensive guide for students, radiologic technologists, and medical specialists seeking a solid foundation in imaging science. This volume consolidates leading-edge information on image formation physics, instrumentation, applied techniques, and safety. Every chapter provides simple-to-grasp explanations, supplemented by examples and illustrations, to help readers develop a sound footing before moving on to more sophisticated issues in later volumes or domains of specialized practice.

Chapter 1 presents the basic physics relevant to medical imaging, beginning with the interaction between radiation and matter. It covers the photoelectric effect, Compton scattering, and pair production, then the production of X-rays and the characteristics of the resulting spectrum. Principles of image formation, like geometric unsharpness and modulation transfer function, are thoroughly discussed. Finally, units of radiation, methods of measurement, image signal-to-noise, and elementary safety principles like ALARA and personal monitoring are touched on.

Chapter 2 covers the detector design and operation as well as the imaging instrumentation. X-ray tube design is covered in the X-ray tube design topic, including discussions of anode materials, anode cooling, focal spot shape and size, and the high-voltage generator. Flat-panel detectors are investigated for indirect- and direct-conversion panels, dynamic range, and detective quantum efficiency. Also covered are image intensifiers, scintillation and photomultiplier detectors, and semiconductor types of detectors as well as key performance factors such as linearity, lag, and modulation transfer function.

Chapter 3 discusses standard radiography techniques used in daily clinical routine. Projectional radiography techniques for chest, abdominal, and skeletal imaging are described, along with concepts of fluoroscopy, including continuous vs pulsed operation and dose control. : The workflow of digital radiography involves acquisition modes, processing algorithms, and archiving. Tomosynthesis techniques, image-quality optimization approaches, and quality-assurance methodologies for day-to-day detector testing and preventive maintenance conclude the chapter.

Chapter 4 addresses computed tomography, from scanner design and gantry mechanics (e.g., slip-ring and patient table design) to data acquisition modes such as axial, helical, and dual-source scanning, contrasted with one another. Image reconstruction techniques range from filtered back projection to iterative and model-based algorithms. Protocol optimization ranges from kVp, mAs, pitch, and rotation time to contrast timing selection. Advanced CT applications, such as dual-energy imaging, perfusion imaging, and CT angiography, are included, as are dose management techniques, including automatic exposure control and dose monitoring.

Chapter 5 depicts the theory of magnetic resonance imaging. The physical principles of nuclear magnetic resonance, including spin dynamics, the Larmor frequency, and relaxation mechanisms, are explained. The physics part describes the main magnet types, gradient systems, and RF coil designs. Principles of pulse sequences like spin-echo, gradient-echo, and inversion recovery are described, followed by an explanation of image contrast mechanisms and artifacts.

Safety considerations explain RF heating, ferromagnetic hazards, and implant-related contraindications.

Chapter 6 summarizes ultrasound physics and equipment. Acoustic wave properties — such as frequency, wavelength, attenuation, and impedance — are reviewed, along with transducer technologies, including piezoelectric materials, array types, and bandwidth issues. Imaging modes like B-mode, Doppler, and M-mode are outlined. Image formation processes, such as beam steering and time-gain compensation, are introduced, as are quantitative ultrasound methods, such as elastography and contrast-enhanced imaging. Safety considerations include mechanical and thermal indices and cavitation concerns.

Chapter 7 covers nuclear medicine, with emphasis on gamma camera design and single-photon emission computed tomography. Techniques for radioisotope production, methods of radiolabeling, and quality control are presented. The gamma camera section covers collimator selection, scintillation crystals, and photomultiplier arrays. Planar imaging protocols, tomographic SPECT acquisition, reconstruction algorithms, and attenuation correction techniques are covered. Quality assurance tests and significant clinical applications, such as cardiac perfusion and bone scintigraphy, conclude the chapter.

Chapter 8 covers the fundamentals of positron emission tomography. The annihilation physics of positrons and the detection of annihilation photons, as well as scanner elements such as scintillation materials and time-of-flight, are explained. Acquisition and reconstruction approaches, quantitative imaging techniques such as SUV calculation and kinetic modeling, and radiopharmaceutical production are covered. Hybrid PET/CT and PET/MRI integration are also covered in the chapter, with an emphasis on attenuation mapping and clinical workflow problems.

Chapter 9 discusses contrast media used in imaging diagnostics, starting with iodinated and gadolinium-containing contrast agents, their preparation, dose calculation, and safety. It also covers ultrasound microbubble contrast, radiopharmaceutical safety, administration, and disposal procedures, and adverse reaction management and pre- and post-procedure patient care, providing practical advice for patient preparation and monitoring.

Chapter 10 covers dosimetry of radiation and concepts of patient safety. It outlines fundamental dose concepts, dose measurement using dosimeters and OSL devices, and dose optimization methods such as protocol adaptation and adaptive exposure control. Regulation policy from international and national bodies are outlined. The chapter concludes with guidelines on risk communication, informed consent, and occupational safety practices, such as shielding practices and personal protective equipment.

Chapter 11 is digital image acquisition and quality control. Sampling and quantization, bit depth, aliasing artifacts, and post-processing techniques such as edge enhancement and noise reduction are some of the topics discussed in this chapter. Monitor calibration and ambient lighting are among the display system considerations. Acceptance testing, routine inspection, and cybersecurity measures, along with quality assurance procedures for their implementation, are discussed, as are workflow automation strategies to reduce errors and improve efficiency.

Chapter 12 provides an overview of picture archiving and communication systems (PACS). Client-server, web-based, and cloud-native PACS solution structures are described. DICOM standard components, security extensions, and integration with hospital information systems are detailed. Data storage methods, disaster recovery planning, and user interface choices such as 2D/3D workplaces and mobile viewers are discussed. System management concerns, such as performance monitoring, backups, and user training, make up the final chapter.

This text is designed for radiology residents, medical physicists, radiologic technologists, biomedical engineers, and clinicians seeking an easy-to-use yet comprehensive review of the principles and applications of diagnostic imaging.

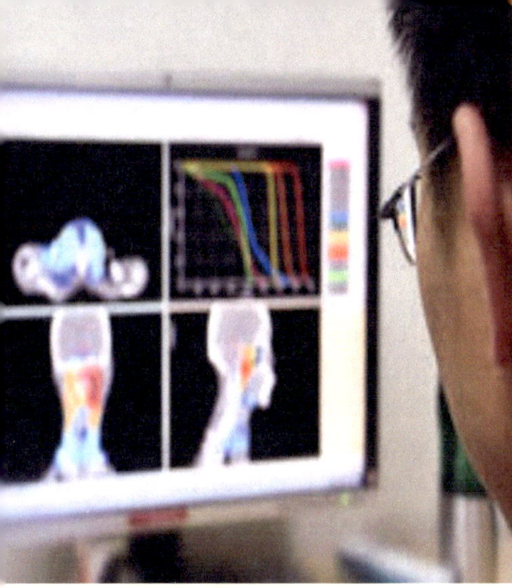

Chapter 1

FUNDAMENTAL PHYSICS OF MEDICAL IMAGING

Contents

Introduction

The discipline of medical imaging is a critical component of modern medicine, serving as an invaluable aid in diagnosis, treatment planning, and disease monitoring. It is crucial to understand the physics of imaging modalities because not only does it encapsulate the science of image formation, but also emphasizes technological progress throughout time. Techniques such as X-ray, Computed Tomography (CT), Magnetic Resonance Imaging (MRI), and Ultrasound leverage fundamental physical principles to produce high-resolution internal images of the human body. Even more so, with today's boom in the application of artificial intelligence in imaging, command of these principles is essential. Without such information, professionals in the field cannot fully realize the technology's potential, thereby limiting patient care and advancements in outcomes (Cobo et al., 2025). The relationship between fundamental physics and medical imaging technologies illustrates how quantum mechanics and other physical sciences provide the foundation for these sophisticated systems. Magnetic Resonance Imaging

(MRI), for instance, relies on nuclear magnetic resonance principles based on quantum mechanics. By exploring the intricate process of image construction, from the beginning with signal generation to the end with image reconstruction, the contribution of physics is underscored correctly. One would understand how even magnetic field and resonance frequency variations can affect image resolution and quality. Also, ignorance of these principles can give birth to the limitation of new imaging techniques, where integration with modern computational techniques remains the mainstay. Thus, fostering an interdisciplinary culture among medical imaging specialists can accelerate further improvements in imaging capability (Islam, 2024). Further, rapid technological advances in artificial intelligence and machine learning have opened new avenues for innovation in medical imaging. While these technologies have immense promise for improving diagnostic accuracy and efficiency, their efficacy depends on a balanced understanding of the underlying physics. By applying physics principles, AI algorithms can be fine-tuned to leverage the strengths and weaknesses of imaging modalities. Convergence fosters a more systematic approach to overcoming challenges such as data availability and image quality. Ongoing pruning of imaging physics, particularly in the context of AI, foreshadows a convergence of disciplines toward eventual enhanced credibility and reliability of medical imaging findings. As medical imaging continues to broaden its horizon, it will be essential to cultivate a symbiotic partnership between technology and physics if breakthrough patient care outcomes are to be realized (Cobo et al., 2025) (Figure 1.1).

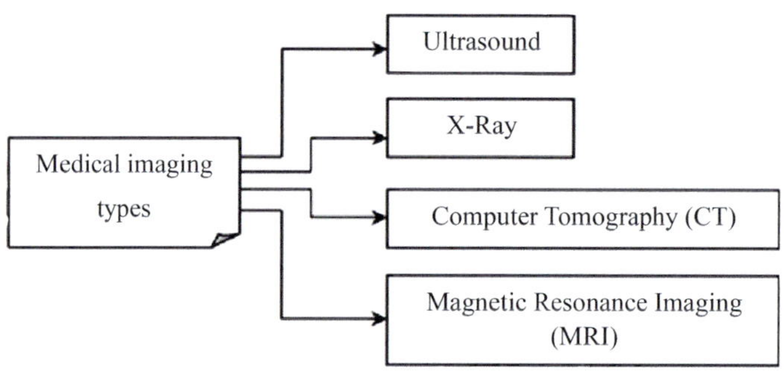

Figure 1.1. Overview diagram of major medical imaging modalities used in clinical diagnostics.

Source: https://www.researchgate.net/profile/M-Hanefi-Calp/publication/344313790/figure/fig35/AS:950761450139674@1603690602666/Block-diagram-of-medical-imaging-types.png.

1.1. Basic Principles of Physics

The basic principles of physics are crucial to the conception and operation of medical imaging modalities. These principles, for instance, electromagnetic radiation, wave-particle duality, and principles of energy transfer, are fundamental to understanding how various imaging modalities function. A case in point is X-ray imaging, one of the most prevalent techniques employed in modern medicine, founded on the interaction of high-energy photons with matter. When these photons pass through the body, they are absorbed differently depending on the density and nature of the tissues they traverse. Differential absorption creates the contrast that makes diagnostic images, demonstrating how physics directly enables the functionality of medical imaging equipment. A thorough grasp of these principles is required to optimize the use of medical imaging while ensuring patient safety, especially regarding radiation exposure, which is currently a significant consideration in medical practice (Hogg et al., 2015). In addition to these fundamental physics principles, however, the role that technology has played and continues to play in medical imaging cannot be overstated. Technological developments have revolutionized the capabilities of imaging techniques such as computed tomography (CT) and magnetic resonance imaging (MRI). For example, the integration of complex photonics-based detection systems into imaging technologies has enabled the production of images with exceptional resolution and clarity (Figure 1.2).

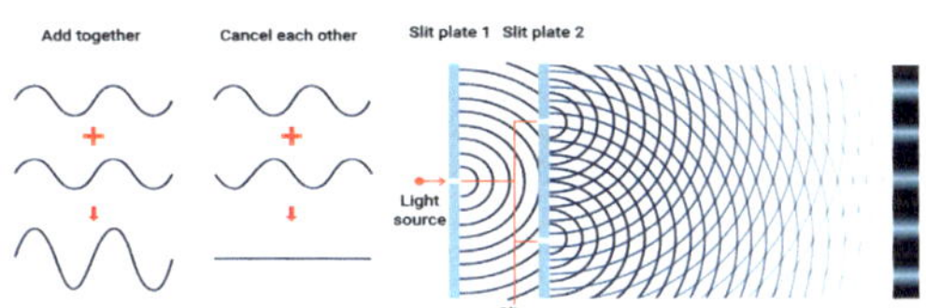

Figure 1.2. Conceptual diagram illustrating wave-particle duality of photons and electrons.

Source: https://photonterrace.net/en/photon/duality/file/276/img01.png.

Boston University Photonics Center's work on creating such technologies also underscores the value of interdisciplinarity in the fields of optics and medical device development (Center TBUP, 2017). Not only do such developments contribute to the diagnostic tools that can be made available to physicians, but they also initiate critical discussions regarding the balance between image quality and radiation protection. As increasingly advanced imaging techniques are developed, an understanding of the physics on which they rely will be crucial for practitioners to apply these technologies effectively and with reduced patient risk. Clinical application of medical imaging technology must further operate within the guidelines of accepted radiation protection and optimized dose. With increasing reliance on X-ray-based imaging, professionals are being asked to reduce patients' radiation exposure more and more, particularly in vulnerable groups such as the elderly and children (Hogg et al., 2015). This necessitates a comprehensive knowledge base of dose-minimizing principles, such as balanced diagnostic requirements and safety measures. Efforts to optimize imaging practice are supported by training that equips radiographers and technologists with essential radiation protection skills. The focus on evidence-based techniques for image quality assessment and lesion visibility underscores the need to integrate principles of physics into clinical practice. With each new advancement in medical imaging, grounding these fields in a solid grasp of physics remains important for ensuring effective diagnosis and patient safety.

1.1.1. Wave-Particle Duality

The duality between waves and particles is a fundamental concept of quantum mechanics of immense significance to the science of medical imaging. It propounds that particles such as electrons and photons exhibit wave and particle characteristics depending on the context in which they are observed. The duality is central to understanding how the various imaging procedures work, particularly those involving electromagnetic waves such as X-rays and MRI. In these modalities, an understanding of the interaction of matter with waves at the quantum level enables enhanced image formation, resolution, and discrimination between tissue types. Medical imaging devices thus leverage this duality to improve diagnostic capability, where an intimate understanding of the underlying physical principles governing wave-particle behavior in imaging becomes critical. Advances in medical imaging technologies are often intertwined with the exploration of wave-particle duality. A case in point is the adoption of terahertz (THz) frequencies in medical imaging, which has underscored the groundbreaking potential produced by the principle. Research has attested that THz waves have unique properties that can penetrate biological tissues, allowing for non-invasive imaging techniques with superior sensitivity towards the detection of various conditions, such as cancerous tissues. Understanding wave-particle duality directs the actions of these THz waves toward cellular structures and subsequently improves diagnostic equipment. It is described in current research that the advances in imaging technology leveraging the potential of THz frequencies can amount to a revolutionary change in medical diagnostics, illustrating how theoretical physics can be directly applied to beneficial medical purposes (Theodore et al., 2019). Further, wave-particle duality is converging with nanomedicine to drive emergent treatment and diagnostic imaging strategies. Engineered nanoparticles, here, are acting as contrast agents that take advantage of wave-particle duality to enhance imaging resolution and accuracy. Nanoparticles can alter the wave properties of incoming radiation, thereby enhancing signal contrast and enabling more precise feedback to facilitate clinician decision-making. The work currently being undertaken in nanomedicine involves nanoscale materials that can be engineered to respond to electromagnetic waves, thereby improving imaging outcomes (Pelaz et al., 2017). Wave-particle duality, thus, extends not only the limits of imaging technologies but also opens up possibilities for the development of new diagnostic devices that could redefine the standard of medical practice.

1.1.2. Electromagnetic Spectrum

The electromagnetic spectrum is a fundamental physical phenomenon with a wide range of frequencies and wavelengths, and is extremely important in medical imaging modalities. The spectrum includes various types of radiation, from radio waves and microwaves to infrared, visible light, ultraviolet, X-rays, and gamma rays. All kinds of electromagnetic radiation interact with matter in distinct ways, making it useful for specific medical procedures. For instance, gamma and X-rays, which are found at the high-energy end of the spectrum, are used primarily in radiology to create images of internal structures (Figure 1.3).

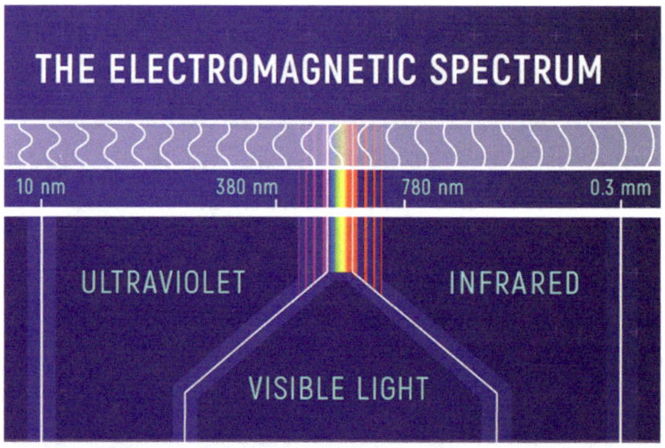

Figure 1.3. Full electromagnetic spectrum highlighting X-rays and gamma rays used in imaging.

Source: https://stsci-opo.org/STScI-01F8QGTR86KAVY61W98CQNH9Z5.jpg.

In contrast, infrared radiation is used in thermal imaging to detect heat differences, an important factor in diagnosing conditions such as inflammation or tumors. Familiarity with the unique properties and responsiveness of such wavelengths is essential in optimizing imaging modalities across most medical applications. Terahertz (THz) radiation, between microwave and infrared wavelengths, is a promising field for future medical imaging. This frequency band reveals unmistakable vibrational fingerprints that are beneficial in biospecimen analysis, thereby enabling label-free imaging technologies without recourse to potentially harmful contrast agents. In recent years, the broader application of THz technology beyond its traditional uses, such as security screening, has become increasingly popular in biomedical fields. For example, the use of THz waves can enable clear images of skin cancers without surgical intervention, thereby increasing patient comfort and diagnostic accuracy. Researchers further noted that THz waves provide a broad spectrum with very low photon energy, which is essential to preserve tissue integrity when imaging. Therefore, exploring THz applications for medical imaging enhances diagnostic quality and provides an opportunity to develop novel non-invasive imaging methods (Lee et al., 2022). The integration of state-of-the-art imaging technologies, including THz radiation, reflects the potential of interdisciplinarity for medical therapy and diagnostics. Terahertz source development and detector advances have widened the technical gap that once limited the range of clinical applications of THz radiation. These advances have led to the advent of more sophisticated algorithms for data processing, including real-time imaging and higher resolution. This increased dependability and sensitivity render THz imaging a vital tool in detecting several medical conditions, including cancers and other tissue abnormalities (Manjappa et al., 2020). Moreover, researchers are currently combining artificial intelligence and machine learning to enhance image interpretation, signaling a revolution in how medical imaging is handled. In short, the broad range of electromagnetic radiation, particularly the potential applications of THz radiation, represents a significant advancement in medical imaging technology, enhancing diagnostic capabilities and patient care.

1.1.3. Interaction of Radiation with Matter

As radiation, especially ionizing radiation like X-rays or gamma rays, travels through living tissues, it interacts with the electrons within the tissues. This may lead to many results, including ionization of atoms, electron excitation, or scattering. The first ionization produces secondary electrons that can ionize adjacent atoms, producing a cascade. Understanding of these interactions is important because it has a direct bearing on the quality of the images created in techniques such as computed tomography (CT) and X-ray imaging, whose resolution and contrast are based on the penetration ability of radiation and the extent of interaction with different tissue densities (Bracco et al., 2010). To this end, the specific mechanisms of interaction between radiation and matter are based on the energy levels of the radiation and the atomic constitution of the matter.

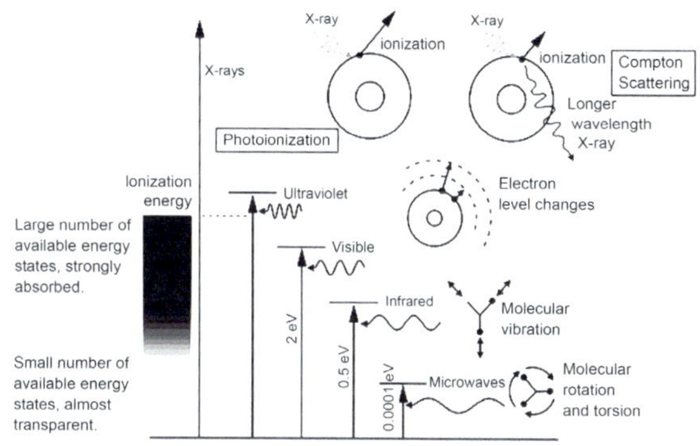

Figure 1.4. The interaction of radiation with matter is a fundamental phenomenon that underlies the principles of medical imaging.

Source: https://lh3.googleusercontent.com/proxy/fquGf0dH7ECsr5b3o76IndkKnKbX57gIlvL1Wm Cn0ZMEb hkrmwcBjdOl byl4tez997WWmUuOOBfCz_u8Hz6lVm9sEnfmIseZEjnlBnk.

For example, low-energy photons typically undergo photoelectric absorption, where they are entirely absorbed by an atom, resulting in heavy ionization. At higher energies, Compton scattering becomes predominant, allowing photons to lose energy through scattering with electrons. Such interactions are always emulated in computer environments employed in medical imaging, such as the J-PET Framework, which provides tools for data reconstruction and analysis based on such fundamental interactions.

Through simulations and understanding of these processes, scientists can optimize imaging procedures better, increasing diagnostic capability and patient care (Figure 1.4).Gajos et al. (2020) state that the knowledge of radiation interactions with matter is also vital in radiation safety and dosimetry, which play a significant role in medical imaging. Medical professionals should understand the potential risks of exposure to ionizing radiation, such as cell damage and carcinogenicity. Adequate dosimetry helps the absorbed patient dose to be measured and controlled throughout the imaging procedure, so the benefit is more significant than the risk of causing harm. Ongoing advances in imaging technology aim to reduce radiation doses while maintaining optimal image quality, calling for ongoing work on the interaction of radiation with matter. The overlap of safety, efficiency, and imaging performance underscores the primacy of physics in the design and application of medical imaging techniques (Bracco et al., 2010).

1.2. X-Ray Imaging

The development of X-ray imaging represents a seminal line of research in medical diagnostics, the interweaving of underlying physics with viable application. First identified in the late 19th century, X-ray technology transformed visual examinations of the human body, enabling the non-invasive inspection of skeletal injuries and pathological conditions. This mode of imaging relies on differential X-ray absorption during passage through body tissues, utilizing differences in tissue density and atomic structure. Bones, being denser, absorb more X-rays than soft tissues and thus generate a contrast that can be used for diagnosis. As technology became more advanced, digital systems integration eventually displaced traditional film-based imaging, offering higher-quality images and allowing immediate analysis. This development not only represents the technological advancement but also accentuates the importance of stringent physical principles in the manufacture and detection of X-rays, which still underlie today's medical practices (Vrdoljak et al., 2024). As much as contemporary X-ray imaging is concerned, the emergence of advanced computational techniques has further enhanced diagnostic capacity. Recent studies show robust synergy between physics and machine learning in developing robust imaging models, particularly through methods such as physics-informed machine learning (PIML) (Ghosh et al., 2024). The approach not only describes the important features of anatomical structures but also respects the underlying physics of X-ray interaction. By incorporating physics-based constraints into machine learning algorithms, the imaging process becomes more interpretable and sensitive, yielding enhanced precision in image reconstruction. These methods are particularly useful in low-dataset situations where traditional techniques may not work. The creation of such algorithms is a prime example of interactive synergy between technology and physics that ultimately supports clinical imaging in radiology and underscores the evolving nature of X-ray imaging strategies in modern medicine. The effect of X-ray imaging extends beyond short-term diagnostic applications, reflecting broader realignments in patient treatment and treatment protocols. The high resolution of X-ray images not only aids in the identification of pathologies but also supports treatment planning, particularly in oncology. The function of medical physicists becomes essential, ensuring safety adherence to protocols and optimizing imaging parameters for minimal radiation exposure, thus providing diagnostic efficacy with patient safety assurance (Vrdoljak et al., 2024). Additionally, research continues to strive to make imaging findings more readable, providing clinicians with more information about patient conditions. The revolutionary nature of X-ray imaging, especially when combined with enlightened processes such as those depicted in current studies, highlights its far-reaching implications within medical diagnosis. Thus, X-ray imaging continues to evolve, cementing its status as a cornerstone of medical imaging (Figure 1.5).

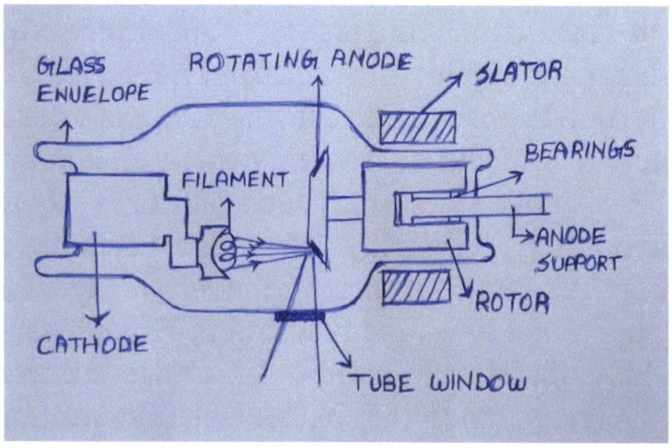

Figure 1.5. Basic components of an X-ray tube and beam filtration system.

Source: https://blogger.go ogleusercontent.com/img/b/R29 vZ2xl/AV vXsEghgXyWxn Ac8V1sx5jmwCyuxiQTbLbdaf697G_ QjBWmamHY TYtGAZ6M 3B2zDvLa1 Vhzjv5G4v8LT7dAkhwlxb eXyIyv3fPCuWlEo2ZuP A8a5k3_7yZTjT3TB27xfwwmTF1L e4XeHbU9aVY/s2048/x+ray+tube.jpg.

1.2.1. Mechanism of X-Ray Production

The production of X-rays is based on the interactions between high-energy electrons and matter, particularly in medical imaging. In an X-ray tube, electrons are created via thermionic emission from a hot filament and subsequently accelerated towards a target usually constructed by tungsten or molybdenum. Upon collision, high-energy electrons undergo two significant processes: characteristic radiation and Bremsstrahlung. Characteristic radiation occurs when an electron dislodges an inner-shell electron from the target atom. An electron from a higher energy level fills the vacancy, and this transition produces the release of energy in the form of an X-ray. Bremsstrahlung radiation occurs due to electrons being deflected by the target atom's nuclear electric fields, resulting in energy loss as X-ray photons. These processes are vital to generate the high-quality images needed in diagnostic radiology. The efficiency of X-ray production highly relies on several factors, such as the energy of the incident electrons, the target material's atomic number, and the operating conditions of the X-ray tube. Electron energy should be more than a critical level to cause characteristic efficiently and Bremsstrahlung radiation. With higher atomic number materials, production of X-rays is enhanced by virtue of a higher probability of interaction of electrons and higher efficiency of photon production, especially in the characteristic radiation process, where the energy of emitted X-ray is specific to the atomic structure of target materials (Figure 1.6).

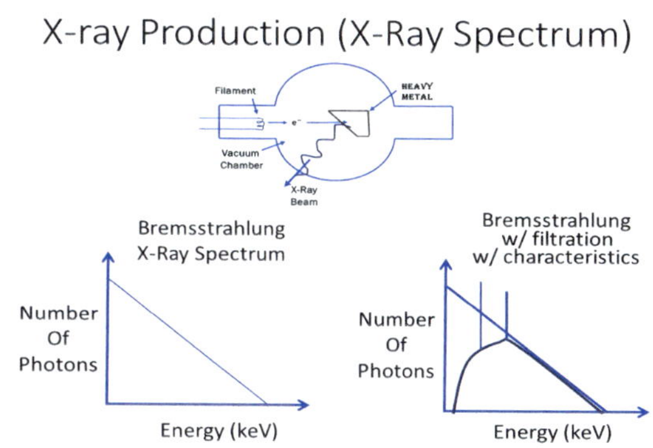

Figure 1.6. Diagram showing Bremsstrahlung and characteristic X-ray generation.

Source: https://cdn.shortpixel.ai/spai/w_1005+q_lossy+ret_img+to_webp/howradiologyworks.com/wp-content/uploads/2019/03/Spectrum-1.gif.

Operational conditions, such as tube current and voltage, also significantly affect the number and quality of emitted X-rays. Understanding these is important to have the best X-ray output with minimal patient exposure, a critical element in the medical imaging industry. Improvements in X-ray production technology continue to enable clinical imaging. Technologies such as digital X-ray detectors and sophisticated collimation techniques allow more precise targeting of X-ray beams, reducing scatter and improving image quality. Computer processing algorithms in X-ray imaging improve the visualization of anatomical features and pathologies, enabling proper diagnoses. As shown in recent studies, this technology has changed the use of X-rays, not just for routine imaging but also for new applications such as dual-energy X-ray absorptiometry for bone density measurement. Continued research into the mechanisms of X-ray production alongside these technological advances promises further simplification of medical imaging practice, with the twin advantages of effectiveness and safety for patients who rely on these diagnostic substances (Collaboration et al., 2024; Collaboration et al., 2025).

1.2.2. Image Formation and Contrast

The image formation process in medical imaging is crucial for obtaining clear, authentic diagnostic information. In imaging modalities such as X-ray computed tomography (CT), images are formed from the differential absorption of X-rays by body tissues. Contrast in the images relies on differences in tissue composition and density, which cause variations in the intensity of the X-rays received. In particular, contrast can be enhanced using an array of methods, some of which utilize contrast agents that increase the X-ray absorptivity of specific regions. This enhancement is crucial for distinguishing between healthy and pathological structures, so that clinicians can make sound decisions. Each new advance in imaging technology provides finer details on how contrast is manipulated, with the ability to greatly affect diagnostic precision as well as patient outcomes. Moreover, the role of noise in image formation cannot be underestimated, as it directly affects the readability and quality of medical images. In conventional absorption-based CT, noise variance scales inversely with the cube of spatial resolution, making it impossible to achieve high-resolution images without increasing noise (Arrizón et al., 2010). The advent of differential phase contrast imaging has offered a new frontier in overcoming these challenges. Interestingly, this approach adheres to an anomalous scaling law for noise variance in differential phase-contrast CT, which is inversely proportional to spatial resolution. This scenario yields substantial increases in image contrast and clarity, enabling better visualization of anatomical detail.

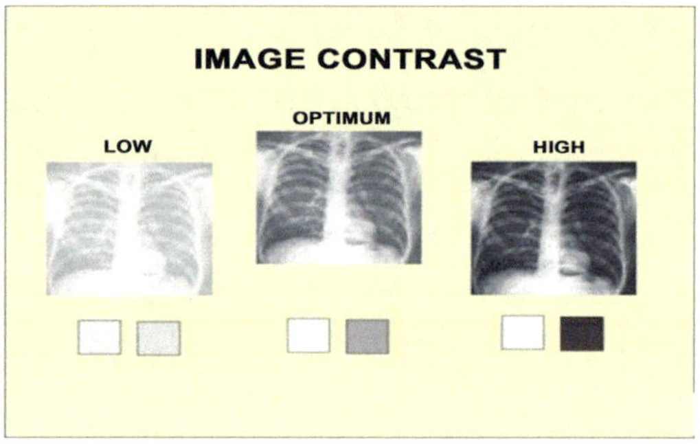

Figure 1.7. Comparison of radiographic images with high and low contrast.

Source: https://lh5.googleusercontent.com/proxy/J6dfh52UKdFyQ-s4dX7Y9MzDzWc5UD7vqzwLpAaXuRLSi9Pgep1Ugnqidiqk3q6zHOpnamd9c1beW_Vk_srW6IbGSmlm6j7WCjxD6PrOHZc.

As medical imaging evolves, it can be used to support diagnostic procedures and facilitate early disease diagnosis. Furthermore, developments in imaging technology hold profound significance for future medical diagnostics. Breakthroughs at facilities such as the Boston University Photonics Center illustrate how application and research converge in imaging technology (Center TBUP, 2017). The ongoing development of cutting-edge imaging technologies, including neurophotonics and biophotonic sensors, shows the prospects for more detailed visualization of complex biological processes. With translational research at the center, translation of these technologies to clinical use has the promise of refining image formation and contrast under dynamic conditions, such as in cancer diagnosis or neurologic testing. With the interdisciplinary research partnership among researchers, clinicians, and engineers still at the center, the future of medical imaging is also exciting, leading the way toward a new era of precision medicine (Figure 1.7).

1.2.3. Applications in Diagnostics

Applications of medical imaging for diagnosis abound and are crucial, yielding unparalleled visualization of the human body that allows for early disease detection and treatment.

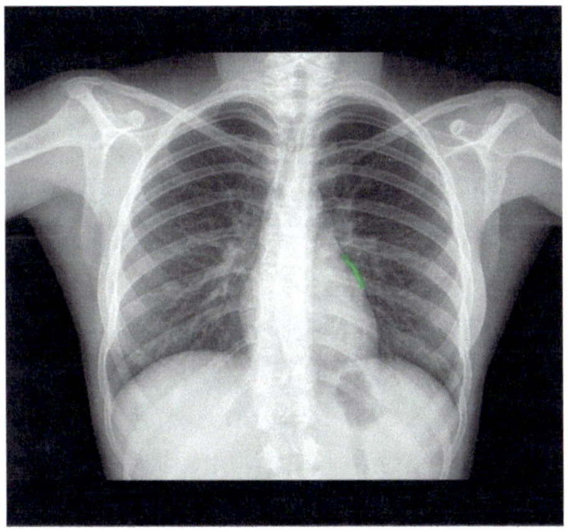

Figure 1.8. Chest X-ray highlighting pulmonary pathology in a clinical case.

Source: https://www.kenhub.com/thumbor/AkXFsw0396y894sLEMWlcDuChJA=/fit-in/800x1600/filters:watermark(/images/logo_url.png,-10,-10,0):background_color(FFFFFF):format(jpeg)/images/library/10851/eXtmE1V2XgsjZK2JolVQ5g_Border_of_left_atrium.png.

Radiology employs a range of imaging methods, grounded in fundamental physics principles, to visualize anatomical structure and physiological function. Techniques such as X-ray imaging and computed tomography (CT) produce high-resolution images that aid in the diagnosis of disease, from fractures to cancer (Figure 1.8).

The interpretive capability of such images is of utmost importance, enabling clinicians to ascertain the presence and extent of disease, which, in turn, informs treatment (Vrdoljak et al., 2024). Additionally, the transition to newer imaging modalities underscores the ongoing incorporation of novel technologies into diagnostic protocols, underscoring the fundamental role that physics plays as a facilitator of better patient outcomes. In recent years, the implementation of machine learning algorithms in diagnostic imaging has been among the milestones towards maximizing the effectiveness of standard imaging modalities. This paradigm is founded on leveraging the physics foundations to develop more advanced and interpretable system matrices within imaging processes, particularly in X-ray uses. By incorporating physics-informed machine learning (PIML) techniques, researchers have merged quantitative imaging information with machine learning algorithms to improve image reconstruction precision and predictive performance. This new approach not only streamlines diagnosis but also accounts for the inherent complexity of medical imaging, which can affect interpretation, thereby enabling higher diagnostic precision and earlier disease detection (Ghosh et al., 2024). The impact of advances in diagnostic imaging, driven by the laws of physics and facilitated by technology breakthroughs, extends beyond the diagnostics themselves. With greater fidelity and more interpretable images, doctors are increasingly able to apply more targeted therapeutic measures with reduced risks of unnecessary interventions and reduced exposure of patients to noxious radiation. Hence, the role of the medical physicist becomes even more significant in ensuring that imaging equipment is meticulously maintained and calibrated to guarantee patient safety. As medical imaging continues to advance, the emphasis on marrying fundamental physical principles with modern technological advances is sure to drive further innovation that will continue to improve diagnostic capabilities, streamline patient treatment, and transform the medical diagnostics landscape (Vrdoljak et al., 2024).

1.3. Computed Tomography (CT)

Computed Tomography (CT) is a medical imaging technology that enables non-invasive visualization of internal body structures with high precision. The principle behind CT is founded on the use of X-rays, which are generated from a rotating source and received by detectors located opposite the source.

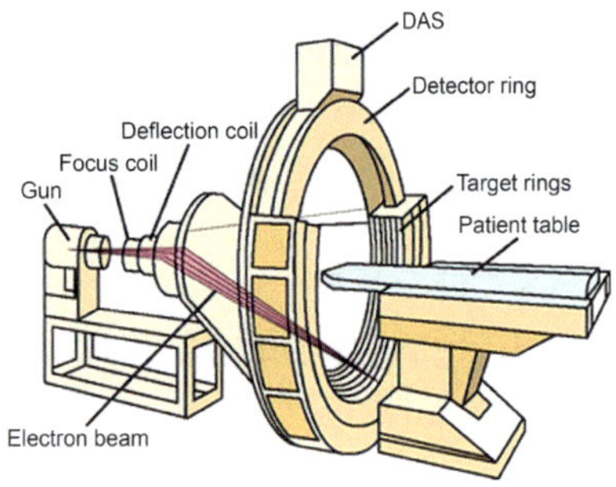

Figure 1.9. Cross-sectional schematic of a CT scanner and gantry setup.

Source: https://radiologykey.com/wp-content/uploads/2016/03/B9780323073233500175_f31-10-9780323073233.jpg.

This rotating mechanism allows acquisition of multiple projections from varied positions, which, when reconstructed by sophisticated algorithms, yield cross-sectional imaging of the body. Notably, technological advancements in CT, such as the addition of polychromatic X-ray sources, have significantly enhanced image quality and reduced scan times, making it an option for clinicians seeking high-resolution anatomical data. CT's clinical applicability extends across a number of fields, such as oncology, assessment in trauma cases, and preoperative evaluation, highlighting its essential position in modern medical diagnostics (Figure 1.9).

The success of the technology's application is also evident in image reconstruction algorithms, which play a significant role in enhancing the quality and accuracy of the resulting images. Techniques such as Filtered Back Projection (FBP) and Maximum Likelihood Expectation Maximization (MLEM) seek to achieve maximum image sharpness while minimizing artifacts and noise. Specifically, these methods improve the contrast-to-noise ratio (CNR), which is central to the detectability of pathologies in complex biological tissues. Experiments have demonstrated that emerging methods, such as polychromatic X-ray fluorescence computed tomography (XFCT) with sheet-beam geometry, can produce faster imaging protocols while preserving high fidelity. These advancements represent ongoing evolution in CT technology that continually enhances its application in clinical practice, a study exploring the feasibility of XFCT systems (Chen et al., 2017) finds. Additionally, advancements in CT imaging extend beyond traditional techniques to encompass sophisticated applications, including functional imaging and hybrid modalities. CT can be combined with other imaging modalities, such as Positron Emission Tomography (PET), to provide simultaneous functional and anatomical information, enhancing diagnosis. Not only is this multi-faceted imaging much more accurate for tumor detection, but it also aids in deriving information regarding metabolic activity, thereby making therapeutic interventions possible. With researchers continuing to explore new imaging techniques, such as those that employ Monte Carlo simulations to enhance reconstruction models, the prospects for CT technology are limitless. The ongoing research and development in this area are a testament to the dynamic character of medical imaging and its incessant pursuit of precision and efficiency in treating patients (N/A, 1993).

1.3.1. Principles of CT Scanning

Computed Tomography (CT) scans have revolutionized medical imaging to the point that it is now possible to see the human body with accurate detail and cross-sectional images.

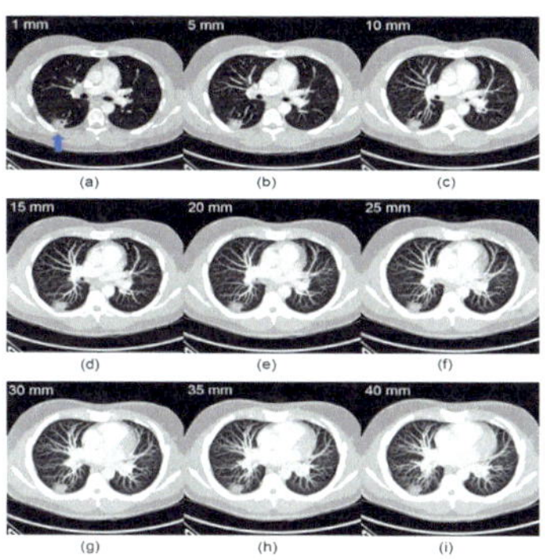

Figure 1.10. Examples of the 1 mm axial section slice and MIP images in various slab thicknesses. From (a) to (i), the slab thickness is 1, 5, 10, 15, 20, 25, 30, 35 and 40 mm, respectively. One nodule is indicated with a blue arrow in the right lower lobe lung. With increase of the slab thickness, the nodule stands more out, whereas vessels are more continues. The nodule still can be seen after (f), although more vessels are projected in this slice. This does not add more value for detection but causes a more crowded image.

Source: https://www.researchgate.net/figure/Examples-of-the-1-mm-axial-section-slice-and-MIP-images-in-various-slab-thicknesses-From_fig1_342346556.

CT scanning relies on the very principles of X-ray technology, using the rotation of X-ray tubes around the patient to capture multiple images from an array of angles. These projections are subsequently computationally reconstructed to generate a whole three-dimensional model of the physical structures. This method not only improves visualization of soft tissues but also provides valuable information regarding various pathological conditions, including tumors and fractures, thereby increasing the accuracy of diagnosis (Figure 1.10).

The significance of understanding the physics behind CT scanning cannot be overstated, as this knowledge is the driving force in developing imaging techniques and technologies in contemporary medicine, enabling practitioners to effectively deploy their strategies in patient care (McKeown et al., 2024). However, despite advances in CT scanning technology, image artifacts and inaccuracies remain prevalent. For instance, the presence of metal objects, such as implantable cardioverter-defibrillators (ICDs), can lead to severe distortion of CT images and obscure significant anatomical information. Researchers are continually seeking new methods to mitigate these issues. An example is a recent study that emphasizes deep learning techniques for the automatic detection and correction of metal artifacts in cardiac CT scans. The development of a two-dimensional U-Net deep learning model demonstrates the application of sophisticated computational processes to improve image quality and enhance segmentation accuracy. By using such sophisticated approaches, clinicians can achieve more reliable imaging results, which ultimately lead to better clinical decision-making (McKeown et al., 2024). The incorporation of a learning component in understanding CT fundamentals is also vital for modern-day medical professionals. An integrated model that incorporates physics and medical practical applications helps maintain a balanced learning experience. The addition of the combination helps students grasp the basic scientific principles that govern medical imaging more effectively. Active learning units have been designed to value this correspondence, with hands-on tutorials and interactive simulations that facilitate the transfer of knowledge from basic physics to advanced imaging techniques. By highlighting the significance of physics in medical imaging, students are more likely to appreciate the subtleties of CT technology, ultimately resulting in more efficient, better-educated healthcare practitioners (Zollman et al., 2010).

1.3.2. Reconstruction Algorithms

Reconstruction algorithms are the core of medical imaging, enabling the transformation of raw data captured by imaging modalities into visualizations that make sense.

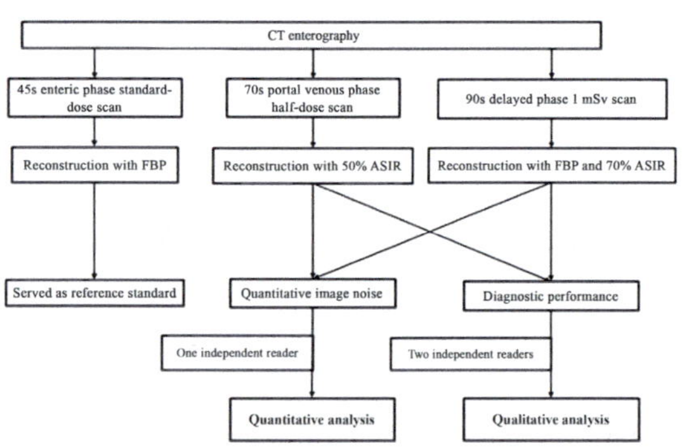

Figure 1.11. Flowchart comparing filtered back projection and iterative reconstruction.

Source: https://www.researchgate.net/publication/320430344/figure/fig2/AS:941410995949583@1601461280358/Flow-chart-of-the-study-process-FBP-filtered-back-projection-ASIR-adaptive-statistical.gif.

The algorithms are particularly vital in techniques such as computed tomography (CT) and magnetic resonance imaging (MRI), where laborious calculations are required on large data sets to produce accurate images. Using mathematical models and the physical principles inherent to each imaging modality, reconstruction algorithms can significantly enhance image quality while minimizing noise and other interference artifacts. As medical imaging becomes increasingly accurate, sophisticated algorithms are playing a critical role, enabling clinicians to achieve more accurate diagnoses from the high-fidelity images they produce. Such developments highlight the importance of combining a solid understanding of the physics behind medical imaging with computational techniques in order to take the fullest advantage of the latest imaging technology (Figure 1.11).

Advances in artificial intelligence (AI) have triggered a revolutionary wave in reconstruction algorithms, boosting efficiency and accuracy. As emphasized in ongoing debates, the union of AI and medical imaging is based on a sound understanding of the physical principles underlying image acquisition protocols. There remains a gap between professionals, and particularly those experts in the field of AI, when it comes to the physics concepts underpinning them, which can limit the efficient application of these technologies. This gap must be addressed, as it will enhance the integrity and trustworthiness of AI reconstruction algorithms. This synergy is employed to deliver enhanced performance under low-data conditions, thereby enabling greater potential for precise diagnostic outcomes and more reliable outcomes in the clinic, as discussed in recent reviews of the potential of AIs in reconstruction methods (Cobo et al., 2025). Among the greatest challenges in medical imaging is noise, which degrades image quality and diagnostic accuracy. Traditional image denoising techniques have been found to lag in the complexity of high-dimensional data and thus fail to deliver optimal results. A new approach hinges on drawing on quantum physics, as proposed in recent reconstruction frameworks. The quantum-inspired techniques analyze medical images in a manner akin to amorphous states of condensed matter physics, such that the distinction between noise and signal is feasible based on a new paradigm. By incorporating mode-resolved localization principles, these algorithms, besides lowering noise, incorporate minimal tuning due to their design aspect, therefore being an extremely efficient standalone solution for optimizing imaging clarity in medical imaging technologies (Hashemi et al., 2024). Such innovations represent a significant breakthrough, uniting sophisticated physics with practical applications in medical imaging to optimize patient outcomes.

1.3.3. Advantages and Limitations

Medical imaging has experienced exponential growth due to a range of technologies that leverage simple principles of physics. One significant advantage lies with the precision provided by modalities such as magnetic resonance imaging (MRI) and computed tomography (CT).

These imaging modalities allow high-resolution visualization of internal anatomy, thereby enhancing diagnostic accuracy. For example, MRI exploits the magnetic susceptibility of atoms to produce high-resolution images without ionizing radiation, as in X-rays. This characteristic is particularly beneficial for the assessment of soft tissues, making MRI an essential component in neurological and musculoskeletal evaluations. However, there are constraints, such as the cost of the technique and the need for sophisticated equipment and trained staff, which may limit availability in certain healthcare settings. Furthermore, the advent of microwave imaging, as has been investigated in more recent studies, provides fresh possibilities and challenges to medicine diagnostics (Figure 1.12).

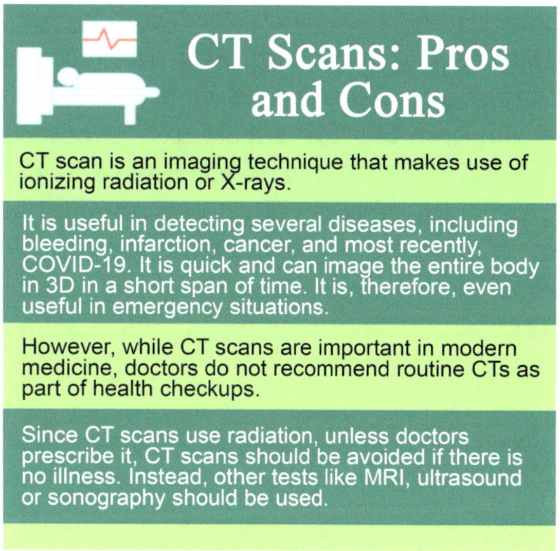

Figure 1.12. Chart outlining CT's strengths and limitations in clinical imaging.

Source: https://financialexpresswpcontent.s3.amazonaws.com/uploads/2021/09/CT-scan-413x413.png?w=374.

Advantages of microwave medical imaging include its non-ionizing nature and the capability to penetrate tissues of various types with the prospect of real-time tumor imaging. The use of varying antenna designs, such as monopole and bow-tie antennas, highlights new approaches for microwave imaging optimization (Busawon et al., 2010). A disadvantage of these advantages is the difficulty of achieving comparable resolution with conventional imaging techniques. The intricacies of antenna operation and design in sophisticated biological media underscore the need for continued research and development in this changing field. At the same time, novel detector technologies and hybrid pixel detectors, in particular, pose encouraging advantages together with necessary constraints. The detectors, used in medical and particle physics, can produce high-resolution images while addressing data processing challenges (Amati et al., 2005). The hybrid architecture allows for higher performance in high-dynamic range imaging, which is beneficial for recording subtle variations in tissue properties. Nevertheless, the sophisticated fabrication processes and the requirement for specialized substrates limit scalability and cost-effectiveness. With the progress of technology, overcoming such limitations and taking advantage of new technology opportunities is a crucial area of interest to enable maximum benefits in medical imaging modalities.

1.4. Magnetic Resonance Imaging (MRI)

Magnetic Resonance Imaging (MRI) is an advanced medical imaging technology founded on the nuclear magnetic resonance principles. Unlike standard imaging modalities such as X-rays or CT scans, MRI exploits the magnetic characteristics of atoms, mostly the hydrogen nuclei from water molecules. When placed in a strong magnetic field, these nuclei align themselves with the field and, when excited by radiofrequency pulses, yield signals that are converted to high-resolution images. The intrinsic contrast of MRI is particularly valuable for imaging soft tissues and is thus extremely useful in neurological, musculoskeletal, and cardiovascular applications. Significant technological advances have improved spatial resolution and imaging speed, allowing real-time testing that maximizes diagnostic effectiveness. The unique ability of MRI to image anatomical structures without ionizing radiation makes it a more patient-friendly modality in cases where patients must be repeatedly imaged (Islam, 2024). Understanding the complex interplay of physical principles is key to advancing MRI technology. MRI physics cannot be separated from concepts in quantum mechanics and electromagnetic fields, which govern how protons behave in a magnetic field. Critical parameters include the strength of the magnetic field, relaxation times (T1 and T2), and pulse sequence timing, all of which control image quality and diagnostic application. Of specific note, T1-weighted images provide tissue composition and anatomy information, and T2-weighted images are important in defining pathological change, e.g, edema or tumors. A precision imaging protocol, with adequate coil selection and patient positioning, guarantees that the optimal images produced are not only diagnostically beneficial but also reproducible from session to session.

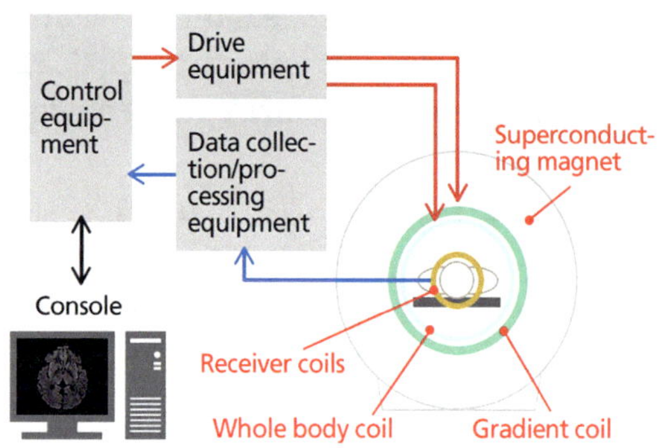

Figure 1.13. MRI scanner layout with labeled coils and magnetic field directions.

Source: https://d18x2uyjeekruj.cloudfront.net/wp-content/uploads/2024/05/mri.jpg.

Hence, the role of medical physicists becomes increasingly important in calibrating devices and confirming imaging protocols (Vrdoljak et al., 2024). The application of MRI in clinical practice has expanded by leaps and bounds, demonstrating its potential to do much more than just structural imaging. Functional imaging with MRI techniques such as diffusion-weighted imaging (DWI) and functional MRI (fMRI) makes the measurement of perfusion and neural activity possible, respectively. DWI has also established its central role in acute stroke imaging by enabling early identification of ischemic changes. fMRI, on the other hand, is a new technique in neuroscience that has the potential to clarify the brain's workings and provide real-time activity mapping. As MRI is increasingly used in preoperative planning and intraoperative navigation in the medical field, one needs to become more familiar with its physics and gain a better understanding of its principles. The knowledge allows clinicians to utilize the full potential of MRI and avoid possible adverse effects of patient exposure to magnetic fields, as understood through the concept of prevention (Islam, 2024) (Figure 1.13).

1.4.1. Basics of Nuclear Magnetic Resonance

The foundation of nuclear magnetic resonance (NMR) is the theory of magnetism and the behavior of atomic nuclei under magnetic fields.

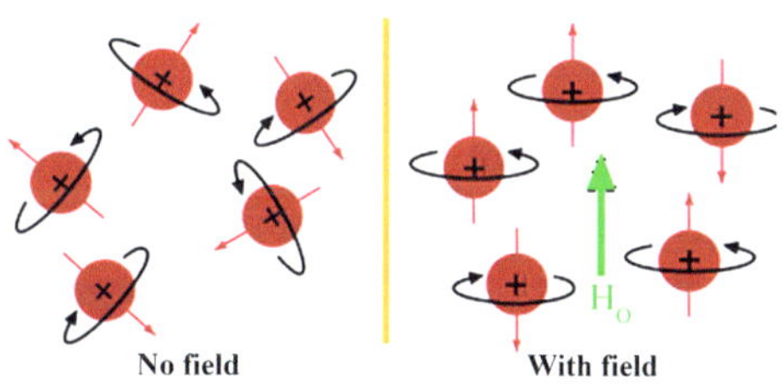

Figure 1.14. Illustration of spin alignment and precession in a magnetic field.

Source: https://i.sstatic.net/7AiK1.png.

When a nucleus is placed in a strong magnetic field, its energy levels split due to the Zeeman effect, thus producing a process called resonance. The most commonly used nuclei in biomedical imaging are hydrogen nuclei, largely because of their prevalence in biological tissues. In NMR, the use of a radiofrequency pulse causes these nuclei to absorb energy and ascend to higher levels of energy. As they relax, they emit radiofrequency signals that can be detected. This signal sensitivity after excitation forms the foundation of NMR imaging techniques, allowing doctors to image internal body structures without invasion (Figure 1.14). Though NMR theory is established, its medical imaging applications continue to advance with improved methods. Magnetic resonance imaging (MRI) utilizes the principles of NMR to generate high-resolution images of soft tissues. Image contrast is caused by tissue variations in relaxation times, which rely on their biochemical surroundings. There have been new advances in enhancing image contrast by applying control-theoretic optimization approaches to MRI, with researchers probing the intrinsic limits of attainable contrast. Besides enhancing diagnostics, these advances provide solid frameworks for building optimized pulse sequences that are robust to experimental flaws, as documented in recent literature (Glaser et al., 2012).

This development underscores the significance of NMR as a basis in the context of medical imaging. In addition, the incorporation of NMR principles into medical imaging has advanced key developments in other fields beyond traditional diagnostics. The applications of NMR span functional imaging, where brain activity is measured by differences in blood oxygen levels, and dynamic imaging, which captures physiological phenomena in real time. NMR techniques' versatility extends to materials science, as studies of molecular structure have broad implications. The progressive advancement of NMR techniques in the field promises to render medical imaging even more precise and reliable. As researchers refine techniques, the future of medical imaging, underpinned by NMR physics, promises to completely transform how clinicians identify and diagnose disease (N/A, 1996). This multidisciplinary focus underscores the central role of NMR as a foundation for future medical diagnosis and scientific investigation.

1.4.2. Image Contrast and Resolution

In medical imaging, image resolution and contrast are essential to enable proper diagnosis and treatment planning. Image contrast refers to the difference in intensity or hue that allows objects to be distinguished from one another in a scan. High contrast is significant because it enables maximum visualization of various anatomical structures and potential abnormalities, allowing radiologists to make informed decisions. Insufficient contrast will lead to subtle abnormalities being missed, with the risk of misdiagnosis. The interaction between contrast and resolution remains fundamental;. However, additional contrast will make things more distinct, it is resolution—the amount of detail in an image that can be perceived—that actually determines the success of medical imaging techniques (Figure 1.15).

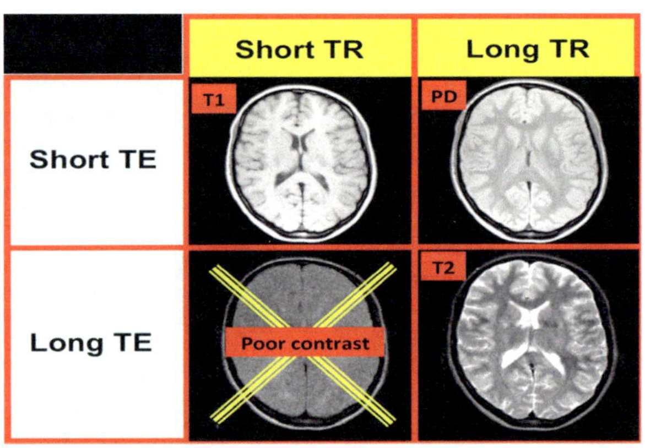

Figure 1.15. T1 vs T2 weighted images showing different tissue contrasts.

Source: https://mriquestions.com/uploads/3/4/5/7/34572113/3310360_orig.gif.

Better resolution allows one to see finer details at a deeper structural level, which is essential for early disease detection, underscoring the importance of these two variables in achieving optimal diagnostic outcomes. Resolution is the smallest detail that can be perceived in a picture and is specifically related to the extent to which one is able to interpret what a scan indicates. In medical imaging, this is particularly important in modalities such as MRI, CT, and ultrasound, where the ability to observe small details can influence patient management regimens. Advances in technology, in the form of enhanced algorithms and image hardware, have been aimed at increasing resolution and contrast. For instance, developments in computer imaging systems have enabled technologies such as more pixels per unit of space and more advanced capture capabilities, enabling higher resolution without distorting contrast. It should be remembered that while resolution can be improved upon with technologies, contrast within images tends to require collaboration from interpreting professionals based on physics, computation, and medical know-how in order to derive the most significant information out of the image data (Manning et al., 2025).

Contrast versus resolution in medical imaging, too, is not strictly technical, as it also involves crossing into human perception and interpretive capabilities. The performance of pictures depends on how medical staff view and perceive visual information, suggesting that the interpreter's effort is no less significant than the imaging technology. Human Inter-interpreter Variability can introduce errors in diagnosis, underscoring the need for stringent training and uniform calibration of imaging devices to deliver optimal contrast and resolution. A more complete understanding of visual decision-making, grounded in multidisciplinary inquiry, is essential to reducing variability in medical imaging (Manning et al., 2025). Moreover, as key components of diagnostic precision, effective innovations in imaging technologies owe an obligation to continue beyond refining the technical terms of resolution and contrast to maximize their effectiveness in clinical practice.

1.4.3. Safety Considerations and Contraindications

In medical imaging, safety is essential, especially when dealing with ionizing radiation. Modalities such as computed tomography (CT) and fluoroscopy release varying levels of radiation, which require a proper understanding of the risks associated with their use. Medical professionals must weigh the diagnostic benefits against potential side effects such as radiation-induced malignancies. The ALARA principle is a guiding rule that urges practitioners to maintain radiation exposure as low as reasonably achievable to produce effective imaging results. The patients need to be informed of these risks, too, thereby again pointing towards informed consent (Figure 1.16).

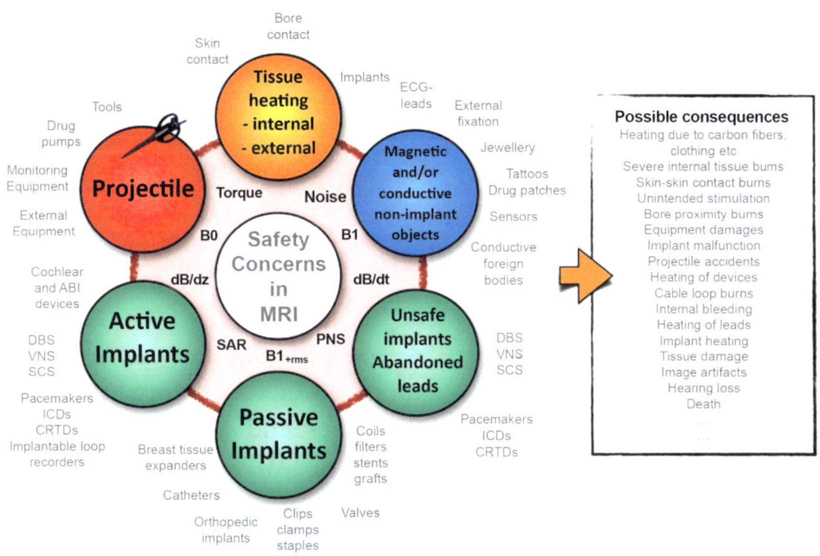

Figure 1.16. Infographic showing MRI safety zones and contraindicated implants.

Source: https://media.springernature.com/lw685/springer-static/image/art%3A10.1007%2Fs00330-024-10999-8/MediaObjects/330_2024_10999_Fig2_HTML.png.

Consequently, the safety of medical imaging extends beyond technology to include ethical considerations regarding patient information and the risks associated with various imaging modalities (Dan et al., 2022). Contraindications are part of the safe use of medical imaging techniques, particularly for certain patient groups. For instance, pregnant individuals are typically advised to avoid ionizing imaging methods unless essential, on the grounds of greater sensitivity of fetal tissue to radiation. Similarly, patients who have had previous allergic reactions to contrast agents can develop serious complications while undergoing such procedures involving such agents, and the use of alternative imaging modalities is necessitated. In addition, certain patients with specific comorbidities may have imaging modalities that are contraindicated; for example, individuals with extreme claustrophobia may experience problems with MRI scans. The in-depth patient assessment of medical history and health status is therefore critical for guiding the selection of an optimal imaging modality that minimizes risks and maximizes diagnostic performance (Weber et al., 2022). The rapid evolution of the field of medical imaging is ever-improving safety protocols by virtue of technological improvement and updated guidelines. Techniques such as digital imaging have reduced radiation exposure while significantly improving image quality. In addition, technologies such as personalized dosimetry in radiation therapy represent pivotal steps towards patient-by-patient safety, offering individualized techniques to optimize therapeutic gain at low risk. These advances include multidisciplinary tumor boards that bring together expertise from multiple medical specialties to determine the most effective and safest imaging modalities for cancer patients. By adhering to current clinical guidelines and respecting each patient's unique needs, medical professionals can enhance the efficacy and safety of medical imaging. Continued research and revision of safety protocols are thus needed to ensure that advances in imaging technology keep pace with patient safety requirements (Dan et al., 2022; Weber et al., 2022).

1.5. Ultrasound Imaging

In the realm of medical imaging, ultrasound imaging stands out for its use of sound waves to image internal structures and is thus an essential resource in the diagnostic and therapeutic fields. The technique employs high-frequency sound waves that travel through tissue and are reflected, capturing various anatomical features based on their acoustic properties. As a non-invasive technology, it offers real-time imaging that enables healthcare providers to observe physiological processes dynamically. Moreover, unlike other imaging modalities such as CT or MRI, ultrasound imaging does not expose patients to ionizing radiation. This characteristic makes it particularly useful in vulnerable populations such as pregnant women and children. As technology advances in the realm of ultrasound, enhanced image processing and resolution strengthen its potential as a diagnostic tool, further cementing its place in modern-day medical practice (Figure 1.17).

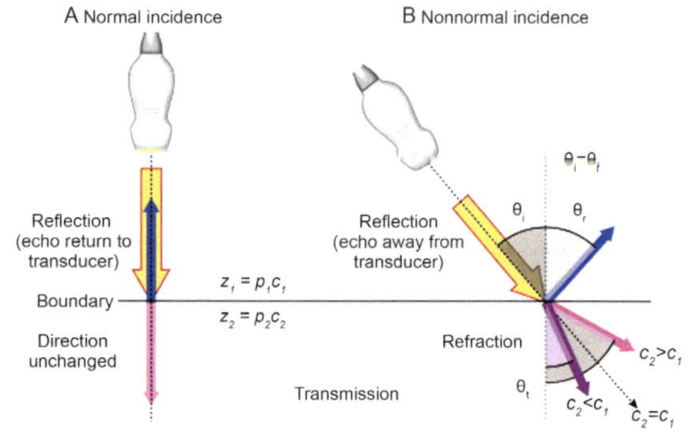

Figure 1.17. Schematic of sound wave propagation and echo reflection in soft tissues.

Source: https://radiologykey.com/wp-content/uploads/2020/03/f01-03-9780323596428.jpg.

Pioneering among ultrasound technologies is the new method, Computed Ultrasound Tomography in Echo mode (CUTE). The new method quantifies the spatial distribution of the speed of sound (SoS) in tissue using handheld pulse-echo ultrasound devices. By detecting phase shifts in generated beams and analyzing data across various transmit and receive angles, CUTE offers revolutionary improvements in quantitative measurements of tissue properties. The inclusion of a better forward model has been proven to be indispensable; it enhances SoS reconstruction accuracy by making up for previously overlooked factors such as phase shift detection and positional reconstruction error. These are particularly valuable in complex diagnostic situations, such as liver imaging, where precise measurements can directly influence patient management and treatment planning. Thus, CUTE is a promising development of ultrasound's diagnostic capability, uniting traditional imaging and sophisticated quantitative analysis (Frenz et al., 2019). As ultrasound imaging advances, it continues to embrace new technologies that enhance its effectiveness and expand its uses. A good example is the increased use of three-dimensional (3D) ultrasound scanning, which allows volumetric analysis with precise measurements of the structures and offers an improved visual overview compared to older two-dimensional systems. The enhanced visualization is particularly valuable in obstetrics and cardiology, where accurate measurement of growth and anatomical anomaly is critical. And finally, the portability of modern ultrasound systems has enabled access to life-saving diagnostic equipment in a variety of settings, from emergency rooms to outpatient clinics. Seamless integration with digital platforms further enhances its convenience, enabling practitioners to easily save and process information. As these technological advances continue to unravel, ultrasound imaging will play an even greater role in providing quick and effective healthcare remedies (N/A, 1987).

1.5.1. Principles of Sound Wave Propagation

Propagation of sound waves is governed by fundamental principles that define how pressure waves propagate through different media, a basic principle in medical imaging. The speed of sound (SoS) in a medium depends on its elasticity and density and therefore changes according to variation in tissue properties along the way. In medical contexts, knowledge of these differences is important because tissues such as muscle, fat, and bone exhibit distinct acoustic properties. Through the interaction of sound waves with these different biological structures, clinicians can visualize internal anatomies. Techniques like ultrasound exploit these ideas, employing high-frequency sound waves to collect echo patterns used for image formation. By analyzing these echoes correctly, doctors can identify structural defects, which contribute to diagnosis, demonstrating the significance of sound wave propagation in medical imaging equipment. Advances in image processes, such as computed ultrasound tomography in echo mode (CUTE), indicate the emerging application of concepts for the propagation of sound waves in medical diagnostics. CUTE facilitates SoS spatial distribution mapping in tissues by leveraging transmit- and receive-angle-varying echo phase shifts. Reconstruction is ensured by a robust forward model possessing specific characteristics, including co-alignment of transmitting and receiving angles around shared mid-angles and accounting for reconstruction-error-caused phase shifts. By enhancing the fidelity of SoS reconstruction, CUTE is a powerful adjunct to conventional ultrasound imaging, extending its diagnostic utility in real-time. This convergence of advanced principles of sound wave propagation in medical imaging represents a significant advance toward improved measurement and patient outcomes, underscoring the relevance of fundamental physics in contemporary healthcare applications (Frenz et al., 2019). With the traditional imaging modalities, new studies of acoustic phenomena such as topologically protected wave propagation (TPWP) reveal promising avenues for future medical imaging research. This concept explores the way sound waves travel through structured media, transforming the understanding of the dynamics of wave interactions. With simpler geometric configurations, researchers were able to delineate conditions under which TPWP can be used to improve imaging contrast. Through systematic tuning of unit-cell geometries, the visibility of Dirac-like cones represented the potential for systematic wave manipulation technologies. This new approach not only advances the fundamental understanding of the original mechanisms of sound propagation but also opens the door to integrating advanced acoustic metamaterials into medical imaging protocols. Applying the principles of sound wave transmission, we should anticipate transformative developments that will significantly influence diagnostic procedures and treatments in healthcare (Khan et al., 2024).

1.5.2. Doppler Effect in Imaging

The Doppler effect is an observed effect in medical imaging that significantly enhances the diagnostic capability by describing the movement of fluids and tissues. When sound waves are emitted from a transducer and reflected from moving targets, such as blood cells, the reflected wave frequency changes with the relative motion of the targets, this alteration can be utilized to determine the velocity and direction of blood flow and is, as such, a critical tool for cardiovascular diagnostics and monitoring. By examining such frequency shifts, health care practitioners can non-invasively quantify conditions such as stenosis, thrombosis, and other vascular diseases. Thus, the Doppler effect is a principle underlying numerous medical imaging modalities, particularly in ultrasound technology, where it adds value to functional information transmitted alongside traditional anatomical details. Continuous-wave and pulsed-wave Doppler techniques are two primary modalities employed in ultrasound imaging. Two transducer elements, one transmitting and the other receiving, use continuous-wave Doppler to continuously monitor the frequency changes of reflected echoes from moving blood cells. This method is better to quantify blood flow at high velocities but is not spatially resolved. In contrast, pulsed-wave Doppler allows measurements from specific points, enabling clinicians to measure flow velocities at set depths. Depth discrimination enables hemodynamic measurements from various cardiac chambers and vessels, thereby enhancing the capacity to diagnose congenital heart disease and valvular disease. Both techniques underscore the importance of the Doppler effect in providing critical physiological information to enhance cardiovascular well-being and expand knowledge of cardiovascular pathology. In addition, the clinical application of Doppler imaging extends beyond cardiology and has a multidisciplinary influence on patient care. The Doppler effect is a significant advantage in obstetrics for tracking fetal health, quantifying circulatory patterns in the placenta, and identifying potential compromises in oxygen supply. Moreover, advanced Doppler ultrasound technology enables detection of microvascular blood flow in tumors, helping oncologists assess tumor perfusion and response to treatment. These responses make reactions not only a cornerstone of medical diagnosis but also an extension of an ongoing physician, furthering the ongoing exploration of physiology. By applying the Doppler effect to imaging modalities, the clinician can produce high-resolution images that drive clinical outcomes, becoming the cornerstone of the development of medical imaging as a discipline (Postema, 2011; Collaboration et al., 2024) (Figure 1.18).

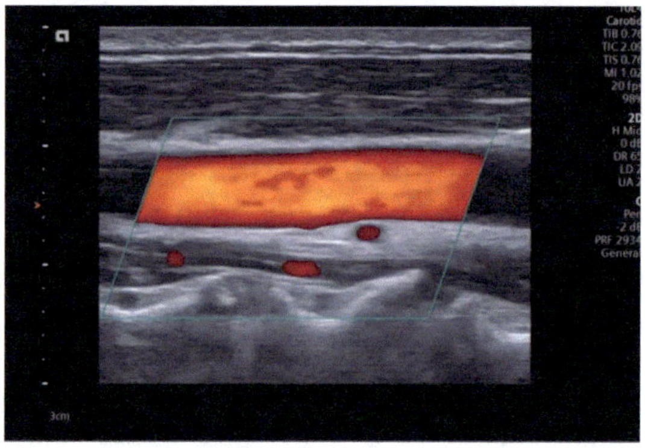

Figure 1.18. Color Doppler ultrasound of the carotid artery showing flow direction.

Source: https://legacy.123sonography.com/sites/default/files/styles/video_thumbnail/public/video/images/5.2Color%20Doppler%20normal.png?itok=7KjX5b9v.

1.5.3. Clinical Applications and Benefits

In the contemporary medical setting, the application of fundamental physics concepts has catalyzed tremendous growth in medical imaging, yielding vast clinical applications and benefits. A good example is the use of nanoinformatics, which has begun to transform medical diagnosis and therapeutic regimens. Using nanomaterials, scientists are developing new devices that promise enhanced imaging and therapeutic benefits. Such clinical potential rivals the revolutionary impact of genomics on targeted therapy, to the extent that information from nanoscience could enable prevention, early diagnosis, and custom-tailored treatment regimens. Thus, understanding the physical foundations of such advancements is necessary to ensure optimal implementation in hospitals and to streamline research and clinical practice at the same time, with regard to the intricacies entailed in clinical information and biological interactions (Anguita et al., 2012). Moreover, photonics development has unveiled novel routes in the field of medical imaging, particularly in non-invasive imaging, which lies at the heart of precise diagnostics. The Boston University Photonics Center illustrates the potential that interdisciplinary projects hold to stimulate innovation in this field. Through research initiatives and significant funding, the center demonstrates advances in optical imaging technologies that enable disease detection at higher resolutions. The focus on such areas as "Optics of Cancer Imaging" illustrates the center's commitment to addressing significant healthcare challenges. These developments not only increase diagnostic precision but also minimize patient discomfort and lower the demand for invasive interventions. As medical imaging with optical technology has advanced, it is important to maintain an uncompromising understanding of the physics underlying this technology to ensure that practical applications translate into significant clinical benefit (Center TBUP, 2017). Moreover, the physics-driven, rapidly evolving field of medical imaging extends to new therapeutic applications. As imaging technologies develop, they enable disease monitoring and treatment outcomes to be viewed in real time, providing clinicians with insights that can lead to improved patient outcomes. For instance, merging imaging modalities such as functional MRI and PET scans has enabled health practitioners to visualize metabolic processes and brain activity, revolutionizing treatment for neurological disorders. Such advanced imaging techniques allow health care practitioners to make informed choices regarding treatment protocols and guide more personalized care plans. For this purpose, a comprehensive understanding of physics concepts is necessary, as they provide the framework for developing imaging methods with significant clinical applications and benefits that ultimately maximize patient care and healthcare systems (Anguita et al., 2012) (Figure 1.19).

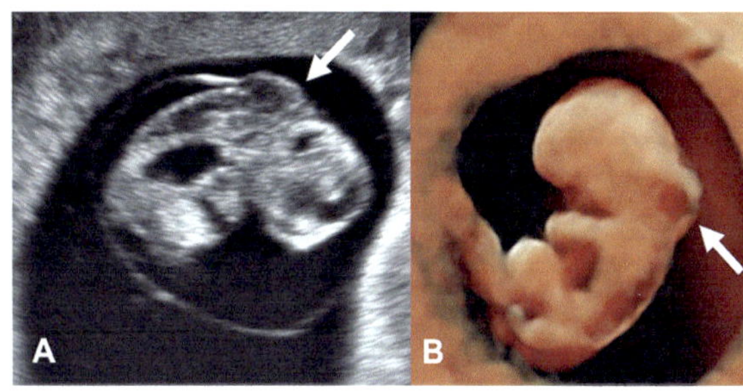

Figure 1.19. Ultrasound images demonstrating fetal development stages.

Source: https://images-glowm.cms.ama.uk.com/img/Obstetrics-V18-C02-31.jpg.

1.6. Nuclear Medicine

In medical imaging, nuclear medicine is a significant application that employs radiopharmaceuticals for the diagnosis and treatment of several medical disorders. The underlying physics in nuclear medicine involves understanding the properties of radioactive material and how these substances interact with biology. Nuclear medicine employs gamma cameras and positron emission tomography (PET) to image and quantify tissue metabolic activity, providing information not readily observable by other imaging techniques. One of the foremost characteristics of nuclear medicine is the delivery of precise radiation dose therapy to the target with minimal exposure to surrounding healthy tissues. These high degrees of precision in diagnostic and therapeutic procedures are the result of advancements in detection systems and a sophisticated understanding of the physics underlying radioactivity and imaging systems. Therefore, the role of medical physicists takes center stage, enhancing patient care and safety in nuclear medicine procedures. Uses of nuclear medicines extend beyond basic diagnostic imaging; they also involve therapeutic treatment such as radioimmunotherapy and targeted radionuclide therapy. This integrative treatment applies concepts from physics, chemistry, and biology to offer individualized medicine strategies that selectively target specific disease processes, such as cancer. The therapeutic agents of nuclear medicine, which release beta or alpha particles, are designed to deliver high doses of radiation selectively to malignancies while sparing normal tissues. Such a targeted application is made possible only by strict adherence to radiation dosimetry, ensuring precisely calculated doses are administered to maximize patient benefit. While nuclear medicine progresses with new radiopharmaceuticals and imaging agents in development, the background in the history of these developments and their value in the broad scheme of medical imaging must be appreciated, as observed in plans for curricula within the field (Burmeister et al., 2022). Also, as nuclear medicine progresses, the addition of new technology in practice is an opportunity as well as a challenge. Such technologies as hybrid imaging systems, which combine functional and anatomical imaging, are transforming patient management and diagnosis. A combination of imaging modalities like PET/CT and PET/MRI creates extensive assessments that transform clinical decision-making approaches. The effective application of such technologies, however, relies heavily on the expertise of medical physicists, who are skilled in ensuring the quality and safety of imaging processes. This requirement for robust training in nuclear medicine underscores the importance of curricular guidelines that integrate fundamental principles of physics with experimental and clinical applications. Continuous upgrading of programs is vital to prepare future practitioners for the evolving realities of nuclear medicine, enabling them to contribute to patient care and navigate the ethical dimensions of their practice (Theodore et al., 2019) (Figure 1.20).

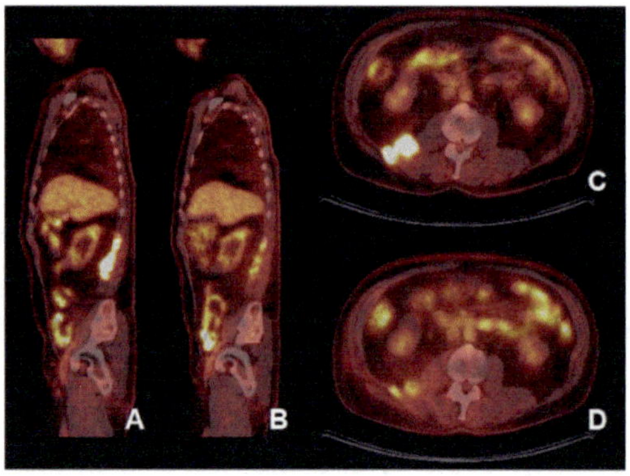

Figure 1.20. PET/CT fusion image showing metabolic activity in oncology.

Source: https://www.researchgate.net/publication/334781402/figure/fig2/AS:786558441500672@1564541554168/PET-CT-scan-images-showing-changes-in-metabolic-activity-at-the-site-of-recurrent-tumor.png.

1.6.1. Principles of Radiopharmaceuticals

The principles of radiopharmaceuticals are firmly established in the union of nuclear medicine with pharmacology and serve as the foundation for radiopharmaceutical diagnostic and therapeutic applications in clinical imaging. Radiopharmaceuticals consist of radioisotopes bound to biologically active molecules, enabling targeted delivery to tissues or organs. It is particularly critical because it enhances diagnostic and therapeutic efficacy while minimizing exposure to adjacent healthy tissues. With mechanisms that include passive targeting via enhanced permeability and retention and active targeting via ligand-receptor interactions, radiopharmaceuticals can penetrate the complex biological milieu of the human body. Recent advancements in radiopharmaceutical research have highlighted their potential for precision medicine, a philosophy poised to be revolutionized by the advent of molecular imaging and targeted therapies (Dhoundiyal et al., 2024). Therapeutic applications of radiopharmaceuticals extend beyond imaging; they involve a variety of therapeutic regimens popularly referred to as theranostics. This dual capability makes radiopharmaceuticals a central part of modern medicine, not just for imaging of diseases but also for the selective destruction of cancer cells. New developments occur continuously, particularly with the use of radio-labeled antibodies and peptide receptor radionuclide therapy for various cancers. These developments rely heavily on concepts from radiation physics to ensure that specific doses are effective but safe. By incorporating radiopharmaceuticals into patient-specific dosimetry, healthcare providers can maximize treatment regimens, potentially enhancing survival rates while reducing side effects (Kögreen Gleisner et al., 2023). The harmony of diagnostic imaging and therapeutic intervention personifies the potential of radiopharmaceuticals in current oncology. With continued research, the integration of safety measures becomes essential for the use of radiopharmaceuticals. Ensuring interventions not only work but are also safe is a top priority for healthcare providers. Rules and regulations, such as the European Council Directive 2013/59/Euratom, help by setting standards for optimizing and verifying radiotherapy and the absorbed dose. The directive emphasizes individualized treatment strategies developed from patient dosimetry to prevent over- and under-treatment hazards. Cross-disciplinary partnerships between researchers, clinicians, and medical physicists are imperative for creating an integrated approach that maximizes patient outcomes. Training programs to enhance knowledge in molecular radiotherapy will be key to a new generation of professionals with a solid foundation in the underlying physics and the clinical application of radiopharmaceuticals, ensuring this active area a firm future (Kögreen Gleisner et al., 2023).

1.6.2. Imaging Techniques: PET and SPECT

Among the various imaging techniques employed in modern medicine, Positron Emission Tomography (PET) and Single Photon Emission Computed Tomography (SPECT) stand out for their unique roles in disease detection. PET utilizes radiotracers that emit positrons that react with electrons in the body to produce gamma rays. This method provides invaluable information on metabolic activity, as it can visualize biochemical alterations in tissues. SPECT, however, functions through the detection of gamma rays produced by radionuclides that have been placed inside the body. Although these two share common principles, the sensitivity and resolution differ between them, which determines their use. For instance, PET typically offers higher spatial resolution than SPECT, making it particularly useful in oncology and neurology, where precise imaging of metabolic function is critical. PET and SPECT imaging modalities have revolutionized diagnostic imaging, particularly in oncology, cardiology, and neurology. The physics underlying these modalities deals with the detection mechanisms of gamma rays and the precise localization of emitted radiation. In recent years, advances in technology have further increased the capabilities of these imaging devices. For example, advances in detector sensitivity and image reconstruction algorithms have improved the accuracy of imaging tracer distribution within the body. Small-animal imaging has become a crucial tool in the design of novel radiotracers and the testing of novel therapies, as is highlighted in the literature (Bankstahl et al., 2015). This capability further underscores the significance of PET and SPECT, which provide both exploratory research and clinical applications, and underscores their key position in the history of medical imaging. Although PET and SPECT differ in their mechanisms and applications, they share a similar foundation in nuclear medicine. This shared foundation underscores the need for understanding radiopharmaceuticals, which are central to both imaging modalities. Design and selection of suitable radiotracers should fulfill definite clinical goals to achieve optimal diagnostic yield. With advances in molecular imaging techniques, investigators are increasingly applying these modalities to develop targeted therapies and individualized medicine. Technical improvements in imaging physics also enable the creation of sophisticated algorithms for image analysis and diagnostic productivity. By integrating new technologies with traditional imaging methods, the future of PET and SPECT is bright, opening avenues for further possibilities in medical imaging (N/A, 1989).

1.6.3. Role in Disease Diagnosis and Treatment

Medical imaging physics plays a key role in the accurate diagnosis and treatment of disease in modern medicine. Imaging techniques such as X-rays, computed tomography (CT), and magnetic resonance imaging (MRI) employ fundamental physical principles to produce high-quality images that assist physicians in diagnosing conditions. Medical physicists play a crucial role in this work, ensuring the safe and effective performance of imaging procedures. They are responsible for quality assurance of imaging equipment, monitoring radiation exposure, and ensuring diagnostic equipment accuracy, thereby increasing patient safety and outcomes. Methods such as Positron Emission Tomography (PET) are key for shedding light on the structural and biological changes in the body and for emphasizing the complementarity between disease management and medical physics (Gambo et al., 2024). Moreover, advances in nanotechnology are revolutionizing disease diagnosis and treatment. The development of multifunctional sensors and new materials, particularly carbon-based nanostructures, emphasizes the intersection of medicine and physics. These materials possess excellent properties that enable them to exhibit high sensitivity and specificity in detecting numerous disease biomarkers, including cancer biomarkers. For instance, certain nanostructured magnetic materials have been reported to have significant potential as drug carriers for targeted drug delivery systems, enabling dual modes of diagnosis and therapy. Also, the application of these new materials in imaging techniques not only maximizes the diagnostic capability but also optimizes treatment outcomes through providing instant feedback on treatment efficacy (Moreira, 2024). This dualistic nature of diagnostics and treatment reflects the revolutionizing influence of physics on clinical practice. The convergence of physics with medical imaging ultimately optimizes the precision of disease treatment plans. In clinical practice, advanced imaging facilitates early diagnosis, accurate staging, and personalized treatment plans tailored to each patient's specific requirements. As medical imaging science evolves, the technology increasingly employs high-level algorithms and artificial intelligence to interpret complex imaging data, thereby further enhancing diagnostic accuracy. The role of the medical physicists in the evolving environment cannot be overstated, given that their service equates to guaranteeing compliance with safety standards and improving imaging techniques. Sustained innovation not only aids in the understanding of diseases in depth but also underscores the central role of solid scientific fundamentals in the development of global healthcare practices and in improving patient outcomes (Gambo et al., 2024).

SUMMARY

In summarizing the fundamentals of physics in medical imaging, it is evident that the convergence of imaging modalities greatly enhances our understanding of biological systems. The convergence of techniques such as MRI, CT, and PET not only improves diagnosis but also the potential for longitudinal studies of disease progression and response to treatment over time. The technological advancement in small-animal imaging devices is a classic case in point, as such technologies enable scientists to monitor complicated interactions at a cellular level, spurring innovations in drug development and targeted medicine. According to Bankstahl et al. (2015), the synergistic combination of various systems enables pioneering experiments spanning experimental boundaries between biology, pharmacology, and medical physics, highlighting the multi-disciplinary nature of modern-day medical research. Besides, the implication of such developments extends beyond imaging diagnosis to therapeutic applications. For instance, emerging techniques such as Receptor-focused Magnetic Resonance anesthesia portend the employment of electromagnetic models to achieve maximum patient benefits with fewer side effects, representing the intersection of imaging and treatment modalities. As argued by Golyanishchev et al. (2016), the advent of high-resolution magnetic resonance technology provides opportunities for personalized therapeutic approaches by enabling the production of a dynamic 3D model of receptor interactions. These advances highlight the importance of tapping into the underlying physics not just to enhance imaging capabilities but also to provide a basis for more efficient, patient-specific medical treatments. Lastly, the physics underlying medical imaging is the foundation upon which future technology integration can offer more comprehensive healthcare solutions. With the continued advancement, subsequent research efforts should target the merging of imaging modalities and the theoretical foundation upon which they rest. In this ongoing quest for improvement, educational and industry players must collaborate to explore new uses of imaging technologies to improve patient outcomes. The future is both ominous and exciting as developments in medical imaging not only enhance our understanding of diseases but also redefine the landscape of healthcare delivery, eventually benefiting+ society as a whole.

CLOSER LOOK

THE PHYSICS BEHIND MEDICAL IMAGING

Medical imaging works because physics gives us ways to look inside the body without cutting it open. Each major imaging method relies on a specific physical principle, and understanding these principles helps explain why different scans reveal different types of information.

X ray imaging uses high energy photons that pass through soft tissue more easily than bone. When the beam travels through the body, dense structures absorb more radiation. This creates contrast on the detector and forms a clear picture of bones and foreign objects. The simplicity and speed of X rays make them a first choice in emergency care.

Computed tomography builds on X ray physics. A rotating tube sends many thin beams through the body from multiple angles. A computer collects the signals and reconstructs them into cross sectional images. This approach gives doctors a three dimensional look at organs, tumors, and internal bleeding with much greater detail.

Magnetic resonance imaging takes a different path. It uses a strong magnetic field to align the hydrogen nuclei in the body. Radiofrequency pulses disturb that alignment, and when the nuclei return to their original state they release energy. The system measures that energy and converts it into images that show soft tissues with remarkable clarity. Because MRI uses no ionizing radiation, it is often preferred for brain, spine, and joint studies.

Ultrasound uses sound waves instead of radiation. A transducer sends high frequency waves into the body. These waves bounce off structures with different densities and return to the probe. The machine interprets the echoes and produces real time images. This makes ultrasound ideal for fetal monitoring and for guiding procedures at the bedside.

Each method has strengths and limits. Together they form a toolkit that lets clinicians see structure and function, track disease, and guide treatment with precision. The physics is the foundation that makes this insight possible.

REFERENCES

1. Ali, I. G. (2024). Advancements and applications of NMR and MRI technologies in medical science: A comprehensive review. https://www.semanticscholar.org/paper/a862648e4e957f18f855b5f9e34920d835c58c9f (accessed on 14th July 2025).
2. Krüger, H. (2005). 2D Detectors for particle physics and for imaging applications. *Nuclear Instruments and Methods in Physics Research Section a Accelerators Spectrometers Detectors and Associated Equipment, 551*(1), 1–14. https://doi.org/10.1016/j.nima.2005.07.037Anguita, A., Pazos, A., Geissbuhler, A., Smith, B., Kim, B. Y., Kulikowski, C., Rosse, C., et al. (2012). Nano informatics: Developing new computing applications for nanomedicine. https://core.ac.uk/download/28969094.pdf (accessed on 14th July 2025).
3. Arrizón, V., David, M., Faris, S., Chen, G. H., Herzen, J., Huang, H., Huang, J., et al. (2010). Anomalous scaling law for noise variance and spatial resolution in differential phase contrast computed tomography. http://arxiv.org/abs/1006.0967 (accessed on 14th July 2025).
4. Bankstahl, J., Belcari, N., Krämer, S., Vandenberghe, S., et al. (2015). Accurate molecular imaging of small animals taking into account animal models, handling, anesthesia, quality control and imaging system performance. https://core.ac.uk/download/55743381.pdf (accessed on 14th July 2025).
5. Bracco, A., Chomaz, P., Gaardhøje, J. J., Heenen, P. H., et al. (2010). Perspectives of nuclear physics in Europe: NuPECC Long Range Plan 2010. https://core.ac.uk/download/19502483.pdf (accessed on 14th July 2025).
6. Burmeister, J., Busse, N. C., Cetnar, A. J., Howell, R. R., Jeraj, R., Jones, A. K., King, S. H., et al. (2022). Academic program recommendations for graduate degrees in medical physics: AAPM Report No. 365 (Revision of Report No. 197). *Journal of Applied Clinical Medical Physics, 23*. https://doi.org/10.1002/acm2.13792 (accessed on 14th July 2025).
7. Busawon, K., Elsdon, M., Fernando, M., Smith, A., et al. (2010). Fundamental issues in antenna design for microwave medical imaging applications. https://core.ac.uk/download/4148450.pdf (accessed on 14th July 2025).
8. Chen, M., Deng, L., He, P., Jiang, Y., et al. (2017). Monte Carlo simulation for polychromatic X-ray fluorescence computed tomography with sheet-beam geometry. https://core.ac.uk/download/188807521.pdf (accessed on 14th July 2025).
9. Cobo, M., Corral Fontecha, D., Silva, W., & Lloret Iglesias, L. (2025). Physical foundations for trustworthy medical imaging: A review for artificial intelligence researchers. https://www.semanticscholar.org/paper/a247332773e841859a414c3ae58e671db1b03151 (accessed on 14th July 2025).
10. Dhoundiyal, S., Srivastava, S., Kumar, S., Singh, G., Ashique, S., Pal, R., Mishra, N., et al. (2024). Radiopharmaceuticals: Navigating the frontier of precision medicine and therapeutic innovation. *European Journal of Medical Research, 29*. https://doi.org/10.1186/s40001-023-01627-0 (accessed on 14th July 2025).
11. Euclid Collaboration, Bhargava, S., Benoist, C., Gonzalez, A. H., Maturi, M., Melin, J., Stanford, S., Munari, E., et al. (2025). Euclid Quick Data Release (Q1): First detections from the galaxy cluster workflow. https://www.semanticscholar.org/paper/e7c8d58ea28a4e233b5e4fae7e8d3b09b6a5c3fe (accessed on 14th July 2025).

12. Euclid Collaboration, Mellier, Y., Abdurro'uf, Barroso, J. A., Ach'ucarro, A., Adamek, J., Adam, R., Addison, G. E., et al. (2024). Euclid. I. Overview of the Euclid mission. *Astronomy & Astrophysics.* https://www.semanticscholar.org/paper/e3e133f6894cf03514a3e626545fbfd46491503e (accessed on 14th July 2025).

13. Frenz, M., Jaeger, M., Kuriakose, M., Stähli, R., et al. (2019). Forward model for quantitative pulse-echo speed-of-sound imaging. https://core.ac.uk/download/343224403.pdf (accessed on 14th July 2025).

14. Gajos, A., Kacprzak, K., Korcyl, G., Krzemien, W., et al. (2020). J-PET framework: Software platform for PET tomography data reconstruction and analysis. https://core.ac.uk/download/344434920.pdf (accessed on 14th July 2025).

15. Gambo, N., & Shehu, M. (2024). The role of diagnostic medical physics in medicine: An overview. *Sahel Journal of Life Sciences FUDMA.* https://www.semanticscholar.org/paper/372a33a3ed2cd5bb3d645657730b8c7801785d41 (accessed on 14th July 2025).

16. Ghosh, S., Varshney, N., Al Hasan, M. M., Roy, A., Craig, P. J., Koppal, S. J., Dalir, H., et al. (2024). Exploring physics-informed machine learning for system matrix formulation in x-ray imaging forward models. *13152*, 131521W–131521W-8. https://www.semanticscholar.org/paper/403d3454d5c42daef3c33f5af3c79895a5316e93 (accessed on 14th July 2025).

17. Glaser, S. J., Janich, M., Lapert, M., Sugny, D., et al. (2012). Exploring the physical limits of saturation contrast in magnetic resonance imaging. http://arxiv.org/abs/1208.5865 (accessed on 14th July 2025).

18. Golyanishchev, M. (2016). Hypothesis of RFMRA development–The receptor-focused magnetic and resonant anesthesia. https://core.ac.uk/download/301580510.pdf (accessed on 14th July 2025).

19. Hashemi, A., Dutta, S., Georgeot, B., Kouamé, D., & Sabet, H. (2024). A novel perspective on denoising using quantum localization with application to medical imaging. *ArXiv.* https://www.semanticscholar.org/paper/120fc9e54e42437c7c88193324fe7baa0cfd032e (accessed on 14th July 2025).

20. Hogg, P., & Lança, L. (2015). *OPTIMAX 2014–Radiation Dose and Image Quality Optimization in Medical Imaging.* https://core.ac.uk/download/47133930.pdf (accessed on 14th July 2025).

21. Khan, M. A. I. (2024). Investigation of topologically protected wave propagation near Dirac-like cones in acoustic metamaterials. https://core.ac.uk/download/640244148.pdf (accessed on 14th July 2025).

22. Lee, G., Lee, J., Park, Q. H., & Seo, M. (2022). Frontiers in terahertz imaging applications beyond absorption cross-section and diffraction limits. *ACS Photonics, 9*, 1500–1512. https://doi.org/10.1021/acsphotonics.1c02006 (accessed on 14th July 2025).

23. Manjappa, M., & Singh, R. (2020). Materials for terahertz optical science and technology. *Advanced Optical Materials, 8.* https://doi.org/10.1002/adom.201901984 (accessed on 14th July 2025).

24. Manning, D. J. (2025). 'Do you see what I see?' Medical imaging: The interpretation of visual information. https://core.ac.uk/download/29421572.pdf (accessed on 14th July 2025).

25. McKeown, T., Gach, H., Hao, Y., An, H., Robinson, C. G., Cuculich, P., Yang, D., et al. (2024). Small metal artifact detection and inpainting in cardiac CT images. *ArXiv.* https://www.

semanticscholar.org/paper/38f9934ae70ba5fd4df41aba9134d85b39d75b3c (accessed on 14th July 2025).

26. Moreira, F. (2024). Ferromagnetic carbon/graphite: From CBRN defense to sensors applied to oncology as a promising way to detect and fight cancer and tumors/neoplasms. *Medical Research Archives*. https://www.semanticscholar.org/paper/b8c83950522d1f2f3eb25d84de1e364ee8778e9c (accessed on 14th July 2025).

27. Pelaz, B., Alexiou, C., Álvarez-Puebla, R. A., Alves, F., Andrews, A. M., Ashraf, S., Balogh, L., et al. (2017). Diverse applications of nanomedicine. *ACS Nano, 11*, 2313–2381. https://doi.org/10.1021/acsnano.6b06040 (accessed on 14th July 2025).

28. Postema, M. (2011). *Fundamentals of Medical Ultrasonics*. https://www.semanticscholar.org/paper/d8eae906c9c9e053d4533bd002e1b06ea33b658a (accessed on 14th July 2025).

29. Rappaport, T. S., Xing, Y., Kanhere, O., Ju, S., Madanayake, A., Mandal, S., Alkhateeb, A., et al. (2019). Wireless communications and applications above 100 GHz: Opportunities and challenges for 6G and beyond. *IEEE Access, 7*, 78729–78757. https://doi.org/10.1109/access.2019.2921522 (accessed on 14th July 2025).

30. Sjögreen Gleisner, K., Flux, G., Bacher, K., Chiesa, C., de Nijs, R., Kagadis, G. C., Lima, T. V. M., et al. (2023). EFOMP policy statement NO. 19: Dosimetry in nuclear medicine therapy–Molecular radiotherapy. *Physica Medica, 116*, 103166–103166. https://doi.org/10.1016/j.ejmp.2023.103166 (accessed on 14th July 2025).

31. Stein, D. J., Shoptaw, S., Vigo, D., Lund, C., Cuijpers, P., Bantjes, J., Sartorius, N., et al. (2022). Psychiatric diagnosis and treatment in the 21st century: Paradigm shifts versus incremental integration. *World Psychiatry, 21*, 393–414. https://doi.org/10.1002/wps.20998 (accessed on 14th July 2025).

32. The Boston University Photonics Center. (2017). *The Boston University Photonics Center Annual Report 2016–2017*. https://open.bu.edu/bitstream/2144/29755/1/Photonics-Center-Glossy-Annual-Report-2017-v5.pdf (accessed on 14th July 2025).

33. Vrdoljak, I., & Bradarić, A. (2024). Medical physics in radiological practice. *Journal of Applied Health Sciences*. https://www.semanticscholar.org/paper/3062f5c5bf3e4222cd2d8fb11e0d706966920462 (accessed on 14th July 2025).

34. Weber, M., Lam, M. G. E. H., Chiesa, C., Konijnenberg, M., Cremonesi, M., Flamen, P., Gnesin, S., et al. (2022). EANM procedure guideline for the treatment of liver cancer and liver metastases with intra-arterial radioactive compounds. *European Journal of Nuclear Medicine and Molecular Imaging, 49*, 1682–1699. https://doi.org/10.1007/s00259-021-05600-z (accessed on 14th July 2025).

35. Zollman, D., McBride, D. L., Murphy, S. K., Aryal, B., Kalita, S., & Wirjawan, J. (2010). Teaching about the physics of medical imaging. *1263*, 3–8. https://www.semanticscholar.org/paper/bd5e9f4c282485fdd81dd978ca16ebc755e39c1e (accessed on 14th July 2025).

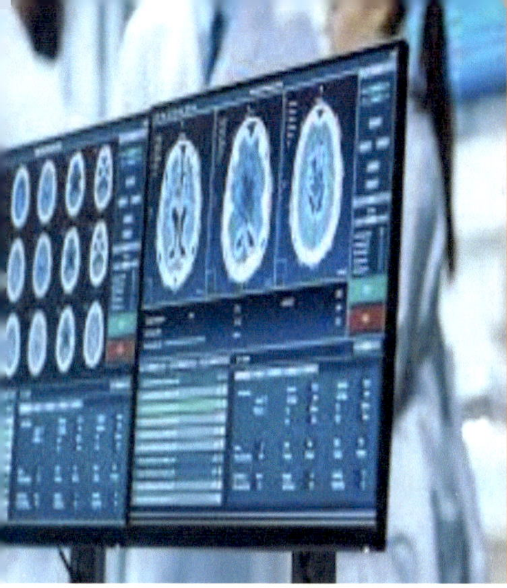

Chapter 2

INSTRUMENTATION AND DETECTOR TECHNOLOGIES IN DIAGNOSTIC IMAGING

Contents

Introduction

The evolution of diagnostic imaging has elevated instrumentation and detector technology to foundational pillars of modern medical practice. With the need for accurate, effective practical imaging comes the demand for technologies that deliver better image quality and reduce patient radiation exposure. Technical innovations in x-ray tube design have been central to driving this trend, making it possible to extract accurate clinical data from minimal invasiveness. Moreover, the interplay between various detector types and their inherent properties determines the scope of applications for imaging modalities. It is crucial that radiologists, along with engineers and scientists dedicated to developing imaging techniques, be familiar with these technical details. Thus, the initial section of this essay will discuss the most important technologies underlying diagnostic imaging and set the stage for subsequent in-depth discussions of x-ray tube design and multiple detector arrays. A crucial component of the advances in diagnostic imaging is the interdependence of hardware development and effective image acquisition. By analyzing the design of the X-ray tube, it is possible to see how advances in anode materials, cooling, and high-voltage generators enhance functional performance. Each piece of hardware serves some particular role in facilitating the generation and manipulation of the X-ray beam to meet maximum performance without compromising on safety standards. Simultaneously, the development of flat-panel detectors and splitting up of indirect and direct conversion technologies revolutionized how images are captured and processed. These detectors not only improve image clarity but also provide a high dynamic range and a high detective quantum efficiency (DQE), significant indicators of their functionality and application. As a means of extensive discovery of these components, the latter sections of the essay discuss the intricate technologies that eventually simplify the diagnostic image formation space. Given technology's continual advancement, the proper integration of both detectors and supporting imaging platforms is increasingly critical. Yet the detector technology selection influences not only the imaging result but also the operational parameters, such as energy resolution and thermal effects. Technologies such as scintillation detectors and semiconductor detectors, such as CdTe and CZT, demonstrate the diversity of what is possible. Such innovations not only enhance spectral imaging capabilities but also address the inherent drawbacks of previous imaging technologies. There is a need for an in-depth understanding of detector performance parameters, including detective quantum efficiency and modulation transfer functions, to discuss the performance of various systems based on their capabilities. These technologies will be discussed in more detail as the essay progresses through the subsequent chapters, their applications, advantages, and disadvantages, in the context of delivering quality diagnostic imaging in medical practice.

2.1. X-Ray Tube Design

The design of X-ray tubes is fundamental to diagnostic imaging, serving as a critical component in generating high-quality images.At the center of their functioning, the anode materials that are used in X-ray tubes play a central role in determining the efficiency of X-ray formation. The choice of typically used materials, such as tungsten and molybdenum, is determined by high atomic numbers and melting points that enable endurance against the thermal and radiative stresses to which they are exposed during use. Efficient thermal dissipation is essential; hence, the incorporation of cooling systems—such as rotating anodes or precision cooling fins—is vital to ensuring the tube operates optimally at its working temperature. The uses extend beyond extending the life of the X-ray tube, as they also optimize image quality at large by minimizing artifacts caused by thermal expansion and mechanical defects, thereby directly impacting diagnosis accuracy and patient safety (Figure 2.1).

In addition to the anode material, the properties of the focal spot also play crucial roles in establishing the resolution and sharpness of images. The focal spot size, or the area where electron beams interact with the anode, determines the amount of detail visible in X-ray images. More minor focal spots produce higher image resolution, allowing radiographers to see subtle anatomical changes that signal disease. But more minor spots generate more heat, so an exact balance between resolution and safe working conditions must be achieved. Dual-focus design engineering provides flexibility to alternate between resolutions as the situation demands for diagnosis. Such flexibility becomes increasingly relevant for high-end imaging modalities where fine detail is essential for proper interpretation. Understanding and optimization of focal spot behavior are hence critical elements of X-ray tube design for optimal diagnostic output. High-voltage generators are an indispensable requirement for energizing the X-ray tube. They supply the necessary voltage to propel electrons to the anode with sufficient energy to produce X-rays. The generators must provide precise voltage control to maintain consistent image quality and minimize patient exposure risk. The technology has progressed to create high-frequency generators that are more efficient and reduce the patient radiation dose. In addition, modern systems generally include onboard software for real-time monitoring and setup, making it easier for operators to control imaging conditions. With changing imaging demands, there is a need for new high-voltage options in X-ray tube designs that have to catch up with the latest advancements in diagnostic imaging technologies. This will support efforts in patient-centered care and safety standards, leading to improved clinical outcomes.

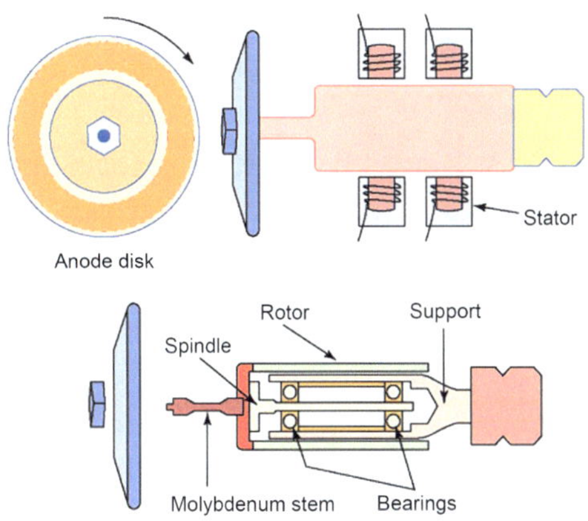

Figure 2.1. Schematic of a rotating anode X-ray tube.

Source: https://radiologykey.com/wp-content/uploads/2021/05/C6-FF13.gif.

2.1.1. Anode Material and Cooling

The evolution of anode materials in medical imaging has become a significant area for improving the performance of X-ray tubes. Material choice plays a key role in influencing the thermal management performance and system effectiveness. Materials with a high atomic number, such as tungsten, are primarily utilized because they possess a greater ability to absorb X-rays, in addition to demonstrating superior thermal conductivity and wear resistance. In this regard, cooling systems further enhance the functioning of such anodes. By using forced-air or oil-cooled systems, producers can prevent overheating, thereby improving the longevity and stability of the X-ray tube.

An efficient cooling system, in its proper functioning form, not only guards the material integrity of the anode but also ensures consistent imaging quality, making it an integral part of the functionality of equipment used for many diagnostic exams. The coupling between the anode material and the cooling technology results in a significant reduction in unwanted fluctuations in X-ray output (Figure 2.2).

	Graphite Laminate	Aluminum 6061	Pure Copper
Density (g/cm^3)	1.33	2.7	8.96
Thermal Conductivity (In-Plane) (W/m•K)	233	180	400
Specific Thermal Conductivity (W•m^2/kg•K)	0.175	0.067	0.045
Thermal Anisotropy	52	1	1

Figure 2.2. Comparative thermal conductivity of common anode materials including tungsten, molybdenum, and graphite.

Source: https://www.researchgate.net/profile/Julian-Norley/publication/3893315/figure/tbl2/AS:652971155140608@1532691863096/Thermal-Conductivity-Comparison-of-Graphite-Laminates-with-6061-and-Copper.png.

Better cooling methods create a more uniform thermal atmosphere, and that is critical since temperature changes can lead to undesirable changes in the electron beams' dynamics. Stable cooling maintains focal spot size, which directly affects image contrast and resolution. Understanding the processes of anode surface degradation through the detection and profiling of elements, such as lithium formation in batteries, is a testament to the complexity of managing heat in energy systems. Through multimodal characterization methods, engineers can design robust cooling systems that efficiently counter thermal challenges, ultimately enabling the operational demands of imaging technologies and the quality diagnostic outputs required for patient care (Partha et al., 2021). Improvements in anode and cooling technologies also signal enhanced design and improved detector systems. Detector performance often relies not only on material composition but also on the integration of precision cooling technologies that render the whole of diagnostic device more operationally effective. For instance, liquid-argon time-projection chambers used in neutrino detection emphasize the importance of stable, low-temperature conditions for effective operation (Acciarri et al., 2017). Similarly, applying such concepts to the X-ray tube industry could help reduce noise and maximize the signal-to-noise ratio of the resulting images. Anodic material innovations coupled with advanced cooling technologies are, therefore, the secret to the further evolution of imaging technology, where reliability and precision must be combined in order to meet the evolving demands of medical diagnostics.

2.1.2. Focal Spot Characteristics

In imaging diagnosis, the character of the focal spot is responsible for determining the sharpness and adequacy of radiographic images. The focal spot, defined as the location on the anode where the electron beam interacts to produce X-rays, directly affects resolution and quality of the image. A smaller focal spot typically allows greater detail and improved spatial resolution, and it is critical for high-precision applications such as mammography. The expense, however, in terms of focal spot size versus heat dissipation, is a significant issue, since a smaller one may cause greater thermal stress on the anode and thus necessitate elaborate cooling systems. Therefore, understanding these characteristics is critical to balancing image quality needs with the operational constraints of the radiographic system (Figure 2.3).

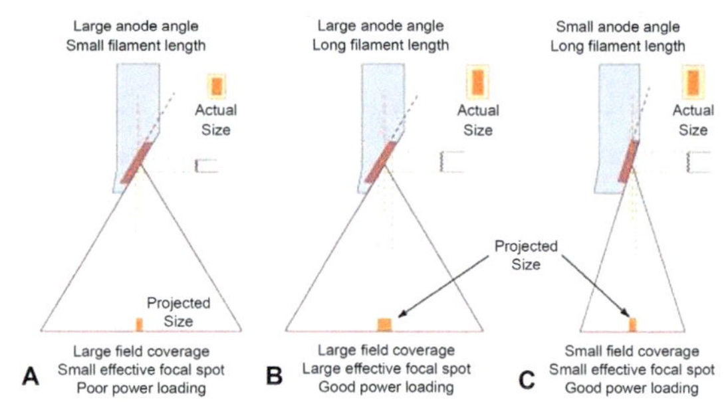

Figure 2.3. Diagram illustrating focal spot size variation with filament current and anode angle. *Source:* https://radiologykey.com/wp-content/uploads/2023/04/C6-FF14.gif.

To enhance the operating efficiency of focal spots, selecting the anode material and configuration is essential. Modern X-ray tubes use tungsten as their anode due to its high melting point and thermal conductivity, enabling better heat management, even during high-energy operations. The anode type—rotating or stationary—also influences the focal spot characteristics. Rotation of the anode provides more even heat distribution and enables the use of small focal spots without compromising tube life. Ultimately, this operating configuration dictates the usability of various imaging protocols, particularly in high-throughput clinics. Technological innovations in anode design and materials are thus necessary to optimize focal spot performance in diagnostic imaging systems. Emerging technologies in diagnostics further enhance the performance of focal spots. Advancements such as broad-tunability, high-brightness laser-based sources, as is being discussed in the case of mid-infrared spectroscopic imaging, illustrate the ability to enhance signal-to-noise ratios and spatial resolution in imaging and offer solutions to some of the age-old problems, such as those caused by conventional thermal sources, which tend to produce poor-quality images due to the lack of signal strength. In addition, the integration of sophisticated algorithms for data processing will further enhance the diagnostic imaging capabilities of imaging modalities by leveraging these improved focal spot characteristics to deliver higher image contrast and resolution. Consequently, these developments indicate an evolving trend towards increasingly accurate and effective diagnostic imaging technology consistent with the overall trend of instrumentation and detector technique in the field (Appleby et al., 2025; McCrow et al., 2011).

2.1.3. High-Voltage Generators

The role of the high-voltage generators in medical imaging is an integral component that enables the operation of X-ray tubes.

These generators supply the x-ray tube with the necessary voltage and current to generate high-energy photons for imaging. High-voltage generators operate on the principle of applying low-voltage AC that is converted into the necessary high-voltage DC for the successful production of X-rays. This function is important because voltage influences the energy and quality of the x-ray beam and thus resolution and detail of the image. Also, improvements in generator technology have increased reliability and efficiency, which are essential for contemporary imaging systems that require consistent performance. Not only is this improvement essential to the safety of the procedure, but it is also crucial in the diagnostic accuracy needed in many medical evaluations. High-voltage generator integration extends beyond functional integration; it also affects the design and technology of the entire X-ray system (Figure 2.4).

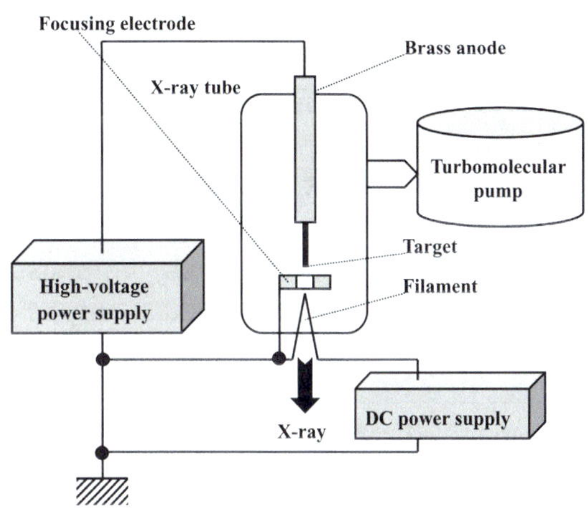

Figure 2.4. Block diagram of a high-voltage generator setup used in diagnostic radiology.

Source: https://www.researchgate.net/profile/Toshiyuki-Enomoto/publication/252653046/figure/fig1/AS:669068294115345@1536529720574/Block-diagram-of-a-characteristic-x-ray-generator.ppm.

Technological advancements in generators, such as the use of digital controls and advanced electronic components, have optimized performance parameters, ensuring accurate, controllable voltage output. Their impacts are achieved through improved image quality in diagnostic images and the provision of various imaging needs. Moreover, these generators are designed to be efficient and use up little space, offsetting the limited spaces typically available in clinical settings. Greater reliability leads to less imaging system downtime, ultimately improving patient throughput and healthcare efficiency. High-voltage generators are thus not only essential from an operational standpoint but also in their role in enhancing the overall utility of diagnostic imaging equipment. In addition, the evolving scenario of medical imaging technology demands continuous high-voltage generation development. This change is viewed in the context of collaboration among industry, academia, and government institutions, as exemplified by efforts such as the NASA SBIR program for innovation development (Gilman et al., 2025). These innovations are imperative in the development of future-generation diagnostic tools that employ high-voltage generators to enhance imaging. Besides, the 2020 NASA Technology Taxonomy emphasizes discipline in technology development, improving communication and coordination among industries that engage in health and technology development (Miranda et al., 2025). The ongoing evolution and fusion of these technologies will continue to position high-voltage generators at the forefront of diagnostic imaging in the future, propelling advancement in more precise and efficient medical diagnostics.

2.2. Flat-Panel Detectors

These advances in imaging technologies have vastly improved diagnostic potential in medical practice, with the flat-panel detectors (FPDs) being a breakthrough factor in this respect. FPDs enable high-resolution imaging with greater efficiency than traditional methods. The evolution of flat-panel detectors, especially cone-beam computed tomography (CBCT), is a prime example of this. While these detectors are multithreaded and multielement and can be applied in various hospital settings, ongoing innovation, such as the dual-layer FPD technology, is aimed at transcending the existing limitations in image quality, particularly for head scans. Quantitative dual-energy imaging could take it to the next level, moving from qualitative checks to more accurate measurements that can make a significant difference in patient care for diagnostics and therapy planning (Wang et al., 2023). The functioning of FPDs relies on two types: indirect and direct conversion panels. Indirect conversion panels use scintillators to convert X-rays into visible light, which is then detected by a photosensitive array. Direct conversion panels eliminate the middleman by converting X-rays into electrical charges, aiming to improve speed and spatial resolution. This difference is crucial in establishing the general performance and suitability of every type of panel to undertake specific imaging missions. The dynamic range and detective quantum efficiency (DQE) of such detectors further determine their ability to produce a wide range of diagnostic images, thereby maintaining maximum performance across different clinical conditions. As demand for high-quality imaging increases, the optimization of FPD parameters underscores the growing need for precise diagnostic tools in current medical practice (Wang et al., 2022). New hybrid methods, particularly in dual-layer FPD configurations, are promising ways to overcome the constraints of conventional systems. The remarkable success of a physics-based material decomposition algorithm enables improved image quality by appropriately exploiting the detected X-ray signals, thereby overcoming issues related to low signal-to-noise. Interestingly, the approach incorporates prior knowledge from imaging physics to enhance material decomposition and enable noise reduction without compromising structural integrity. Since studies show significant improvements in quantification precision—for example, reduced error in iodine quantification—these developments underscore the foundational role of flat-panel detectors in defining imaging methods. Such sophisticated methods not only enhance current applications but also open doors for future studies in targeted and improved diagnostic imaging modalities (Wang et al., 2023).

2.2.1. Indirect Conversion Panels

Advances in imaging technology have revolutionized the diagnostic imaging industry, particularly with the introduction of flat-panel detectors. Indirect conversion panels are a significant component of this new technology, as they convert X-ray photons entering the system into visible light through a two-step process, then detect the light as an electronic signal. The efficiency of their design, comprised primarily of materials such as cesium iodide (CsI), significantly increases spatial resolution and sensitivity.

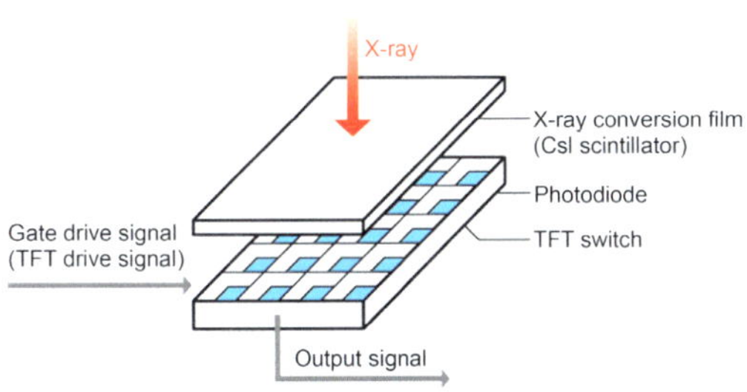

Figure 2.5. Structure of an indirect conversion flat-panel detector with scintillator layer and photodiodes.

Source: https://www.matsusada.com/product/uploads/images/app/fpd.png.

By employing phosphor materials, indirect conversion panels can advance X-ray signals and support better imaging of anatomical structures relevant for diagnosis. Such improved performance is vital in clinical settings, where the need to register subtle changes in soft tissues prevails. Thus, the transition from traditional film-based technology to the latest indirect conversion panels is a significant step towards digital radiography, which equips practitioners with tools to facilitate proper diagnostics within a reasonable time. One of the key advantages of indirect conversion panels is their ability to reduce patient radiation dose while maintaining high image quality. The phosphor layer's ability to fluoresce ensures that even low X-ray doses can be used effectively to produce diagnostically beneficial images (Figure 2.5).

This is particularly useful in sensitive applications, such as pediatric imaging, where radiation dosage should be minimized. Furthermore, the dynamic range and Detective Quantum Efficiency (DQE) of the indirect conversion panels enhance their clinical application. The ability to image a wide range of densities in the image results in high- and low-contrast structures being well visualized. This trait yields higher image quality, enabling medical practitioners to identify early disease signals, ultimately leading to better patient outcomes and informed clinical decisions. In the face of sustained demand for top-quality diagnostic imaging, indirect conversion panels are spearheading advancements in medical imaging technology. Further studies and the advancement of the materials used in such detectors, such as those under study by the SYRMA-3D project, have very serious implications for enhancing image quality. Signal-to-noise ratio-oriented research and the discovery of new applications, such as enhanced breast imaging, all underscore the importance of indirect conversion technology to diagnostic imaging today. Further, their integration into clinical procedures not only hastens and facilitates imaging processes but also strengthens the possibility of intraoperative imaging use. Thus, as diagnostic imaging continues to develop as a discipline, the role of indirect conversion panels remains as crucial as ever, continuing to leave its indelible mark on research and clinical use in healthcare facilities around the globe.

2.2.2. Direct Conversion Panels

Advances in imaging technology have emphasized the significant advantages of direct conversion panels for diagnostic imaging. Direct conversion panels convert X-ray photons to electrical signals, minimizing delay and improving signal quality, which is essential for efficient imaging procedures. At the heart of advances in flat-panel detector technology, direct-conversion panels use materials such as cadmium telluride (CdTe) and cadmium zinc telluride (CZT). These semiconductors enhance imaging performance by providing high resolution and enabling higher detective quantum efficiency (DQE), which is inversely proportional to radiation dose and associated with improved image quality across modalities such as computed tomography (CT) and mammography. Utilization of direct conversion technologies facilitates a shift toward safer imaging through lower patient exposure to ionizing radiation while simultaneously boosting the confidence level of diagnosis. In diagnostic imaging applications, particularly in mammography, moving toward direct-conversion panels is a milestone. In comparison to traditional indirect conversion schemes, which require an intermediate scintillator material, direct conversion panels streamline the process by eliminating this middle step, thereby providing better spatial resolution. The continuous development of direct-conversion photon-counting detectors continues to advance imaging modalities by enabling the differentiation of single-photon events, thereby enhancing detection capacity, especially in tissue-dense environments. The technology has shown recent promise for breast imaging, where overlying tissues can exclude visualization. Advancements in image resolution and diagnostic potential are set to transform breast diagnostics for non-palpable lesions, in line with the community's demand for better screening practices that ensure patient safety while maximizing diagnostic effectiveness (Karellas, 2016). Research into direct conversion panels also confronts the requirement for constant innovation across image modalities. Whereas previous mammography devices were constrained by 2D projections, which created false positives in dense breast tissue, direct conversion technology has opened the door to high-definition three-dimensional imaging solutions. Such an evolution focuses not just on the possibility of better microcalcification visualization but also points to the need for attention to radiation dosage in the design of breast CT and other technologies. The flexible nature and high-performance mode of direct conversion panels are instrumental in overcoming previous technological obstacles, paving the way for assured clinical outcomes. As such, further study is necessary to realize the full potential of direct conversion materials and their application to more holistic diagnostic imaging paradigms, ultimately enhancing patient treatment and diagnostic accuracy in clinical practice (Shaji et al., 2024) (Figure 2.6).

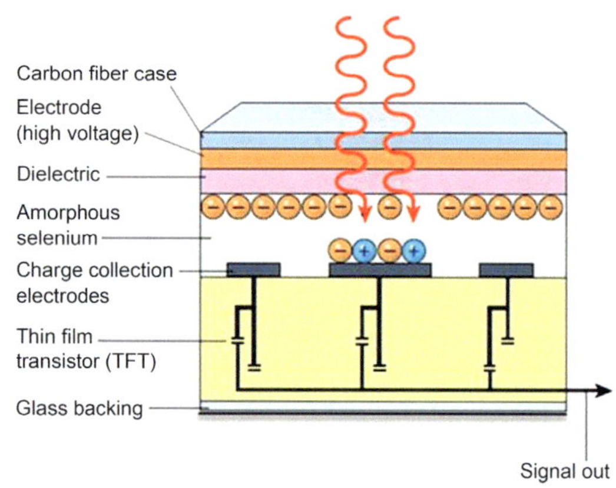

Figure 2.6. Cross-sectional view of a direct conversion detector using amorphous selenium.

Source: https://blogger.googleusercontent.com/img/b/R29vZ2xl/AVvXsEhXVrDMXfnrp8QGvOrLGTaWOgcsVqfT-dXd1cYRuLhb5N4ph9AMNpEZqgwR0GjhkHFPDKeEibvfkwKkVxPsCqinATboilFFJVNsOGAa8edaTKNO7C67FxEZ7UmzHFrdk9eqcArCwBqknYYw/s1600/direct+conversion.JPG.

2.2.3. Dynamic Range and DQ

Detective quantum efficiency (DQE) and dynamic range have the most important relationship in optimizing the performance of diagnostic imaging devices. Dynamic range is the range of exposure levels that can be detected by an adequate detector with a high degree of precision, enabling meaningful information about low and high signal levels to be brought into view. This property is imperative for diagnostic definition because it enables the identification of subtle variations in imaged tissue without saturating the detector. Within the context of DQE, or the ability of a detector to convert X-ray photons into useful image information, a wide dynamic range can significantly improve image quality using minimal radiation dose to patients (Figure 2.7).

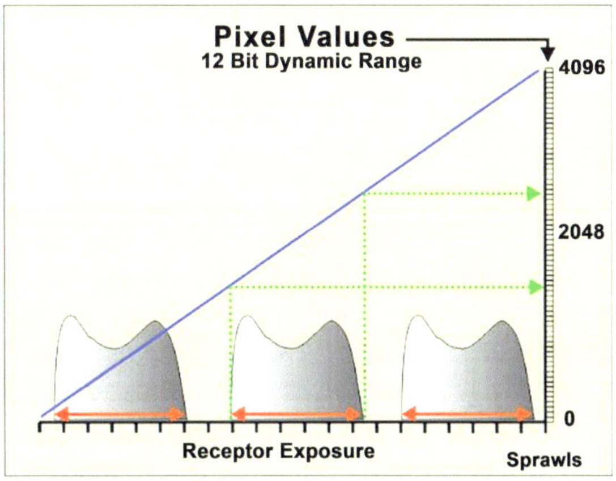

Figure 2.7. Graph showing dynamic range comparison across digital detector types.

Source: https://lh5.googleusercontent.com/proxy/A_aRCmSyzKJyRIQQOKLfnVoGIXKSgZUld3clHEcCrx6Lxv37gn9Q7bZji2jH00sbzWWZNX2gp2ptfVGJMYgjcxKAGvYFs6C-jg.

Optimization and the value of such parameters in clinical practice can considerably influence diagnostic confidence and patient safety, underscoring the importance of the synergy between DQE and dynamic range in emerging imaging modalities. The clinical role of DQE cannot be overstated, as it serves as a benchmark for detector imaging efficiency. It is crucial for establishing the extent to which a system provides diagnostic data while minimizing radiation exposure. The non-linear nature of processed image data, which can distort accuracy, has resulted in challenges in measuring DQE, particularly in routine clinical environments. Despite such challenges, recent advancements have promoted methodologies for the estimation of DQE from processed data, enabling the ability to provide routine quality assurance in the clinic. This trend is significant, as the inclusion of such tests within standard procedures would ensure that imaging devices perform optimally under varying conditions and thus permit healthcare practitioners to make informed decisions through proper image assessment. Lastly, the necessity for routine DQE testing in clinical settings has a synergy with the broader goal of maximizing patient outcomes while also ensuring safety. As understood from the present research, computer-aided DQE measurement systems are becoming concrete alternatives to address the technical issues typically burdened on end-users in clinical environments (Escartin et al., 2017). The evolving perception of DQE requires a rational approach to its use in daily routines, with a focus on its status as an important quality control indicator. This integrated method is supported by evidence showing that measuring DQE provides information on the degree to which imaging systems operate in real clinical practice environments, influencing patient care quality and determining health outcomes (McDonald et al., 2012).

2.3. Image Intensifiers

The use of image intensifiers in diagnostic imaging is the peak of the combination of utility and innovation in medical devices. Essential to improving poor lighting, they amplify electron emission via the photoelectric effect, as light photons collide with the photocathode coating. The resulting photoelectric effect creates a significant increase in brightness, allowing for better visualization of radiographic structures. This increase is critical in applications where exposure time must be minimized to limit radiation hazards, thus making image intensifiers a core technology for real-time imaging modalities. In addition, advances in photocathode materials have enabled broader spectral responses, enhancing detection of low-light levels in most medical applications, including fluoroscopy and angiography. These developments underscore the crucial role of image intensification in improving diagnostic precision and patient management productivity. In image intensifier technology, minification gain can be seen as a fundamental feature in optimizing the quality of output visual data. Minification gain has been described as the capacity of image intensifiers to focus a larger proportion of input light into a smaller, intensified output image without reducing resolution. When light photons bombard the photocathode, subsequent photon-to-electron conversion is further regulated in a progression of microchannel plates that enhance brightness and resolution without sacrificing spatial integrity. The focus of this light highlights the value of diagnostic imaging, particularly for dynamic studies requiring high temporal resolution. Hence, gain minification not just provides improved visibility under poor imaging conditions but also serves as a driving force for exploring advanced imaging techniques involving high accuracy, such as interventional radiology. While they do offer advantages, the operating complexities of image intensifiers pose problems, mainly distortion and lag. Distortion undermines the geometric fidelity of images—essential for proper diagnoses—by warping shape and proportions in the visual display. Lag, with trailing images left after the source of activation is withdrawn, further complicates dynamic image interpretation in real time. Better designs and calibration methods are therefore essential to offset these challenges, thereby yielding clearer, more consistent pictures. The application of image intensifiers is therefore still contingent on continuous technological improvement and close attention to their inherent limitations. According to calibration studies of high-technology detector systems, as discussed in (Castaneda et al., 1999) and (Desorgher et al., 2003), optimal image intensifier performance is essential for achieving better diagnostic outcomes in contemporary imaging practices (Figure 2.8).

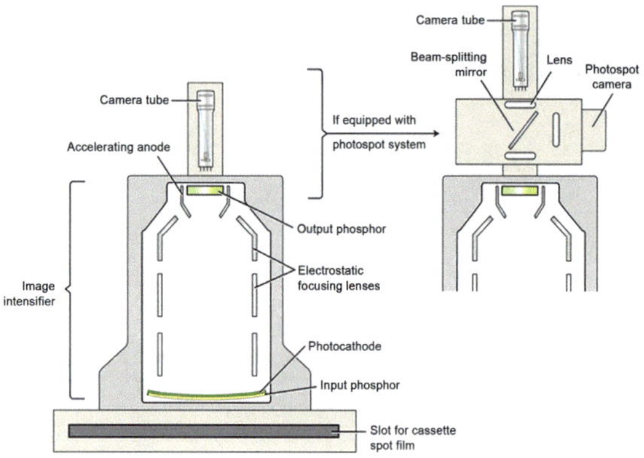

Figure 2.8. Image intensifier assembly highlighting input phosphor, photocathode, and output screen. *Source:* https://radiologykey.com/wp-content/uploads/2016/02/B9780323069748100141_f14-03-9780323069748.jpg.

2.3.1. Photocathode Operation

The role of photocathodes in image intensifiers is critical, particularly for operational performance and sensitivity. Image intensification technology uses photocathodes to convert incident light into electrons, a process that is most important for amplifying low-light images. The materials possess high quantum efficiency, thus capable of converting photons to photoelectrons effectively, thus amplifying the signal before it reaches the following imaging devices. The choice of material for the photocathodes is of paramount importance, as their characteristics directly influence the overall performance of the imaging system. New developments have demonstrated that the deposition of optimized coatings can significantly enhance the quantum efficiency of such photocathodes, making them extremely important for achieving high-quality imaging in diagnostics. Research prioritizes temporal stability and minimizing drifts during use, which is paramount for accurate diagnostics (Lumpkin et al., 2012). Moreover, the design of photocathodes affects their integration into advanced imaging systems. The work on photocathode technology development addresses how future techniques can enhance detector performance in general. UV technology improvements, for instance, show that photocathode materials can be engineered to achieve quantum efficiencies above 50%, thereby increasing the detectable signal spectrum and image quality. These improvements pertain to the requirements for improved detector technology in diagnostic imaging, as they provide concrete solutions for low-light image processing. Coalescence of topmost levels of coatings and layered structures in the photocathodes is also essential, indicating a cooperative process that improves detection and imaging fidelity in the medical imaging process (Martin et al., 2012). With the advancement of imaging, continuous optimization of the photocathode function remains central to effective diagnostic performance. The developments in the photocathode technologies enhance not only the response time and sensitivity but also broaden the dynamic range of the imaging systems. By focusing on improving photoconductive materials and their configurations, researchers are laying the foundation for next-generation advances in imaging devices. These advancements would deliver breakthroughs in the production of compact, efficient image intensifiers, which are an integral part of clinical diagnostic processes. Therefore, the evolution of photocathode function has a direct impact on the reliability and efficiency of diagnostic imaging technology to meet rising medical practitioners' needs (Lumpkin et al., 2012).

2.3.2. Minification Gain

Improvements in diagnostic imaging technology have brought fundamental changes in the way doctors view and detect disease. Among those advances is the concept of Minification Gain in image intensifiers, a critical metric of enhancing image quality and system performance. By minimizing the output image's size relative to the input, Minification Gain enables higher brightness and contrast, essential characteristics for examining complex anatomical structures (Figure 2.9).

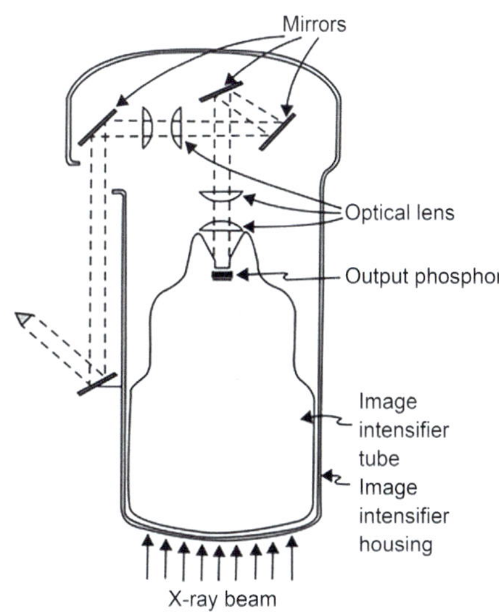

Figure 2.9. Illustration of minification gain through electron beam compression inside the intensifier tube.

Source: https://d45jl3w9libvn.cloudfront.net/jaypee/static/books/9788184482140/Chapters/images/187-1.jpg.

This light amplification enables radiologists to perceive finer details that are otherwise lost in conventional imaging systems, conferring enormous value for clinical diagnosis, especially in high-risk environments such as surgery and emergency medicine. A closer look at Minification Gain reveals its mechanisms and engineering principles serving to amplify this effect. Image intensifiers employ a series of operational layers, such as photocathodes, which convert incoming photons into electrons. The produced electrons are converged through a series of steps before being re-emitted as an enhanced image. Both the design of the photocathode and the minifying optics geometry dominate the determination of the amount of Minification Gain achieved. With optics optimized to capture as much light as possible and maximize image sharpness, technologies in this area deliver a startling boost to diagnostic capability, yielding more detail and greater visual distinction in the images produced. Beyond increased image sharpness, the influence of Minification Gain has far-reaching implications: it renders imaging systems overall more efficient in patient care. As may be evident from recent breakthroughs in developing detectors of high resolution, such as those in the INSERT project, which is sensitivity-in-system-focused, having Minification Gain in the equation helps to balance the demand for both sensitivity and spatial resolution in complex imaging environments such as MRI scanners. Integrating these technologies not only highlights the importance of Minification Gain but also complements ongoing efforts to improve diagnostic equipment. New collimator designs, such as techniques for gamma-shielding control and enhanced spatial resolution, augment Minification Gain synergistically in extending the boundaries of what diagnostic imaging can accomplish in contemporary medicine (Salvado et al., 2017).

2.3.3. Distortion and Lag

The overall quality evaluation of diagnostic images is closely related to awareness of the idiosyncrasies of lag and distortion in instrument design, particularly in image intensifiers. These technologies play a significant role in enhancing the quality of images generated from X-ray and other radiation modalities. Distortion is typically presented as a geometric aberration that undermines the validity of clinical diagnoses, in that images fail to accurately reflect the underlying anatomical structure due to departures in the optical path or in the electronic processing of signals. Such distortion, if left uncorrected, can undermine the correct interpretation of patient conditions and even have a bearing on treatment outcomes. Technological advancements in detector design to reduce distortion are important, as they are primarily responsible for the overall reliability of diagnostic imaging systems; thus, it is necessary to continue research and development in this area (Anuskiewicz et al., 2025) (Figure 2.10).

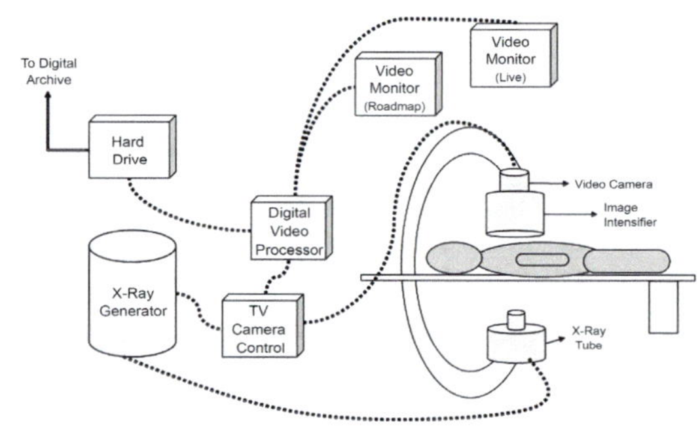

Figure 2.10. E X-ray image intensifier – an overview.

Source: https://ars.els-cdn.com/content/image/1-s2.0-S073510970401959X-gr5.jpg.

Lag —the delay in the imaging system's response to varying amounts of input radiation —is another parameter that must be carefully considered. Lag leads to image blurring or smearing, particularly in dynamic measurements such as tracing moving anatomical structures. Effective control of lag is required for ensuring good temporal resolution in imaging systems.

Investigation of detector algorithms and processing techniques aims to mitigate lag effects, thereby enhancing the diagnostic capability of imaging instruments. Progress in minimizing lag is critical to providing sharper images, which will give clinicians greater temporal information on which to make their decisions (Bautz et al., 2025). As imaging technology evolves, combating lag will be central to achieving the highest diagnostic value from new equipment. The marriage of advanced designs and technologies to minimize both lag and distortion is opening new frontiers in diagnostic imaging. As health care demands escalate and the complexity of the imaging situation increases, it becomes imperative that researchers and engineers find solutions to these two challenges. By making the improvement of image intensification systems the top priority, the possibility of higher-fidelity images becomes increasingly within sight. This effort not only enhances the overall effectiveness of diagnostic imaging but also enhances patient outcomes through improved accuracy in diagnostic procedures. Consequently, continuous progress in noise reduction, signal processing, and materials science becomes essential for further refining the operational capabilities of imaging modalities, prompting further analysis of these aspects in future studies (Anuskiewicz et al., 2025; Bautz et al., 2025).

2.4. Photomultiplier and Scintillation Detectors

The evolution of imaging systems is bound to influence diagnostic medicine, and photomultiplier tubes (PMTs) and scintillation detectors play critical roles across various modalities, including Positron Emission Tomography (PET). Scintillation material detectors use scintillation materials that emit light when exposed to ionizing radiation. The choice of scintillator material makes a significant difference in performance; common scintillators include sodium iodide (NaI) and bismuth germanate (BGO). Each material has varying properties of light output, decay time, and energy resolution and hence affects the quality and reliability of detected signals. This heterogeneity necessitates a rigorous selection process to optimize diagnostic imaging equipment for specific applications, such as accurately capturing metabolic activity in oncology, enhancing detection sensitivity in neurology, and facilitating the delivery of tailored therapies and improved patient outcomes (Lamprou et al., 2021). In conjunction with scintillation materials, the operating efficiency of PMTs is essential to the efficiency of these detection systems. Photomultiplier tubes work by converting scintillation light into an electrical signal via a cascade of photoelectrons, amplifying it to a level detectable and analyzable. High energy resolution, something which allows for a clear distinction between gamma-ray energies, is one of the significant challenges PMT design must endure. PMT performance depends on working voltage and temperature conditions, which must be controlled to function optimally. Improved energy resolution also means improved image quality because noise and artifacts in the output diagnostic images are reduced, a factor critical for such applications requiring precise contrasts, for example, PET scanning (Cherry et al., 2008). Against the backdrop of developments in combined imaging technology, the complementarity between photomultiplier technology and scintillation detectors remains fundamental. Current research focuses on the fusion of both technologies into hybrid PET and MRI systems, a rapidly growing trend in diagnostic imaging towards multi-modality. Convergence enables the simultaneous collection of complementary data sources, leading to a more comprehensive understanding of patient conditions. Nevertheless, achieving artifact-free images requires ongoing innovation in detector design and calibration methods. With ongoing developments in the field, a good understanding of the operational fundamentals of scintillation detectors and PMT systems remains essential for the development of more sophisticated imaging modalities to advance diagnostic accuracy and therapeutic interventions in modern medicine (Lamprou et al., 2021).

2.4.1. Scintillator Materials

Development in scintillator materials has deeply influenced diagnostic imaging technology, particularly in the performance and efficacy of detector technology. Scintillators are critical materials that convert ionizing radiation into visible light utilized and quantified for the generation of diagnostic images. Various materials are used for scintillation, each offering specific properties such as light yield, decay time, and energy resolution. For example, inorganic scintillators such as sodium iodide (NaI) and lanthanum bromide (LaBr3) are favored for their high light output and fast response time, which are ideal for medical imaging. The ability of such materials to provide accurate spectral information results in improved image contrast and resolution, hence enhancing the diagnostic capability. The interface between scintillating material and detection technologies unlocks the possibility of innovation in non-invasive imaging modalities, with profound implications for patient care and outcomes. Furthermore, the integration of next-generation scintillator materials into detector systems has addressed outright problems in diagnostic imaging. Background noise suppression is paramount, especially in applications such as gamma-ray detection and high-energy imaging. By applying novel materials such as LaBr3, which offers superior speed and energy resolution, imaging system sensitivity can be readily improved. This is useful for minimizing the impact of undesirable neutron-induced gamma rays that may impair diagnostic visibility, as highlighted in recent studies (Bancroft et al., 2010). The performance of existing detectors can also be improved through innovative designs that incorporate pulse-shape discrimination and higher timing resolution, thereby enhancing overall imaging capability and reliability in medicine. Recent developments have emphasized the role of scintillator technology in advancing medical imaging. The design of scintillator-based detectors, such as those that use deuterated organic scintillators in combination with LaBr3, represents one cohesive effort to reduce internal background emissions and thus improve signal clarity and detection accuracy (Bancroft et al., 2009). Beyond facilitating improved imaging results, these advancements also provide access to the utilization of diagnostic technology in areas previously compromised by background noise. The constant evolution of scintillator materials thus finds ideal congruence with the ultimate goal of maintaining maximum diagnostic efficacy while ensuring patient safety. With continued research and development in the field, the future implications for diagnostic imaging technology remain deep, promising a new generation of precise and effective medical imaging (Figure 2.11).

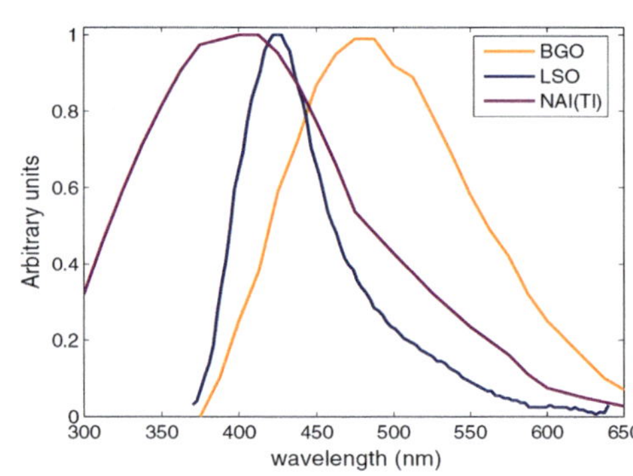

Figure 2.11. Common scintillator materials and their emission spectra.

Source: https://www.researchgate.net/publication/320217811/figure/fig3/AS:11431281208806376@1701442092416/Emission-spectra-of-three-examples-of-common-scintillators-LSO-BGO-and-NaITl.jpg.

2.4.2. Photomultiplier Tube Functioning

The ability to sense and quantify low-light intensities accurately is critical in diagnostic imaging, where accuracy prevails. Photomultiplier tubes (PMTs) are essential components of most imaging instruments, particularly in scintillation detector-containing applications. The operation of such equipment is a multi-step process in which incident photons first strike a photocathode or photosensitive surface. This is followed by the emission of photoelectrons, which are then accelerated and amplified in a series of electrodes known as dynodes (Figure 2.12).

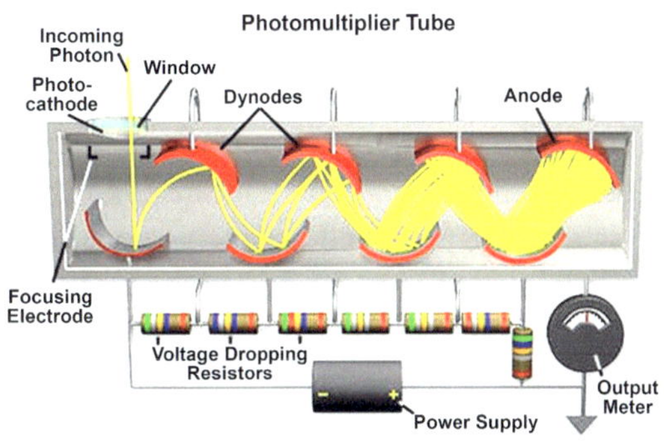

Figure 2.12. Internal structure of a photomultiplier tube with dynode stages and voltage divider.

Source: https://evidentscientific.com/en/microscope-resource/knowledge-hub/digital-imaging/concepts/media_1508aefa8c365f5aedac84d0926c6ca6a3c001fbe.png?width=1200&format=pjpg&optimize=medium.

Each dynode stage amplifies the electrons, thereby increasing the original signal considerably. One incident photon may thus lead to the generation of thousands of electrons at the output, boosting the sensitivity and overall performance of imaging systems. Amplification is crucial in high-precision applications, and PMTs are thus an essential tool in modern diagnostic technologies. In scintillation detection, photomultiplier tubes work well with scintillator materials. Scintillator crystals transform the incident radiation into visible light, which is then detected by PMTs. The scintillator material has a significant impact on the system's efficiency and sensitivity. Phases such as sodium iodide doped with thallium (NaI(Tl)) have been widely used and have worked well due to their excellent scintillation properties.

The operation of PMTs enables the accurate measurement of light intensity, permitting the quantification of radiation absorbed by the scintillator. This interaction between scintillation materials and PMTs provides greater imaging capabilities, allowing the detection of faint variations in tissue contrast and ultimately improving diagnostic accuracy in medical imaging. The operational efficiency of photomultiplier tubes also depends on features such as detection efficiency and energy resolution. These factors directly influence the accuracy with which imaging devices capture and interpret diagnostic data. For instance, improved energy resolution in PMTs can make a more precise distinction between different radiation energies, which is very essential in PET and gamma cameras. In addition, variables such as dark current, noise, and temperature stability significantly contribute to the operational efficiency of PMTs. The evaluation of these variables maximizes detector performance for targeted medical applications, thereby enhancing diagnostic imaging technology. With the evolving profile of diagnostic imaging, the seamless integration of photomultiplier tube technology with next-generation detection methods remains at the forefront of advancing clinical imaging, ultimately enabling more precise patient diagnoses.

2.4.3. Energy Resolution

In the context of diagnostic imaging, measurement accuracy largely depends on the capability of various detector technologies to distinguish between two different energy levels. Such a capability is generally referred to as energy resolution and is crucial for distinguishing gamma-ray and x-ray photons whose energies are very close to each other.

The energy resolution of scintillation and photomultiplier detectors is primarily determined by the inherent properties of the scintillator materials used. Better energy resolution enables these detectors to produce more informative and clearer scans, improving diagnostic accuracy. The performance of such detectors is critically assessed by their ability to detect minute differences in spectral data, enabling more targeted interventions in patient management in imaging technologies (Figure 2.13).

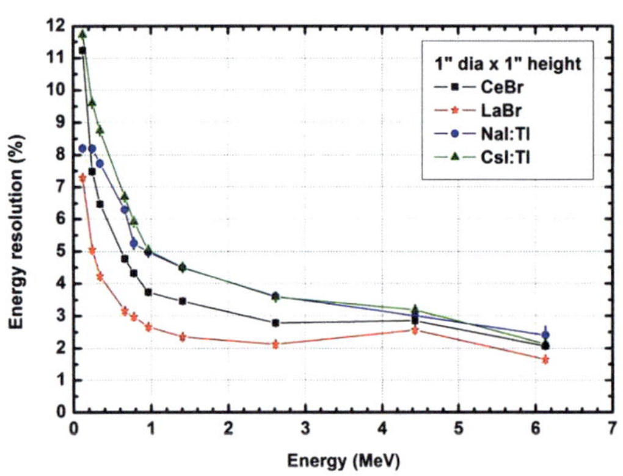

Figure 2.13. Graph showing energy resolution measured for NaI:Tl, CsI:Tl, LaBr 3 :Ce and CeBr 3 scintillators for γ-ray energies in the range between 0.1 and 6.1 MeV.

Source: https://www.researchgate.net/profile/Aneta-Gojska/publication/323891517/figure/fig4/AS:606477735694349@1521606968712/Energy-resolution-measured-for-NaITl-CsITl-LaBr-3-Ce-and-CeBr-3-scintillators-for.png.

Further, advances in scintillator technology have led to the manufacture of materials with improved energy resolution, thereby decreasing the effects of noise that may disrupt significant signals. For instance, interaction between incident radiation and a scintillator may yield light that is later amplified via photomultiplier tubes. Here, photon collection efficiency and scintillator decay time are significant variables in determining overall energy resolution.

Improvements here have been aimed at maximizing these parameters to the level where even small energy changes are measured and utilized for diagnostic purposes. Such improvements are particularly important in those imaging applications that require precise discrimination between pathological and non-pathological tissue, thus enhancing the efficiency of imaging modalities for clinical use. In addition, the increasing demand for real-time imaging and the use of complex spectral imaging technologies further underscore the importance of energy resolution in diagnostic equipment. Infrared spectroscopic imaging, for instance, is highly dependent on high-energy resolution to provide both morphological and biochemical information about tissues, particularly in cancer diagnosis.

With high-brightness laser sources, it is possible to augment the signal-to-noise ratio, thereby boosting energy resolution and operational efficiency, which are crucial for delivering quick and accurate diagnoses. As technology advances, sustained focus on detector technologies and energy-resolution collaboration will remain important, enabling future medical diagnostic imaging innovations and eventually contributing to better patient care in medical practice (McCrow et al., 2011; Benford et al., 2013).

2.5. Semiconductor Detectors

The use of semiconductor detectors in diagnostic imaging has become imperative due to their ability to directly convert incident radiation into electronic signals. The procedure is imperative in many imaging modalities, where the precision and reliability of the output data significantly impact diagnostic conclusions. Two of the more prevalent semiconductor materials used are cadmium telluride (CdTe) and cadmium zinc telluride (CZT), which can provide better energy resolution and sensitivity than standard detection methods. The ability to produce spectral imaging with these materials enables more selective discrimination between different types of radiation, which is particularly valuable for distinguishing and quantifying several distinct pathological processes. Due to their small size and ability to convert signals instantaneously, semiconductor detectors are becoming increasingly integral components of modern imaging systems, improving diagnostic effectiveness and overall patient care. The performance of semiconductor detectors in imaging, however, is impacted by various factors, including temperature. Stability during use is critical to ensure consistent imaging results, particularly in environments where temperature fluctuations can occur. When the temperature is altered, the electronic properties of semiconductor materials can be altered, which leads to degradation of energy resolution and increased levels of noise in the detected signal. Countermeasures such as incorporating temperature control systems into imaging devices and developing high-level signal-processing algorithms that can reverse the impact of temperature alterations are being embraced. This ongoing research indicates the need for continued development in detector technology so that semiconductor detectors remain effective and dependable under various conditions and solidify their roles in diagnostic imaging. Another significant advantage of semiconductor detectors is that they can enhance diagnostic efficiency of imaging modalities by enabling greater detective quantum efficiency (DQE). The ability of an imaging system to efficiently transform incoming radiation into a signal that may be exploited is defined by this measure. Higher DQE is implied by improved performance, allowing for the use of lower radiation dosages without compromising image quality. This has specific use in medical imaging, where it is necessary to minimize the patient's exposure to hazardous radiation. The use of semiconductor detectors in most imaging techniques helps achieve higher DQE values, allowing for better-quality images and diagnoses. Thus, it is all the more crucial that semiconductor detector technology continue to be developed and implemented, as it not only affects the efficacy of diagnostic imaging practice but also the further development of patient safety and quality of care (Daynene et al., 2009; Farshidfar et al., 2020).

2.5.1. CdTe and CZT Detectors

In the evolving situation of diagnostic imaging, advancements in detection technologies play a crucial role in enhancing image quality and resolution. Cadmium telluride (CdTe) and cadmium zinc telluride (CZT) detectors are among the most notable developments, which have been in the spotlight due to their superior performance compared to traditional silicon- and germanium-based detectors. These semiconductors have high detection efficiency and performance at room temperature, enabling the development of compact, rugged detection systems. CdTe and CZT material research continues to seek to capitalize on their unique properties, thereby improving device characteristics and enhancing material performance (Figure 2.14).

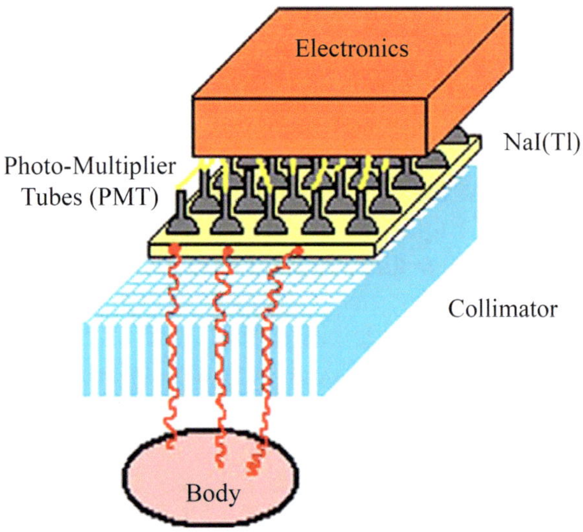

Figure 2.14. Crystal structure of CdTe and CZT semiconductor materials used in imaging.

Source: https://www.mdpi.com/sensors/sensors-09-03491/article_deploy/html/images/sensors-09-03491f23-1024.png.

With greater dependency on precise imaging modalities for diagnostic imaging, the role of CdTe and CZT detectors assumes a critical significance in scientific as well as in clinical applications, especially in medical imaging and astrophysics where the detection of gamma rays and X-rays must be exact (Abbene et al., 2009). The practical advantages of CZT detectors in X-ray imaging are a prime example of their application in contemporary diagnostic technology. Characterized by superior charge-transport properties, CZT detectors offer enhanced electron mobility and lifetime, which are essential for genuine imaging under fluctuating flux conditions. Over the past few years, progress in CZT materials has led to the development of low-flux (LF-CZT) and high-flux (HF-CZT) varieties, each tailored to specific uses and sensitivity requirements. The novel structural architectures, particularly sub-millimeter-pixel structures, also enhance performance to a greater extent by enabling improved charge collection and reducing the effects of charge-sharing events. Experimental procedures have shed light on energy spectra and charge-sharing correction techniques, which, in turn, help mitigate challenges related to incomplete charge collection. These advances together facilitate the integration of CZT technology into energy-resolved X-ray scanners and the expansion of their applications in medical diagnosis and industrial non-destructive testing (Abbene et al., 2022). Further pursuit of resolution and efficiency leads to the integration of CdTe and CZT detectors in more integrated diagnostic image schemes and is a significant development in the field. It is the relationship between material properties and detector performance parameters, such as detective quantum efficiency and spectral imaging, that makes these semiconductor detectors so promising. Understanding the effect of temperature fluctuations on their performance is also crucial because it affects the design and operation of systems under various conditions. Ongoing R&D work is focused not just on improving the intrinsic characteristics of these detectors but also on making them robust and compatible in hospital settings. CdTe and CZT detectors, therefore, can continue to be basic components of imaging technologies in the future, contributing towards enhanced patient care and diagnostic accuracy.

2.5.2. Spectral Imaging Capability

In the evolution of diagnostic imaging devices, the addition of spectral imaging functionality has been a groundbreaking advancement, greatly enhancing their diagnostic capabilities. With the utilization of semiconductor detectors, including cadmium telluride (CdTe) and cadmium zinc telluride (CZT), the ability to acquire and process spectral information allows for nuanced distinctions in various tissue structures and disease states. These materials enable the breakdown of detected photons into distinct energy levels and facilitate more effective material differentiation than conventional imaging modalities. The richness of information afforded by spectral imaging positions it as a central force in distinguishing between numerous tissues and in detecting and characterizing disease, particularly in oncology and cardiology. Beyond mere image acquisition, application in diagnostics is underscored by its ability to provide quantitative data regarding tissue properties. This is a result of the unique interaction between radiation and biological tissues, in which each material exhibits a distinct set of spectral signatures. Consequently, spectral imaging makes it easier to generate advanced algorithms to augment image reconstruction and analysis. These advances allow clinicians not only to visualize but also quantify tissue composition. Applications range from cancer detection to quantifying treatment efficacy. Lastly, this advancement in imaging data analysis is a step toward precision medicine, in which nuanced imaging data can yield bespoke treatment plans. Furthermore, the ongoing advancement of detector technology significantly affects the efficacy of spectral imaging. Advancements in detector resolution and sensitivity are critical for the increased precision needed in high-throughput applications, such as those outlined in the treatment of high-throughput UV spectroscopy and wide-field imaging by the Ultraviolet-Optical Working Group (Baum et al., 1999). These technological developments should also account for temperature effects, which can cause variations in detector performance —a critical aspect identified in the new study (Appleby et al., 2025). As the imaging ecosystem transforms, the complementary synergy between advanced detector technologies and highly developed spectral imaging will more than likely revolutionize diagnostic imaging, leading to improved outcomes and transforming clinical paradigms (Figure 2.15).

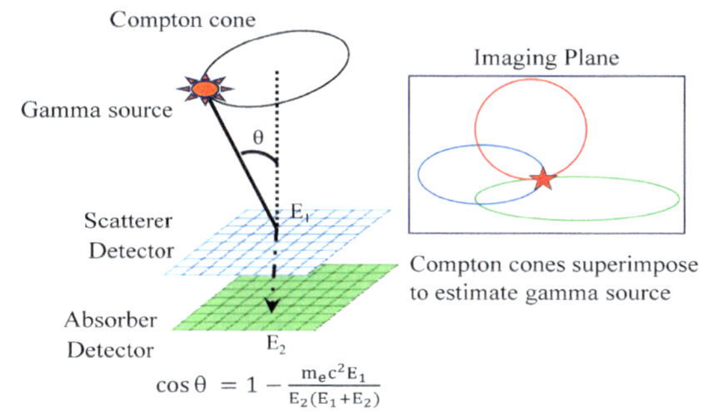

Figure 2.15. Spectral imaging results from CZT detector arrays for multi-isotope differentiation. Source: https://www.mdpi.com/sensors/sensors-24-00725/article_deploy/html/images/sensors-24-00725-g008.png.

2.5.3. Temperature Effects

The multifaceted interplay between temperature and semiconductor detector operation is critical in diagnostic imaging. Variations in temperature can have a significant influence on the electrical properties of semiconductor materials such as Cadmium Telluride (CdTe) and Cadmium Zinc Telluride (CZT), which are pivotal in spectral imaging. Variation in temperature affects carrier concentration and mobility, which directly affects the energy resolution and efficiency of the detectors. Specifically, a temperature rise can cause elevated noise levels, diminishing the signal-to-noise ratio. This is why optimal temperatures must be maintained to ensure accuracy and efficacy in imaging processes, underscoring the need for advanced thermal management techniques in detector design and operation. Thus, it is crucial to understand these temperature effects to improve diagnostic devices and streamline the quality of medical images they render. In addition, the detector design must include robust temperature stabilization to prevent adverse effects on imaging performance. For instance, the inclusion of a cooling apparatus can be utilized to guarantee an optimal operating temperature, thus the integrity of the detectors' functional properties. Research in advanced materials and coatings has also shown promise for enhancing thermal efficiency, with innovation at the materials science and engineering interface. Findings from workshops, such as those NASA has held in the past, point to the need for technological innovation to address the temperature issues facing detectors used in space and Earth imaging missions (Appleby et al., 2025). As research continues to advance, renewed efforts to improve temperature control will be core to the reliability of diagnostic imaging technologies.

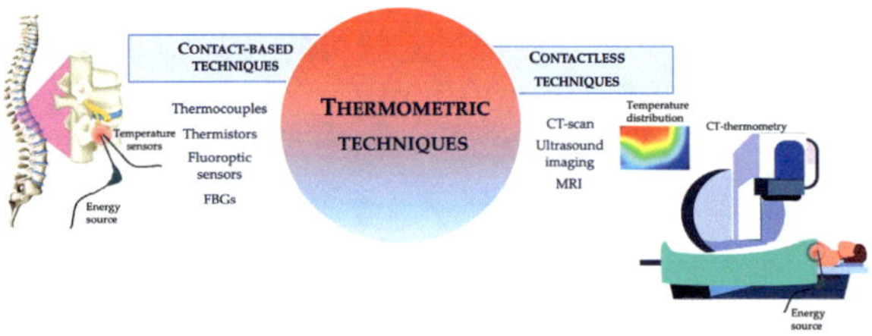

Figure 2.16. Temperature monitoring in hyperthermia treatments of bone tumors.

Source: https://pub.mdpi-res.com/sensors/sensors-21-05470/article_deploy/html/images/sensors-21-05470-g001-550.jpg?1628853560.

Ultimately, the effects of temperature impacts go beyond short-term performance measurement; they carry real-world implications for patient outcomes and diagnostic accuracy. Diagnostic accuracy can be compromised by misinterpretation and possibly harmful effects on patients when imaging systems are operating below optimal temperatures. By describing the specifics of temperature-dependent variations in detector technologies, the medical imaging community can more effectively schedule maintenance and upgrade procedures to ensure that imaging systems are always functioning optimally. In addition, research funded under initiatives such as NASA's SBIR program is necessary in obtaining insight into how to develop new technologies that efficiently counteract these challenges (Gilman et al., 2025). In this evolving setting, the need to understand and manage the influence of temperature will continue to promote the quality of care in diagnostic imaging (Figure 2.16).

2.6. Detector Performance Indicators

In diagnostic imaging, detector performance characteristic testing is of utmost importance for delivering the best image quality and diagnostic effectiveness. One of these measures of importance is the Detective Quantum Efficiency (DQE), which is a measure of a detector's ability to create an image in relation to the amount of radiation it is subjected to. This is a key measurement, as higher DQE indicates that less radiation exposure is needed to achieve diagnostic-image quality, and therefore is safer for the patient. Furthermore, DQE combines both the detector's spatial resolution and its ability to preserve contrast, and as such is a core part of assessing detector performance. With the continued evolution of imaging technology, it is important to emphasize these performance parameters, since they are intrinsically tied to the practical usage and clinical efficiency of various imaging modalities in modern healthcare centers (Abu-Shawareb et al., 2022). The second important component of detector performance parameters includes the Modulation Transfer Function (MTF), which characterizes the spatial resolution of the imaging system. MTF indicates the extent to which a detector can replicate the spatial frequencies present in an object and, in this way, shows the system's capability to represent delicate structures. A greater MTF value indicates the detector's potential to depict complex structures within the area of interest accurately, and this is critical for successful diagnosis and treatment planning. Also, MTF has a universal application for comparing detector technologies and provides an objective standard for measuring progress in imaging systems.

For this reason, MTF knowledge is not only essential for optimizing diagnostic imaging techniques but also for guiding technological advancements that improve image quality in clinical applications (Meryem et al., 2021). Finally, linearity and lag testing of detector response further streamline the use of imaging technologies in diagnosis. Linearity is the consistency of detectors' responses to varying amounts of radiation, ensuring that images reflect real exposure levels. This aspect is most critical, as a non-linear response can lead to inaccurate interpretation and misdiagnosis. Similarly, lag, or a trailing signal that results from an exposure, can severely compromise the temporal integrity of dynamic imaging scenarios. By assessing these characteristics of detector performance, radiologists can be certain that imaging findings are correct and consistent, ultimately leading to better patient outcomes. Therefore, ongoing research and development have been aimed at maximizing these indices to further strengthen the diagnostic quality and working performance of imaging technologies in practice (Abu-Shawareb et al., 2022).

2.6.1. Detective Quantum Efficiency

In diagnostic imaging, understanding the efficiency of various detectors is crucial to ensure maximum patient safety and care. Detective Quantum Efficiency (DQE) is a critical parameter that outlines the efficiency with which the incident X-ray photons are utilized by the imaging system in order to achieve a good-quality image. This measure is particularly significant within the theme of decreased exposure of radiation to patients, which is a significant factor as dental and medical radiography constitutes a major component of man-made radiation exposure in the populace. Application of the DQE in clinical settings can enhance the efficacy of x-ray imaging while reducing unnecessary radiation exposure, leading to improved diagnostic outcomes and patient protection (Hamann et al., 2019). Hence, a firm grasp of DQE enables experts to select and optimize imaging systems adequately so that patients can receive the maximum diagnostic benefit with minimum risks. Advances in detector technologies have enhanced DQE performance (Figure 2.17).

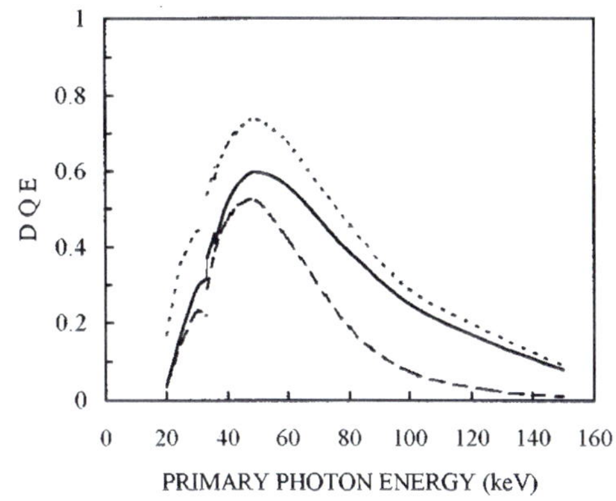

Figure 2.17. Chart illustrating detective quantum efficiency (DQE) for different imaging modalities. *Source:* https://www.researchgate.net/profile/Jerry-Thirlwall/publication/30509398/figure/fig4/AS:309979757203459@1450916341501/The-detective-quantum-efficiency-of-x-ray-image-intensifiers-with-CsI-input-phosphors.png.

fine acceptable illustration is the development of X-ray detector fold structures that leverage the advantage of single-crystal and polycrystalline material properties. These advances aim to maximize the direct conversion of X-ray photons into electric charge, thereby improving the sensitivity and performance of imaging systems across a range of photon energies. The manufacturability enabled by thin-film technology makes inexpensive yet effective designs feasible that, based on analytical modeling and simulations, demonstrate sensitivities comparable to those of conventional single-crystal detectors. Such advancements hold tremendous potential for folded detectors to affect DQE and the overall quality of imaging, representing huge breakthroughs in detector technology for diagnostic imaging applications

(Hamann et al., 2019). With the continuous expansion of DQE applications in clinical use, there is a need to solve measurement problems. Complications in clinical environments make it hard to conduct accurate DQE measurements, which rely on advanced equipment and technical expertise. Recent efforts at mechanizing DQE measurement processes aim to de-mystify this critical endeavor, making clinical end-users receive accurate DQE ratings promptly. By meeting regulatory requirements, this automation reduces the burden of experiments and makes access to this vital parameter more democratic. Such innovations enable the inclusion of DQE testing in quality control and assurance programs, ultimately resulting in a stronger paradigm for diagnostic imaging that prioritizes accuracy and patient safety (Escartin et al., 2017). This visionary synergy of practice and technology serves to reinforce the applicability of DQE in the continued evolution of diagnostic imaging protocols.

2.6.2. Modulation Transfer Function

In image diagnosis, image quality evaluation is based mainly on quantifiable parameters with the ability to represent a system's performance adequately. Among these, the Modulation Transfer Function (MTF) is the key concept, as it measures the degree to which an imaging system reproduces the contrast of various spatial frequencies in an input signal. Such ability is essential in medical diagnosis, where higher fidelity in replicating details enables more accurate pathology detection. The MTF can provide information on the resolution capability of imaging devices, such as X-ray machines and CT scanners, where the ability to discriminate between healthy and diseased tissues can be a primary determinant of patient outcomes. Thus. Knowing and optimizing. MTF is becoming increasingly significant in the design and development of high-performance detectors that underlie advanced imaging systems (Figure 2.18).

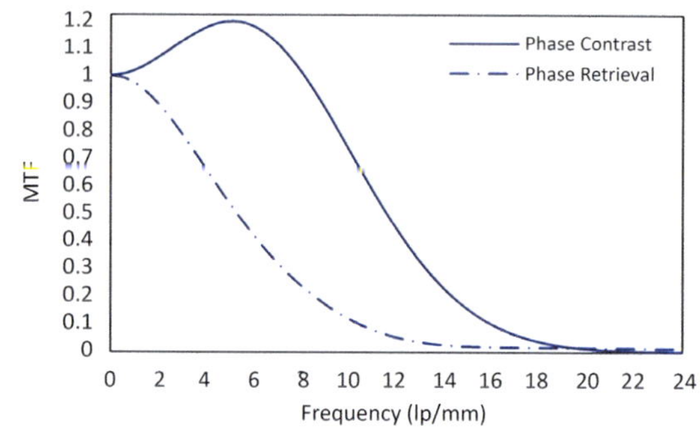

Figure 2.18. Modulation transfer function (MTF) curves demonstrating spatial resolution limits.

Source: https://www.researchgate.net/publication/331291039/figure/fig4/AS:729315276767234@1550893720639/Modulation-transfer-function-MTF-curves-for-the-phase-sensitive-and-phase-retrieved.ppm.

The Modulation Transfer Function is not merely an indicator of resolution but is also associated with other performance parameters, such as Detective Quantum Efficiency (DQE). The MTF values differ across imaging technologies and reflect the unique characteristics of flat-panel detectors, digital X-ray systems, and other modalities. For instance, while conventional film-based systems may have some limitations in MTF, digital detectors with advanced algorithms can fine-tune image quality by compensating for distortions and optimizing the spatial frequency response. Determination of the MTF for various detector types illuminates the trade-off between spatial resolution and image noise and informs the continued evolution of detector technologies. Methods for MTF measurement typically involve specific test patterns and strict measurement protocols to ensure accuracy and reproducibility of results. Emerging detector technologies, such as integrated optics and segmented planar imaging, have driven advances in MTF, enabling higher-quality images with more compact designs and smaller resource footprints (Chen et al., 2021). As new imaging technologies emerge in the clinical setting, ongoing efforts to enhance MTF measurement techniques will be essential. Not only will this continue to enhance image quality, but it will also advance diagnostic imaging, enabling health care practitioners to diagnose and treat patients more effectively (Welsch, 2018).

2.6.3. Linearity and Lag

A practical understanding of linearity and lag concepts is equally required in evaluating the diagnostic imaging systems performance. Linearity refers to the direct proportionality between the intensity of input signals and the resultant output signal, a characteristic relevant to ensuring accurate image representation.

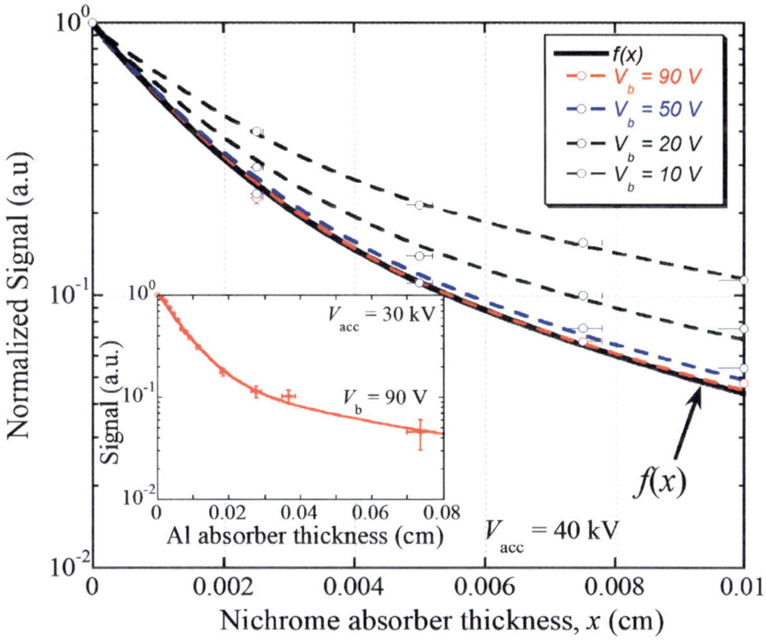

Figure 2.19. Linearity testing of detector response versus incident X-ray dose.

Source: https://www.mdpi.com/crystals/crystals-11-01258/article_deploy/html/images/crystals-11-01258-g003.png.

The perfect detector would be one that delivers a fixed output regardless of input level, ensuring that imaging setting variations do not taint the clinical interpretation of the information. This is particularly critical in applications such as X-ray and MRI imaging, where accurate diagnostic data can dictate treatment plans. Failure to achieve linear responses can lead to images that reflect the actual anatomical structures or pathologies incorrectly, ultimately impacting patient care (Figure 2.19).

Lag, on the other hand, introduces additional complexity in the description of the output response delay of a detector to changes in incident radiation levels. Such an effect may lead to chronic artifacts in images, especially in dynamic studies where signal intensity changes rapidly, such as with fluoroscopy or with real-time imaging applications. Lag may also distort temporal resolution and obscure valuable information about anatomical motion or functional processes. The magnitude of lag varies with factors such as detector material properties and the image processing method employed. Both these dimensions of lag must be known and addressed to ensure temporal accuracy and general reliability in diagnostic findings so that clinicians can make decisions confidently based on imaging data. In the case of current diagnostic imaging, linearity and lag are directly associated with technological advancements in detectors. With the development of systems, particularly the utilization of advanced materials such as semiconductor detectors, compliance with these metrics has become imperative. Innovations in detector design, for instance, improvement of Detective Quantum Efficiency (DQE) and Modulation Transfer Function (MTF), directly influence linearity and lag characteristics. Lag compensation is addressed by optimization of readout operations and sophisticated use of algorithms in image reconstruction. By attending to these conditions, clinicians and scientists can improve imaging techniques and eventually provide better diagnostic accuracy, as seen through the persistence of workshops and initiatives that strive to improve biophotonic technologies and detector engineering so that diagnostic imaging continues to be of high quality and efficacy (Baum et al., 1999; Brownstein et al., 2007) (Figure 2.20).

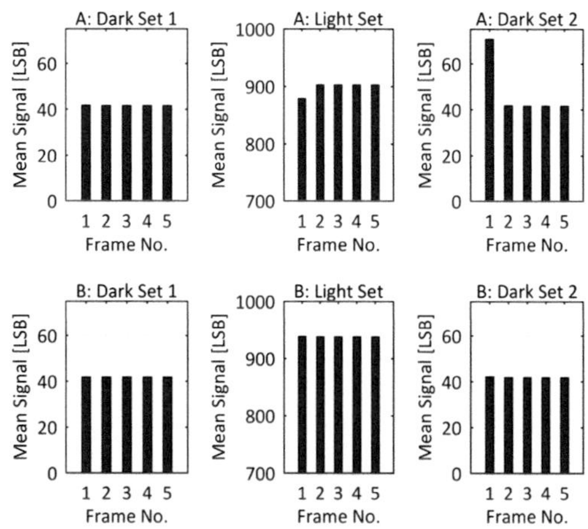

Figure 2.20. Comparative lag measurements under pulsed exposure conditions for various detector types.

Source: https://www.researchgate.net/profile/Orit-Skorka/publication/326717279/figure/fig4/AS:1128190055579658@1645992878359/Lag-measurement-on-two-sensors-using-the-pulsed-LED-method-Sensor-A-which-has-a-PD.ppm.

SUMMARY

The culmination of developments in instrumentation and detector technologies has a tremendous impact on the efficacy of diagnostic imaging. The evolution from traditional methods to sophisticated methodologies has not only enhanced image quality but also enhanced diagnostic accuracy. As highlighted throughout the discussion, continuous innovation of detector performance metrics, such as Detective Quantum Efficiency (DQE) and Modulation Transfer Function (MTF), is central to diagnostic precision achieved in the clinic. With each advancement, there is improved spatial resolution and image quality, which are critical for detecting subtle pathology. The integration of new technologies, including spectroscopic imaging, represents a new frontier capable of enhancing diagnostic potential, as part of a broader strategy to overcome limitations in existing strategies. As demonstrated by data gathered through workshops and research studies, biophotonic devices hold vast potential for cellular and tissue diagnostics. Organizational initiatives, in this case, by the National Institute of Standards and Technology, reflect an increase in emphasis on measurement equipment central to the assessment of biological systems. The ongoing need to address measurement requirements further underscores the need for collaborative structures that support technology development. Provided that there is a well-formulated plan for enhancing measurement capability, the incorporation of developing technologies into mainstream clinical practice becomes increasingly feasible. Furthermore, as the discussion demonstrates, it is important to understand the intricate dynamics of biological interactions and photon-based measurement systems in order to advance the field. Emerging technologies, particularly in mid-infrared spectroscopic imaging, offer promising opportunities for cancer diagnosis. Using high-brightness, broadly tunable lasers, it becomes possible to circumvent the historical limitations of conventional imaging techniques. The trend of incorporating Quantum Cascade Lasers (QCLs) reflects a continuous effort to improve signal-to-noise ratios and overall image capture efficiency. The results of current research point towards the application of these reliable technologies in real diagnostics. As increasingly sophisticated studies continue to identify optimal configurations for tapping into such resources, we stand at the threshold of an enormous shift in diagnostic technology, which will bear on early diagnosis and improved patient outcomes in the treatment of cancer. The diagnostic imaging of the future thus hangs on the implementation of these new technologies in routine clinical practice, enabling a higher order of care for patients.

CLOSER LOOK

REVOLUTIONIZING DIAGNOSTICS THROUGH NEXT-GENERATION IMAGING AND DETECTION SYSTEMS

The spectacular advances in detection technology and instrumentation have revolutionized the diagnostic imaging industry, reflecting the profound impact of innovation on health outcomes. As we advance toward personalized medicine, these technologies have become increasingly vital for proper diagnosis and successful treatment planning. Advancements in high-quality imaging technology, such as next-generation X-ray tubes and flat-panel detectors, have enabled previously unimaginable detail and clarity in images. Not only do these advancements contribute to greater visibility of anatomical structures, but they also contribute to safety for the patient by reducing exposure to radiation. Furthermore, advancements such as dynamic range optimization and high-resolution detectors enable more precise measurements and analyses, which are essential for diagnosing complex conditions. As such, ongoing improvement and enhancement of these technologies represent key concerns to facilitating the healthcare industry's continued growth and demands of modern medicine. In parallel with progress in imaging capability, progress in detection technology has also been key to the diagnostic imaging landscape. Techniques such as X-ray microscopy are increasingly significant in nanoscale material analysis, yielding information crucial to scientific research as well as practical uses in medicine. Tracking the discharge of batteries in modern medical devices, facilitated by advanced X-ray imaging methods, is one example of the need for reliable technologies that ensure diagnostic machinery functionality. As technology keeps improving, the incorporation of various detection technologies—for example, semiconductor detectors and photomultiplier tubes—provides clinicians and researchers with the tools to collect complete data at various imaging modalities. The multi-aspect design not only enhances diagnostic efficiency but also enables effective management of patient treatment pathways, demonstrating that technical improvements in instrumentation and detection are a valuable resource in today's healthcare systems. A future of revolutionary diagnostic imaging is envisioned with the impending interfacing of sophisticated instrumentation and detection sciences. The vision articulated by scientific organizations underscores the pressing need for sustained research investment, particularly in areas such as UV detectors and imaging systems (Baum et al., 1999). Such advances aim not only to provide theoretical astrophysical answers but also to resonate in a broader scientific environment in which precise imaging and detection technologies are embedded. Furthermore, significant research into new technology and materials like those that go into the production of high-performance lithium-ion batteries for diagnostic purposes illustrates instrumentation and novel application interdependence (Gelb et al., 2017). Such innovation in research areas opens new avenues for designing diagnostic approaches, leading to improved, more effective healthcare solutions. With growing demands for precision medicine, such technological development cannot be more critical.

REFERENCES

1. Buttacavoli, A., Principato, F., Gerardi, G., Cascio, D., Raso, G., Bettelli, M., Zappettini, A., Seller, P., Veale, M. C., & Abbene, L. (2022). Incomplete charge collection at Inter-Pixel gap in Low- and High-Flux Cadmium Zinc telluride pixel detectors. *Sensors, 22*(4), 1441. https://doi.org/10.3390/s22041441Abbene, L., Caroli, E., Mancini, A. M., Sordo, S., et al. (2009). Progress in the development of CdTe and CdZnTe semiconductor radiation detectors for astrophysical and medical applications. https://core.ac.uk/download/pdf/8692622.pdf (accessed on 14th July 2025).
2. Abu-Shawareb, H., Acree, R. L., Adams, P. A., Adams, J. J., Addis, B., Aden, R., Adrian, P. J., et al. (2022). Lawson criterion for ignition exceeded in an inertial fusion experiment. *Physical Review Letters, 129*. https://doi.org/10.1103/physrevlett.129.075001 (accessed on 14th July 2025).
3. Acciarri, R., Adams, C., An, R., Aparicio, A., Aponte, S. A., Asaadi, J., Auger, M., et al. (2017). Design and construction of the MicroBooNE detector. *Journal of Instrumentation, 12*, P02017–P02017. https://doi.org/10.1088/1748-0221/12/02/p02017 (accessed on 14th July 2025).
4. Anderson, R. C., Rubin, L. F., Swain, D. M., Trucco, A., et al. (2025). Visualization of hydrogen injection in a scramjet engine by simultaneous PLIF imaging and laser holographic imaging. https://core.ac.uk/download/pdf/42810411.pdf (accessed on 14th July 2025).
5. Anuskiewicz, T., Johnston, J., Leavitt, W., Zimmerman, P., et al. (2025). Technology applications. https://core.ac.uk/download/pdf/85232549.pdf (accessed on 14th July 2025).
6. Appleby, J. F. (2025). Workshop on advanced technologies for planetary instruments, part 1. https://core.ac.uk/download/pdf/42806195.pdf (accessed on 14th July 2025).
7. Bancroft, C., Bloser, P. F., Julien, M., Kippen, R. M., et al. (2010). A fast scintillator Compton telescope for medium-energy gamma-ray astronomy. https://core.ac.uk/download/72048981.pdf (accessed on 14th July 2025).
8. Bancroft, C., Bloser, P. F., Julien, M., Kippen, R. M., et al. (2009). A new low-background Compton telescope using $LaBr_3$ scintillator. https://core.ac.uk/download/72049115.pdf (accessed on 14th July 2025).
9. Baum, S. A., Clarke, J. T., Dupree, A. K., Hasan, H., et al. (1999). The emergence of the modern universe: Tracing the cosmic web. http://arxiv.org/abs/astro-ph/9907101 (accessed on 14th July 2025).
10. Bautz, M. W., Bock, J. J., Kilbourne, C. A., Reid, P., et al. (2025). Physics of the Cosmos (PCOS) Program Technology Development 2018. https://core.ac.uk/download/pdf/161998267.pdf (accessed on 14th July 2025).
11. Benford, D. J., Neff, S. G., Perez, M. R., Scowen, P. A., et al. (2013). Scientific objectives for UV/Visible astrophysics investigations: A summary of responses by the community (2012). https://core.ac.uk/download/pdf/42723648.pdf.
12. Brombal, L. (2020). X-ray phase-contrast tomography: Underlying physics and developments for breast imaging. https://core.ac.uk/download/287861738.pdf (accessed on 14th July 2025).
13. Brownstein, M., Dowell, M. L., Gaigalas, A. K., Hoffman, A. S., et al. (2007). Biphotonic tools in cell and tissue diagnostics. https://core.ac.uk/download/323070689.pdf (accessed on 14th July 2025).

14. Castaneda, C., Cutlip, H. H., Li, W., Macri, J. R., et al. (1999). A scintillating plastic fiber tracking detector for neutron and proton imaging and spectroscopy. https://core.ac.uk/download/72048942.pdf (accessed on 14th July 2025).

15. Chen, T. Y., Zeng, X., Bai, Y., Zhang, Z., Wang, Y., Zhang, F., & Zhang, X. (2021). Sparse-aperture photonics-integrated interferometer (SPIN) imaging system: Structural design and imaging quality analysis. *Optics Express, 29(24)*, 39256–39270. https://www.semanticscholar.org/paper/4684d9235233cc28d642064f82093d812bd1d33c (accessed on 14th July 2025).

16. Cherry, S. R., Jacobs, R. E., & Louie, A. Y. (2008). The integration of positron emission tomography with magnetic resonance imaging. https://core.ac.uk/download/4877286.pdf (accessed on 14th July 2025).

17. Desorgher, L., Flückiger, E. O., Macri, J. R., McConnell, M. L., et al. (2003). SONTRAC: An imaging spectrometer for solar neutrons. https://core.ac.uk/download/72048943.pdf (accessed on 14th July 2025).

18. Escartin, T. R. (2017). Determining the detective quantum efficiency (DQE) of X-ray detectors in clinical environments. https://core.ac.uk/download/129546030.pdf (accessed on 14th July 2025).

19. Farshidfar, N., & Hamedani, S. (2020). The potential role of smartphone-based microfluidic systems for rapid detection of COVID-19 using saliva specimen. *Molecular Diagnosis & Therapy, 24*, 371–373. https://www.semanticscholar.org/paper/03135f77d6751985914d2217f58136f128e0d0db (accessed on 14th July 2025).

20. Gajos, A., Kacprzak, K., Korcyl, G., Krzemien, W., et al. (2020). J-PET framework: Software platform for PET tomography data reconstruction and analysis. https://core.ac.uk/download/344434920.pdf (accessed on 14th July 2025).

21. Gelb, J. D. (2017). A 3D framework for characterizing microstructure evolution of Li-ion batteries. https://core.ac.uk/download/85001245.pdf (accessed on 14th July 2025).

22. Gilman, J. A., Paige, J. B., & Schwenk, F. C. (2025). NASA SBIR abstracts of 1990 phase 1 projects. https://core.ac.uk/download/pdf/42808250.pdf (accessed on 14th July 2025).

23. Gilman, J. A., Paige, J. B., & Schwenk, F. C. (2025). NASA SBIR abstracts of 1991 phase 1 projects. https://core.ac.uk/download/pdf/42806098.pdf (accessed on 14th July 2025).

24. Hamann, E., Lemmer, U., & Mescher, H. (2019). Simulation and design of folded perovskite x-ray detectors. https://core.ac.uk/download/197480890.pdf (accessed on 14th July 2025).

25. Klimenk, A., Zych, A., Zoglauer, A., Hoover, A., Phlips, B., et al. (2006). The Advanced Compton Telescope. https://core.ac.uk/download/72054708.pdf (accessed on 14th July 2025).

26. Lamprou, E. (2021). Development and performance evaluation of high resolution TOF-PET detectors suitable for novel PET scanners. https://riunet.upv.es/bitstream/10251/162991/1/Lamprou%20-%20Development%20and%20Performance%20Evaluation%20of%20High%20Resolution%20TOF-PET%20Detectors%20Suitable%20fo....pdf (accessed on 14th July 2025).

27. Lesco, D. J. (2025). Research and development of optical measurement techniques for aerospace propulsion research: A NASA Lewis Research Center perspective. https://core.ac.uk/download/pdf/42817201.pdf (accessed on 14th July 2025).

28. Lumpkin, A., Maxwell, T., Piot, P., Ruan, J., et al. (2012). Synchronization and characterization of an ultra-short laser for photoemission and electron-beam diagnostics studies at a radio

frequency photoinjector. http://arxiv.org/abs/1203.1657 (accessed on 14th July 2025).

29. Martin, D. C., Nikzad, S., & Schiminovich, D. (2012). Enabling technologies for next generation ultraviolet astrophysics, planetary, and Helio physics missions. https://core.ac.uk/download/211388429.pdf (accessed on 14th July 2025).
30. McCrow, A. (2011). Laser based mid-infrared spectroscopic imaging–Exploring a novel method for application in cancer diagnosis. https://core.ac.uk/download/1592070.pdf (accessed on 14th July 2025).
31. McDonald, M. C. (2012). A method to measure the detective quantum efficiency of radiographic systems in clinical setting. https://core.ac.uk/download/61632636.pdf (accessed on 14th July 2025).
32. Miranda, D. (2025). 2020 NASA technology taxonomy. https://core.ac.uk/download/pdf/286392574.pdf (accessed on 14th July 2025).
33. N/A. (2025). Preliminary applications and evaluation results. *Lixiscope: Proceedings of the Lixiscope Conference*. https://core.ac.uk/download/pdf/42867100.pdf (accessed on 14th July 2025).
34. N/A. (2025). Small business innovation research. Abstracts of completed 1987 phase 1 projects. https://core.ac.uk/download/pdf/42824003.pdf (accessed on 14th July 2025).
35. Nguyen, H. H., Park, J., Kang, S., & Kim, M. (2015). Surface plasmon resonance: A versatile technique for biosensor applications. *Sensors, 15*, 10481–10510. https://doi.org/10.3390/s150510481 (accessed on 14th July 2025).
36. Paul, P. P., McShane, E. J., Colclasure, A. M., Balsara, N. P., Brown, D. E., Cao, C., Chen, B. R., et al. (2021). A review of existing and emerging methods for lithium detection and characterization in Li-ion and Li-metal batteries. *Advanced Energy Materials, 11*. https://doi.org/10.1002/aenm.202100372 (accessed on 14th July 2025).
37. Prusti, T., de Bruijne, J. H. J., Brown, A. G. A., Vallenari, A., Babusiaux, C., Bailer-Jones, C. A. L., Bastian, U., et al. (2016). The *Gaia* mission. *Astronomy and Astrophysics, 595*, A1–A1. https://doi.org/10.1051/0004-6361/201629272 (accessed on 14th July 2025).
38. Salvado, D. S. A. S. (2017). SPECT system design optimization for a simultaneous SPECT/MRI clinical scanner. https://core.ac.uk/download/111022627.pdf (accessed on 14th July 2025).
39. Shaji, A., Fidha, A. F., Kumari, S., Dabholkar, A., & Gaonkar, O. (2024). Recent advancements in CT detectors: A comprehensive review. *Journal of Clinical and Diagnostic Research*. https://www.semanticscholar.org/paper/a243ac8945b32475f2eb44e6640ac06eccc2fa54 (accessed on 14th July 2025).
40. Vykoukal, D. M., Stone, G. P., Gascoyne, P., Alt, E., & Vykoukal, J. (2009). Quantitative detection of bioassays with a low-cost image-sensor array for integrated microsystems. *Angewandte Chemise, 48(41)*, 7649–7654. https://www.semanticscholar.org/paper/ab564b9875aa112ac3814de5456af46cb6157e30 (accessed on 14th July 2025).
41. Wang, Z., Zhou, H., Gu, S., & Gao, H. (2022). Dual-energy head cone-beam CT using a dual-layer flat-panel detector: Physics-based material decomposition. *12304*, 123041R–123041R-6. https://www.semanticscholar.org/paper/d124080ff6ab0fbf60686164a9a2fe93265f8633 (accessed on 14th July 2025).

42. Wang, Z., Zhou, H., Gu, S., Xia, Y., Liao, H., Deng, Y., & Gao, H. (2023). Dual-energy head cone-beam CT using a dual-layer flat-panel detector: Hybrid material decomposition and a feasibility study. *Medical Physics*. https://www.semanticscholar.org/paper/1a4b60e47dadee65344d1a0f6d32ef0d38f5ff9c (accessed on 14th July 2025).

43. Welsch, C. (2018). Enhancing hadron therapy through OMA. https://www.semanticscholar.org/paper/9626625e18315f9e45afe7d7e3c40a0c6bc83298 (accessed on 14th July 2025).

44. Yücel, M. A., von Lühmann, A., Scholkmann, F., Gervain, J., Dan, I., Ayaz, H., Boas, D. A., et al. (2021). Best practices for fNIRS publications. *Neurophotonics, 8*. https://doi.org/10.1117/1.nph.8.1.012101 (accessed on 14th July 2025)

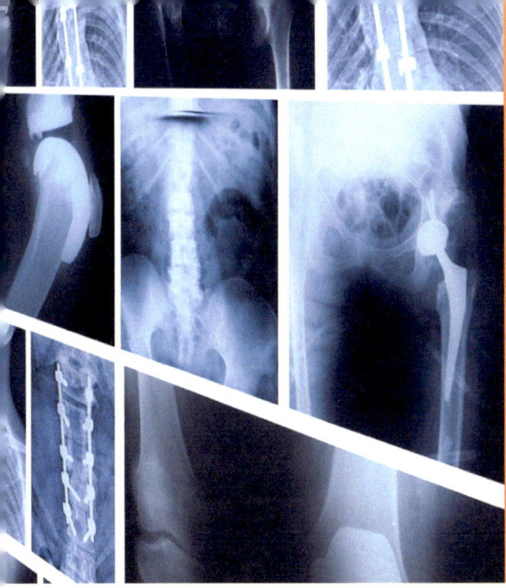

Chapter 3

CONVENTIONAL RADIOGRAPHY TECHNIQUES

Contents

Introduction

The evolution of radiographic devices has transformed medical imaging to a large degree, leading to more accurate diagnostics and patient management. Conventional radiographic examinations, along with a wide range of modalities, remain the backbone of medical imaging despite the availability of advanced systems such as CT and MRI. Such conventional methods provide critical visualizations of internal anatomical organization, which assist physicians in diagnosing disease. In particular, the comparison of two-dimensional images obtained via conventional means with three-dimensional imaging modalities facilitates exhaustive evaluation of the patient. As medical imaging continues to advance, understanding the core principles of conventional radiography is increasingly vital for both students and professionals. Various approaches under conventional radiography warrant careful examination, especially given their extensive application in various medical settings. Of all these, projectional radiography is the foundation of most imaging regimes, enabling a vast array of examinations from chest and abdominal screenings to bone studies. In addition, advancements in digital radiography have revolutionized traditional image-making processes by delivering a new level of image quality and enabling rapid retrieval. The Amperometric imaging techniques have progressed to enable improved dose management, a crucial aspect of ensuring patient security. Therefore, a deep understanding of these conventional methods is imperative for health professionals determined to employ the entire range of radiography in diagnosis. With the ongoing application of traditional radiography, there is a need for quality assurance procedures to ensure standards of imaging. Maintaining consistent image quality through rigorous protocols, such as daily detector calibration and phantom imaging, is vital to peak performance in radiographic units. Also, the application of robust image quality optimization techniques ensures that clinicians can have confidence in the consistency and reliability of the diagnostic data obtained. The integration of advanced methodologies into conventional practices is an assertion of their durability and relevance in current diagnostics, despite the relentless evolution of technology. As the chapter unfolds, further details about these pivotal techniques and how they work will showcase their ongoing use in radiographic imaging.

3.1. Projectional Radiography

Projectional radiography remains important in most areas of medical imaging, offering a uniform process for capturing anatomical images as a series of two-dimensional projections. This method uses X-ray beams focused on the body, with images recorded on radiographic film or digital detectors, enabling visualization of internal structures. One main benefit of projectional radiography is that it can give instantaneous results, making it possible to make a diagnosis in a timely fashion in clinical environments. For example, implementing specialized protocols in chest radiography will maximize visualization of pulmonary or cardiac disease, enabling key information to be presented in a functionally immediate way to medical workers. As a base for diagnostic imaging, projectional radiography continues to have applicability, evolving to incorporate new developments in technology while continuing to be a requirement for many clinical applications, including emergency care and general screening. In abdominal radiography, experts use projectional techniques to assess a range of gastrointestinal illnesses. By employing specific angles of projection and patient positioning, radiologists can project the required structures, such as the liver, spleen, kidneys, and gastrointestinal tract. With this specialized imaging process, diagnostic accuracy is enhanced, enabling medical practitioners to recognize issues such as obstructions, perforations, and masses. With advanced digital radiography systems, experts can achieve improved image quality and lower radiation doses compared to older methods. Notably, studies comparing projections for radiographic imaging show that conventional planar digital X-ray imaging provides high diagnostic utility, particularly in challenging settings such as archaeological inspections, confirming its continued relevance even amid advancing technologies (Seiler et al., 2018). The examination of skeletal structures using projectional radiography is beneficial in the diagnosis of dislocations, fractures, and degenerative conditions. Radiographic use here is based on a systematic approach, emphasizing proper positioning, collimation, and exposure to achieve high-quality images. The high-tech imaging capability allows specialists to identify minor pathologies, thereby improving patient care. Additionally, recent innovations have demonstrated the technical feasibility of using traditional radiography to quantify three-dimensional joint kinematics, particularly in studies of total knee arthroplasty, with clinically applicable benefits in real-world environments (Seslija et al., 2012). These breakthroughs constitute a significant achievement in the field, where projectional radiography's inherent quality is balanced with increasing demand for precise diagnostic imaging, influencing patient outcomes in the majority of healthcare fields.

3.1.1. Chest Radiography Protocols

The use of chest radiography protocols is directly related to radiation safety and optimal imaging practices. Protocol compliance guarantees that diagnostic efficacy is optimized while minimizing patient exposure to ionizing radiation. Protocols typically specify appropriate patient positioning, the type of imaging technology, and the determination of exposure parameters. For instance, an adult patient is typically instructed to obtain a posterior-anterior (PA) view, which reveals the lungs and heart in their entirety. Additionally, the choice of protocol must be informed by the physician's question, as it is clinically relevant because tailored imaging can lead to higher diagnostic accuracy. Systematic use of these protocols is critical to early diagnosis of potential pathologies such as pneumonia or lung nodules, ultimately determining patient outcomes profoundly. Therefore, chest radiography protocols, their interpretation, and their implementation are the foundation of practice in clinical radiography (Figure 3.1).

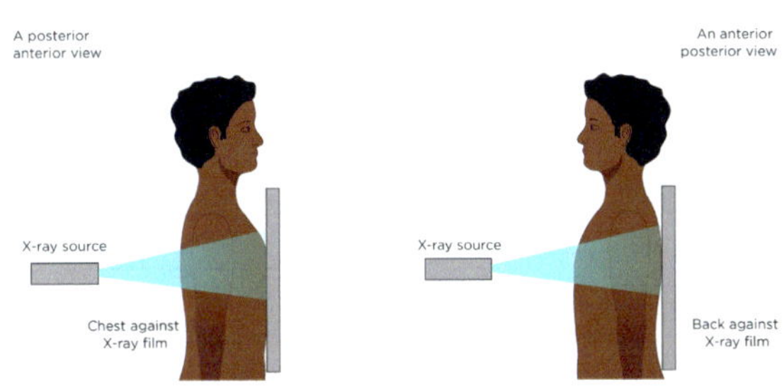

Figure 3.1. Standard setup for posterior-anterior chest radiography.

Source: https://cdn.ps.emap.com/wp-content/uploads/sites/3/2024/05/Fig-1.-Patient-positioning-scaled.jpg.

In children, chest radiography protocols need to be rigorously evaluated to account for their unique physiological features. Children are much more sensitive to the deleterious effects of ionizing radiation. Therefore, the justification and optimization principles are most crucial in such scenarios to restrict unnecessary radiation exposure. American College of Radiology standards suggest that pediatric protocols should include measures such as adjusting technique factors based on the patient's size and age. Furthermore, shielding techniques, such as thyroid and gonadal shielding, offer a secondary level of protection against radiation. Recent research indicates that optimized radiographic protocols can significantly reduce unnecessary examinations, thereby minimizing exposure risks without compromising diagnostic quality (Mhezi et al., 2024). Optimal scripting of the protocols is thus pivotal in ensuring the development of a secure imaging environment for pediatric patients. Among recent chest radiography protocol advancements is the use of advanced imaging technology, such as artificial intelligence (AI). The application of AI to the processing and analysis of chest radiographs has yielded promising results in enhancing diagnostic accuracy. Deep learning algorithms can be utilized for the early diagnosis of conditions such as COVID-19, thereby creating a need for policies that integrate these new solutions with prevailing practices. For instance, studies indicate that CNNs can improve diagnostic performance, achieving high sensitivity and specificity in detecting pneumonia and other pathologies on chest radiographs (Ullah et al., 2024). As this technology evolves, protocols for chest radiography must incorporate AI-based decision-making into their implementation while continuing to comply with current clinical guidelines. This change has the potential to revolutionize conventional radiography techniques, making chest imaging safer and more convenient for patients.

3.1.2. Abdominal Radiography

In the context of diagnostic imaging, abdominal radiography is an essential modality of assessment for various pathologies that are found within the abdominal cavity. Abdominal radiography relies on standard X-ray projections, primarily in the erect and supine positions, to provide full visualization of organs such as the spleen, liver, kidneys, and intestines. One of the significant advantages of this radiographic investigation is the ability to assess for abnormalities like obstructions, perforation, or foreign body.

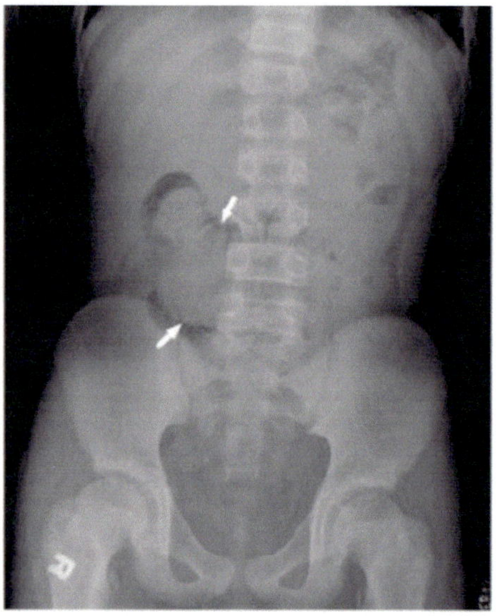

Figure 3.2. Supine radiograph of the abdomen shows a nonobstructive bowel gas pattern and a paucity of gas (almost gasless) in the left half of abdomen. The cecum and ascending colon could not be delineated. An intraluminal soft tissue density (arrows) was delineated with gas over the transverse colon.

Source: https://www.researchgate.net/figure/Supine-radiograph-of-the-abdomen-shows-a-nonobstructive-bowel-gas-pattern-and-a-paucity_fig1_40774468.

In addition, correct patient positioning is essential in an attempt to avoid superimposing of structures and conceal significant findings and also make diagnosis difficult. Cost-effective and uncomplicated, abdominal radiography remains a vitally crucial first-line imaging tool in both emergency and routine clinics, attesting to its continued applicability to contemporary practice. Accurate communication of abdominal radiography results is fundamental to the diagnostic process. Physicians and radiologists need to collaborate to interpret imaging findings, as existing research has indicated, underscoring the increasing frequency of using imaging modalities to diagnose neonatal abdominal abnormalities. For instance, in a Romanian-language retrospective study, concordance between clinical suspicion and radiographic diagnosis was observed at an estimated rate of 52.35%, underscoring the need for heightened collaboration among medical staff to achieve greater diagnostic accuracy (Ciurea et al., 2009) (Figure 3.2).

Furthermore, imaging technologies have enabled the visualization of more delicate anatomical details, enhancing diagnostic confidence. All these findings reiterate the importance of constant professional training for clinicians and radiologists to maintain pace with the evolving abdominal imaging setting. Beyond its diagnostic application, abdominal radiography is an integral component of therapeutic procedures. Conventional procedures enable one to identify not only operative emergencies but also preoperative screening that informs clinical decision-making. The ability to use radiography to detect pathologies can lead to better, more targeted treatment options. Radiography can, further, serve as a non-invasive tool for tracking the evolution of known conditions, so that intervention is initiated in good time where required. In this context, the use of abdominal radiography for tracking chronic condition management demonstrates its value within patient care regimes. With research on radiological techniques for drug concealment highlighting the methodology's flexibility, further integration of conventional radiographic techniques into clinical practice is more than justified (Zammit et al., 1992).

3.1.3. Skeletal Radiography

Skeletal radiography is a fundamental area of projectional radiography, primarily to assess the bones and joints for a variety of conditions, including fractures, degenerative diseases, and infections.

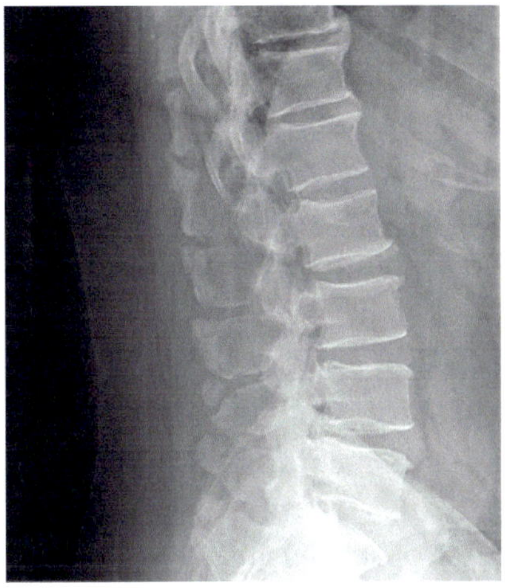

Figure 3.3. Lateral view of the lumbar spine using skeletal radiography.

Source: https://www.researchgate.net/figure/Lumbar-spine-radiography-lateral-view_fig1_273786248.

The technique uses X-rays to produce high-resolution images of the skeletal system, enabling clinicians to analyze structural abnormalities and pathologic changes. Among the important advantages of skeletal radiography is its ability to image bone integrity and density, and thus it plays a vital role in the diagnosis of conditions like osteosarcoma and osteoporosis. Moreover, advancements like digital radiography have improved the quality and diagnostic imaging of bones, especially in visualizing fine structures within bones. Its application in clinical practice streamlines patient care, enabling timely intervention and treatment planning for musculoskeletal disorders, thereby enhancing patient care. The technique is applicable to a range of clinical scenarios, with some protocols suitable for addressing various diagnostic requirements. For example, weight-bearing projections may be used to assess joint alignment and stability, particularly in suspected ligamentous pathology (Figure 3.3).

In addition, accurate collimation and positioning techniques are critical for optimizing image quality while minimizing radiation exposure to overlying structures. Gridding and sophisticated digital algorithms also enhance image contrast and resolution, enabling radiologists to accurately interpret images. As defined in recent reports, the use of new imaging modalities, such as dual-energy CT, presents promising outcomes relative to the traditional methods, especially in their diagnostic sensitivity to detect crystal deposition diseases in patients, again reflecting the need for new methods in skeletal radiography (Chen et al., 2016). Quality control in skeletal radiography remains important in generating accurate, high-quality images on a regular basis. To ensure compliance with the standards offered, regular equipment checks, phantom testing, and maintenance procedures are essential features that professionals must keep up with. Such procedures validate any differences in image performance and help avert potential issues that may impact patient care. Detector checks are also required at regular intervals to validate imaging system consistency and accuracy, particularly in challenging clinical environments. Finding the appropriate balance between image quality and patient safety remains an issue, as adequate exposure techniques have a direct impact on the likelihood of successful diagnosis.

Sharpening techniques in skeletal radiography enables medical practitioners to achieve better patient outcomes while successfully combating the evolving state of conventional radiographic techniques (Martini et al., 2017).

3.2. Fluoroscopy Basics

The use of fluoroscopy within conventional radiography techniques is a significant step forward in image methodology. It is a technique that plays a vital role in generating dynamic, real-time images of internal structures, which are essential for diagnosis and treatment. Fluoroscopy operates using a real-time X-ray beam that passes through the body to create an image moving across a screen, and is most beneficial in applications where motion analysis is required, for example, the gastrointestinal tract, and when interventional procedures are being conducted. Separating pulsed and continuous fluoroscopy allows professionals to choose the method that best fits specific clinical applications (Figure 3.4).

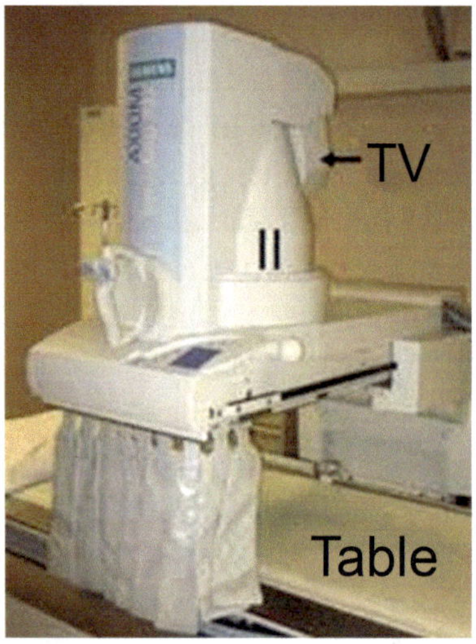

Figure 3.4. Basic fluoroscopy unit with image intensifier in use.

Source: https://encrypted-tbn0.gstatic.com/images?q=tbn:ANd9GcRxmvwustKHmN5F_LGJrEd7PDeiqYcjmPyYKg&s.

Continuous fluoroscopy provides continuous visualization, while pulsed fluoroscopy offers intermittent imaging, thereby reducing radiation exposure —a feature common to radiographic imaging, especially in pediatric patients and those who need a series of follow-up tests (Tomaihi et al., 2024). Some of the requisites of fluoroscopy include dose management, a process aimed at reducing radiation exposure to patients and medical staff to achieve optimal image quality. This dual focus is especially critical due to the prolonged exposure to radiation common with fluoroscopic procedures. Technology has enabled numerous dose-saving features, including pulsed fluoroscopy and automatic brightness control, which adjust tube output based on each patient's anatomy. Persistent training and adherence to clearly defined protocols are necessary in the provision of safety and efficiency during the procedure.

The personnel responsible must be cautious regarding cumulative patient dose, actively employing equipment such as personal dosimetry and optimizing procedure duration to reduce the hazards posed by high radiation exposure (Ronkainen et al., 2007). Image intensifier usage is included in optimizing the quality and utility of fluoroscopic images. These devices amplify the incoming X-ray signal, producing a high-contrast, bright image that can be seen in real time.

Image intensifiers accomplish this by converting X-ray photons into visible light, thus enabling clearer visualization of anatomical structure. Their effectiveness is particularly significant in diagnostic examinations, as better image quality has direct implications for clinical practice. The continuous advancements in this technology, including flat-panel detectors, enable improved resolution and lower radiation doses through more efficient image acquisition. As healthcare continues to evolve, the optimization of image quality through exposure control is central to advancing patient safety and diagnostic effectiveness in fluoroscopic procedures (Tomaihi et al., 2024).

3.2.1. Continuous Versus Pulsed Fluoroscopy

The choice between pulsed and continuous fluoroscopy is instrumental in optimizing patient safety and diagnostic efficiency in radiographic examinations. Continuous fluoroscopy produces a constant stream of X-rays, providing continuous real-time imaging of anatomy and physiology. However, the mode poses a greater radiation risk to patients, a significant consideration for health effects.

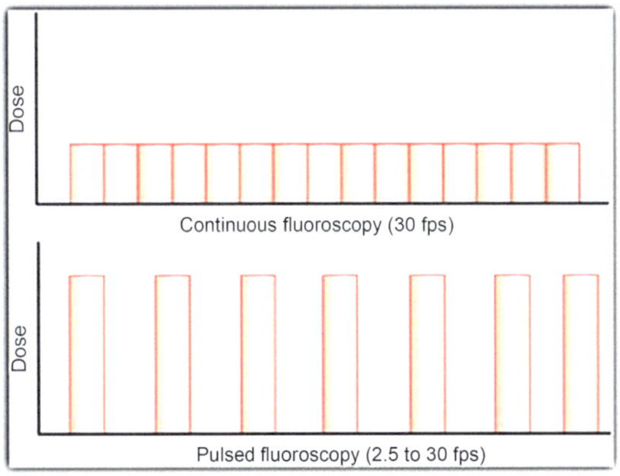

Figure 3.5. Continuous versus pulsed fluoroscopy waveform comparison.

Source: https://d45jl3w9libvn.cloudfront.net/jaypee/static/books/9789350904978/Chapters/images/229-1.jpg.

On the other hand, pulsed fluoroscopy involves an intermittent sequence of pulses of X-rays that reduces radiation dose without image quality compromise for clinical evaluation. This is a critical distinction for the procedural application, in which extensive fluoroscopic guidance is necessary, thereby requiring a prudent decision on the mode of delivery based on the clinical situation. Moreover, the development in pulsed fluoroscopy technology has facilitated the implementation of a sequence of dose management solutions for practice based on the ALARA principle. For instance, the implementation of automated exposure controls and image processing algorithms has enhanced practitioners' approach toward balancing image quality with radiation dose. Clinical studies have established that the pulsed method does not compromise diagnostic outcomes when properly calibrated and utilized, again attesting to its growing utilization in gastrointestinal examinations, where the benefits of reduced radiation exposure are most applicable (Figure 3.5).

The proper application of these techniques in the pediatric setting, as highlighted in recent literature, shows that they minimize risk while optimizing imaging results (Diamond et al., 2006). Practitioners must be educated within the education and training model for the implications of choosing either of these two modalities. Continuing education on the difference between continuous and pulsed fluoroscopy optimizes radiographers' skills and patient safety. Evidence shows that radiographic professionals can manage fluoroscopic procedures effectively by mastering these techniques with strict safety measures in place, as implemented in the United Kingdom approach to gastrointestinal radiology (Hogg et al., 2007). Such general knowledge not only benefits in the guarantee of patient-centered practice but also improves the practice of fluoroscopy in general within the context of conventional radiography practices.

3.2.2. Dosage Management

In traditional radiography, the optimization of dose management cannot be overstressed. Ensuring that patients receive the lowest effective dose of radiation for obtaining high-quality diagnostic images is imperative in minimizing the potential for long-term risks from radiation exposure. Factors influencing dose management include radiographic technique, patient positioning, and the selection of appropriate imaging protocols. Understanding these factors helps radiologists and technologists strike a balance between image quality and patient safety. Further, regular training of radiological staff in the principles of dose management is advocated, with an environment that permits the implementation of safety measures to minimize excessive patient and worker radiation exposure (Figure 3.6).

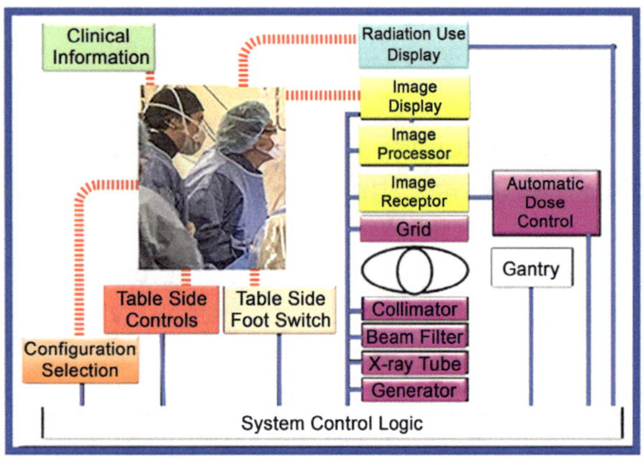

Figure 3.6. Real-time dose monitoring panel during fluoroscopic procedures.

Source: https://radiologykey.com/wp-content/uploads/2021/05/C9-FF1.gif.

Standardization of dose management across various radiographic methods significantly enhances the efficacy of imaging. Standardization can be achieved through policies that encourage the deployment of protective devices, such as lead aprons or thyroid shields, thereby reducing exposure during fluoroscopic examinations. In addition, advances in digital technology have substantially contributed to dose management, particularly in fluoroscopy, enabling the strategic use of continuous and pulsed modes. The use of real-time feedback mechanisms that monitor radiation dose based on image quality can help the operator make real-time adjustments to guarantee the resulting image is diagnostic while minimizing radiation exposure to the extent possible. Such modalities reflect the continued focus on patient safety in radiology. Ongoing monitoring and optimization of dose management methods are the norm for optimal results in conventional radiography. Implementation of quality assurance programs, including rigorous quality control checks of imaging equipment and strict adherence to protocols, facilitates dose management by ensuring consistency in radiation protection and image quality. Of particular interest, data obtained through these quality assurance processes can identify areas for improvement, revealing abnormalities or trends that may necessitate adjustments in technique or equipment. Lastly, adopting dose management principles as part of the general radiographic practice supports a culture of safety and responsibility such that technological improvements result in tangible patient care benefits without diluting safety standards, as evidenced by ongoing research in treatment regimens (Reisig et al., 2025; Wargantiwar et al., 2025).

3.2.3. Image Intensifier Operation

In fluoroscopy, image intensifiers are pivotal in enhancing the visibility of anatomical structures. These devices achieve this by converting low-intensity X-ray photons to a more visible range of light, thus boosting the image quality of tests. It operates on a sequence of operations: incident X-rays strike a photocathode, releasing electrons. These electrons are then sped up and focused onto a fluorescent screen, producing a much brighter image. This amplification process allows for real-time observation of moving processes within the body which is essential for diagnosis. In addition, the utility of image intensifiers is demonstrated by their capacity to reduce patient radiation doses without compromising image quality, a significant consideration in standard radiographic procedures (Heindel et al., 2011). In addition to enhancing clinical efficacy, a profound understanding of image intensifier function also addresses the crucial issue of dose control in radiographic examinations. Such devices enable a balance between the need for high-quality images and the common responsibility to minimize patients' exposure to ionizing radiation. With the utilization of image intensification, radiologists are able to utilize lower doses of X-rays while still achieving resolution in the resultant images. With this, it becomes a critical consideration in procedural uses, such as orthopedic assessments or gastrointestinal exams, where close visualization is required (Figure 3.7).

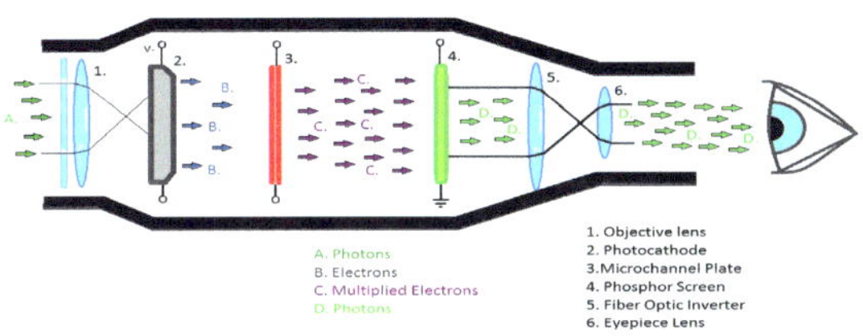

Figure 3.7. Internal layout of an image intensifier tube.

Source: https://rongland.co.uk/cdn/shop/articles/Image_intensifier_diagram1.jpg?v=1494787239.

The balance between technical competence and knowledge of image intensifier operation enables practitioners to achieve optimal imaging protocols and adhere to safety protocols, resulting in improved patient outcomes and diagnostic consistency. This innovation in fluoroscopy is a remarkable advancement in conventional radiography that opens the path for future innovations (Molina Gómez et al., 2018). Furthermore, the integration of advanced technologies into image intensifier systems remains at the forefront of conventional radiography applications. With ongoing developments, the design of image intensifiers has evolved to include more complex functions such as digital conversion, which streamlines processes and enhances image processing. All these developments have transformed the way radiologists capture and view images, yielding greater flexibility in diagnostic applications. The shift to digital systems not only improved image quality but also facilitated archiving and retrieval, making images readily accessible for comparison and review. As traditional radiographic techniques evolved into these new technologies, the role of image intensifiers remains critical in ensuring that diagnostic imaging is efficient, effective, and safe for patients (Heindel et al., 2011; Molina Gómez et al., 2018).

3.3. Digital Radiography Workflows

In radiography, the transition from conventional film-based to digital workflows is a milestone development in image acquisition, processing, and management. Digital radiographic workflows enable greater access to high-quality images and streamline the diagnostic process. One of the essential aspects of digital workflows is the variety of image-acquisition modes they offer, including direct and indirect radiography systems. These modes of acquisition include the utilization of digital detectors that are employed to detect and digitize x-ray data into digital images, facilitating real-time visualization and immediate analysis. Rapid access to imaging enables more timely clinical decision-making and better patient outcomes, as medical professionals can respond more quickly to diagnostic needs. Combined with other technological advances, these modes of acquisition represent a revolutionary step in medical imaging (Beck et al., 2024). Secondly, digital radiography's performance is highly enhanced by high-level image processing algorithms that improve image quality, contrast, and diagnostic information. By using high-level algorithms, image characteristics can be controlled to reduce noise and highlight critical anatomical details. These algorithms allow image functions like filtering, edge detection, and artifact reduction, which are necessary to obtain clinically effective images in various diagnostic procedures. Notably, such algorithms' automated processing reduces the need for repeated imaging, thereby lowering patients' radiation exposure. The breakthroughs thus not only improve diagnostic quality but also foster a better imaging environment that prioritizes patient safety (Pera et al., 2023). Digital image processing in radiographic procedures is another example of efficiency gained through the use of this technology. Archiving and retrieval systems are essential in guaranteeing that images acquired are securely archived and quickly available when needed. Digital images are stored in Picture Archiving and Communication Systems (PACS), which enable complex data management, rapid retrieval, and dissemination to health professionals. This type of system is significantly different from the cumbersome physical storage of legacy film, which can take time and risk loss or damage. Thus, the incorporation of cloud storage solutions enhances availability and facilitates remote consultation and second opinions, thus optimizing the potential for collaborative care. Overall, simplified archiving and retrieval operations highlight the profound impact of digital radiography workflows on the efficiency and effectiveness of radiologic practice (Beck et al., 2024).

3.3.1. Image Acquisition Modes

In digital radiography, the modes of image acquisition play a pivotal role in determining the quality and utility of the resulting images. The two primary modes are direct and indirect acquisition. Direct acquisition uses detectors that convert X-ray photons into electrical signals, enabling immediate image formation. In contrast, indirect acquisition employs materials such as scintillators to convert X-ray photons into visible light, which is then captured by a complementary metal-oxide-semiconductor (CMOS) sensor. This distinction not only impacts image clarity and detail but also influences workflow efficiency (Figure 3.8).

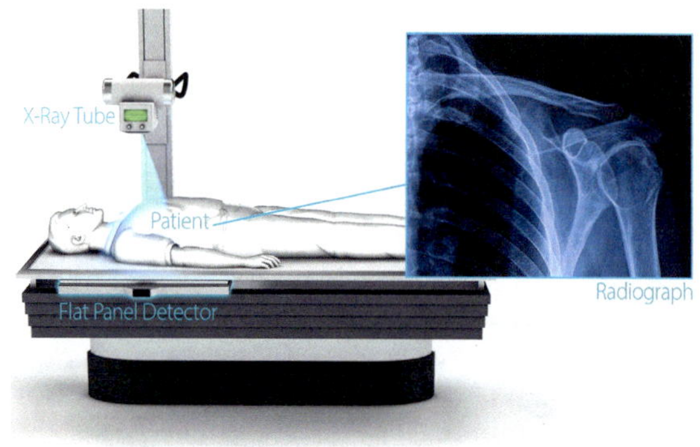

Figure 3.8. Flat panel detector capturing digital radiograph.

Source: https://www.mavenimaging.com/hs-fs/hubfs/Digital_X-ray_Systems_1390x956.jpg?width=1390&height=926&name=Digital_X-ray_Systems_1390x956.jpg.

Knowledge of these modes of acquisition facilitates image-quality optimization with minimal radiation exposure, thereby enabling optimal patient safety and best-practice care. Advances in imaging acquisition technologies have further diversified the methods to be used in radiographic imaging. For instance, digital time-delay integration (TDI), as implemented in novel instrument designs, enables continuous image collection with improved signal-to-noise ratios (SNR) by synchronizing the sensors' readouts to the subject's motion. The technique significantly enhances the ability to collect high-quality images in conditions where motion would compromise traditional methods. Effective integration of various imaging modalities ensures that clinical needs are met, from high-resolution anatomical examinations to functional imaging, thereby increasing the usability of conventional radiographic techniques. Second, the use of sophisticated image processing algorithms enables various modes of image acquisition by enhancing image quality and increasing diagnostic confidence. Algorithms designed to tackle problems like contrast enhancement and noise reduction are instrumental in converting raw detector data into readable images. Coupled with optimized acquisition methods, the ability to efficiently process and store these images is part of what enables enhanced diagnostic routines. For example, initiatives such as integrating machine learning frameworks can streamline the analysis of large volumes of imaging data, enabling traditional radiography to meet the requirements of modern medical imaging (Leonarski et al., 2025; Livens et al., 2025). Through integration, radiographic imaging is made more sophisticated to cope with today's healthcare challenges.

3.3.2. Image Processing Algorithms

The function of image processing algorithms in digital radiography procedures is becoming increasingly vital as algorithms enhance the diagnostic value and quality of medical images. Algorithms for image processing operate by altering digital photos to enhance visibility and minimize noise so that subtle pathologies can be identified. Elaborate techniques such as filtering, segmentation, and image reconstruction are what take images into analysis. Furthermore, computer-assisted diagnosis (CAD) methods incorporated into practice demonstrate the revolutionary impact of such algorithms, through which radiologists are able to identify anomalies that might not otherwise be detected successfully. Of paramount significance, algorithm design and optimization are necessary to maximize the use of high-resolution images, thereby optimizing the overall efficacy of conventional radiographic techniques in practice, as seen in the preceding sections on image acquisition modes and archiving approaches. In breast imaging, particularly digital mammography, image processing algorithms have shown great promise (Figure 3.9).

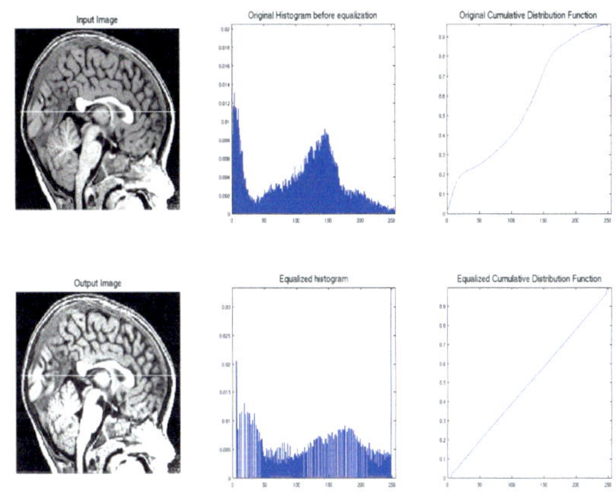

Figure 3.9. Histogram equalization during digital image processing.

Source: https://www.sci.utah.edu/~acoste/uou/Image/project1/images/test_MRI_equilized.png.

The requirement for sophisticated processing is due to the images created, which are mostly complicated in nature and end up forming large data sets that need proper management. Noise suppression and enhancement algorithms are central to improving image quality without reducing diagnostic effectiveness, thereby helping healthcare personnel make precise decisions. Compression methods are also important in this regard, as large volumes of data must be stored and communicated efficiently. Practitioners must therefore understand the trade-off between virtually lossless and lossy compression methods so that accessibility can be provided with sufficient detail for adequate diagnostics (Blaine et al., 2025). Expanding the application range of image processing algorithms, the employment of Cone Beam Computed Tomography (CBCT) is yet another field where improved algorithms enhance diagnosis. CBCT, initially intended for dental imaging, is now gaining popularity in musculoskeletal disorders, where image quality is a matter of utmost importance. The algorithms employed provide high spatial resolution and effective image processing, enabling a more extensive evaluation of complex anatomical structures. CBCT's ability to outperform conventional radiography in delineating structures obscured by superimposition reflects advances in image processing algorithms. With further advancement in its implementation, their role in improving diagnostic images will likely expand and address more of the disparity between conventional methods and modern imaging machines, as posited in the musculoskeletal imaging methodology discourse (Desimpel et al., 2018).

3.3.3. Archiving and Retrieval

The process of digital radiography archiving and retrieval is a cornerstone to effective patient management and correct diagnosis. With the transition from radiographic to digital images, the need for efficient archiving systems becomes increasingly evident. Digital images produced through various modalities must be archived in an orderly fashion so that they are easily retrievable and accessible for clinical assessment and teaching. Adoption of Picture Archiving and Communication Systems (PACS) has replaced the traditional ways, replacing tedious file storage with efficient computer-based databases. These systems not only enhance availability but also facilitate easier comparison of previous examinations, enabling the continuity of care required for decision-making in the clinical setting. Advances in archiving technology streamline workflows, reduce wait times for image availability, and ultimately improve patient outcomes. Such convergence of technology illustrates substantial developments noted in literature that describe contemporary practice within the radiography practice (Guzman et al., 2002) (Figure 3.10).

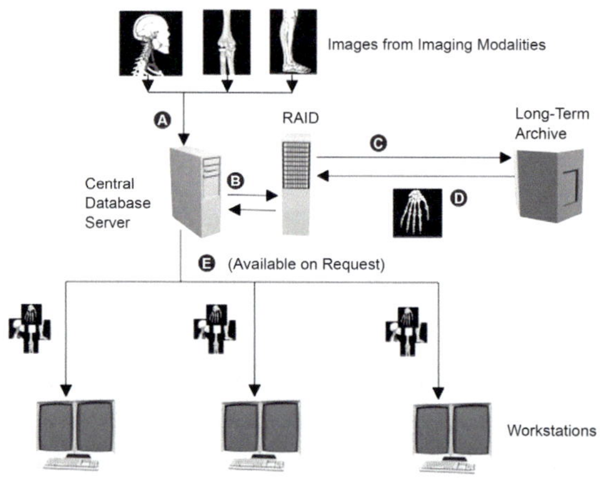

Figure 3.10. PACS interface showing image archiving and retrieval screen.

Source: https://ars.els-cdn.com/content/image/3-s2.0-B0123868602007760-gr2.jpg.

At the core of any effective archiving system is the need for firm protocols that govern retrieval, with the highest degree of precision and effectiveness. Organizations will have to develop standardized procedures for handling the disparate forms of images and information generated by various radiographic techniques. The retrieval of chest radiographs, for instance, might involve different considerations than those for skeletal or abdominal images and thus necessitate a tailored approach. This also suggests an urgent need to train technical personnel and radiologists in the effective use of these systems, since understanding has a direct bearing on their capacity to meet clinical demands in a timely manner. Successful archiving and retrieval systems must also include metadata tagging that enhances searchability, so that relevant image sets can be identified immediately. The combination of advanced technology and strategic protocols is employed to facilitate the central goals of enhancing diagnostic performance and expedient patient care (Guzman et al., 2002). Additionally, the convergence of retrieval and archiving practices across conventional radiography and emerging technologies underscores the imperative for ongoing refinement and regulatory compliance. The move from analogue procedures to computer systems offers the potential to reduce miscommunication and loss of vital patient data, making the quality control of these systems of paramount concern. Regular mandatory audits and reviews of archiving systems are necessary in order to identify inefficiencies or where improvement can be made, with the view to maintaining systems in line with best practice and legislative frameworks. With the evolving nature of medical imaging, adaptive archiving solutions capable of embracing emerging innovations, becoming a part of them, become critical in providing high levels of services in radiology departments. This is consistent with the continued emphasis on quality and efficiency, aligned with current developments in medical imaging to improve patient care standards in the health system (Abonyi et al., 2022).

3.4. Tomosynthesis Principles

In the radiographic imaging, it is essential to understand the principles of tomosynthesis for improved diagnostic accuracy and optimization of patient care. The new technique allows the formation of multiple images with varied angles and the creation of three-dimensional anatomical reconstructions. With the formation of a sequence of thin slice images, tomosynthesis minimizes superimposition, as is predominantly encountered in traditional two-dimensional radiography. Such clarity is particularly useful in detecting minute pathologies, where the overlying of structures obscures vital details. In comparison with conventional imaging modalities, the research has indicated that it provides considerable improvement in terms of sensitivity and accuracy, particularly in challenging cases such as caries detection near restorations. The incorporation of tomosynthesis in the standard clinical workflow is a significant development in radiological imaging, since it aids in making informed clinical decision (Hilton et al., 2019). Underpinning tomosynthesis is the use of advanced angle-acquisition methodologies that influence how images are acquired and reconstructed. This is a process in which the X-ray source and detector are positioned strategically to acquire a sequence of projections at a range of angles, which are subsequently reconstructed to form an overall image of the target anatomy. Several angulation techniques can be applied depending on the desired diagnostic requirements, offering varying flexibility for addressing a range of clinical issues. In addition, advances in digital imaging technology enabled the efficient processing of such projections into high-resolution multiplanar reconstructions. The precision and flexibility offered by these acquisition methods not only enhance the visibility of thin anatomic details but also make an invaluable contribution towards maximizing the diagnostic value of tomosynthesis in clinical application (Jadidi et al., 2019). Clinical applications of tomosynthesis span diverse medical fields and hold vast potential to optimize patient outcomes by providing better imaging capabilities. Its use is especially beneficial in breast imaging, where it has been very effective in detecting breast cancers that can be masked under conventional mammography. Also, tomosynthesis has been explored for application in areas such as pulmonary imaging, where it will reduce the need for more invasive techniques by revealing lung lesions better. As the technique advances, further studies are needed to determine its diagnostic performance relative to traditional modalities. The integration of tomosynthesis into routine diagnostic procedures not only reflects its increasing popularity among radiologists but also underscores the need for ongoing research to continually assess its contribution to enhancing healthcare efficiency and patient safety (Jadidi et al., 2019).

3.4.1. Angle Acquisition Strategies

In the area of tomosynthesis principles, angle-acquisition methods play a vital role in enhancing image sharpness and diagnostic reliability. By acquiring images in varying angles, it is possible for radiologists to create a three-dimensional representation of the anatomical structures involved.

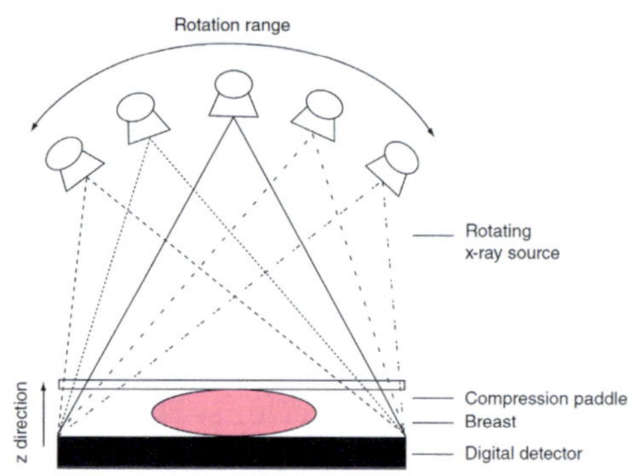

Figure 3.11. Typical digital breast tomosynthesis system. The x-ray source rotates around the compressed breast within a limited angle range and projection images are formed on the detector. The projection images are then reconstructed into slices through the volume of the breast along the z direction.

Source: https://www.researchgate.net/profile/Ehsan-Samei/publication/269483791/figure/fig1/AS:616350099705875@1523960723935/Typical-digital-breast-tomosynthesis-system-The-x-ray-source-rotates-around-the.png.

This is unlike in conventional radiography, where images are usually acquired with a single projection, as a general rule that results in superimposed structures that can potentially hide vital details. With modern imaging technology, the ability to capture images from multiple views allows for better definition of pathologies because overlapping tissues are minimized or eliminated. Such methods thus are not only important for the accurate diagnosis but also the design of effective therapy protocols based on a better understanding of the three-dimensional patterns of seen abnormalities (Figure 3.11).

The effectiveness of angle acquisition methods depends on the accurate selection of angles when taking images, as this choice directly affects the quality and interpretability of the resulting images. Scientists have found that capturing images at incremental angles—typically between 15 and 30°—can significantly enhance the visibility of features that in normal two-dimensional images would be hidden. Additionally, the use of computer algorithms supports the generation of reconstructed images from multiple-angle captures, as well as enabling radiologists to visualize structures in different orientations. This multidimensional approach enhances not only diagnostic yield but also supports disease progression tracking, further cementing its significance in contemporary radiographic practice. Apart from their technological use, angle acquisition schemes also need strict adherence to image quality optimization protocols. Parameters such as exposure indexing, grid selection, and proper collimation directly affect the overall image quality of tomosynthesis images derived from acquisitions at different angles. For instance, exposure parameter optimization is essential to ensure that single or multiple images are neither under-exposed nor over-exposed, and those scenarios can adversely affect interpretability. In addition, the use of focused collimation minimizes unnecessary radiation exposure while increasing contrast resolution in the obtained images. Therefore, the integration of angle acquisition methods into the total image quality management framework not only strengthens the accuracy of conventional radiography processes but enhances patient safety and outcomes as well.

3.4.2. Reconstruction Filters

The sophisticated processes of tomosynthesis rely significantly on reconstruction filter performance, which is pivotal in diagnostic image quality and interpretability. During image reconstruction, reconstruction filters are employed to appropriately transform raw projection data into a three-dimensional representation of anatomical structures. By modifying image data, reconstruction filters enhance certain features and suppress noise, thus diagnostic enhancement. Their use is particularly significant in situations where delicate details must be clarified, such as in breast scans or complex skeletal studies, to detect lesions or fractures that would otherwise go undetected. Optimization of these filters has a significant impact on image quality and can enhance diagnostic value in radiology (Figure 3.12).

Understanding the various reconstruction filters is crucial for optimizing radiographic results in conventional radiography techniques. Filters can be linear or non-linear, and each is suited for a specific clinical application. Linear filters, such as the Wiener filter, are primarily used for noise reduction and are trained to handle pixel values comparably. Non-linear filters, like the median filter, perform better in preserving edges while still performing well in noise reduction. The choice of an appropriate filter matters because it will not only affect the visual quality of images but also the subsequent diagnostic process. With growing technology, there is a need to explore new filtering methods in order to enhance the efficiency of radiographic exams and deliver quality care to patients. Also, the use of reconstruction filters is intertwined with digital radiography advancements, such that image processing algorithms must take into account the special needs of each modality of imaging. Reconstruction filters' interaction with digital imaging systems underpins a core revolution in the processing of radiographic data. The implementation of computer-aided diagnosis (CAD) systems is yet another manifestation of this synergy, emphasizing methods for image noise elimination and recovery, as discussed in recent studies (Blaine et al., 2025). In this way, integration facilitates accurate radiologic diagnoses with higher confidence. Moreover, with ongoing improvements in imaging technologies, ongoing optimization of reconstruction filters is required to continue addressing emerging challenges in radiographic imaging efficacy and efficiency, delivering robust clinical outcomes for diverse patient populations (Alimin et al., 2001).

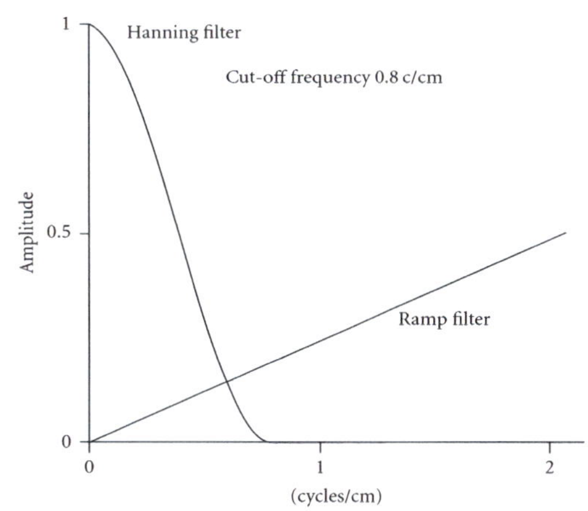

Figure 3.12. Use of ramp and hamming filters in tomographic reconstruction.

Source: https://www.researchgate.net/publication/51494115/figure/fig5/AS:213408751329285@1427892019960/Hanning-filter-and-Ramp-in-FBP-reconstruction.png.

3.4.3. Clinical Applications

New diagnostic imaging technologies have placed greater emphasis on tomosynthesis in the clinical arena, particularly in radiography. The technology enables the acquisition of multiple images at multiple angles, which are subsequently reconstructed into a three-dimensional image of the anatomy.

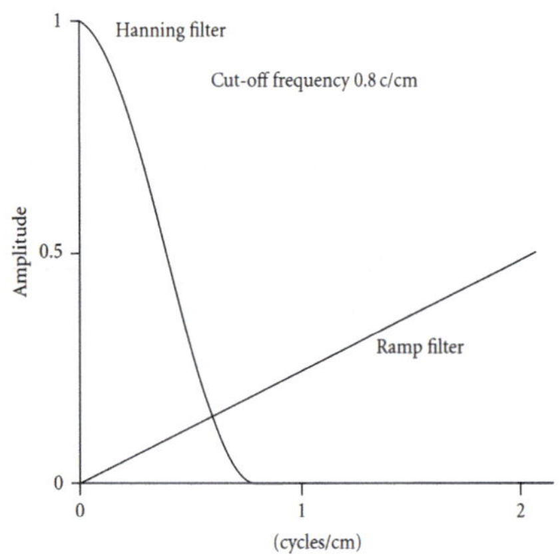

Figure 3.13. Digital breast tomosynthesis image of microcalcifications. *Source:* https://www.researchgate.net/publication/51494115/figure/fig5/AS:213408751329285@1427892019960/Hanning-filter-and-Ramp-in-FBP-reconstruction.png.

The development of image-processing algorithms is the most important factor in rendering tomosynthesis clinically optimal. More advanced algorithms enhance the resolution of reconstructed images, enabling improved visualization of anatomical structures and disease. Algorithms also reduce the usual difficulty in the detection of low-contrast objects and so generally improve the diagnostic performance of radiographic devices. Specifically, algorithms for noise reduction and detail enhancement enable clinicians to detect small changes in tissue structure. The clinical advantage of employing such sophisticated imaging modalities becomes evident, as they lead to correct diagnoses and reduced false positives and negatives. This is particularly important when it comes to diseases like cancer, where timely and accurate detection can be a significant advantage in deciding the treatment plan and the patient's prognosis. As the health care landscape continues to evolve, inclusion of cutting-edge image processing techniques will be crucial to reaching the full clinical potential of tomosynthesis. Furthermore, application of tomosynthesis in endodontics represents a growing convergence between radiographic technologies and clinical approaches. Recent research has investigated the use of other materials to obturate root canals, emphasizing the enhanced capabilities of modern imaging modalities. For instance, application of nanodiamond alongside digital radiography has provided accurate visualization of the root canals during treatment, improving accuracy in endodontic treatments. Improved imaging capabilities enable comprehensive planning and treatment execution, resolving issues commonly encountered with conventional materials. Such advances form a paradigm shift in endodontic treatments, where new materials can potentially reverse issues like leakage and reinfection caused by traditional use of gutta-percha. This shift represents the broader pattern of clinical applications of conventional radiographic techniques, while stressing continued emphasis on maximizing patient benefit through technological advancement in diagnostic imaging (N/A, 2010Ho et al.,; 2015).

3.5. Image Quality Optimization

In traditional radiography, maximizing image quality is crucial to facilitate accurate diagnosis while reducing radiation dose. Exposure indexing is one of the most important parameters that determine image quality. It allows a radiologist to determine whether the radiation dose used in an imaging procedure is proportionate to the body region being imaged. Providing feedback on image quality, exposure indexing helps technicians refine their procedures to enhance diagnostic effectiveness. More importantly, it helps in patient safety by preventing unnecessary radiation doses. With advances in digital radiography systems, proficiency in interpreting and understanding exposure indices is increasingly valuable. Overall, optimizing the exposure index improves overall radiograph quality and maximizes the potential for precise diagnoses, thereby increasing the level of care in medical image protocols. The use and selection of grids are key factors in maximizing image quality, as they directly impact radiographic contrast. Grids are intended to capture scattered radiation, which can degrade image quality; thus, their efficient application has the potential to significantly improve diagnostic results. In routine radiography, knowledge of the correct grid ratio and its proper positioning relative to the x-ray tube is crucial. Grids can differ in design, and improper application can result in artifacts or underexposures in the image. Besides, the employment or omission of a grid is also determined by the anatomical region being scanned, body part thickness, and anticipated scatter levels. Technicians must be well-trained in the appropriate use of grids to maximize image quality and enable healthcare providers to make clinical decisions based on reliable information, thereby improving patient diagnosis and treatment procedures. In addition to grid utilization and exposure indexing, precise collimation and proper patient positioning are keystones in achieving quality radiographs. Collimation serves to limit the X-ray beam to the area of concern, minimizing unwanted radiation exposure to tissues outside and increasing image sharpness. This technique not only promotes patient health but also helps eliminate scatter, which lowers image quality. Adequate alignment is also important, as misalignment produces distorted images that are difficult to interpret. A good understanding of anatomy and imaging protocols on the part of the radiologic technologist is necessary to apply proper collimation and positioning. As discussed by Barai et al. (2022), digital radiography technology provides scope to enhance these rudimentary techniques, allowing more images of quality at reduced doses and making the diagnostic process efficient along with being safe. All this focus on detail in these disciplines is key to improving the overall effectiveness of routine radiographic procedures.

3.5.1. Exposure Indexing

Maximal image quality of conventional radiography demands meticulous exposure indexing. The procedure measures the radiation exposure to the digital detector and provides radiologists with useful feedback on the adequacy of the exposure achieved during imaging procedures.

A correct exposure index (EI) enables radiographers to make good decisions, maximizing the diagnostic quality of images while minimizing unnecessary patient radiation exposure. By using exposure indicators, health practitioners can determine whether images are overexposed or underexposed and make adjustments accordingly to align with the ALARA (As Low as Reasonably Achievable) best-practice principle. This is particularly important in scenarios where patient safety is a top priority, helping achieve high-quality imaging without endangering patient welfare through excessive radiation dosage. Beyond the straightforward measurement, effective use of exposure indexing is a significant aspect of workflow optimization in digital radiography (Figure 3.14).

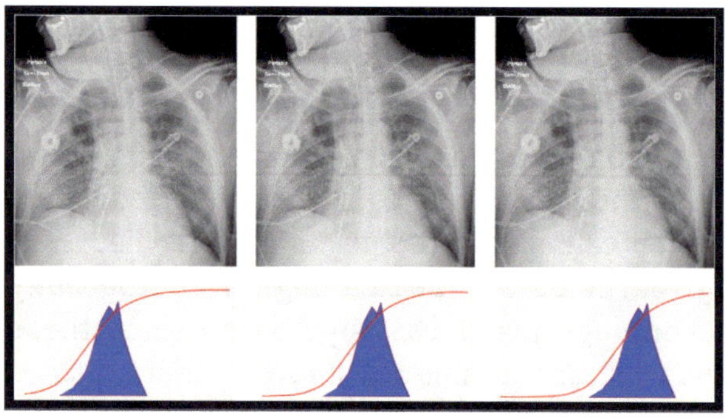

Figure 3.14. Visual comparison of exposure index variations in chest imaging.

Source: https://ajronline.org/cms/10.2214/AJR.12.8678/asset/images/12_12_8678_01b_cmyk.jpeg.

This approach not only aids patient exposure monitoring but also enhances systematic evaluation of imaging quality across different radiographic modalities. In practice, regular evaluation of exposure indices allows radiographers to be aware of rejection and repeat rate patterns, hence directly supporting quality assurance procedures in medical imaging sections. Through reject analysis and the implementation of exposure-indexing results, institutions can effectively address the economic and health ramifications of repeat imaging caused by suboptimal exposure. Furthermore, the systematic approaches provide a solid foundation for newly entering radiography practitioners to understand fully the role of exposure values in maintaining high exposure standards for patient treatment and diagnostic effectiveness (Atkinson, 2017). Apart from its role in quality assurance, exposure indexing has stimulated the evolution of imaging technologies to superior methods of data processing and interpretation. Digital radiography has transformed medical imaging, with prospects for automated feedback loops that optimize exposure parameters and image quality in real time. These developments do not only assist with triaging imaging studies but also enhance the overall workflow of the radiology department, thereby playing a role in better clinical outcomes. Using data from exposure indices, experts can continuously refine their imaging protocols, ensuring each acquisition is clinically relevant and ethically sound. This commitment to enhancing the quality of imaging through exposure indexing highlights the connection between technology, safety for the patient, and effective practice in contemporary radiological practice (Coorens et al., 2024).

3.5.2. Grid Selection and Use

In conventional radiography, achieving optimal image quality depends on numerous technical factors, including the judicious choice and use of grids. Grids have a significant function in that they limit scattered radiation, which can drastically lower image contrast and sharpness. By introducing a grid between the patient and the image receptor, radiographers can enhance the clarity of anatomical structures and gain more explicit diagnostic images. This technology is particularly beneficial in such examinations with greater depth of tissues, where scatter radiation is more apparent—such as in pelvic or abdominal radiography. Care should be taken, however, since incorrect grid use can unnecessarily increase patient radiation exposure and also make imaging more difficult. The decision to select a grid must thus be made based on clinical expertise and knowledge of the anatomical region to be imaged. Understanding of different types of grids is essential for effective radiography grid selection. Grids are further classified into two categories: stationary grids and moving grids. Stationary grids do not change position, making them more straightforward to apply but also causing some loss in image quality due to scatter. In contrast, moving grids, which generally make use of oscillation or reciprocation, achieve high image quality by actively eliminating the effect of scatter (Figure 3.15).

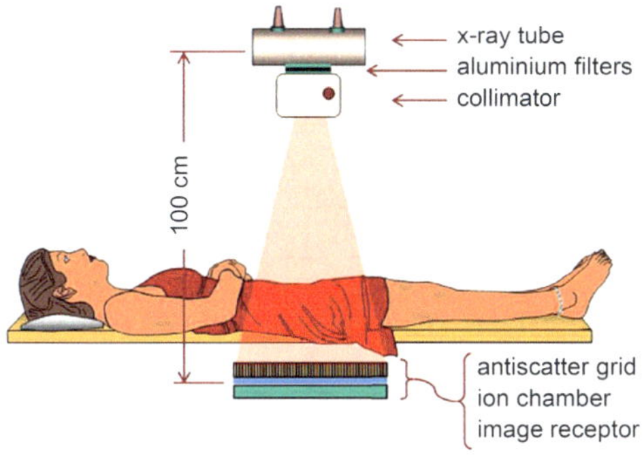

Figure 3.15. Parallel grid used to reduce scatter in radiographic imaging.

Source: https://radiologykey.com/wp-content/uploads/2023/04/C7-FF10.gif.

The choice between the two relies, to some degree, on the specific imaging requirements and technology at hand. For example, moving grids are generally favored in high-level imaging devices to achieve maximum image quality with a lower radiation dose. Promoting a clear understanding of the two types, along with their individual merits and drawbacks, enables radiographers to select the most appropriate grid configuration for each imaging case. Moreover, grid ratio is a significant parameter in the selection process, influencing both patient exposure levels and the quality of the resulting image. Grid ratio, or the lead strip height to distance between strips, is a dominant factor in determining the degree of scatter that can be successfully reduced. Higher grid ratios, while being more effective at lowering scatter, may also necessitate increased exposure settings in an effort to offer adequate film density. This is a delicate balance that practitioners must handle through both clinical experience and technical know-how. In addition, advances in imaging systems and methods, such as the inclusion of algorithms for digital image processing, could further impact the choice of grid by allowing post-processing compensation for some scatter effects. Thus, continuing education and adaptability in acquiring new technologies are the solution for radiographers to get the most out of grid-based applications, achieving improved image quality while ensuring patient safety and comfort during diagnosis.

3.5.3. Collimation and Positioning

Collimation and proper positioning are the main concepts in obtaining the best results with conventional radiography techniques. Radiographic imaging inherently involves a fine balance between image quality and patient radiation dose.

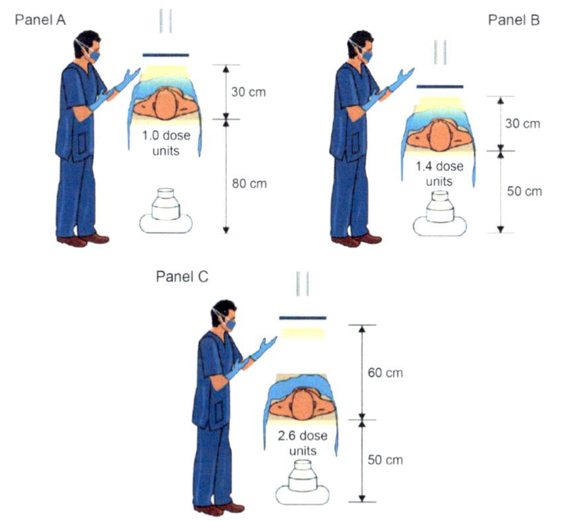

Figure 3.16. Proper collimation technique for minimizing patient dose.

Source: https://www.researchgate.net/profile/Georgios-Christakopoulos/publication/283975887/figure/fig1/AS:296599436709904@1447726224530/Example-of-optimal-table-positioning-to-minimize-patient-dose-The-patient-should-be.png.

Collimation is adequately utilized to restrict the x-ray beam to the area of concern, which minimizes unnecessary exposure of the surrounding tissue. In such situations, rectangular collimation has been found to significantly reduce radiation doses relative to circular collimators but can also increase exposure errors, particularly due to cone cuts. These are emphasized as a reminder of the importance of technicians acquiring the skill of collimation as a way of improving diagnostic outcomes under strict observance of safety protocols, such as the ALARA principle, which is still a guiding principle in radiography practice (AlAli et al., 2013; Avelãs et al., 2013). Interestingly, accurate positioning is also as important for successful radiography tests. This necessitates that the anatomical structure of interest be positioned in the optimal location in the collimated field (Figure 3.16).

Radiographers must use established positioning protocols that vary depending on different imaging procedures, for example, chest, abdomen, or skeletal radiography. Poor patient positioning can lead to distorted images or the need for repeat exposures and higher radiation doses. Furthermore, the use of digital technologies has enabled better positioning techniques through improved imaging performance and immediate feedback. This technology enables radiographers to assess positioning errors on the spot and adjust accordingly, further optimizing diagnostic image quality and supporting ongoing patient safety (Avelãs et al., 2013). Last but not least, positioning and collimation have the most significant relationship in traditional radiography. Understanding collimation principles allows radiographers to manage the X-ray beam effectively, minimizing overall exposure to radiation while ensuring maximum image quality. Accurate patient positioning also ensures that diagnostic images depict the anatomical areas of concern and thus fulfill the goals of medical imaging. Owing to the continually evolving nature of radiology and technological advancements, constant training on collimation techniques and positioning is continuously important. This not only conforms to ideal practices for patient safety but also supports achieving maximum efficiency in radiologic procedures in clinical practice and realizing the utmost health benefits (Avelãs et al., 2013; AlAli et al., 2013).

3.6. Quality Assurance in Radiography

In conventional radiography, implementing an effective quality assurance (QA) program is essential to ensure maximum image quality and minimum radiation exposure. Quality assurance is a series of systematic processes conducted to maintain and ensure the performance of radiographic equipment and procedures. Some essential QA elements in radiography include daily detector testing, which assesses the functionality and calibration of imaging equipment. Aside from aiding early detection of malfunctions, these tests help ensure consistent diagnostic output, enabling accurate patient assessments. This watchful regimen plays a significant role, with a large influence over the reliability of radiographic diagnosis and ultimately improving health outcomes. Another extremely significant component of radiography quality assurance procedures is phantom testing. It involves the use of calibrated test items that mimic body tissue to quantify the performance of imaging equipment. This regular checkup allows radiographers to measure various quality factors, including spatial and contrast resolution and noise levels, thereby enabling the detection of potential shortcomings in equipment performance. Moreover, regular phantom checking provides a culture of continuous improvement and compliance with accepted standards, thus enhancing the general efficiency of radiographic examinations. This approach has been instrumental in the evolution of radiographers' roles, as evidenced by the success of GI radiographers in the United

Kingdom, who established their competence in providing high-quality examinations efficiently (Hogg et al., 2007). Preventive maintenance is a cornerstone of effective quality assurance, ensuring radiographic equipment remains in optimal condition for long-term operation. Scheduled maintenance may involve regular inspections, calibration, and overhauls to prevent equipment breakdown and extend the lifespan of the system. Far from causing downtime, this proactive approach promotes a culture of responsibility among radiography personnel, who are attuned to the importance of equipment reliability. Moreover, the cost of implementing extensive preventive maintenance programs is justified by the increased patient safety outcomes and better operational effectiveness they yield. By looking at the historical context of comparable models —for example, that of GI radiographers —lessons can be learned that emphasize the importance of quality assurance measures in upgrading the level of care delivered through traditional radiography procedures (N/A, 1996).

3.6.1. Daily Detector Checks

Radiographic image quality relies heavily on the stable operation of the equipment; therefore, daily detector quality checks are included in quality control programs in conventional radiography. They detect any changes in imaging detector function, which are crucial for accurate diagnosis.

By performing a routine checkup on detectors, radiologic technologists can verify the image quality and the levels of radiation dose delivered to patients so that both are within safety limits. This proactive approach not only guarantees high standards of care but also increases health professionals' confidence in their ability to diagnose, effectively bridging the gap that may have resulted from equipment overuse or gradual degradation (Figure 3.17).

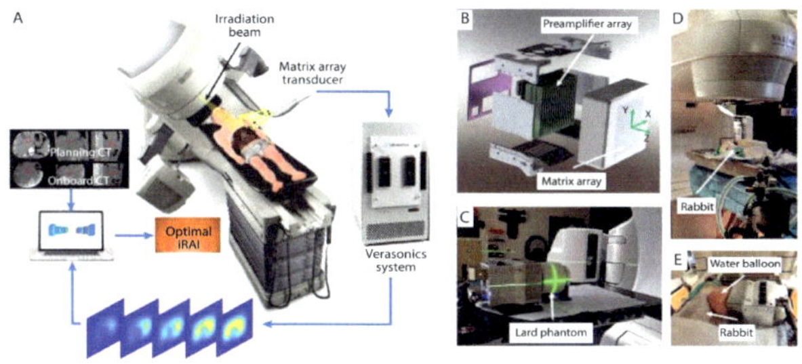

Figure 3.17. Daily quality assurance checklist for digital detectors.

Source: https://media.springernature.com/lw685/springer-static/image/art%3A10.1038%2Fs41587-022-01593-8/MediaObjects/41587_2022_1593_Fig1_HTML.png?as=webp.

Radiographic detectors should be regularly checked and calibrated to achieve optimal performance and limit patients' radiation exposure. Defective detectors will produce poor images, which might lead to misdiagnosis or re-imaging, exposing patients to unnecessary radiation. The addition of daily testing will allow fault detection such as image deformation, signal loss, or machine malfunction. These congruent processes enable thorough checks within health systems, particularly in settings classified as overburdened or under-resourced, as indicated by the need for new equipment and the effective use of resources (Silva et al., 2022). Regular detector check, therefore, becomes a cornerstone of maintaining requirements necessary to ensure quality management in medical imaging. In addition, adherence to daily detector testing has long-term, forward-looking benefits for image quality and patient safety; it is an expense-avoidance measure to offset the cost of operational inefficiency. Radiographic equipment is expensive to repair, and minor malfunctioning can lead to widespread disruption in diagnostic imaging. With a daily inspection and a standardized quality assurance program, healthcare facilities can detect future problems before they become major issues, thus ensuring operational effectiveness and reducing repair costs. With limited budgets, these measures are essential to provide an industry level of care and patient expectation (Martin et al., 2007). Thus, regular detector-check practice is an example of the emphasis on quality and sustainability in conventional radiography techniques.

3.6.2. Phantom Testing

Phantom application is vital to implementing quality assurance procedures for conventional radiography and heavily relies on phantom testing, one of the most significant aspects of performance assessment of imaging systems. Phantom testing is the final step, using standard test objects called phantoms that simulate the characteristics of human tissue. With phantoms, radiologists can assess how well imaging systems capture and store images under standardized conditions, thereby maintaining uniform diagnostic quality.

The testing of this sort is essential to detecting possible malfunctions in radiographic systems, such as fluctuations in contrast resolution, spatial resolution, and dose efficiency. Phantom testing also has greater applicability when placed within the realm of regulatory compliance, as it aligns with the prescribed standards for the safety and accuracy of medical imaging practice. It is a critical practice through which healthcare facilities can become skilled in meeting high practice standards in radiological practice. Building on the critical testing of radiographic equipment, phantom testing enables imaging procedures to be fine-tuned with the essential provision of feedback. Feedback from this process could help modify protocols to improve image quality and reduce patients' radiation exposure (Figure 3.18).

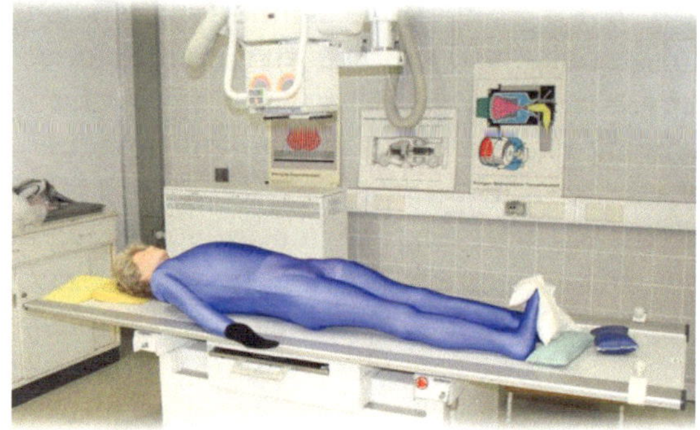

Figure 3.18. Use of anthropomorphic phantom in radiography QA testing.

Source: https://quart.de/sites/default/files/styles/page_width_50_lg/public/2017-05/Quart%20full-body-phantom-1.jpg?h=f6664cea&itok=yMZC3EdS.

As radiology advances towards newer technologies, phantom testing remains applicable, particularly for assessing the impact of digital technology on image quality. Employing standardized phantoms, doctors are able to compare the effectiveness of different modes of imaging, such as traditional X-rays versus newer digital technology. Apart from that, various research studies have established that phantom-based systematic assessments enhance patient care by promoting adherence to best practices in image quality optimization and dose management at every imaging cycle. The continued use of phantom testing highlights its basic role in maintaining radiographic excellence. Phantom testing also has applications in training and education, providing trainee radiologists with hands-on experience and essentially bridging the gap between a book and clinical practice. Phantom testing allows students to mimic various imaging modalities and compare their outputs against set standards, gaining a deeper appreciation of the challenges involved in creating high-quality radiographs.

Additionally, phantom testing can be highly useful in research, where it helps develop new imaging methods and enhance existing technologies. Current developments such as statistical image reconstruction methods demonstrate the potential for incorporating phantom testing alongside cutting-edge research projects (Parker et al., 2014; Brown et al., 2019). By repeatedly testing imaging systems with phantoms, the radiology community enhances its educational framework and enables iterative improvement of conventional radiography techniques.

3.6.3. Preventive Maintenance

The foundation of effective preventive maintenance in conventional radiography relies mostly on the regular inspection of equipment performance and reliability. The goal of this proactive measure is to minimize downtime and improve imaging quality, which is an important factor in maintaining accurate diagnosis and treatment planning.

Grease Trap or Interceptor (A)			Grease Trap or Interceptor (B)			
Date	Initials	% removed of grease & settled solids	Date	Initials	% removed of gease & settled solids	Date

Figure 3.19. Maintenance log sheet for digital imaging systems.

Source: https://images.sample.net/wp-content/uploads/2021/11/Standard-Equipment-Maintenance-Log.jpg.

With a regular check-and-service program, facilities can address minor issues before they develop into major defects that compromise patient care. Regular checks ensure radiographic equipment operates within its parameters, preventing equipment breakdown and the potential for poor-quality images. These processes demonstrate the necessity of regular checks and evaluation of radiographic equipment to ensure safety standards and the integrity of diagnostic findings, rendering preventative maintenance a vital component of quality assurance practices in radiography departments. A key element of success in preventive maintenance is careful construction. The procedures to be executed with caution are a mixture of manufacturer instructions and organizational standards applicable to specific radiographic technologies (Figure 3.19).

Effective preventive maintenance programs typically include daily, weekly, and monthly tasks, ranging from quick visual inspections to comprehensive performance measurement through phantom testing. These measurements allow for the identification of any changes in image performance, thereby ensuring radiographic machines are calibrated and functioning at the highest level. By integrating these systematic inspections into routine work processes, radiologic technologists and equipment managers can systematically eliminate the risk of equipment-related errors, thereby optimizing overall operational efficiency and ensuring patient and staff safety in radiology facilities. Advanced monitoring technologies that have emerged have further made it easier to traverse the horizon of preventive maintenance in radiography. The integration of machine learning and data analytics into traditional maintenance processes opens new horizons for optimizing equipment performance. For instance, live data can be used to predict impending failures by analyzing past performance patterns, enabling early intervention and reducing surprise downtime. This aligns with the mathematical models used in predictive maintenance across various industrial applications, as evidenced by research on ball bearing systems, which indicate the efficacy of such data-driven approaches (Farooq et al., 2024). Thus, the emergence of preventive maintenance practices towards a data-driven approach guarantees not only the longevity of radiographic equipment but also the high-quality delivery of imaging services on an ongoing basis, paving the way for improved patient outcomes in conventional radiography.

SUMMARY

The evolution of conventional radiography techniques has led to unprecedented advancements in diagnostic imaging, with enhanced clarity, speed, and safety. Integrating technologies such as digital radiography, fluoroscopy, and tomosynthesis has revolutionized how doctors view and analyze anatomical information. Each technique has a unique clinical application, from precise evaluation of chest and abdominal X-rays to the dynamic studies provided by fluoroscopy. Furthermore, research emphasizes ongoing refinement of techniques to optimize image quality, reduce radiation dose, and improve overall diagnostic accuracy, ensuring patients receive the best possible benefit. With advancing technology, the demand for efficient teaching systems and quality assurance protocols in radiography is increasing, laying the foundation for excellence in diagnostic imaging. In examining the evolution and current practice in conventional radiography, it is equally crucial to recognize the ubiquitous need for robust research and development. Introduction of new diagnostic modalities such as dual-energy computed tomography (DECT) and ultrasound has added to the diagnostic armamentarium, particularly in conditions such as calcium pyrophosphate crystal deposition disease (CPPD), where conventional radiography is insufficient. The comparative sensitivity of such methods to traditional ones underscores the necessity of continuous evaluation of diagnostic tests and standards. Traditional methods will remain a foundation, but their efficacy can be supplemented by integration with newer imaging technologies. A balance between conventional and newer methodologies will maximize the potential for accurate, early diagnosis and improved patient outcomes. Reflecting on the development of traditional radiography, quality assurance becomes a must-have in clinical practice. Strict daily detector inspections, phantom testing, and routine preventive maintenance ensure the life of radiographic equipment while safeguarding patients' health through ideal image quality. Systematic practice in healthcare facilities is the largest requirement for providing an environment of quality and safety. Whenever new technology emerges, a review of these protocols to improve them could offer enhanced reliability in imaging findings. In the end, the course of conventional radiography is one of adjusting to the emerging technologies and keeping a resolute commitment to quality assurance, paving the way for the next advance in diagnostic imaging.

CLOSER LOOK

LIFELONG LEARNING IN RADIOGRAPHY: ENSURING SAFETY, PRECISION, AND PROFESSIONAL GROWTH

Advancements in conventional radiography techniques are a testament to the necessity for professionals to ensure ongoing training and education. With technological advancements rewriting the book on medical imaging at breakneck speed, professionals must adhere to the latest methodologies and protocols to deliver effective and safe results. For instance, in projectional radiography, expertise in the finer aspects of chest, abdominal, and skeletal imaging is critical, but periodic refreshing of such knowledge through formal training courses is essential. This type of education maintains radiographers proficient in handling next-generation imaging equipment, enhances their diagnostic skills, and improves safety in dealing with patients. Apart from being a method for sharpening technical skills, ongoing education also instills a culture of continuous improvement, which is vital in an environment where accuracy affects patient outcomes. Thus, a culture of lifelong learning is an epicenter in professional development for radiologic professionals, facilitating better delivery of care. Also, the integration of digital radiography workflows has underscored the importance of ongoing training on sophisticated imaging systems. Advancements like acquisition modes of images and algorithms for processing require personnel to stay updated with the latest best practices and standards. By participating in ongoing educational experiences, radiologic technologists can better manage archiving and retrieval systems, making patient care and data management more convenient. Furthermore, such participation not only enhances each individual's ability but also improves interprofessional practice among healthcare teams. Fostering an active learning environment allows healthcare practitioners to respond effectively to evolving clinical situations and, therefore, improves patient care overall. For this reason, integrating comprehensive training programs into radiology's professional development process can improve diagnostic precision and safety measures. Finally, the need for quality assurance in radiography is yet another indication that ongoing education and training are essential in the profession. Regular inspections, such as on-site detector tests and phantom scanning, highlight the need for professionals to be well-versed with quality management methods. By using ongoing learning procedures, professionals can be aware of the underlying principles that enable the achievement of optimum image quality and safety compliance. These educational programs not only help reduce risks associated with radiation exposure but also contribute to an active process of identifying and resolving potential workplace issues. As the healthcare profession becomes increasingly complex, ongoing education for radiologic technologists is very important for ensuring quality assurance measures are in place and continually improved. Thus, including extensive and continuous training is crucial in ensuring high standards in conventional radiography procedures.

REFERENCES

1. Njoku, J. N., & Abonyi, C. (2022). A Review of Medical Imaging Innovations that Impacted Patient Care in Recent Decades as Link to Future Trends. *Journal of Radiography and Radiation Sciences*, *33*(1). https://doi.org/10.48153/jrrs.v33i1.223069AlAli, T. (2013). A comparison of rectangular vs. circular radiographic collimation during simulated endodontic therapy. https://core.ac.uk/download/51289982.pdf (accessed on 14th July 2025).
2. Alimin, A. J., Hushim, M. F., Mohd Rohi, N., Muslim, M., et al. (2001). Kajian motivasi ekstrinsik di antara pelajar lepasan sijil dan diploma Politeknik Jabatan Kejuruteraan Awam KUiTTHO. https://core.ac.uk/download/12007369.pdf (accessed on 14th July 2025).
3. Atkinson, S. (2017). Student conference ePosters. *64*, 106–110. https://www.semanticscholar.org/paper/8f0e5c9b7cce7f58c23625120b368111613c2097 (accessed on 14th July 2025).
4. Avanzo, M., Wei, L., Stancanello, J., Vallières, M., Rao, A., Morin, O., Mattonen, S. A., et al. (2020). Machine and deep learning methods for radiomics. *Medical Physics, 47*. https://doi.org/10.1002/mp.13678 (accessed on 14th July 2025).
5. Avcı, O., Abdeljaber, O., Kıranyaz, S., Hussein, M. F. M., Gabbouj, M., & Inman, D. J. (2020). A review of vibration-based damage detection in civil structures: From traditional methods to machine learning and deep learning applications. *Mechanical Systems and Signal Processing, 147*, 107077. https://doi.org/10.1016/j.ymssp.2020.107077 (accessed on 14th July 2025).
6. Avelãs, R., De Francesco, S., Ferreira, C., Martins, A., et al. (2013). Visual grading analysis of image quality in pediatric abdominal images acquired by direct digital radiography and computer radiography systems. https://core.ac.uk/download/15570354.pdf (accessed on 14th July 2025).
7. Barai, J., Tivaskar, S., Sable, A., & Luharia, A. (2022). Dose optimization and image quality in digital radiography: A review article. *Journal of Pharmaceutical Negative Results*. https://www.semanticscholar.org/paper/5554700810b2288617bab5d533f849f1ebdecaf7 (accessed on 14th July 2025).
8. Beck, F., Zupancic Cepic, L., Lettner, S., Moritz, A., Ulm, C., Zechner, W., & Schedle, A. (2024). Clinical and radiographic outcomes of single implant-supported zirconia crowns following a digital and conventional workflow: Four-year follow-up of a randomized controlled clinical trial. *Journal of Clinical Medicine, 13*. https://www.semanticscholar.org/paper/37564e0200b2563fa952ee92beb961792d439154 (accessed on 14th July 2025).
9. Blaine, G. J., Brown, G. S., Clarke, L. P., Doi, K., et al. (2025). Digital mammography, cancer screening: Factors important for image compression. https://core.ac.uk/download/pdf/42807614.pdf (accessed on 14th July 2025).
10. Blakey-Milner, B., Gradl, P., Snedden, G., Brooks, M. J., Pitot, J., López, E., Leary, M., et al. (2021). Metal additive manufacturing in aerospace: A review. *Materials & Design, 209*, 110008. https://doi.org/10.1016/j.matdes.2021.110008 (accessed on 14th July 2025).
11. Brinkbäumer, K., Dresel, S., Hahn, K., Höpfner, M., et al. (2004). Preoperative imaging of Charcot neuroarthropathy in diabetic patients: Comparison of Ring PET, hybrid PET, and magnetic resonance imaging. https://core.ac.uk/download/12175339.pdf (accessed on 14th July 2025).
12. Brown, J. M. C., Garbe, U., & Pelliccia, D. (2019). Statistical image reconstruction for high-throughput thermal neutron computed tomography. http://arxiv.org/abs/1806.02741 (accessed on 14th July 2025).

13. Chen, K., Terkeltaub, R., & Wu, Y. (2016). Systematic review and quality analysis of emerging diagnostic measures for calcium pyrophosphate crystal deposition disease. https://core.ac.uk/download/323065310.pdf (accessed on 14th July 2025).

14. Ciurea, A., Botar-Jid, C., Ciortea, C. A., Bolboacă, S. D., & Dudea, S. M. (2009). Cost analysis on imaging diagnostic techniques in cerebral and abdominal neonatal pathology. https://core.ac.uk/download/pdf/26798124.pdf (accessed on 14th July 2025).

15. Coorens, N., Janssen, N., Daemen, J. H., Franssen, A. J., Hulsewé, K. W., Vissers, Y., & de Loos, E. D. (2024). Advancements in preoperative imaging of pectus excavatum: A comprehensive review. *Journal of Thoracic Disease, 16*, 696–707. https://www.semanticscholar.org/paper/8b4a1448dff46a735687f23070e337888958d9c8 (accessed on 14th July 2025).

16. de Molina Gómez, C. (2018). Advanced capabilities for planar X-ray systems. https://core.ac.uk/download/288500045.pdf (accessed on 14th July 2025).

17. Desimpel, J., Posadzy, M., & Vanhoenacker, F. (2018). Cone beam CT of the musculoskeletal system: Clinical applications. https://core.ac.uk/download/147045015.pdf (accessed on 14th July 2025).

18. Diamond, D. A., Ron, E., Hall, E. J., Mandell, G. A., Boland, G. W. L., Hahn, H., et al. (2006). Patient dose reduction during voiding cystourethrography. https://core.ac.uk/download/pdf/8274425.pdf (accessed on 14th July 2025).

19. Farooq, U., Ademola, M., & Shaalan, A. (2024). Comparative analysis of machine learning models for predictive maintenance of ball bearing systems. *Electronics*. https://www.semanticscholar.org/paper/af0298afd665871ae8e7d747f0b24b5a6aff7e1d (accessed on 14th July 2025).

20. Farooqi, A. H. (2024). Innovative solutions for grout edge lifting identification, causes, and mitigation through best practices and reinforcement techniques. *International Journal on Science and Technology*. https://www.semanticscholar.org/paper/2a4215e817ec1378741fefbff2be194dd8f5af65 (accessed on 14th July 2025).

21. Foote, P., Hollstein, K., Jolly, M. R., Prabhakar, A., et al. (2015). Review of non-destructive testing (NDT) techniques and their applicability to thick-walled composites. https://core.ac.uk/download/74410705.pdf (accessed on 14th July 2025).

22. Gielen, I., van Bree, H., & Van Ryssen, B. (2012). Diagnostic imaging of the canine stifle. https://core.ac.uk/download/55823299.pdf (accessed on 14th July 2025).

23. Guzman, D. N. (2002). Curriculum guide to teach computed radiography at El Camino College. https://core.ac.uk/download/153384852.pdf (accessed on 14th July 2025).

24. Heindel, T. (2011). A review of X-ray flow visualization with applications to multiphase flows. https://core.ac.uk/download/38936136.pdf (accessed on 14th July 2025).

25. Hilton, R. (2019). Detection of caries adjacent to tooth-colored proximal restorations using stationary intraoral tomosynthesis. https://core.ac.uk/download/225545831.pdf (accessed on 14th July 2025).

26. Ho, D., Hong, C., Kang, M. K., Kim, H., et al. (2015). Nanodiamond-Gutta Percha composite biomaterials for root canal therapy. https://core.ac.uk/download/323080327.pdf (accessed on 14th July 2025).

27. Hogg, P., & Nightingale, J. (2007). The role of the GI radiographer: A UK perspective. https://core.ac.uk/download/1663999.pdf (accessed on 14th July 2025).

28. Hwang, H. (2017). Knowledge, attitude and perception on radiation imaging among children's caregivers in the pediatric dental clinic. https://open.bu.edu/bitstream/2144/23797/5/Hwang_bu_0017N_12842.pdf (accessed on 14th July 2025).

29. Jadidi, M. (2019). The dependency of image quality on acquisition protocol and image processing in chest tomosynthesis. https://core.ac.uk/download/225136004.pdf (accessed on 14th July 2025).

30. LeBoff, M. S., Greenspan, S. L., Insogna, K., Lewiecki, E. M., Saag, K. G., Singer, A., & Siris, E. S. (2022). The clinician's guide to prevention and treatment of osteoporosis. *Osteoporosis International, 33*, 2049–2102. https://doi.org/10.1007/s00198-021-05900-y (accessed on 14th July 2025).

31. Leonarski, F., & Wang, M. (2025). Enabling kilohertz data acquisition and analysis for the Swiss Light Source 2.0. *Structural Dynamics*. https://www.semanticscholar.org/paper/5b1d7b81989be12952d023480d0573e207998a9d (accessed on 14th July 2025).

32. Lewis, W. H., & Pless, W. M. (2025). Space shuttle: Structural integrity and assessment study. https://core.ac.uk/download/pdf/42890475.pdf (accessed on 14th July 2025).

33. Livens, S., Nuyts, D., Dries, J., Collaud, X., Di Paola, R., Bastin, C., Moreau, V., et al. (2025). A small hyperspectral satellite mission designed for improved image quality. *Proceedings of SPIE, 13546*, 135461L–135461L-12. https://www.semanticscholar.org/paper/a350f4531a2effe4a02db20043ef7e947bc3ef64 (accessed on 14th July 2025).

34. Low, W. C. S., Chuah, J. H., Tee, C., Anis, S., Shoaib, M., Faisal, A., Khalil, A., et al. (2021). An overview of deep learning techniques on chest X-ray and CT scan identification of COVID-19. *Computational and Mathematical Methods in Medicine, 2021*. https://www.semanticscholar.org/paper/a5a993eb35858c2adfb645d2a82b5e6bf64b763c (accessed on 14th July 2025).

35. Macovski, A. (2025). Radiographic applications of spatial frequency multiplexing. https://core.ac.uk/download/pdf/42858477.pdf (accessed on 14th July 2025).

36. Martin, C. J. (2007). Optimization in general radiography. https://core.ac.uk/download/pdf/8566929.pdf (accessed on 14th July 2025).

37. Martini, K., Baessler, M., Baumueller, S., Frauenfelder, T., et al. (2017). Diagnostic accuracy and added value of dual-energy subtraction radiography compared to standard conventional radiography using computed tomography as standard of reference. https://www.zora.uzh.ch/id/eprint/136513/1/ZORA136513.pdf (accessed on 14th July 2025).

38. Mhezi, V., Nkrumbih, Z., Kisukari, J. D., Hadi, Y., & Lyimo, F. (2024). Enhancing radiation safety and justification of imaging in pediatric chest radiography: Insights from a tertiary hospital in Tanzania. *Saudi Journal of Radiology*. https://www.semanticscholar.org/paper/0957bdbed0f757b65db193834bb664c3c1545ab6 (accessed on 14th July 2025).

39. N/A. (1996). *Focal Spot*, Fall/Winter 1996. https://core.ac.uk/download/129069303.pdf (accessed on 14th July 2025).

40. N/A. (2010). *Focal Spot*, Spring/Summer 2010. https://core.ac.uk/download/129069380.pdf (accessed on 14th July 2025).

41. Pandey, R., Kamble, R., & Kanani, H. (2024). Revolutionizing smiles: Advancing orthodontics through digital innovation. *Cureus, 16*. https://www.semanticscholar.org/paper/ca35f9f68b6562640d025586c2dcc7c53dbdb93e (accessed on 14th July 2025).

42. Parker, D. J., Esposito, M., Evans, P. M., Ferrari, A., Poludniowski, G., Goethals, P. E., Nieto-Camero, J., et al. (2014). Proton-counting radiography for proton therapy: A proof of principle using CMOS APS technology. https://core.ac.uk/download/20321159.pdf (accessed on 14th July 2025).

43. Pera, F., Pesce, P., Bagnasco, F., Pancini, N., Carossa, M., Baldelli, L., Annunziata, M., et al. (2023). Comparison of milled full-arch implant-supported frameworks realized with a full digital workflow or from conventional impression: A clinical study. *Materials, 16*. https://www.semanticscholar.org/paper/081e3b5e09db456d90f744dc9757985861a24aef (accessed on 14th July 2025).

44. Ponikowski, P., Voors, A. A., Anker, S. D., Bueno, H., Cleland, J. G. F., Coats, A. J. S., Falk, V., et al. (2016). 2016 ESC guidelines for the diagnosis and treatment of acute and chronic heart failure. *European Heart Journal, 37*, 2129–2200. https://doi.org/10.1093/eurheartj/ehw128 (accessed on 14th July 2025).

45. Rayyani, A. A., Shalalni, A. A., Radwan, A. H., Shibli, K. A., Jabin, J. Y., Mokli, M. A. Y., Mabuj, J. M., et al. (2024). Digital X-ray imaging: Emphasis can be placed on developments in digital X-ray technologies and their applications in diagnosis and treatment. https://core.ac.uk/download/616775625.pdf (accessed on 14th July 2025).

46. Reisig, D., & Huseth, A. (2025). Establishing best practices for insect resistance management: A new paradigm for genetically engineered toxins in cotton expressing Mpp51Aa2. *Journal of Economic Entomology, 118*, 1–8. https://www.semanticscholar.org/paper/5d0d9335d0d0539e2134a686cf71fe5d706929e6 (accessed on 14th July 2025).

47. Ronkainen, J. (2007). Costs in today's radiology: ABC analysis of typical situations in the transitional period. https://core.ac.uk/download/628859998.pdf (accessed on 14th July 2025).

48. Saavedra-Lozano, J., Falup-Pecurariu, O., Faust, S. N., Girschick, H., Hartwig, N., Kaplan, S. L., Lorrot, M., et al. (2017). Bone and joint infections. *The Pediatric Infectious Disease Journal, 36*, 788–799. https://doi.org/10.1097/inf.0000000000001635 (accessed on 14th July 2025).

49. Schaefer-Prokop, C., & Klein, J. S. (2003). Digital chest radiography. *Journal of Thoracic Imaging, 18(3)*, 123. https://www.semanticscholar.org/paper/c6cbeae5791287720d0827737baf36d5cf69fdec (accessed on 14th July 2025).

50. Seiler, R., Eppenberger, P., & Rühli, F. (2018). Application of portable digital radiography for dental investigations of ancient Egyptian mummies during archaeological excavations: Evaluation and discussion of the advantages and limitations of different approaches and projections. *Imaging Science in Dentistry, 48*, 167–176. https://www.semanticscholar.org/paper/40de758b2472fab23fbbb47d779122e30269e10d (accessed on 14th July 2025).

51. Seslija, P., Teeter, M., Yuan, X., Naudie, D., Bourne, R., MacDonald, S., Peters, T., et al. (2012). Measurement of joint kinematics using a conventional clinical single-perspective flat-panel radiography system. *Medical Physics, 39*(10), 6090–6103. https://www.semanticscholar.org/paper/61a0c45e363b3ec9601f3815e79d6c5abf3e6479 (accessed on 14th July 2025).

52. Silva, J. F. S. da. (2022). Assessment of innovative technologies application in medical imaging in Portugal. https://core.ac.uk/download/491650676.pdf (accessed on 14th July 2025).

53. Spahn, D. R., Bouillon, B., Černý, V., Duranteau, J., Filipescu, D., Hunt, B. J., Komadina, R., et al. (2019). The European guideline on management of major bleeding and coagulopathy

following trauma: Fifth edition. *Critical Care, 23.* https://doi.org/10.1186/s13054-019-2347-3 (accessed on 14th July 2025).

54. Tomaihi, B. H., Sabai, H. A., Aqeli, M. A., Moafa, M. A., Qusairy, A. M. G., Khawaji, M. N., et al. (2024). Development of X-ray imaging techniques to improve image quality. https://core.ac.uk/download/616775623.pdf (accessed on 14th July 2025).

55. Ullah, R. S., Masud, F., Bashir, M. K., & Ali, A. (2024). Utilization of deep learning models for the early diagnosis of COVID-19 through chest radiography. *Review of Applied Management and Social Sciences.* https://www.semanticscholar.org/paper/ab7235ffa78a1814176dffce86b65a2b95846419 (accessed on 14th July 2025).

56. Wargantiwar, S., Bhattacharya, S., & Kanugo, A. (2025). Surgical advancements, immunotherapy, targeted and conventional therapies, biopsy, colposcopy, and Pap smear integration in the management of cervical cancer. *Current Medicinal Chemistry.* https://www.semanticscholar.org/paper/9f1a916b0fdc8d7e5d3b2170fa2618224620927a (accessed on 14th July 2025).

57. Zammit, A. (1992). Apprehending narcotic smugglers in Malta. https://core.ac.uk/download/46601790.pdf (accessed on 14th July 2025).

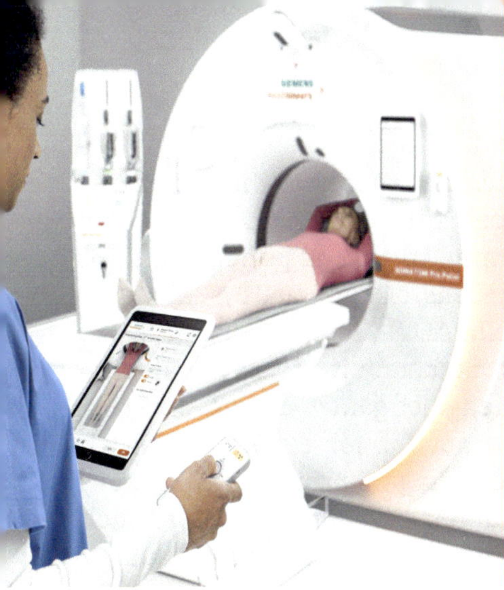

Chapter 4

COMPUTED TOMOGRAPHY: PRINCIPLES AND PROTOCOLS

Contents

Introduction

Medical imaging has been revolutionized, and computer-assisted tomography (CT) is a transformative technology that has changed diagnostic techniques. The peculiar ability of CT to provide cross-sectional images facilitates accurate visualization of complex anatomical structures and enhances clinical decision-making. The following introductory discussion outlines the fundamental principles and protocols behind its use, which is crucial in inpatient management in a wide range of medical specialties. Combining physics and advanced engineering in CT technology not only enables even better image quality but also demands an understanding of its technical structure, data-acquisition practices, and reconstruction algorithms. Furthermore, the addition of advanced techniques such as dual-energy CT and perfusion imaging further augments diagnostic potential while maintaining patient safety through strict radiation dose control. As we delve deeper into the intricacies of CT technology, it is essential that we understand CT scanner design, beginning with gantry design. This crucial component enables rotation of the x-ray tube and detector, which is necessary for acquiring high-quality images. Slip-ring technology has transformed image acquisition protocols by enabling continuous gantry rotation, resulting in significantly improved scanning speed and patient comfort. These advances make possible the accommodation of various patient needs, expanding CT's utilization across healthcare settings, from emergency rooms to outpatient clinics. No less important is the design of patient tables, which must provide stability along with adjustability to accommodate the diverse demands of CT procedures. Such comprehensive knowledge of gantry design, slip-ring technology, and patient table systems rounds out the background needed for expert use of CT. Additionally, success in CT in the clinical setting relies on optimized imaging protocols consistent with specific diagnostic requirements. An accurate understanding and control of parameters such as kilovolt peak (kVp) and milliampere-seconds (mAs) aid in achieving optimal image quality while minimizing radiation burden. Knowledge of pitch and rotation time, too, is critical to attain the optimal spatial resolution and scanning time. The introduction of CT protocols also includes contrast timing, which is crucial for demonstrating vascular structures and maximizing tissue differentiation. As these principles and protocols are investigated, it is apparent that mastering CT is critical to improving imaging professionals' proficiency, ultimately contributing to the field's development and enhancing patient outcomes.

4.1. Basic Principles of Computed Tomography

In the context of biomedical imaging, an in-depth understanding of the architectural composition of CT scanners is essential. At the center of this design is the gantry, which houses the X-ray tube and detectors. This equipment determines the scanners' ability to produce high-quality images by optimizing positioning and stiffness during rotation. Among the required design components of modern gantries is the use of slip-ring technology, which enables the free, unbroken rotation of the X-ray unit without interference from cables. This technology improves image acquisition speed and enables uninterrupted data transfer, thus making scanning more efficient in the long run. Moreover, patient table mechanics also contribute significantly towards patient comfort as well as accurate imaging because it must accommodate variable body sizes while providing proper alignment for repeatable results. All these architectural elements together create a synergistic environment conducive to the production of high-resolution tomographic images. The CT scanning methods of data collection significantly influence diagnostic outcomes. The two most frequently employed methods are axial and helical scanning. Axial, or conventional, or slice-by-slice scanning scans in distinct sections, while helical, or spiral, scanning collects continuous information as the patient moves through the scanning apparatus. The second method enhances image quality by the reduction of motion artifacts and provision for volumetric data creation, which provides more adaptable image reconstruction. Dual-source techniques are also revolutionizing CT imaging by using two X-ray sources and detector arrays, accelerating acquisition time and delivering improved temporal resolution. As such, these newer modalities of data acquisition not only mechanize the imaging process but also augment the clinician's capacity to interpret subtle diagnostic nuances within the imaged anatomy. One of the foundations of computed tomography is image reconstruction, the process that transforms raw data into diagnostically useful images. Filtered back projection is the most common technique employed, wherein mathematical filters are applied to the received data, thereby enhancing image quality. But this technique is susceptible to artifacts, so iterative reconstruction methods have been developed that progressively refine images based on successive projections and corrections.

Model-based algorithms are a new method that employs accurate mathematical models of imaging to reduce noise and increase precision. These advances in imaging reconstruction not only improve diagnostic capabilities but also facilitate the optimization of protocols—trading off factors such as radiation dose, image quality, and scanning time. Understanding these reconstruction principles is essential to optimize CT protocols and deliver effective patient care across diverse clinical contexts, underscoring the significance of advances in this field (Ketten et al., 2008; Kitsiou et al., 2013).

4.1.1. X-ray Production and Detection

In X-ray production, there are certain fundamental principles involved in the production of high-quality images in computed tomography (CT). It is concerned with the interaction between high-energy photons and matter. X-ray production is the rapid deceleration of electrons when they collide with a target material, typically composed of tungsten.

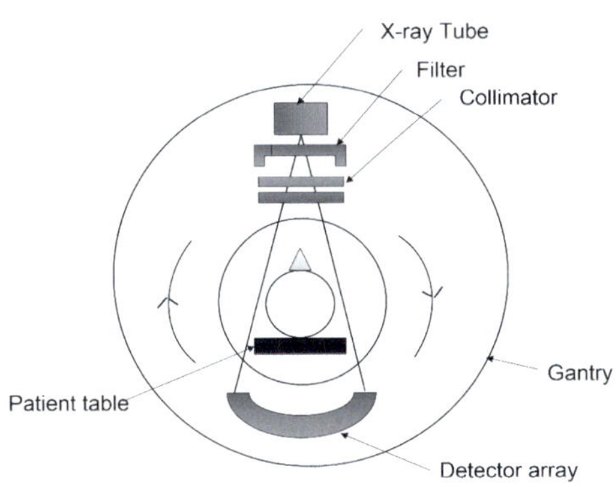

Figure 4.1. Schematic representation of X-ray tube and detector array in a CT scanner.

Source: https://cdnintech.com/media/chapter/80151/1512345123/media/F6.png.

It generates two types of radiation: characteristic radiation, due to individual electron transitions between energy levels in target atoms, and bremsstrahlung radiation, resulting from the slowing of electrons near atomic nuclei. The efficiency of X-ray generation depends on various factors, including the kilovoltage peak (kVp), which determines the energy and penetration of the generated X-rays and consequently influences the contrast and quality of the resulting images, which are necessary for proper diagnosis in clinical practice (Figure 4.1).

The detection of X-ray photons is an essential process in imaging, and the need for accurate conversion of absorbed radiation into a visible spectrum is necessitated. Scintillator detectors and digital detectors are essentially used in CT systems. Scintillation detectors emit light when struck by X-rays, which is then converted into an electric signal by photodetectors to create an image. On the other hand, computer detectors employ direct conversion methods, in which X-rays are directly converted into processable electrical charge in the form of an image. Understanding detection mechanisms is pivotal for evaluating image quality and determining appropriate settings during scanning protocols. Also, technological advancements in detector technology continuously enhance sensitivity and spatial resolution, thereby improving overall diagnostic capabilities of CT imaging in a clinical environment, especially when applying developed scanning modes like Dual-Energy CT or CT Angiography. The principles of X-ray production and detection are the basis for optimizing CT imaging protocols to ensure both image and patient safety. Accurate calibration of mA, kVp, and exposure time is vital to provide proper imaging without unnecessary radiation exposure. Current advancements in radiation dose management, including automatic exposure control systems and organ dose estimation algorithms, improve optimization of imaging protocols according to individual patient needs.

Continuous evaluation of imaging approaches, based on empirical data from phantom models that approximate human anatomy, contributes to improved clinical practice. Anthropomorphic phantom studies have shown promise in quantifying X-ray attenuation and adjusting imaging parameters to maximize image quality and minimize radiation exposure (Ekaterina et al., 2024). Along the way, computed tomography draws closer to achieving greater diagnostic efficacy without compromising patient safety and technological harmony.

4.1.2. Image Reconstruction Methods

The evolution of image reconstruction techniques in computed tomography (CT) has greatly enhanced diagnosis in the clinical setting. Filtered back projection is among the oldest techniques and yet widely used due to its simplicity of implementation and its high processing speed for projecting data. It operates by reversing the mathematically projected data to produce cross-sectional images. Nevertheless, it is becoming increasingly clear that filtered back projection is less than optimal for controlling noise and reducing artifacts compared to newer techniques. Increasingly advanced computing capabilities have provided the impetus to explore iterative reconstruction techniques that employ sophisticated algorithms to improve image quality in real time. Through the reduction of noise and enhancement of contrast resolution, these techniques produce sharper images while potentially reducing radiation exposure, presenting a thrilling future direction for CT technology that can have a significant impact on patient outcomes and safety. Alternately, iterative reconstruction is already a groundbreaking technique in CT imaging that has made significant advancements over traditional methods. By employing iterative algorithms, the approach facilitates repeated refinement of image information, leading to significantly enhanced image quality through noise removal and artifact correction (Figure 4.2).

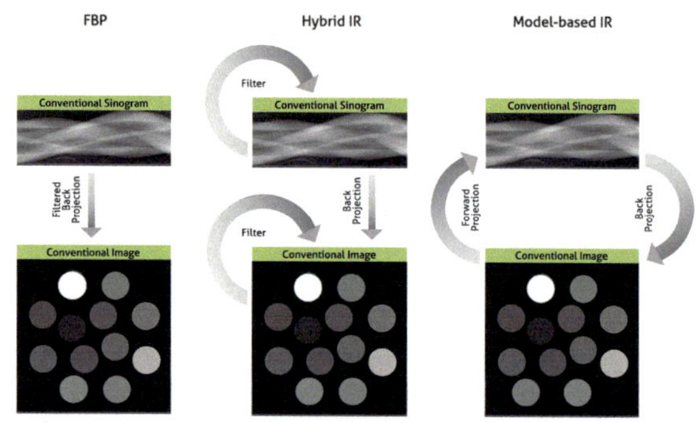

Figure 4.2. Comparison of filtered back projection and iterative reconstruction methods.

Source: https://media.springernature.com/lw1200/springer-static/image/art%3A10.1007%2Fs00330-018-5810-7/MediaObjects/330_2018_5810_Fig1_HTML.png.

Significantly, several high-profile publications have validated the clinical efficacy of iterative reconstruction across various settings, demonstrating its promise to reduce radiation doses without sacrificing diagnostic performance. The algorithms can tailor themselves to the unique nature of the acquired data and are therefore very effective across all imaging tasks. Their use is a key step towards maximizing radiographic outcomes, particularly for the pediatric and other susceptible populations where radiation dosage must remain minimized (Bastarika et al., 2015). Besides iterative reconstruction, model-based algorithms are another cutting-edge advancement in image reconstruction, maximizing the characteristics of next-generation CT technology. These applications use a model of the imaging system's physics and geometry during reconstruction to achieve more accurate representations of the scanned anatomy. The ability to enhance image quality while reducing radiation dose is particularly beneficial across a broad range of clinical applications, including oncologic imaging and vascular assessment. Fresh evidence highlights the use of model-based techniques in complex imaging scenarios, yet another testament to protocol optimization in the clinical environment. These breakthroughs not only improve diagnostic confidence but also reflect the dynamic nature of CT imaging as it opens up to embrace more complex cases, ensuring that radiologists and doctors have tools at their disposal to provide complete patient care (Kussman et al., 2007).

4.1.3. Contribution of Algorithm to CT Imaging

Algorithmic innovation has significantly advanced the application of computed tomography (CT) scanning, particularly in image reconstruction. A key innovation is iterative reconstruction (IR) algorithms that have augmented traditional filtered back-projection methods.

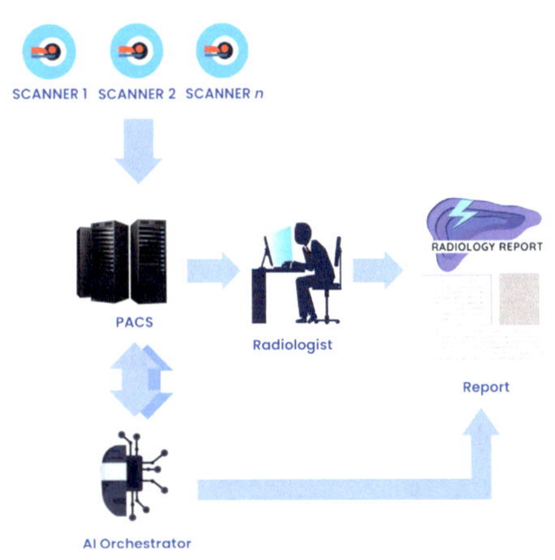

Figure 4.3. Simplified workflow showing algorithmic processing in CT imaging.

Source: https://media.springernature.com/lw1200/springer-static/image/art%3A10.1007%2Fs10278-024-01200-z/MediaObjects/10278_2024_1200_Fig1_HTML.png.

IR methods enhance image quality by iteratively refining image data to produce better noise reduction and fewer artifacts. As clinical adoption of these algorithms increases, their potential to reduce radiation doses without compromising diagnostic quality is becoming increasingly apparent. The possibility of IR to improve image contrast makes a strong argument for its use, as shown in studies that compared this method with traditional approaches, which emphasized IR's efficiency in reducing some common drawbacks of conventional methods (Bastarika et al., 2015). The unending development of these algorithms is the pivotal fulcrum around which the future of CT imaging will turn (Figure 4.3).

The role of algorithms extends beyond image reconstruction to encompass significant aspects of CT imaging protocol optimization. Specific selected parameters, such as kVp and mAs, can significantly impact both patient safety and image quality when controlling radiation dose. Advanced algorithms can dynamically adjust these parameters in accordance with clinical requirements while safeguarding patients from hazardous radiation exposure. For example, the use of lower kVp values with specialized filters on reconstruction has been shown in recent studies to reduce exposure by a large degree without reducing the diagnostic quality (Faggioni et al., 2012). This adaptability points to the importance of algorithms, as they not only simplify CT protocols but also enhance patient care by reducing potential hazards from radiation exposure, thereby optimizing the imaging process. Besides, algorithms play an important role in the development of new CT imaging technologies such as dual-energy CT and perfusion imaging. These new techniques leverage the power of sophisticated algorithms for data collection and processing acquired at different energy levels to develop improved discrimination between materials and visualization of anatomy. In dual-energy CT, algorithms aid in the investigation of the relative materials' attenuation, which can be very beneficial for assessment of several conditions, including vascular illnesses. Furthermore, incorporating algorithms into perfusion imaging facilitates quantification of tissue blood flow, providing critical information on conditions such as ischemia or tumors. By improving diagnostic capability and increasing functional application of CT imaging, algorithms propel the development of CT technology so that clinicians are equipped with the devices they require for complete assessment of patients.

4.2. CT Scanner Parts

In computed tomography, the complex architecture of CT scanners is the foundation for effective acquisition of diagnostic images. Central to this design is a gantry configuration that houses the X-ray tube and detectors, enabling rotation to acquire cross-sectional images of the body. Gantry designs control parameters, such as rotational speed and stability, that directly affect image quality. Gantry systems of high-end can be equipped with motorized motions and variable angles, leading to enhanced imaging flexibility and less patient motion artifacts. Furthermore, the weight and size of the gantry can affect the spatial volume of the scanning area and, in turn, the volume of data collected per scan. Overall, the gantry design strength is a crucial parameter for optimizing imaging performance and obtaining high-quality images required for proper diagnostics. Close to this comes the revolution in slip-ring technology, which has revolutionized data transmission in CT scanners. Unlike traditional systems that require time-consuming cable runs, slip-ring technology enables unlimited rotation of the gantry and reliable, untethered data transmission from detectors to the imaging system. This innovative mechanism is essential to helical (spiral) scanning, significantly reducing scan time and increasing patient throughput. In addition, the effectiveness of slip-rings has driven advances in image reconstruction algorithms, facilitating faster and more accurate processing of acquired data. In turn, this technology not only enhances the quality of the images obtained but also minimizes the radiation burden on patients by optimizing scanning protocols and improving the overall safety of CT examinations. The patient table mechanics is another essential factor that dictates the imaging process and patient comfort during CT scanning. The operation and design of the patient table can bring about an impact on the positioning accuracy, which is responsible for the image quality outcome. Modern patient tables are usually motorized and adjustable with the capacity to travel accurately in accordance with scanning protocols. This mechanization is crucial, particularly for accurate alignment, such as when imaging areas with intricate anatomy. The weight capacity of tables and the materials used can contribute to patients' safety and comfort during scans. By integrating ergonomics with advanced mechanics, the patient table is an important contributor to facilitating seamless interactions between the CT scanner and patients without jeopardizing the integrity of each test's imaging protocol.

4.2.1. Gantry Design and Operation

The gantry is the central unit in a computed tomography (CT) scanner that enhances the efficacy and accuracy of imaging procedures. The gantry is generally made round or ellipsoidal in shape to hold rotating X-ray detectors and tubes. The gantry is primarily designed to facilitate the movement and positioning of the elements that generate high-quality images. Such an arrangement allows for multiple slices of cross-sectional images to be captured as the patient moves across the aperture, thus significantly enhancing diagnostic capability. Additionally, design elements such as the gantry's rotation and tilt capabilities are important in maximizing image-acquiring angles, thus enhancing visualization of the anatomical structures under investigation. The smooth integration of these capabilities increases the overall operational productivity of CT technology, ensuring imaging quality that meets clinical specifications for accurate diagnoses. Contemporary CT systems have been developed mainly to advance gantry technology, enabling swift imaging and effective radiation dose management (Figure 4.4).

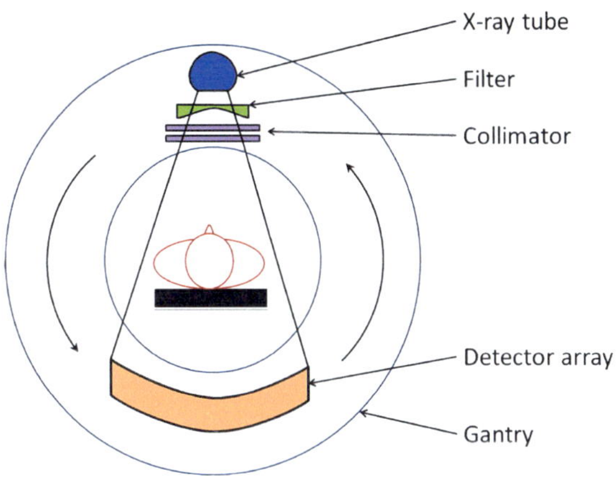

Figure 4.4. Cross-sectional view of a CT gantry highlighting major components.

Source: https://radiologycafe.com/wp-content/uploads/2021/04/ct-equipment-machine.png.

The incorporation of slip-ring technology is a significant advancement in gantry design, enabling continuous rotation without interruption and speeding up and optimizing image acquisition. With the ability to support continuous electrical contact, the gantry can rotate continuously while the X-ray tube and detectors are in motion. This technological advancement supports advanced scanning modalities, such as helical (spiral) scanning, which improve patient comfort by enabling shorter scan times and better image quality. As stated, the importance of radiation dose management cannot be overstated; research on gantry and imaging technologies must be complemented by adherence to the ALARA principle to safeguard the patient (Kärnä et al., 2018). This safety-versus-innovation balance reinforces the need for careful gantry design in CT scanners. The equilibrium between gantry design and patient positioning is crucial in the achievement of optimal imaging outcomes. Some mechanical aspects of the gantry, such as the mechanics of the patient table, directly influence how patients are positioned in the scanning region. An appropriately designed patient table can provide fast, accurate positioning while accounting for a variety of patient requirements, resulting in a smoother workflow in the clinical setting. In addition, contemporary gantry designs also incorporate features for greater patient comfort and ease of use, such as greater openings and height adjustment. These are particularly applicable to patients with mobility issues or who require special attention due to their clinical condition. Higher gantry designs, which prioritize patient comfort, ultimately drive compliance during imaging, yielding improved-quality images critical for effective diagnosis and treatment (Baronette et al., 2018). Gantry design is thus a critical factor underlying the success of CT technologies, with ramifications for the future of diagnostic imaging.

4.2.2. Detector Types and Impact on Image Quality

Advancements in detector technology have had a profound effect on performance as well as on the effectiveness of computed tomography (CT) imaging, with direct influence on image quality. Modern detector systems, such as multi-detector rows, facilitate the collection of sufficient data within a shorter time interval, significantly enhancing spatial resolution and reducing motion artifacts. All of these improvements allow for sharper anatomical visualization, which becomes essential for sound diagnosis and treatment planning. As pointed out, contemporary systems utilize both gas and scintillation detectors, and each possesses other advantages when sensitivity and image precision are taken into account. The use of dual-source CT technologies also mirrors this, as they enable simultaneous operation of two x-ray tubes and are particularly useful in dynamic exams, such as perfusion imaging, where temporal resolution is of great concern. A closer examination of how image quality and various kinds of detectors interact reveals that optimization has direct association with the used scanning protocols (Figure 4.5).

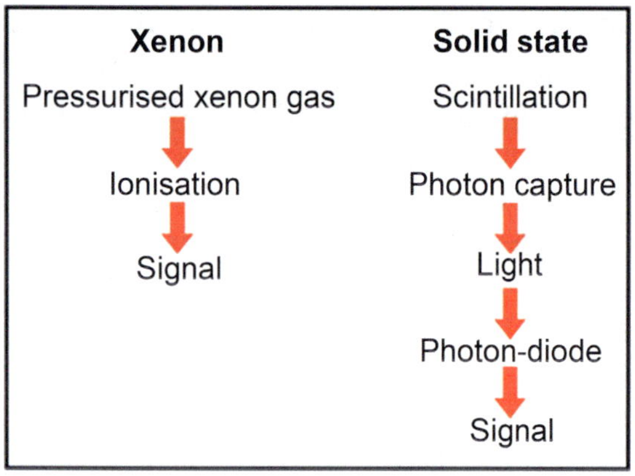

Figure 4.5. Overview of solid-state and gas ionization detectors used in CT.

Source: https://d45jl3w9libvn.cloudfront.net/jaypee/static/books/9788180614804/Chapters/images/21-1.jpg.

Careful adjustment of parameters such as kilovolt peak (kVp) and milliampere-seconds (mAs) is responsible for the creation of the desired image contrast and the reduction of noise. In different clinical applications, proper alignment of detector technology with standard operating procedures ensures concordance with guidelines, such as those by the American College of Radiology (ACR). Recent studies have highlighted the importance of adhering to dose management principles to maintain image quality, while accounting for heightened radiation sensitivity in younger patients, who require adequate justification and optimization (Bithell et al., 2014). In the long term, developments in detector types and their impact on image quality must be carefully monitored and incorporated into CT protocols to ensure the best possible patient care. Regular revision and evaluation of imaging protocols, as well as continuous education for technologists, are recommended to ensure alignment with technological advancements and regulatory guidelines. Results of recent surveys across various healthcare environments indicate that compliance with ACR and European Commission (EC) recommendations can improve patient outcomes and safety (Eghlidospoor et al., 2018). With advancing imaging technology, the obsessive focus on detector performance in clinical CT applications continues to be top of the agenda, underlining the need for careful consideration of both image quality and patient protection in practice today.

4.2.3. Patient Positioning Systems

Patient positioning systems are a critical element of computed tomography (CT) imaging optimization, where accuracy and comfort are the most important requirements. Advanced patient positioning systems ensure correct and safe positioning of patients for optimal imaging without creating artifacts or compromising diagnostic quality. Proper positioning of patients is particularly crucial in complex studies, wherein minor discrepancies can lead to severe misinterpretations of results, thus impacting patients' treatment strategies. Modern systems include adjustable tables and supports that accommodate a wide range of body sizes and support diagnostics, demonstrating ergonomic and technological strides in the imaging arena. Furthermore, awareness of the patient's anatomy within the plane of imaging helps technicians in appropriately using such positioning systems and thus enhancing workflow efficiency and patient safety (Figure 4.6).

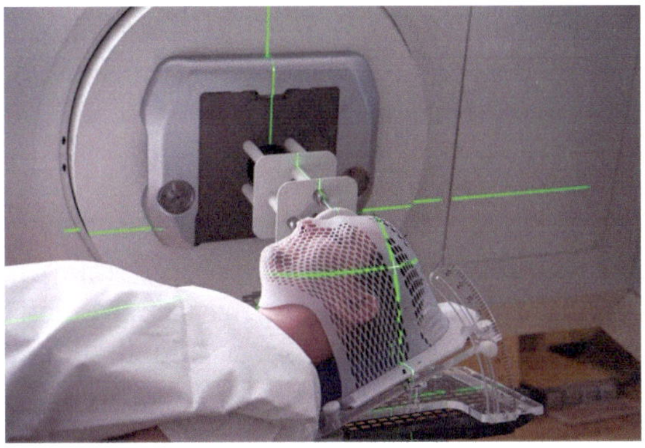

Figure 4.6. Patient table and laser alignment system for accurate positioning.

Source: https://www.prophotonix.com/wp-content/uploads/2017/12/Patient_Positioning.jpg.

The integration of patient positioning systems with cutting-edge CT technologies also allows for innovations in imaging protocols. For instance, while performing dual-energy CT scans, precise positioning is especially important due to the high rate of image acquisition at different energy levels, enabling discrimination of tissues based on their material characteristics. As outlined in more recent studies, the enhanced imaging potential of these systems is significant to the diagnosis of diseases such as pancreatic cancer, where the low-energy monoenergetic decompositions are able to create enhanced tissue contrast (Alvarez et al., 2018). The success or failure of patient positioning systems is directly related to the accuracy of these advanced images, enabling clinicians to identify subtle imaging features that may impact treatment pathways. Thus, ongoing innovation within patient positioning systems continues to play a crucial role in meeting the evolving technology landscape of diagnostic systems. In addition, the position that patient comfort occupies in positioning systems cannot be overestimated since it dictates direct cooperation during the procedure as well as imaging result quality. Proper positioning of patients not only minimizes discomfort and stress but also facilitates improved image quality by removing motion artifacts. Techniques and methods, such as the use of supportive pillows or adjustable wedges, have been used to enhance patient comfort while maintaining desired anatomical alignment during scanning procedures. This patient-wellness-centered focus on patient care is in accord with modern patient-centered practices, improving compliance and satisfaction in diagnostic imaging settings. Along with that, with mounting emphasis being placed on minimizing radiation exposure and maximizing diagnostic efficiency, advanced positioning devices can play a key role in achieving the optimal imaging parameters and hence supporting the necessity of constant innovation in patient positioning devices (Bove et al., 2013).

4.3. CT Imaging Protocols

In CT scanning protocols, selection of variables such as kilovoltage peak (kVp) and milliamperes-seconds (mAs) plays a vital role in obtaining the best image quality without maximizing radiation exposure. They directly determine image contrast and resolution, thereby aiding in precise diagnosis. The relationship between kVp and mAs also governs the effective dose that impinges on the patient during scanning. Correct calibration of these settings is important; higher kVp values tend to reduce contrast in soft tissues but maximize quality of penetration, a feature of enormous advantage in detecting heavy structures. With a delicate balance, medical practitioners can administer the treatments with maximum possible diagnostic importance at minimal health risk occasioned by radiation exposure. Moreover, the application of protocols intended for specific patient groups, such as children, emphasizes the need for systemic adjustments in kVp and mAs settings, as described by Kussman et al. (2007). Optimization of the CT imaging protocol also involves the adjustment of pitch and rotation time, which have important effects on image quality and acquisition time. One can adjust pitch—the speed of table motion to the collimation distance—so that spatial resolution can be traded off against fitting patient anatomical variations and specific diagnostic requirements. Higher pitches allow for faster scans required in emergency cases, while lower pitches are preferable for high-sensitivity exams. In addition, rotation time—the duration of a complete scan—remains linked with image quality as well as patient safety. Reducing rotation times raises temporal resolution and lowers motion artifacts but may lead to increased doses of radiation. It is therefore important to optimize pitch and rotation time by using targeted protocols to achieve the required quality while considering radiation safety guidelines, as applied in research on specialized imaging conditions (Ketten et al., 2008). A vital component of CT imaging protocols also involves proper contrast timing, which is of fundamental importance to effective imaging of vascular organs and structures. Contrast material administration directly impacts the enhancement of diagnostic images, enabling improved visualization of complex anatomical structures. Implementation of appropriate timing techniques guarantees a precise peak of contrast at optimal intervals in relation to the imaging sequence, facilitating enhanced diagnostic accuracy. Radiologists must consider the rate of contrast injection and timing between administration and imaging, adjusting such factors to the clinical indications and patient groups. Further, advances in dual-energy CT hardware have opened new opportunities for better imaging protocols, allowing the discrimination of materials based on atomic number and enhancing diagnostic potential. Adoption of advanced contrast protocols is a reflection of evolving CT imaging horizon and its commitment to maximizing diagnostic performance with the least patient risk.

4.3.1. Standard Protocols for Different Body Regions

In computed tomography (CT) imaging, adherence to standardized protocols ensures optimal imaging effectiveness and diagnostic accuracy. Each region of the body requires specifically tailored protocols that address various anatomical structures and physiological functions, thereby optimizing imaging quality. For instance, abdominal CT typically uses specific kilovolt peak (kVp) and milliampere-seconds (mAs) settings, as these parameters significantly affect image clarity and patient safety.

CT Protocols

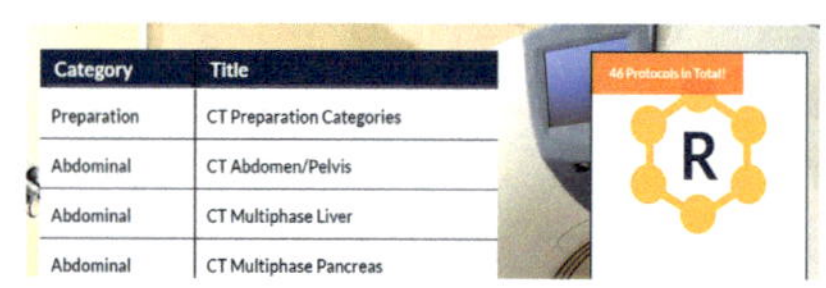

Figure 4.7. CT scan protocols for brain, chest, abdomen, and pelvis.

Source: https://static.wixstatic.com/media/ef1c01_62cc9840aae344deb40bc079a0341663~mv2.jpg/v1/fill/w_973,h_384,al_c/ef1c01_62cc9840aae344deb40bc079a0341663~mv2.jpg.

Tuning of rotation time and pitch is also essential; shorter rotation times in helical scanning can decrease motion artifacts and increase temporal resolution. Such meticulous calibration, tied to specific patient needs as well as the involved organelle system, is the building block for current state-of-the-art imaging technologies, which allow for more precise diagnostic interpretation and timely clinical decision-making. When one reads the guidelines for different parts of the body, chest CT has a set of rules that address special thoracic anatomy. Standard protocols often incorporate parameters such as low-dose techniques that reduce radiation exposure but still maintain diagnostic quality. Dual-energy CT scanning can also improve the visibility of vascular structures and pulmonary pathology. New developments, including iterative reconstruction algorithms, provide improved image quality with reduced dose—a necessary factor in radiation-sensitive patient groups (Figure 4.7).

Thus, protocol analysis in this manner improves diagnostic performance not only at the patient level but also in accordance with broader public health objectives that act to constrain radiation exposure across a variety of demographic parameters, ultimately toward seeking a balance between diagnostic requirements and patient protection. In addition, standard protocol application is extended to specialty applications such as CT angiography (CTA), which provides accurate information concerning vascular anatomy. Iodinated contrast agent administration is central in such protocols to provide the best visualization of blood vessels. As recent studies show, optimally adjusted contrast timing and flow rates can significantly improve image quality while concurrently reducing iodine and radiation doses. All these are a reflection of continuous innovation in contrast medium administration protocols to enable clinicians to provide optimal diagnoses without risky exposures. Moreover, innovations such as the single-breath-hold method illustrated in SBH-PACT for breast imaging illustrate the zeal for creating technologies that promote patient comfort without recourse to ionizing radiation in any form, and indicate a significant direction towards safer imaging procedures in contemporary healthcare systems (Albrecht et al., 2017; Appleton et al., 2018).

4.3.2. Contrast Injection Techniques

Investigating the nuanced realm of contrast administration techniques emerges as a vital factor for the enhancement of diagnostic efficacy in computed tomography (CT) scans. It encompasses the techniques by which iodinated contrast materials are administered into the patient's body to enhance image quality. Maximum rate, volume, and timing of contrast delivery are key choices, as they are recognized to contribute significantly to both the display of anatomical detail and overall image interpretability. For instance, maximum contrast enhancement is often a function of sustaining an optimal ratio between the rate of injection and patient vascular characteristics in order to deliver adequate perfusion within the area of interest. This meticulous adjustment not only aims to maximize the signal intensity of vascular structures but also to improve tissue differentiation on imaging, indicating the importance of patient-specific contrast injection protocols tailored to specific diagnostic requirements (Figure 4.8).

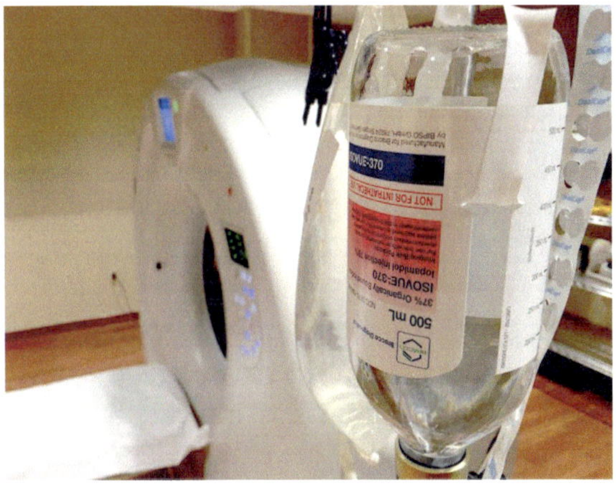

Figure 4.8. Example of iodinated contrast media injection setup.

Source: https://www.dicardiology.com/sites/default/files/styles/content_feed_large/public/field/image/Iodine_Contrast_LOW_RES_CT_Aquilion_one_CDH_Staff_DF.jpg?itok=KpoVd_2Y.

In addition to the general contrast administration principles, the goal is to maximize iodine dose to maximize resolution of images without being restricted by side effects.

Recent research sheds further light on the use of reduced tube voltages in combination with high-iodine-signal algorithms, thereby allowing reduced radiation exposure, as documented by Albrecht et al. (2017). Practically speaking, these techniques enable radiologists to ascertain appropriate image quality as they adjust the flow rates and injected volumes of contrast media to reduce patient risks. This method is most evident in cases where patients are contraindicated for standard contrast dose injections, for example, renal insufficiency patients, and highlights the imperative connection between contrast dosing protocols and patient safety. Moreover, through contrast protocol optimization, radiologists can enhance diagnostic accuracy in a variety of applications in CT imaging, hence ensuring improved patient outcomes. With the trend in CT imaging continuing to evolve, the integration of cutting-edge methodologies in contrast administration practices signals the onset of highly personalized approaches to imaging. Dual-energy CT is a step in this direction, wherein contrast media can be analyzed at varying energy levels to provide more precise information regarding tissue composition and pathology. This application puts radiologists in a position to benefit from comparative analysis of various iodine-based contrast agents and, accordingly, guide subsequent diagnosis. Furthermore, research has indicated that the employment of such advanced methods can result in further reductions in the amount of contrast used without compromising on image quality, a line of development that holds promising potential for enhancing protocols for the safety of patients to be employed in potential allergic reactions or renal adverse effects, as exemplified in (Badal et al., 2013). Through systematic improvements in contrast injection methods, the science of CT imaging is poised to achieve greater efficiency and push the limits of diagnostic accuracy.

4.3.3. Protocol Tailoring for Individual Patient Requirements

In the realm of computed tomography (CT), individualizing protocols to meet specific patient needs is more than a technical adaptation; it is a fundamental part of patient-centered care. Because medical professionals rely on the nuances of CT technology, they must consider many variables such as patient anatomy, clinical use, and radiation sensitivity. Tailoring protocols can be achieved by adjusting parameters like kilovolt peak (kVp) and milliampere-seconds (mAs) to achieve the highest image quality at minimum exposure to radiation. In pediatric patients or patients who have a history of prior exposure to radiation, selection of lower doses of radiation is essential in order to succeed with imaging while safeguarding the patient's health. Innovation of automated exposure control technologies supports tailored imaging practices and thus enhances diagnostic accuracy without compromising patient protection (Zeppenfeld et al., 2022) (Figure 4.9).

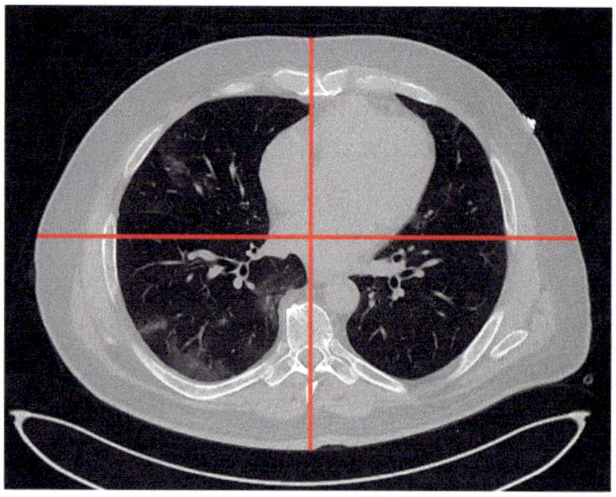

Figure 4.9. Personalized CT protocol adjustments based on patient BMI and pathology.

Source: https://pub.mdpi-res.com/bioengineering/bioengineering-11-00207/article_deploy/html/images/bioengineering-11-00207-g001.png?1708940060.

Also, the function of protocol tailoring extends beyond the integration of patient-dependent variables such as age, habitus, and previous illnesses. Evidence-based modifications are needed to the protocol because omitting consideration of patient demographic differences could lead to suboptimal imaging outcomes. For instance, research shows that patients with pre-existing osteoporosis, the most prevalent metabolic bone disease, have greater fracture risks in standard imaging protocols (Meryl et al., 2022). Under these circumstances, it is crucial to adjust CT protocols to ensure appropriate visualization of bone structures without increasing the likelihood of unnecessary radiation exposure. Consequently, by identifying individual factors and applying enhanced imaging techniques, healthcare professionals can engineer protocols that counter threats to specific conditions and enhance overall diagnostic effectiveness.

Compliance and patient comfort are also primary features of successful protocol personalization in CT imaging. Screening procedures will most likely need to include accommodations that address the needs of anxious or claustrophobic patients, and they should not be compromised as part of the experience. These can involve modifications to the scanning time, the use of wider gantries, or the use of specialized patient-positioning aids to provide a less problematic experience. Patient education can also help reduce anxiety and minimize non-compliance, thereby improving image quality outcomes. Through the understanding of the necessity of having a customized approach while designing CT protocols, professionals can deliver improved patient care, monitor following imaging guidelines, and ultimately obtain more efficient diagnostic outcomes in a clinical setting (Zeppenfeld et al., 2022).

4.4. Control of Radiation Dose in CT

In contemporary computed tomography (CT) imaging, effective control of radiation dose is a key consideration for maintaining patient safety while preserving diagnostic image quality. A chief tactic that is required is the deployment of Automatic Exposure Control (AEC) systems, which change radiation dose dynamically based on the unique requirements of the patient and the region of the body being imaged. AEC technologies utilize real-time feedback during scanning to modify exposure parameters to reduce unnecessary radiation without compromising image quality. This sophisticated method adheres to radiological society recommendations in favor of ALARA (As Low As Reasonably Achievable) principles, reflecting a commitment to safeguarding patient health while successfully acquiring required diagnostic information. As such, adding AEC to CT protocols greatly enhances the radiation safety to diagnostic efficacy ratio. The second fundamental component of dose management for radiation includes the reliable estimation of organ doses to reduce exposure to radiation while maximizing diagnostic yield. Monte Carlo simulation methods and advanced packages of software can provide reliable estimates of organ doses of radiation during CT scanning. This ability to estimate organ dose contributes to the detection of high-risk populations, such as children, who are most susceptible to radiation effects, and thus enables the adoption of special protocols. Furthermore, accurate organ dose estimation is central to well-informed professional decision-making, enabling the advantages of CT imaging to overwhelmingly outweigh the risks. By fostering a culture of awareness of organ doses, hospitals can further instill a sense of responsibility for appropriate imaging practices, thereby promoting patient safety. The importance of reporting and tracking radiation doses cannot be overlooked, as it facilitates ongoing quality improvement in imaging practices. By systematically documenting the radiation doses of various CT protocols, health institutions are able to establish trends, assess adherence to dose standards established, and make informed changes in imaging protocols where appropriate. These dose-monitoring initiatives can enhance patient outcomes by enabling earlier detection of outliers and inefficiencies during imaging. Moreover, open reporting systems enhance radiology department accountability in a manner that patients receive optimum care with minimal risk of exposure. In sum, thorough dose reporting and monitoring are key to the new paradigm of radiation safety for CT scanning, establishing a basis for enhanced best practices centered on the health and welfare of the patient.

4.4.1. Understanding Levels of Radiation Exposure

An understanding of radiation exposure levels is increasingly critical in the contemporary world of medical imaging, even more so in CT where technological developments have been coupled with higher doses that accompany diagnostic interventions.

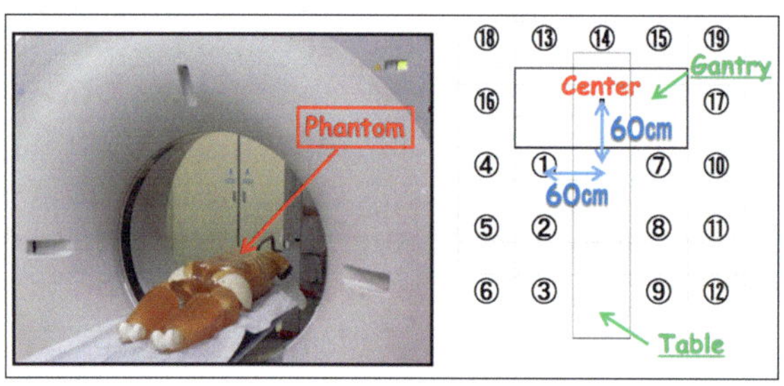

Figure 4.10. Occupational radiation dose to eye lenses in CT-guided interventions using MDCT-fluoroscopy.

Source: ICRP (International Commission on Radiological Protection).

As computed tomography becomes a routine diagnostic intervention, implications for patient safety escalate to a level of paramountcy. For instance, patients undergoing CT coronary angiography (CTCA) are subjected to varying amounts of exposures up to 20 mSv when specific techniques such as retrospective ECG-gating are applied. However, by modifying parameters such as tube voltage and implementing low-noise reconstruction filters, scientists have achieved a dramatic reduction in radiation dose. Particularly, lower tube voltages like 100 kV can cut down effective doses by as much as approximately 7.43 mSv without compromising or enhancing the diagnostic image quality (Figure 4.10).

This highlights the significance of practitioners optimizing protocols to enhance image quality and reduce patient exposure (Faggioni et al., 2012). In addition to optimizing imaging protocols, the discovery and adoption of iterative reconstruction (IR) technologies have transformed radiation dose management in CT. These algorithms reduce the radiation dose to patients by improving image quality through advanced noise reduction and artifact suppression. The use of IR allows diagnostic images to be obtained with fewer radiation doses than with traditional methods such as filtered back projection. IR algorithms' ability to provide high-quality images with less needed radiation exposure is particularly beneficial in challenging situations where precise imaging is critical. As medical science keeps evolving, the significant advantages of IR over the conventional methods will ensure its application at a scale never before seen, illuminating a milestone into our practice in regards to patient care and radiation safety (Bastarrika et al., 2015). Understanding radiation exposure levels and dynamics requires ongoing research and the development of sound policies that prioritize patient protection. Regular monitoring and reporting of radiation doses are essential components of developing an accountability culture in radiology departments.

These include implementing automatic exposure control methods that respond in real time to individual patient characteristics, ultimately administering the right dose to every patient. Moreover, emphasis on organ dose estimation enables practitioners to identify areas most likely to be at increased risk of radiation-induced complications. Together, these advances are part of a larger strategy for minimizing radiation exposure without compromising the diagnostic utility of CT interventions. At a time of accelerated technological advancement in imaging, the balance between the benefits of enhanced diagnostic performance and the need for radiation protection remains a central imperative.

4.4.2. Techniques for Dose Reduction

Techniques of Reducing Dose in Computed Tomography (CT) are essential to improving patient safety with medical imaging without detracting from its diagnostic efficacy.

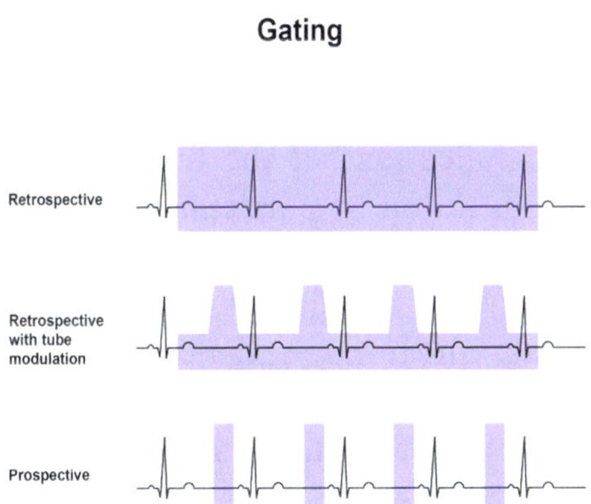

Figure 4.11. Use of automatic tube current modulation for dose reduction.

Source: Siemens Healthineers.

One key way to reduce radiation dose is through the use of Automatic Exposure Control (AEC) systems. They also adjust the radiation dose dynamically based on the size of the individual patient and the specific imaging task. The repeated alteration of exposure parameters makes it possible to significantly limit unnecessary radiation while producing images of sufficient quality for the diagnosis. At a time when multidetector row computed tomography (MDCT) makes imaging faster, the precision of AEC becomes a necessity, further decreasing the cumulated assignment dose required for successful imaging interventions, creating a dose optimization culture in the clinical setup (Kussman et al., 2007) (Figure 4.11).

With advances in imaging technology, the application of iterative reconstruction algorithms is becoming increasingly important for dose management. Their application, as discussed in the recent reviews, can drastically enhance image quality, simultaneously providing an opportunity for dose reduction. Compared to traditional filtered back projection methods that may worsen image noise using lower radiation, iterative reconstruction methods have excellent suppression of this noise by employing repeated processing cycles that enhance the clarity of the image. Such a capability not only maintains diagnostic quality but also allows practitioners to administer reduced doses of radiation per scan, thus avoiding potential radiation-related risks to patients (Bastarrika et al., 2015). Therefore, the implementation of these newer reconstruction techniques is an important step toward the optimization of patient safety in CT imaging. Protocol optimization also complements such dose-reducing maneuvers, offering an organized approach to managing radiation exposure. Accurate kilovolt peak (kVp) and milliampere-seconds (mAs) corrections are also crucial for reducing radiation exposure while ensuring optimal image quality. Having protocols in place to prescribe the correct pitch and rotation time is also extremely significant, since both entities directly influence the volume of data scanned and, by proxy, the total dose administered. By systematically modifying these variables, health-care practitioners can achieve considerable reductions in radiation exposure without sacrificing the diagnostic utility of CT scans, leading to better patient outcomes and more appropriate utilization of imaging resources in the health-care environment.

4.4.3. Patient Safety and Education Importance

From a practice standpoint, patient education and safety are an integral component of medical imaging practice, particularly in the practice of computed tomography (CT). Increased utilization of CT scans for diagnosis necessitates robust safety protocols to offset radiation hazards. Well-informed patients about the procedures they undergo promote openness and trust between healthcare providers and patients. A variety of organizations, such as the American Association of Physicists in Medicine (AAPM), facilitate open communication regarding benefits and potential risks of treatment so that patients are empowered to make sound health care decisions (Figure 4.12).

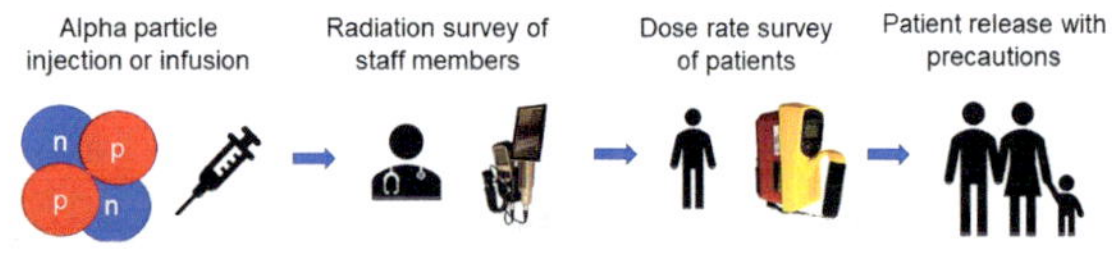

Figure 4.12. Educational chart on CT safety principles and informed consent.

Source: https://encrypted-tbn0.gstatic.com/images?q=tbn:ANd9GcRzj7YNLkjp8nN5j7cDYL5Dr1WN42tcBlmSNg&s.

This emphasis on education not only facilitates patient understanding but also enforces compliance with safety protocols critical to sound diagnosis and treatment in CT uses, and maintains laser-like focus on patient care at all points in the imaging chain. Parallel with the educational is the critical function of implementing rigorous safety protocols in the CT setting. These evidence-based practice guidelines serve as a radiation dose management guide and an overall imaging efficiency guide. For example, AAPM has set clear practice guidelines to ensure that medical physicists have the appropriate skill sets and competencies to guarantee imaging protocols are optimized for patient safety. Such compliance further directly affects the quality of care, as it minimizes unnecessary exposure while ensuring maximum diagnostic quality. Furthermore, the appropriate selection of parameters such as kilovolt peak (kVp) and milliampere-seconds (mAs) is paramount in order to achieve a balance between low doses and efficient imaging, which emphasizes the intersection of education, optimal protocol usage, and patient safety concerning CT scanning. Patient engagement must be conceived as a multi-dimensional process, including not only procedure instruction but also the ramifications of imaging findings.

Because CT scans can yield substantial health data, accurate information about potential outcomes, follow-up treatment needs, and the implications of the treatment plan is crucial. Education is particularly critical due to the dynamic nature of technologies such as dual-energy CT and iterative reconstruction algorithms, which may enhance the diagnostic accuracy but also need a firm understanding of their application and limitations, both by medical personnel and patients. By integrating patient education and safety into the fabric of their practice, professionals can significantly enhance the experience of imaging, having patients feel well-informed and assisted during the procedure, and ultimately contributing to improved health outcomes and patient satisfaction.

4.5. Computed Tomography Image Quality

In CT technology, the integrity of the quality of images can assure correct diagnosis. Advanced imaging procedures depend on the efficiency of the scanner hardware, which directly affects image detail and resolution output. Among the significant factors in this position is the gantry design holding the X-ray tube and detectors. Technologies such as slip-ring technology enable uninterrupted rotation and data collection, with minimal gaps in image collection to achieve maximum resolution of detail. Patient table mechanics are also important; they are designed to ensure stability and precision during the scan, thereby producing the highest-quality image by suppressing motion artifacts. Collectively, these considerations point to the importance of CT scanner architecture as a foundation for achieving high image quality (Eghlidospoor et al., 2018). Modes of data acquisition used in scanning techniques are equally important for improving image quality. Axial and helical scanning each has its own benefits; whereas axial scanning involves the sequential acquisition of slices, helical (spiral) scanning generates continuous data that allows volumetric analysis to be more robust. This capability, together with dual-source approaches, increases temporal resolution, a critical parameter in dynamic process imaging. Choice of acquisition mode could have a profound impact not only on image detail and quality but also on radiation dose administered to patients. Optimal imaging depends on a thorough understanding of these modalities and their implications for diagnostic confidence and patient safety, particularly amid increasing pressures to use CT in clinical settings (Eghlidospoor et al., 2018). Secondly, methodologies applied in image reconstruction directly influence overall image quality. Traditional processes, such as filtered back projection, have been supplemented or supplanted by advanced iterative reconstruction (IR) algorithms that significantly enhance image resolution while potentially reducing radiation exposure. IR algorithms enable detailed manipulation of the data, leading to refined noise reduction and artifact reduction, ultimately delivering clearer images to facilitate accurate diagnosis. Emerging trends also hint at model-based algorithms, which employ state-of-the-art computational methodologies for further image output optimization. The application of these modern reconstruction methods is a transformative step in CT imaging, exemplifying the ongoing commitment to optimizing diagnostic utility without compromising patient safety, as evidenced by numerous clinical applications.

4.5.1. Factors Affecting Image Quality

The quality of the computed tomography (CT) image is of utmost importance for accurate diagnosis and effective treatment planning. Many factors influence the quality of images, and among them are the technical scan process parameters.

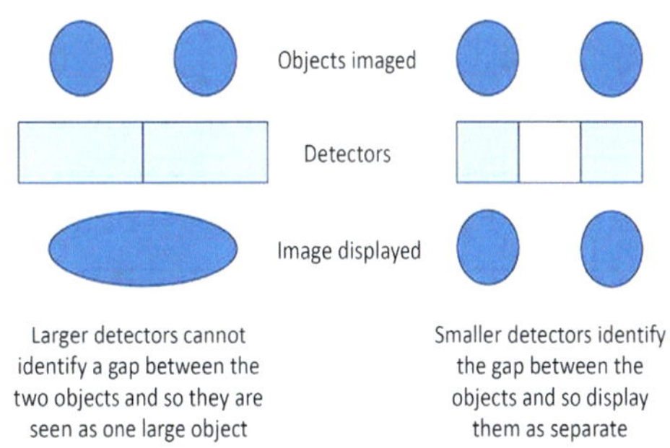

Figure 4.13. Factors such as resolution, noise, and motion artifacts affecting CT image quality.

Source: https://www.radiologycafe.com/wp-content/uploads/2021/04/ct-image2-resolution.png.

Among all those factors, the selection of kilovoltage peak (kVp) and milliampere-seconds (mAs) are of great significance.

Choosing an appropriate kVp impacts contrast and penetration of X-rays in varying tissue densities, while mAs regulates the quantity of photons emitted and thus image brightness and noise. The interrelationship between the two parameters is complex because more mAs will improve image quality by reducing noise, but at the cost of increased exposure to radiation. Therefore, such parameters must be selected to deliver acceptable image quality while adhering to the ALARA principle (Badal et al., 2013). In addition to kVp and mAs levels, the scanning technique employed is also a factor in determining image quality (Figure 4.13).

Various modes of acquisition, such as axial and helical scanning, both have specific strengths and weaknesses. Axial scanning, while conventionally integral, can be susceptible to motion artifacts due to longer scan time. In contrast to axial scanning, helical (spiral) scanning enables rapid acquisition with less motion-induced blurring, thinner slices, and higher spatial resolution. Dual-source techniques further improve image quality by enabling faster data collection and higher temporal resolution. However, such advanced techniques can complicate protocol optimization, which requires careful balancing between speed, resolution, and patient safety (Badal et al., 2013). Therefore, a solid grasp of data-collection modes is critical for clinicians seeking to optimize image fidelity. Finally, the techniques used during image reconstruction play an important role in determining the final image quality radiologists see. Classic filtered back-projection methods have been the standard; they are not always ideal in dealing with artifacts or noise, though. More recent methods, such as iterative reconstruction, have provided exciting new avenues to enhance image quality with noise reduction and improved contrast. Newer algorithms leverage computational capabilities to denoise images without increased radiation doses while maintaining diagnostic quality. With the growth of the discipline, radiologists and technologists must stay updated on advancements in reconstruction methods to achieve maximum image quality and patient safety in computed tomography (Ismail et al., 2023).

4.5.2. Quality Control Measures

Application of quality control procedures in computed tomography (CT) is necessary to ensure optimal image quality while minimizing patient risk. A structured quality assurance program would include many factors, each for maintaining CT scanner performance as well as diagnostic accuracy. For instance, regular calibration of the CT system should be performed to ensure it meets predetermined standards. This involves monitoring image noise, contrast resolution, and spatial resolution, all of which are required for accurate imaging. Further, practitioners must perform ongoing education of technologists to guarantee adherence to best practices in imaging protocols (Figure 4.14).

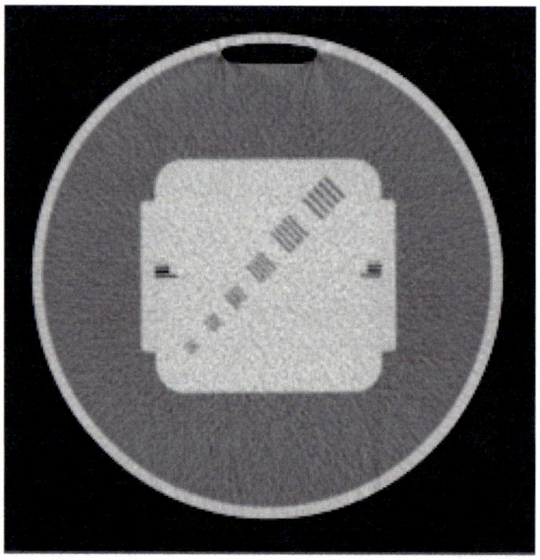

Figure 4.14. Phantom image used for routine CT quality assurance checks.

Source: https://help.imageowl.com/hc/article_attachments/4403113323923.

In these aspects, regular audits and adherence to standards set by organizations such as the American College of Radiology (ACR) and the European Commission (EC) help decrease the risk of mistakes that can lead to excessive exposure to radiation or misdiagnosis, as substantiated in the evidence from Eghlidospoor et al. (2018). In addition, CT protocol optimization must be addressed, with attention to scanning parameters such as kilovoltage peak (kVp), milliampere-seconds (mAs), and contrast timing. Optimization is not merely a technical endeavor but also a clinical endeavor, adapting imaging protocols to the specific needs of varying patient populations. As experiments demonstrate, variation in protocol among institutions can significantly affect patient dose as well as image quality. For example, experience across several Iranian hospitals revealed adherence to the ACR guidelines in the vast majority of cases and a trend towards protocol standardization. Such results underscore the importance of active quality control mechanisms in CT, creating an environment in which technological and technical progress may be balanced by high standards of safety and efficacy (Eghlidospoor et al., 2018).

Besides, quality control measures are used in radiation dose management, an essential feature in the era of advanced imaging modalities. Automatic exposure controls, for instance, help deliver maximal radiation doses and adapt to patients' body sizes and clinical needs. Accurate estimation of organ doses and dose-reporting processes are other ways to ensure transparency in patient safety practices. Continuous monitoring of these factors ensures CT facilities stay compliant with regulatory standards while encouraging the safe use of radiation. With new technologies such as dual-energy CT gaining popularity, comprehensive quality control remains a must, ensuring that both image acquisition and patient safety are prioritized in tandem.

4.5.3. Evaluation of Image Quality Indicators

Quantification of image-quality parameters in computed tomography (CT) is important for achieving maximum diagnostic performance while minimizing patient radiation exposure. Traditionally, spatial resolution, a metric of the capacity to detect minute details, and contrast resolution, a measure of the capacity to differentiate between two different densities in the area under scan, have been fundamental parameters monitored.

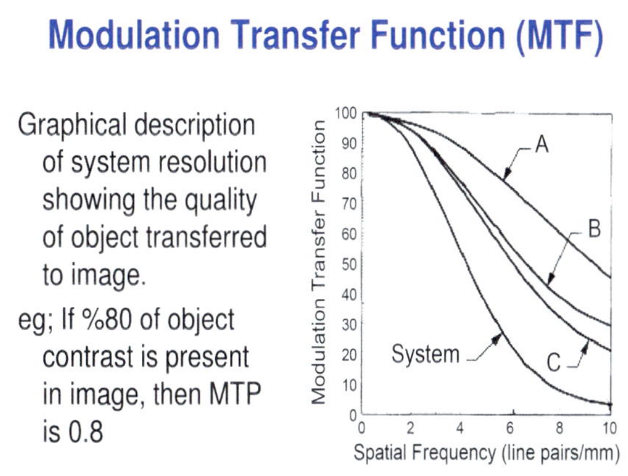

Figure 4.15. Graph of modulation transfer function (MTF) for CT systems.

Source: https://image5.slideserve.com/9437743/modulation-transfer-function-mtf-l.jpg.

Image quality directly affects diagnostic confidence and decision-making. As CT technology continues to advance, measurement requirements that account for noise and artifact reduction become increasingly important. For instance, applications of protocols such as those reported by Badal et al. (2013) demonstrate that dose-reduction strategies can influence the detectability of signals from concentrated features, underscoring the importance of careful evaluation methods in CT imaging. The means to gauge image quality may rely heavily on statistical models and algorithms, thereby influencing the interpretation of the measures (Figure 4.15).

Iterative reconstruction techniques have been shown to be of monumental advantage over conventional filtered back projection methods in effectively suppressing noise and enhancing clarity. The utilization and development of model-based algorithms are also remarkable, as they improve the accuracy of anatomical portrayal by accounting for physical limitations. These advancements can potentially produce improved diagnostic capability, especially under challenging conditions such as coronary artery evaluations. For example, literature (Bastarrika et al., 2015) supports that the transition toward iterative reconstruction improves performance in critical measurements. This indicates greater recognition of advanced measures that take into account not just visual characteristics but also quantifiable outputs on diagnostic efficacy. Sensitive evaluation of such measures is central to optimizing CT protocols to balance image quality and patient safety. As medical imaging practices continue to be refined by healthcare practitioners, applying a range of metrics allows for a better understanding of the strengths and limitations of each method. Quantitative and qualitative techniques, such as signal-to-noise ratio and observer studies, enable an even-handed approach to image quality assessment. The findings from several comparative research studies confirm the view that metrics should be closely linked to clinical tasks to support personalized imaging approaches tailored to specific diagnostic needs. In this case, findings from Badal et al. (2013) illustrate subtle impacts of alternative imaging algorithms on detectability measures, hence guiding clinicians on the best way to utilize the best available protocols, enhancing diagnostic accuracy as well as patient care.

4.6. Advanced Applications of CT

The area of high-end computed tomography (CT) applications has expanded massively, touching many areas of medical specialties. Dual-Energy CT has been the most groundbreaking development so far, employing two X-ray energies to produce images capable of differentiating between materials with different atomic numbers. The technique enhances diagnostic quality by enabling radiologists to better assess tissue composition, especially in defining tumors and evaluating vascular conditions. Additionally, dual-energy imaging will also reduce the need for other imaging modalities, thereby streamlining patient management and decreasing total radiation exposure. As a result, such advanced technology not only optimizes diagnostic accuracy but is also crucial in personalized medicine, where treatment is rendered more individualized based on accurate imaging results obtained with this technology. Perfusion Imaging is yet another sophisticated application of CT technology that yields vital information regarding patterns of blood flow in various tissues and organs. By observing perfusion parameters, doctors are better able to diagnose conditions such as stroke, cancer, and cardiovascular disease. Perfusion imaging techniques, such as dynamic contrast-enhanced CT (DCE-CT), use rapid image acquisition after contrast agent administration to measure and detect blood flow in real time. This allows for precise measurement of organ perfusion and can help in the definition of ischemic brain areas or the assessment of tumor response to treatment. Also, ongoing developments in image reconstruction algorithms, including iterative and model-based algorithms, ensure that these perfusion studies are more precise and dependable. With these advanced uses, CT continues to solidify its position as a quintessential modality in modern diagnostics and treatment planning. CT Angiography has revolutionized the evaluation of vascular structures and cardiac diseases by providing high-resolution, three-dimensional imaging of the blood vessels. It is an uninvasive procedure in which the arterial and venous systems are visualized in detail, and stenosis, aneurysms, and vascular malformations are diagnosable. CT angiography is less invasive and even quicker than conventional angiography, especially useful in life-threatening conditions. The use of newer technology in CT angiography, such as the use of automatic exposure control and optimum timing of contrast, significantly improves image quality with optimal radiation dose management. In addition, studies have shown that the combination of CT angiography with advances in dual-energy modalities will enhance detection of vascular occlusions and enable improved assessment of perfusion to critical organs. By optimal integration of imaging methods, CT angiography is further refining the method for evaluating complex vascular pathology, thereby facilitating improved patient care.

4.6.1. CT Angiography and Its Clinical Importance

Clinical assessments increasingly depend on sophisticated imaging modalities to enable accurate diagnoses and treatment planning. Among these, CT Angiography or CTA has emerged as a crucial tool, particularly in vascular disease diagnosis. By creating images of blood vessels with high resolution, CTA allows radiologists to harness the diagnostic capability to detect abnormalities like stenosis, aneurysm, and thrombosis. The technique makes use of contrast materials to add conspicuity so clinicians can differentiate between normal and pathologic vasculature effortlessly. This is particularly important in the environment of acute clinical practice, such as emergency medicine, where efficiency in diagnosis could have a dramatic effect on patient outcomes. CTA not only enables rapid clinical decision-making but also plays a significant role in long-term management plans for cardiovascular patients. Additionally, the clinical utility of CT Angiography is not limited to diagnosis alone; it is also important for monitoring the progression of vascular disease and assessing the effectiveness of treatment (Figure 4.16).

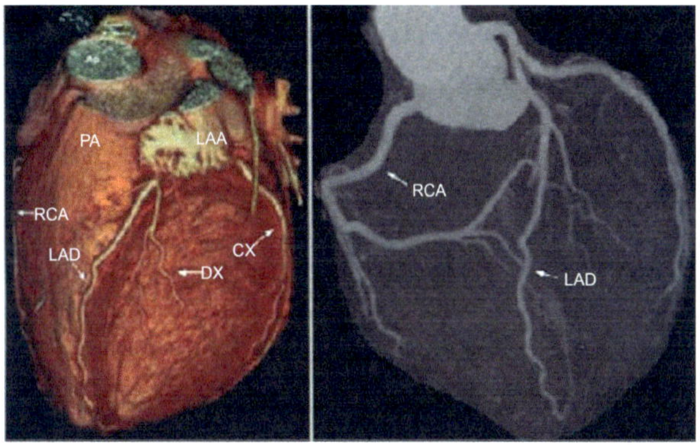

Figure 4.16. CT angiography scan showing coronary arteries in high resolution.

Source: https://www.researchgate.net/figure/CT-Angiography-showing-normal-Coronary-Arteries_fig5_23235742.

Serial CTA imaging also allows clinicians to assess the success of treatments, such as stent placement or operative correction, and detect any post-procedure complications. Moreover, developments in imaging technology and dual-energy CT have improved the specificity of CTA so that differential diagnosis of multiple vascular diseases can be made. To that effect, enhanced visualization techniques assist in reducing the rate of invasive procedures as CTA is capable of providing sufficient information to guide clinical management. Comparisons of the diagnostic ability of CTA with traditional invasive methods support its role in patient management, highlighting its importance in today's radiological practice. The use of CT Angiography in clinical practice demands adherence to optimized protocols for the management of radiation dose without compromising image quality. Radiologists must be aware of the use of correct parameters, including kVp, mAs, and contrast timing, to allow safe and effective CT examination. Radiation dose reduction strategies such as Automatic Exposure Control and tailored imaging strategies further instill patient safety. Since CT Angiography is increasingly employed, dose management research and image reconstruction techniques are becoming ever more important. Novel algorithms, as reported in the literature, can potentially enhance diagnostic accuracy while minimizing radiation exposure hazards (Biondi-Zoccai et al., 2017; Moudi et al., 2014). CT Angiography is thus ever-changing crossroads of technology, medical practice, and patient-centered care in modern medicine.

4.6.2. Oncology Role of CT

Computed tomography (CT) development has had a profound influence on oncology diagnosis and treatment monitoring. CT imaging is indispensable in clinical practice, providing vital information on tumor size, shape, and location, thereby facilitating accurate cancer staging. The imaging technique's ability to provide high-resolution cross-sectional images enables the clinician to determine the extent of disease spread, thereby guiding treatment decisions. For instance, CT accuracy may be used to distinguish benign from malignant lesions, with direct implications for patient care. Coordination of emerging technologies, such as dual-source techniques, enhances image acquisition rate and quality, enabling better visualization of complex anatomical structures. With the expanding uses of personalized medicine, the use of CT in oncology also expands, providing critical information for individually tailored therapeutic intervention, thereby enhancing patient outcomes and optimizing care protocols. In addition to diagnosis and staging, the role of CT in therapy planning and monitoring cannot be overestimated (Figure 4.17).

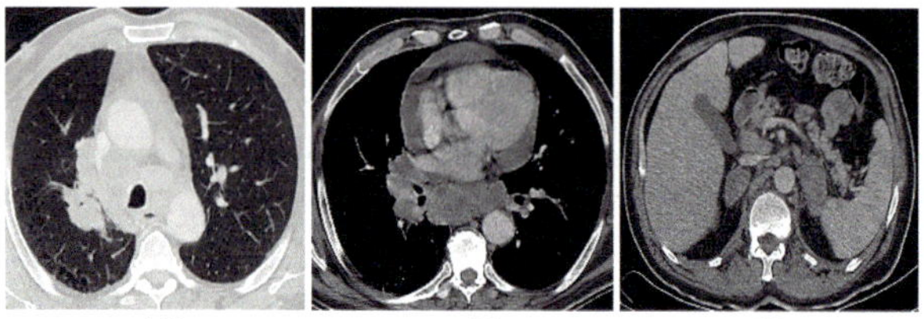

Figure 4.17. Staging of lung cancer using contrast-enhanced chest CT.

Source: https://www.mdpi.com/bioengineering/bioengineering-09-00493/article_deploy/html/images/bioengineering-09-00493-g001.png.

Therapeutic modalities, like chemotherapy and radiotherapy, tend to require precise localization of tumors to optimize treatment efficacy with minimal damage to surrounding healthy tissues. CT's precision in estimating tumor response to therapy enables oncologists to assess efficacy and make timely changes to therapeutic interventions. Post-therapy surveillance with CT scans is also necessary for early detection of recurrence. This real-time monitoring ensures that any alteration in patient status is immediately addressed, substantiating CTs irreplaceable role in the continuum of cancer treatment. In particular, technological advances in radiotherapy, such as those in CT, including iterative reconstruction algorithms, further enhance the treatment planning process by allowing improved accuracy in the calculation of doses, thus optimizing patient safety and treatment regimen. Optimizing the CT protocols is of utmost value to maximize its efficacy while keeping radiation exposure balanced, especially in oncology. Proper selection of kilovolt peak (kVp) and milliampere-seconds (mAs) settings is essential to achieve optimal image quality and reduce dose for serial examinations. Also, the application of advanced techniques, such as dual-energy CT, facilitates improved tissue characterization and contrast resolution, which are essential for differentiating tumor types and evaluating treatment response. Hence, radiation dose management strategies such as automatic exposure control are key to ensuring patient safety without compromising diagnosis quality. This approach not only commends the growing emphasis on patient-centered care but also attests to the profession's dedication to adhering to guidelines developed by organizations such as the American Association of Physicists in Medicine (Seibert et al., 2018). Maximizing CT protocol through prioritization guarantees that healthcare workers have high-quality care while fostering a culture of ongoing improvement within oncology practice.

4.6.3. Functional and Molecular Imaging Innovations

Improvements in molecular and functional imaging technologies have significantly changed the field of medical diagnosis, particularly in the field of computed tomography (CT). Further innovation is enabling more precise imaging of physiology at the cellular and molecular levels, not just facilitating better detection of disease, but also monitoring of therapy. For instance, techniques such as Positron Emission Tomography (PET) with CT imaging have emerged as a powerful oncology modality, allowing clinicians to image tumor metabolism and track therapy response. Furthermore, novel image reconstruction algorithms, such as iterative reconstruction methods, have the potential to reduce radiation dose while improving image quality, providing the patient with a safer diagnostic experience. With improvement in healthcare, these developments serve as evidence of the paramount role of interdisciplinary approaches in maximizing diagnostic imaging along with treatment effectiveness (Kitsiou et al., 2013) (Figure 4.18).

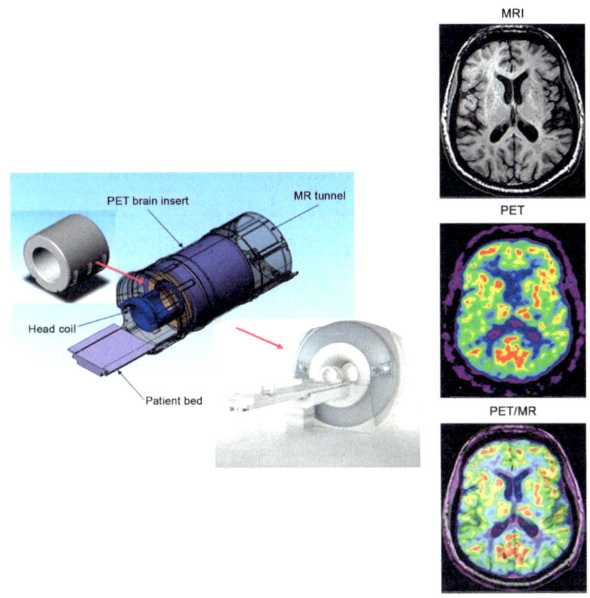

Figure 4.18. Fusion image of CT with PET for molecular imaging applications.

Source: https://ars.els-cdn.com/content/image/1-s2.0-S1556859809000091-gr2.jpg.

The application of dual-energy CT represents a significant improvement in diagnostic capability, particularly in distinguishing materials based on atomic number. It allows for improved specificity in the assessment of different tissues, such as distinguishing between different kidney stones or determining tumor composition. Aside from this, advances in perfusion imaging are allowing for regional blood flow to be measured, which is valuable in a variety of clinical applications, including stroke assessment and cancer staging. With the use of dynamic contrast enhancement and sophisticated algorithms, physicians are now able to elucidate tissue hemodynamic status and help determine viability and disease staging. These new technologies emphasize the transition towards more personalized medicine, with imaging protocols highly matched to individual patient needs and treatment strategies (N/A, 2006). With advancing medical imaging, issues with managing radiation dose come to the forefront. Technologies such as automatic exposure control systems play a pivotal role in protecting patients without compromising image quality. These systems actively adjust the radiation dose delivered based on specific imaging requirements and patient considerations, delivering the lowest possible dose that remains adequately diagnostic. Furthermore, new protocols for estimating organ dose are under development, enabling clinicians to more accurately calculate radiation dose to sensitive organs during CT scans. The commitment to dose optimization, along with the advances in imaging technologies, embodies a shared purpose in radiology: improving patient outcomes and minimizing the side effects of imaging tests. These developments together embody the continual efforts towards maximizing the effectiveness, safety, and customization of computed tomography in clinical use.

SUMMARY

The evolution of computed tomography (CT) technology has significantly increased diagnostic capabilities in medicine. With a focus on enhanced imaging protocols, clinicians are now able to diagnose a wide range of health disorders, ranging from traumatic injury to intricate diseases. These developments have been driven by gantry design innovation, which provides optimal patient positioning and comfort, together with the integration of slip-ring technology to ensure uninterrupted data transfer during scanning. Therefore, the transition from the previous to the new imaging approaches is essential for efficient and effective patient care. Optimization of these protocols is key to improving image quality while minimizing exposure to radiation, as the subsequent health risks from higher doses are an ongoing clinical concern. Furthermore, the inclusion of iterative reconstruction algorithms has transformed image rendering and processing. Traditional filtered back-projection methods are complemented or replaced by iterative algorithms that improve image quality with reduced radiation doses, addressing the call for dose control. The actions towards the application of automatic exposure control and assessment of organ dose estimation have further stressed the call for radiation dose management. Institutions are beginning to add dual-energy CT and other newer imaging modalities to enhance diagnostic capability and improve patient safety. The integration of these newer technologies and protocols has a strong role in the future of medical imaging, making it possible to create more subtle evaluations of complex conditions and diseases. Finally, CT protocol optimization is of utmost importance. As noted, the careful selection of variables such as kilovolt peak (kVp) and milliampere-seconds (mAs) is essential to achieving diagnostic efficacy while maintaining safety. Aside from this, timing of contrast administration can make a significant difference to image quality as well as patient tolerance to scanning. New literature consolidates the role of iodinated contrast agents in making low-radiation-dose scans feasible, especially when combined with newer techniques for contrast injection. New approaches based on these concepts, as introduced in the case of nephrolithiasis treatment, demonstrate the potential for innovation in patient care enabled by optimized CT practice (Bove et al., 2013; Albrecht et al., 2017). Hence, the convergence of technological, procedural, and strategic innovation in CT provides a sound foundation for enhancing diagnostic accuracy while minimizing patient risk.

CLOSER LOOK

MODERN CT IMAGING: INNOVATIONS DRIVING HIGH-RESOLUTION, LOW-DOSE DIAGNOSTICS

The incorporation of Computed Tomography (CT) into medicine has revolutionized diagnosis, enabling complete evaluation that is not typically possible with other imaging modalities. CT, as a multimodal imaging modality, has the capability to generate high-resolution images, enabling clinicians not only to establish the presence of disease but also to dissect anatomical structures in detail. In particular, technological advances within CT, such as helical scanning and dual-source imaging, have hastened imaging while enhancing resolution. Such innovations have practical implications for patient care, enabling rapid diagnoses in emergency cases and informative monitoring of complex health states. Further, the transition to iterative reconstruction methods has optimized image quality while reducing radiation exposure, underscoring once again the relevance of CT as a safe and effective diagnostic tool in modern medicine. The advent of newer CT technologies, such as dual-energy CT and perfusion imaging, has further solidified the technology's position in medicine. Dual-energy CT enables improved tissue characterization, enabling differentiation between pathological conditions and healthy tissues. This is particularly critical in oncology, where accurate tumor delineation defines treatment protocols. CT angiography is another major imaging modality for the assessment of vascular diseases, enabling noninvasive visualization of vessels. The continuing evolution of CT protocols also reflects the commitment to optimizing diagnostic performance and minimizing side effects, as embodied in recent proposals for low-radiation-dose studies with the use of iodinated contrast media. Such a focus on optimizing image quality and safety is necessary in the ever-evolving patient treatment environment. Furthermore, effective management of radiation dose remains a top priority with growing CT use. An important advancement toward ensuring patient safety is the real-time adjustment of radiation dose in accordance with certain parameters of the patient using automatic exposure control systems. Healthcare stakeholders are increasingly recognizing radiation dose reduction strategies as evidenced by the combination of low kilovolt peak (kVp) and iterative reconstruction techniques. These methods reduce radiation burden while maintaining diagnostic efficacy, thereby aligning with current healthcare goals for patient-centered care. Lastly, the current advances in CT technology aimed at improving diagnostic performance while maintaining patient safety consolidate its central role in contemporary healthcare delivery (Kitsiou et al., 2013; Albrecht et al., 2017).

REFERENCES

1. Drees, R., Johnson, R. A., Stepien, R. L., Del Rio, A. M., Saunders, J. H., & François, C. J. (2015). QUANTITATIVE PLANAR AND VOLUMETRIC CARDIAC MEASUREMENTS USING 64 MDCT AND 3T MRI VS. STANDARD 2D AND M-MODE ECHOCARDIOGRAPHY: DOES ANESTHETIC PROTOCOL MATTER? *Veterinary Radiology & Ultrasound*, *56*(6), 638–657. https://doi.org/10.1111/vru.12269Al Moudi, M. Z. (2014). Diagnostic value of nuclear cardiology in coronary artery disease. https://core.ac.uk/download/195631955.pdf (accessed on 14th July 2025).
2. Albrecht, T., Aschoff, A. J., Catalano, C., Kirchin, B., et al. (2017). Low radiation dose in computed tomography: The role of iodine. https://core.ac.uk/download/98341308.pdf (accessed on 14th July 2025).
3. Alvarez, R., Chen, Y., Feng, Y., Frellessen, C., Hardie, R., Herfarth, K., Johnson, D., et al. (2018). Technical note: Enhancing soft tissue contrast and radiation-induced image changes with dual-energy CT for radiation therapy. https://core.ac.uk/download/228028478.pdf (accessed on 14th July 2025).
4. Appleton, C. M., Hu, P., Li, L., Lin, S., et al. (2018). Single-breath-hold photoacoustic computed tomography of the breast. https://core.ac.uk/download/212867848.pdf (accessed on 14th July 2025).
5. Arsanjani, R., Berman, D. S., Dharmakumar, R., Fish, M., et al. (2017). Impact of incomplete ventricular coverage on diagnostic performance of myocardial perfusion imaging. https://core.ac.uk/download/323079904.pdf (accessed on 14th July 2025).
6. Badal, A., Kyprianou, I., Popescu, L. M., Rupcich, M., et al. (2013). Reducing radiation dose to the female breast during CT coronary angiography: A simulation study comparing breast shielding, angular tube current modulation, reduced kV, and partial angle protocols using an unknown-location signal-detectability metric. https://core.ac.uk/download/213089556.pdf (accessed on 14th July 2025).
7. Baronette, R. (2018). Quantitative analysis of three-dimensional cone-beam computed tomography using image quality phantoms. https://core.ac.uk/download/215386638.pdf (accessed on 14th July 2025).
8. Bastarrika, G., De Cecco, C. N., Geyer, L. L., Laghi, A., et al. (2015). State of the art: Iterative CT reconstruction techniques. https://core.ac.uk/download/54522078.pdf (accessed on 14th July 2025).
9. Belyakova, E. D., Nasibullina, A. A., Bulgakova, J. V., Vlasova, O., Grebennikova, V. V., Omelyanskaya, O., Petraikin, A., et al. (2024). Medical phantom of the knee joint for computed tomography studies. *Digital Diagnostics*. https://www.semanticscholar.org/paper/43f806f9bedfc105617757f0a02ba4e571138493 (accessed on 14th July 2025).
10. Biondi-Zoccai, G., Frati, G., Iskandrian, A. E., Nudi, F., et al. (2017). Diagnostic accuracy of myocardial perfusion imaging with CZT technology: Systematic review and meta-analysis of comparison with invasive coronary angiography. https://core.ac.uk/download/153369775.pdf (accessed on 14th July 2025).
11. Bithell, J., Darragh, P., Elliott, A., Evans, R., et al. (2014). Patient radiation dose issues resulting from the use of CT in the UK. https://core.ac.uk/download/33451683.pdf (accessed on 14th July 2025).

12. Bove, P., Finazzi Agrò, E., Kim, F. J., Miano, R., Micali, S., Rosa, M., & Usai, P. (2013). Recent findings and new technologies in nephrolithiasis: A review of the recent literature. https://core.ac.uk/download/pdf/54580708.pdf (accessed on 14th July 2025).
13. Chang, E. F., Jetté, N., & Kwon, C. S. (2020). Cost-effectiveness of advanced imaging technologies in the presurgical workup of epilepsy. https://core.ac.uk/download/323063036.pdf (accessed on 14th July 2025).
14. Eghlidospoor, M., Mahdavi, M., & Rahimi, S. (2018). Evaluation of some spiral and sequential computed tomography protocols of adults used in three hospitals in Shiraz, Iran with American College of Radiology and European Commission guidelines. https://core.ac.uk/download/160736723.pdf (accessed on 14th July 2025).
15. Faggioni, L. (2012). CT coronary angiography with 100 kV tube voltage and a low noise reconstruction filter in non-obese patients: Evaluation of radiation dose and diagnostic quality of 2D and 3D image reconstructions using open-source software (OsiriX). https://core.ac.uk/download/14703676.pdf (accessed on 14th July 2025).
16. Hernandez, A. M., Chen, A. F., Ghatpande, O. A., Omary, R. A., Woolen, S. A., Jung, Y., & Fananapazir, G. (2024). Reducing the energy consumption of magnetic resonance imaging and computed tomography scanners: Integrating eco-design and sustainable operations. *Journal of Computer Assisted Tomography, 49*, 191–202. https://www.semanticscholar.org/paper/d4f5267a98ce5c21c4a8767adda8b30cd29a8825 (accessed on 14th July 2025).
17. Heume, C., Dzieciol, K., Wolf, N., Treutlein, L., Javed, A., Poc, J. P., Rein, L., et al. (2024). Unraveling a novel degradation mechanism in industrial scale PEM electrolytic cells by multimodal analysis based on X-ray computed tomography. *ECS Meeting Abstracts*. https://www.semanticscholar.org/paper/0b05a8cef47e037884238a287c7bfaf47513fa8d (accessed on 14th July 2025).
18. Ismail, S. N., Mahmud, M. H., Nayyef, Q. T., Tajuddin, N., et al. (2023). Knowledge and practices of computed tomography exposure parameters among radiographers. https://core.ac.uk/download/588018421.pdf (accessed on 14th July 2025).
19. Kärnä, R. (2018). Laadunvalvonnan ja potilasannosten seurannan menetelmät tietokonetomografiassa. https://core.ac.uk/download/159158574.pdf (accessed on 14th July 2025).
20. Ketten, D. R., & Montie, E. W. (2008). Imaging procedures for stranded marine mammals. https://core.ac.uk/download/4167104.pdf (accessed on 14th July 2025).
21. Kim, E., Park, Y., Zhao, T., Laugeman, E., Zhao, X., Hao, Y., Chung, Y., et al. (2024). Image quality characterization of an ultra-high-speed kilovoltage cone-beam computed tomography imaging system on an O-ring linear accelerator. *Journal of Applied Clinical Medical Physics, 25*. https://www.semanticscholar.org/paper/b8c8fd354c6abc0cbffe9c80bd6f7be956549ec7 (accessed on 14th July 2025).
22. Kitsiou, A., Caforio, A. L. P., Porta-Sanchez, A., Vahanian, A., Iung, B., Carrera, C., Szymanski, C., et al. (2013). *ESC Core Curriculum for The General Cardiologist (2013)*. https://core.ac.uk/download/55756305.pdf (accessed on 14th July 2025).
23. Kussman, B. D., Owens, C., Young, C., Owens, C. M., Heyer, C. M., Papaioannou, G., Hoppe, H., et al. (2007). Multidetector row CT for imaging the pediatric tracheobronchial tree. https://core.ac.uk/download/pdf/7622724.pdf (accessed on 14th July 2025).

24. LeBoff, M. S., Greenspan, S. L., Insogna, K., Lewiecki, E. M., Saag, K. G., Singer, A., & Siris, E. S. (2022). The clinician's guide to prevention and treatment of osteoporosis. *Osteoporosis International, 33*, 2049–2102. https://doi.org/10.1007/s00198-021-05900-y (accessed on 14th July 2025).

25. Meloni, A., Maffei, E., Positano, V., Clemente, A., De Gori, C., Berti, S., La Grutta, L., et al. (2024). Technical principles, benefits, challenges, and applications of photon counting computed tomography in coronary imaging: A narrative review. *Cardiovascular Diagnosis and Therapy, 14*, 698–724. https://www.semanticscholar.org/paper/cedacb89c36ed454b05f51079c585fd85ca8836a (accessed on 14th July 2025).

26. N/A. (1975). *Focal Spot, Spring 1975*. https://core.ac.uk/download/129069210.pdf (accessed on 14th July 2025).

27. N/A. (1978). *Focal Spot, Spring 1978*. https://core.ac.uk/download/129069222.pdf (accessed on 14th July 2025).

28. N/A. (2000). *Focal Spot, Fall/Winter 2000*. https://core.ac.uk/download/129069319.pdf (accessed on 14th July 2025).

29. N/A. (2006). *Focal Spot, Winter 2005/2006*. https://core.ac.uk/download/129069348.pdf (accessed on 14th July 2025).

30. Seibert, A., Baird, C. T., Clements, J. B., de Boer, S. F., et al. (2018). AAPM medical physics practice guideline 10.a.: Scope of practice for clinical medical physics. https://core.ac.uk/download/286729023.pdf (accessed on 14th July 2025).

31. van Westendorp, S., Robben, S. H. M., van Hooft, M. A. A., Dierckx, S. A. A., & Maas, H. A. A. M. (2024). The clinical implications of using a low threshold for computed tomography scans in older patients presenting with a proximal femur fracture. *European Geriatric Medicine, 15*, 1081–1089. https://www.semanticscholar.org/paper/1f8507307220256e36e3c117c3be2e5bbbb02814 (accessed on 14th July 2025).

32. Zeppenfeld, K., Tfelt-Hansen, J., Riva, M., Winkel, B. G., Behr, E. R., Blom, N. A., Charron, P., et al. (2022). 2022 ESC guidelines for the management of patients with ventricular arrhythmias and the prevention of sudden cardiac death. *European Heart Journal, 43*, 3997–4126. https://doi.org/10.1093/eurheartj/ehac262 (accessed on 14th July 2025).

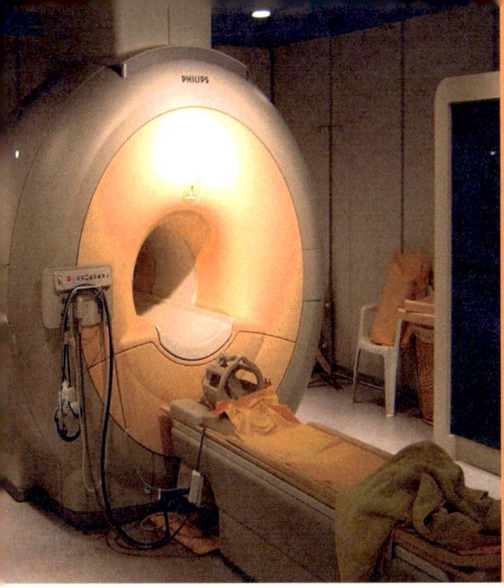

Chapter 5

MAGNETIC RESONANCE IMAGING FUNDAMENTALS

Contents

Introduction

Magnetic Resonance Imaging (MRI) is a non-surgical imaging test that uses strong magnetic fields, radio waves, and a computer to produce detailed images of internal body structures. Unlike ionizing radiation-based imaging, such as X-rays or CT scans, MRI offers a safe but exact method of imaging soft tissues, organs, joints, and the central nervous system. It works by detecting signals emitted by hydrogen atoms in the body when exposed to a strong magnetic field and then stimulated by radiofrequency pulses. It translates the signals into cross-sectional or three-dimensional images that enable clinicians to make diagnoses with accuracy and clarity.

MRI has revolutionized medical imaging with its unmatched contrast resolution, particularly for the brain, spinal cord, muscles, ligaments, and internal organs such as the liver and heart. It is sufficiently accommodating to offer a host of specialized imaging protocols, such as functional MRI (fMRI), diffusion tensor imaging (DTI), and magnetic resonance angiography (MRA), each with a distinct diagnostic purpose. With its ability to create high-definition images without surgery or radiation exposure, MRI is today a ubiquitous feature of modern diagnostic radiology, facilitating the early detection, treatment planning, and follow-up of many diseases and illnesses.

5.1. Basic Principles of MRI

An understanding of the basic principles of Magnetic Resonance Imaging (MRI) is key to realizing its full diagnostic potential. Essentially, MRI is based on nuclear magnetic resonance (NMR), which results from the behavior of atomic nuclei in magnetic fields. Under the influence of an applied external magnetic field, specific nuclei—particularly hydrogen—tend to orient with the external field due to their spin and magnetic moment. This alignment leads to the Larmor frequency, which determines the precession rate of the nuclei's magnetic moments. The radiofrequency (RF) pulse irradiation causes these nuclei to absorb energy and subsequently relax to their original positions via relaxation mechanisms, producing the MR signal used for imaging. T1- and T2-weighted MRI images enhance contrast by separating tissue properties and pathology. With progressing MRI technology, including concepts like molecular imaging, diagnostic capability is being augmented, highlighting its growing applicability in clinical settings (Tarighatnia et al., 2021; Mason et al., 2024).

5.1.1. The Magnetic Field in MRI

The intricate interaction between the magnetic fields and the principles of Magnetic Resonance Imaging (MRI) is at the heart of its functioning and usefulness as a diagnostic tool for medicine. An important aspect of the process is the alignment of the hydrogen nuclei, achieved by applying a strong, homogeneous magnetic field that causes them to adopt specific positions. Exposure to radiofrequency (RF) pulses can drive aligned nuclei into resonance via processes governed by the Larmor frequency, a function of the magnetic field strength. Subsequent relaxation processes, such as T1 and T2, allow the nuclear magnetization to recover and emit signals that are used to derive MRI images. As technology continues to advance, say, by incorporating superparamagnetic iron oxide nanoparticles (SPION) for improved imaging capability, the role of magnetic fields remains at the forefront in shaping the direction of the future of MRI and its utilization in the treatment of cancer (Vangijzegem et al., 2023) and in the node assessment of rectal cancer (Borgheresi et al., 2022) (Figure 5.1).

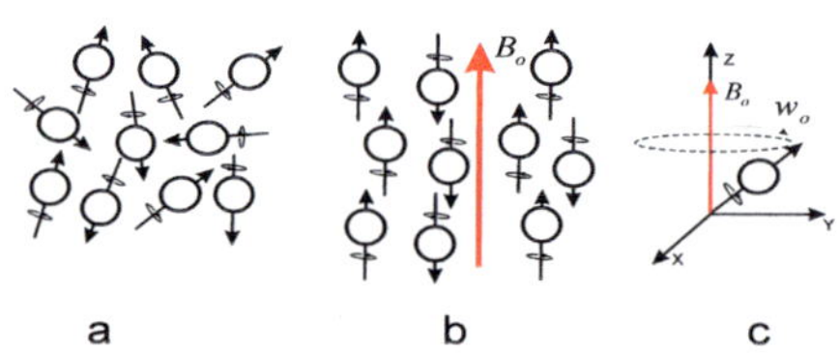

Figure 5.1. Diagram illustrating alignment of hydrogen protons in a magnetic field.

Source: https://www.researchgate.net/profile/Natalia-Florez/publication/50838612/figure/fig9/AS:669388881547271@1536606154839/Alignment-of-protons-with-the-B-o-field-a-Without-external-magnetic-field-hydrogen.jpg.

5.1.2. Hydrogen Atoms and Their Significance in Imaging

The location of hydrogen protons in magnetic resonance imaging (MRI) is better because of their unique properties, which make them ideal for creating high-resolution images. Hydrogen's nuclei, which are single protons and the most abundant element in the human body, have a great magnetic moment. This characteristic makes them highly susceptible to magnetic alignment in a magnetic field when subjected to radiofrequency pulses. The contrast between T1 and T2 relaxation times is mainly accounted for by the reaction-diffusion of the hydrogen atoms throughout the process, influencing the contrast as well as image visibility obtained (Waseem et al., 2018). Besides, variations in hydrogen density in different tissues contribute significantly towards establishing contrast mechanisms required to distinguish various diseases (Waseem et al., 2018). Thus, understanding hydrogen-atom behavior is crucial for optimizing MRI techniques and image quality, ultimately improving patient care in medical imaging (Figure 5.2).

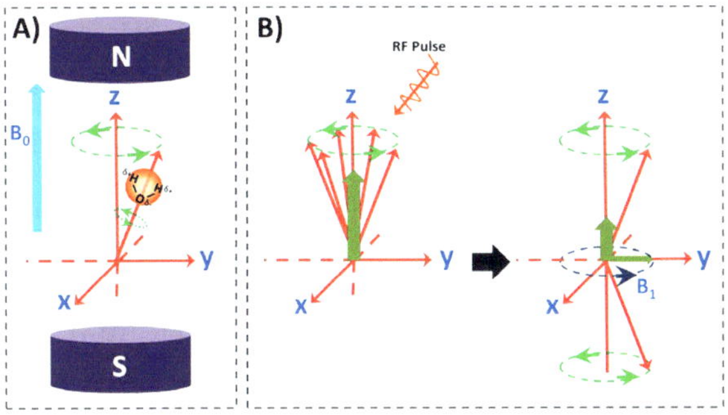

Figure 5.2. Illustration of hydrogen nuclei precession in a magnetic field. A) hydrogen nuclei are processing about the external magnetic field axis B_0. B) The schematic shows how RF pulses decrease longitudinal magnetization M z to form transverse magnetization M xy. Nuclear spins then return to equilibrium M z through relaxation.

Source: https://www.researchgate.net/profile/Dr-Anita-Peacock/publication/364315641/figure/fig4/AS:11431281089437784@1665575592422/Magnetic-resonance-theory-A-hydrogen-nuclei-precessing-about-the-external-magnetic.png.

5.1.3. The Process of Nuclear Magnetic Resonance

In medical imaging, the nuances of NMR are at the heart of MRI understanding. At its most elementary level, NMR is based on atomic nuclei' magnetic moments and their influences on an external magnetic field. The procedure begins with aligning these magnetic moments, which, upon irradiation with radiofrequency (RF) pulses, absorb energy and then release it as they return to their normal state. This energy release occurs at specific rates, or Larmor frequencies, that depend on the type of nuclei excited (Bian et al., 2024).

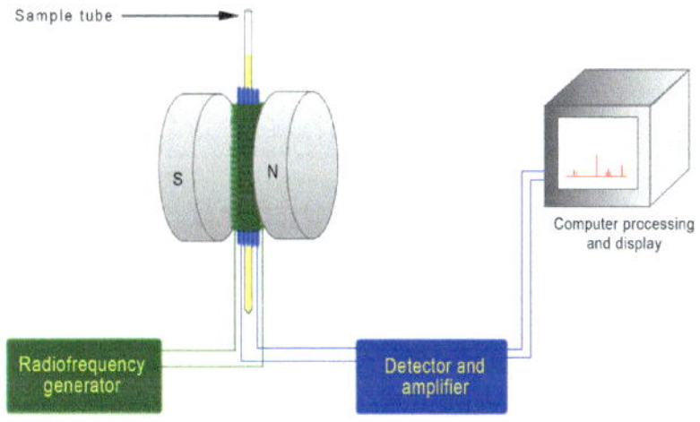

Figure 5.3. Schematic representation of nuclear magnetic resonance signal generation.

Source: https://chem.libretexts.org/@api/deki/files/12647/nmr-4.png?revision=1&size=bestfit&width=627&height=314.

These resultant signals are then processed to yield high-resolution images, using relaxation mechanisms to image tissue properties. Furthermore, NMR innovations like automated processing techniques, such as those in MagMet, facilitate quick and accurate metabolite quantification from biofluids, demonstrating the extensive applications of NMR aside from its conventional imaging and augmenting the clinical application of MRI technologies (Rout et al., 2023) (Figure 5.3).

5.1.4. Radiofrequency Pulses and Their Function

The physics of magnetic resonance imaging (MRI) depends on the application of radiofrequency (RF) pulses, which are the foundation for generating diagnostic signals from body tissues. Under the influence of a strong magnetic field, nuclear spins in body tissues line up along the field's direction, but are temporarily offset by RF pulses.

These pulses excite protons, which then resonate and emit energy as they return to their equilibrium state. The emitted signals are picked up by RF coils, helping to form images. The resolution and quality of the images received are highly dependent on the signal-to-noise ratio (SNR), which can be enhanced by technologies such as bioresorbable implants designed to optimize RF pulse interactions (Lee et al., 2023). Moreover, understanding the mechanisms and operations of RF pulses will become imperative to develop tailored pulse sequences that optimize imaging performance and deliver maximum diagnostic potential in clinical practice (Berry et al., 2024) (Figure 5.4).

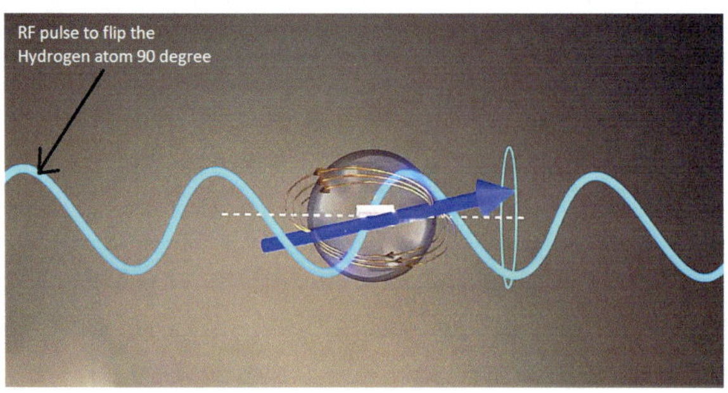

Figure 5.4. Example of an RF pulse altering spin orientation.

Source: https://i.sstatic.net/96sBi.jpg.

5.1.5. Image Formation and Signal Processing

The intricate relationship of magnetic resonance theory and signal processing nuances is an essential component of high-grade image creation in MRI. Manipulation of radiofrequency pulses and magnetic fields is at the center of this process and induces resonant effects in body hydrogen atoms, resulting in signal emission. This radiated signal is then picked up and digitized for reconstruction into high-resolution photographs, a process that relies heavily on sophisticated algorithms that optimize clarity and contrast. Of central importance to this process, sophisticated techniques such as digital downconversion and filtering are employed to transform the acquired data into usable forms for analysis (Jiang et al., 2024). In addition, merging imaging data with non-imaging information improves diagnostic efficiency, providing a comprehensive picture of biopsychological systems (Yadav et al., 2024). The combination of image formation and signal processing is hence vital in advancing MRI technology and its uses in the clinical setting (Figure 5.5).

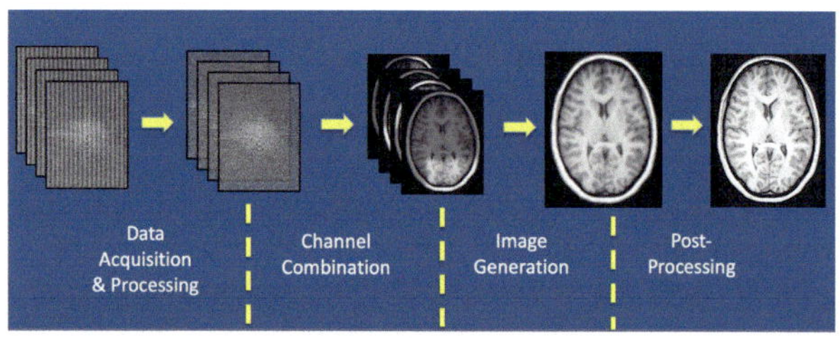

Figure 5.5. Steps in signal reception and image reconstruction from MRI.

Source: https://mriquestions.com/uploads/3/4/5/7/34572113/dl-spots-in-pipeline_orig.png.

5.1.6. The Importance of Relaxation Times (T1 and T2)

In the medical imaging domain of Magnetic Resonance Imaging (MRI), it is necessary to understand the nuances of the relaxation times, T1 and T2, to create high-quality images that accurately represent underlying tissue properties. The relaxation times provide essential information about how tissues respond to the magnetic field and radiofrequency pulses and consequently impact image contrast. T1 relaxation or longitudinal relaxation reflects the time it takes for protons to align after the magnetic field has been excited, and T2 or transverse relaxation is the time it takes for protons to lose phase coherence among the spins. With this knowledge, clinicians can use the best imaging protocols to match specific tissues or pathologies, improving diagnostic accuracy. Moreover, studies indicate that the T1 and T2 changes also correspond to meaningful biological transformations, for example, atherosclerosis treatment outcomes and cheese ripening processes with prevailing structural transformation, thereby establishing their broader applicability in clinical and research applications (Pńczura et al., 2024; Segura et al., 2024) (Figure 5.6).

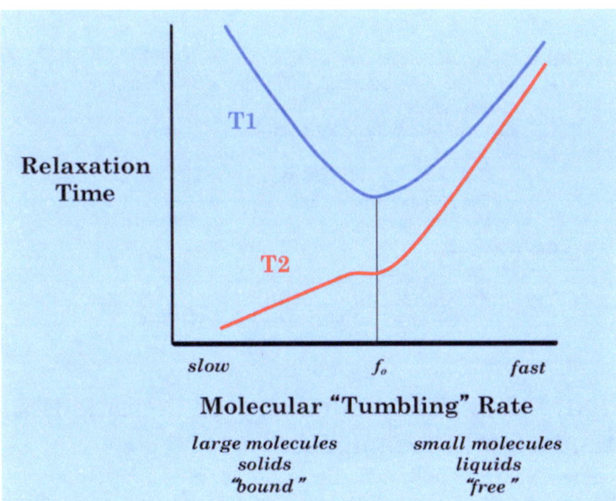

Figure 5.6. Comparison of T1 and T2 relaxation processes.

Source: https://mri-q.com/uploads/3/4/5/7/34572113/molecular-tumbling-rate_1_orig.png.

5.1.7. Spatial Encoding and the Role of Gradients

The intricacies of magnetic resonance imaging (MRI) primarily rely on the effectiveness of spatial encoding, which is a decisive factor in generating high-resolution images of internal body structures. By using gradient fields generated by specific coils, MRI technology achieves spatial signal localization, enabling signal separation by anatomical region.

These gradients function by a variation in the field strength of the magnet in the area of the imaging volume, which converts spatial data into the resonant frequency of the body's nuclei. MRI operation can be readily undermined by factors such as field inhomogeneities and low signal-to-noise ratios, rendering spatial resolution and precision challenging (Schmidt et al., 2020). Furthermore, developments such as multi-spoke RF pulse techniques have been shown to efficiently correct artifacts relative to traditional acquisition processes, thereby enhancing the spatial encoding process itself (Huang et al., 2017). A good understanding of gradients is thus an important aspect in enhancing image acquisition and diagnostic effectiveness in general (Figure 5.7).

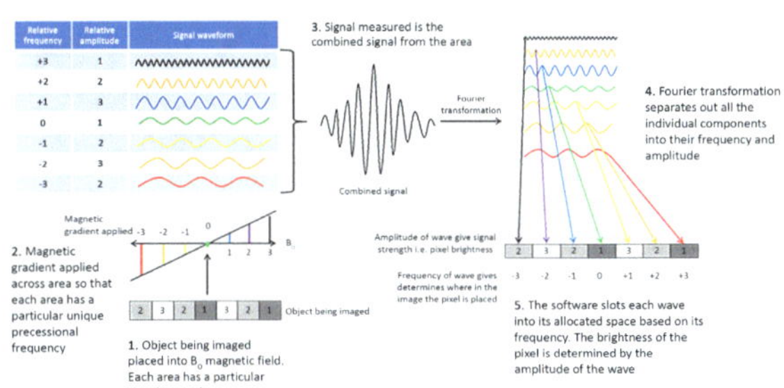

Figure 5.7. Diagram showing gradient application in spatial encoding.

Source: https://www.radiologycafe.com/wp-content/uploads/2021/04/mri-spacial-encoding.png.

5.1.8. The Concept of Voxel in MRI Imaging

In Magnetic Resonance Imaging (MRI), voxel is a simple building block for encoding three-dimensional spatial information. Voxel is linked with an individual volume element in the imaging space, integrating signals from numerous atomic spins within it to produce an image. The technique allows spatial localization and quantification of various tissue parameters and thereby contributes significantly to diagnostic accuracy and image quality. In addition, advances in acquisition techniques, such as functional MRI and diffusion MRI, employ voxel-based analyses to comprehend complex brain networks and connectivity patterns. With connectivity fingerprint mapping, researchers can assess functional integration between brain regions, and the growing importance of voxel-based approaches in neuroscience and medical diagnostics is evident. Thus, the voxel not only serves as a structural feature in MRI imaging but also significantly enhances our understanding of physiological processes (Rogier et al., 2018; Shen et al., 2017) (Figure 5.8).

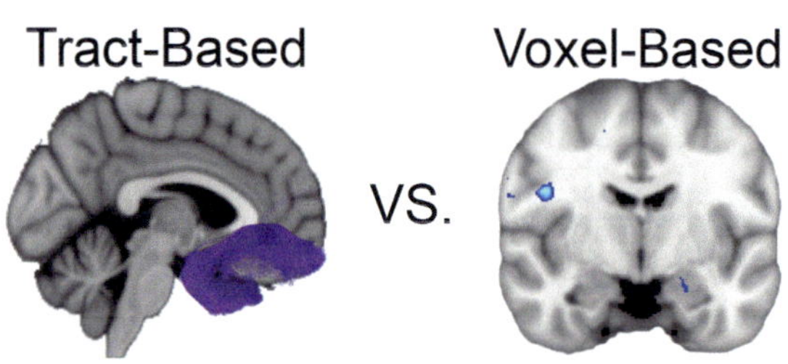

Figure 5.8. 3D voxel structure used in MRI imaging representation.

Source: https://blogger.googleusercontent.com/img/b/R29vZ2xl/AVvXsEhYWsVRok_6znPdw7d6RPRZQl81LMOocFMAiXzSCt7oqfnFx8uJrRErouWMH5-UhNoS8Ae5w6zdNyCmrWoywua-zJGQBptnT3lVcx9gkrpEu-VEG6xIDA51Q67tPv3JnSxVpkpGrZv6_2I/s1600/Voxel-basedvsTract-based.png.

5.1.9. Limitations of Basic MRI Principles

The advanced principles of Magnetic Resonance Imaging (MRI) bring significant benefits but also significant limitations that can influence diagnosis. For instance, the application of nuclear magnetic resonance physics poses inherent image-quality and resolution challenges, which can complicate the interpretation of many medical conditions (Bhuiyan et al., 2023).

Tissue homogeneity, necessary for sharp MRI images, is often disrupted by patient motion and magnetic susceptibility heterogeneity, leading to artifacts that may obscure clinical findings. In addition, while diffusion MRI illuminates tissue's microscopic architecture, scaling up these advanced techniques to clinical scanners remains difficult due to hardware constraints, making accurate estimation of parameters such as axon radius *in vivo* (Aboitiz et al., 2016). Hence, understanding these limitations is essential for clinicians so that they can master MRI diagnostics judiciously (Figure 5.9).

Advantages

- Improved lesion detection, delineation, differentiation from normal tissues
- Improved lesion characterization
- No ionizing radiation
  - Can be performed in pregnancy (2nd trimester onwards) and young children
  - More repeatability

Disadvantages

- Longer scan times
- More expensive
- Machine construction may induce claustrophobia
- Noisier due to RF pulse generation

Figure 5.9. Visual summary of limitations in standard MRI techniques.

Source: https://www.researchgate.net/profile/Chinmay-Nagesh/publication/354915185/figure/tbl1/AS:1073239170248709@1632891566180/MRI-Advantages-and-Disadvantages.png.

5.2. MRI Equipment and Technology

The engineering of MRI technology is a significant factor in advancing medical imaging. Magnetic Resonance Imaging relies on an equipment consisting of several highly engineered components, including the main magnet, gradient coils, and radiofrequency (RF) coils, that come together to facilitate the creation of high-definition anatomy images. The primary magnet creates a homogeneous, intense magnetic field required for aligning the body's hydrogen nuclei, with gradient coils controlling the spatial encoding of signals. RF coils amplify transmitted radio waves needed for excitation and subsequent signal capture, ultimately producing high-contrast images reflective of tissue properties. The architecture of such elements plays a significant role in imaging performance, with an understanding of T1 and T2 relaxation times central to optimizing image quality and diagnostic efficacy across diverse clinical applications (Gaeta et al., 2024; Saito et al., 2024). This wide-spectrum architecture not only optimizes diagnostic performance but also extends MRI applications to an extensive array of medical specialties.

5.2.1. Components of an MRI Machine

The intricate design of an MRI machine consists of several key components that work together to produce detailed images of the human body. Central to this design is the central magnet, which generates a strong and uniform magnetic field required for the alignment of nuclear spins in the bodys hydrogen atoms. Gradient coils accompany the primary magnet, spatially encoding the magnetic field radiated by hydrogen atoms to modulate the signal, enabling precise localization of the imaging data. Other radiofrequency (RF) coils used to transmit and receive RF pulses necessary for exciting hydrogen nuclei and recovering signals that contribute to the construction of final images are also present. This extremely sensitive technology is a premier indicator in diagnostic imaging, enabling physicians to see the interior of the body with unprecedented sensitivity and clarity, as evidenced by studies on the utility and prognostic significance of advanced MRI analysis techniques (Nagawa et al., 2024; Voineskos et al., 2024) (Figure 5.10).

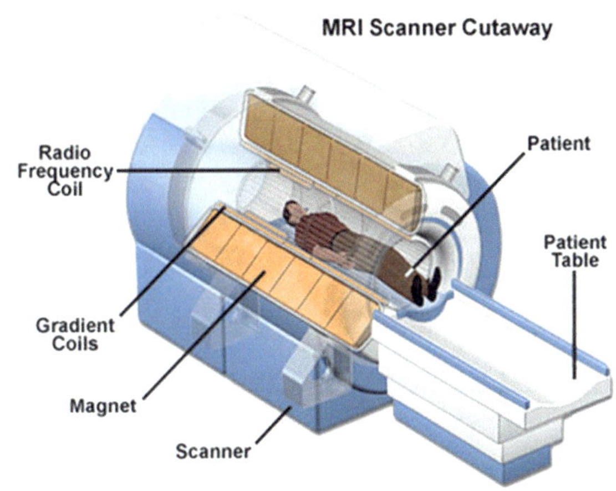

Figure 5.10. Components of a standard closed-bore MRI machine.

Source: Siemens MAGNETOM System Guide.

5.2.2. Types of MRI Scanners (Closed Versus Open)

The MRI technology market is primarily dominated by the design of its scanners, which can be classified as closed- and open-type scanners. The closed MRI scanners are in the shape of a cylinder, with greater magnetic field strength and improved image resolution due to the high signal-to-noise ratio, which is a key parameter for accurate diagnosis. Contrarily, open MRI scanners, with a bigger opening and less body restraining structure, are more comfortable for patients, reducing anxiety levels, especially in children undergoing the test. Open-bore systems are also known to significantly reduce RF heating significantly, implying lower risks to patients with certain medical implants, thereby enhancing overall safety during imaging procedures (Vu et al., 2024). Nevertheless, while their comfort and safety advantages are undeniable, open MRI systems tend to sacrifice image quality relative to the closed system, resulting in a difficult trade-off between patient comfort and diagnostic effectiveness (Runge et al., 2024) (Figure 5.11).

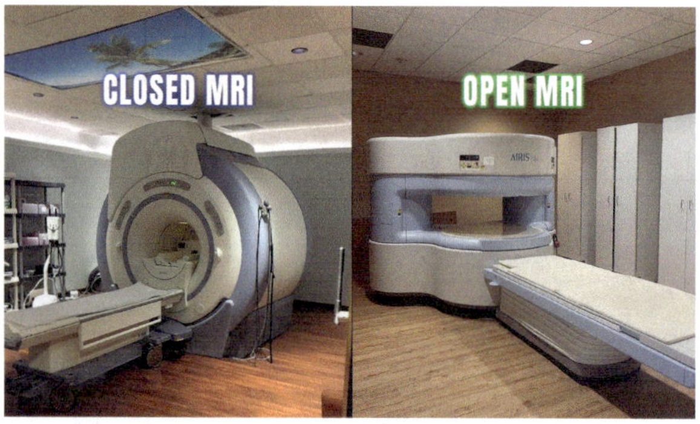

Figure 5.11. Closed versus open MRI scanner image.

Source: https://lakezurichopenmri.com/wp-content/uploads/2024/09/2-image-showing-Open-MRI-machine-vs-Closed-MRI-machine.webp.

5.2.3. Magnet Types and Their Characteristics

In MRI, understanding several types of magnets is essential because they are integral to the overall imaging process. The strongest superconducting magnet is most commonly used in MRI because it provides uniform magnetic fields that are essential for creating high-quality images. These superconducting magnets, typically made from niobium-titanium alloys, are crucial because they operate at low temperatures with zero resistance. Thus, they ensure better magnetic stability (Akbarzadeh et al., 2012). Permanent magnets, though less commonly utilized in practice, are valued due to their convenience and lower operational costs, but yield weaker magnetic fields. Aside from this, experimental technologies employing antiferromagnetic materials are in the pipeline, which can revolutionize the face of MRI magnet design towards greater efficiency and new uses, underscoring the necessity of further research in this field (Baltz et al., 2018). Overall, the choice of magnet directly influences the effectiveness and quality of MRI treatments (Figure 5.12).

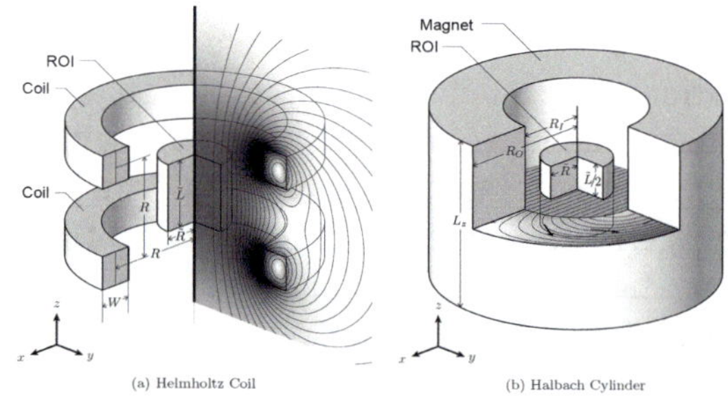

Figure 5.12. Comparison of superconductors and permanent magnets for small-scale magnetic resonance.

Source: https://media.springernature.com/lw685/springer-static/image/art%3A10.1007%2Fs00723-020-01202-4/MediaObjects/723_2020_1202_Fig1_HTML.png.

5.2.4. Radiofrequency Coils and Their Applications

In Magnetic Resonance Imaging (MRI), the role of radiofrequency (RF) coils is paramount, as they serve as transmitters and receivers of RF signals central to image formation. RF coils, designed to be optimized for specific targets such as the head or knee, improve signal reception, thereby enhancing image detail and clarity. The new technologies developed in the past in RF coil technology have led to specially designed coils capable of addressing particular issues, such as B1 field inhomogeneity and increased susceptibility to artifacts at higher field strengths, particularly in 7 Tesla systems. With applications ranging from musculoskeletal imaging to cardiac examinations, a massive improvement in diagnostic accuracy is anticipated through the incorporation of specially designed RF coils in clinical practices. Hence, with improvements in research, particularly related to the deployment and utilization of 7 T MRI, the efficacy of such coils in enhancing patient benefit remains a core focus (Cameron et al., 2018; Nanz et al., 2023) (Figure 5.13).

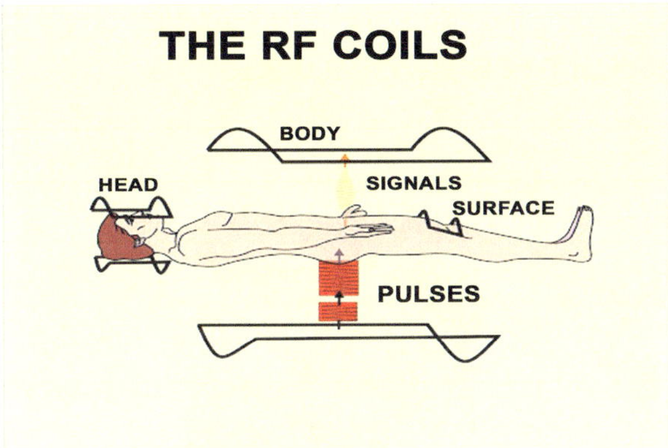

Figure 5.13. Selection of RF coils used for different body parts.

Source: https://lh3.googleusercontent.com/proxy/-y9odx50mIZGNsZwwqDpCJXrf0KuEG7DI9mVMld6MPxeQaG_Fg-6KuprZk9Vb2N2Y7ovMCIeFx_fe0gsgLqrJSohZMo.

5.2.5. Gradient Systems and Their Importance

In the intricate MRI system, gradient systems play a crucial role in determining image quality and resolution. Gradient coils form the gradient system, which is vital for encoding space so that MRI can differentiate signals originating from various points within the body. Using control of magnetic field strength along different axes, gradients enhance contrast and resolution of images, and hence can improve the detection of subtle pathological changes. Advances in gradient echo sequences in recent years, for instance, have expanded the scope of MRI use in diagnosing neuromuscular diseases, as seen in their application to motor unit MRI (MUMRI), (Heskamp et al., 2024). Besides, the application of optimized gradient systems with contrast agents such as Gd-EOB-DTPA has shown potential for detecting alterations in liver function, underscoring the utility of these systems in clinical MRI (Wan et al., 2024). Gradients are not mere devices, then; they form the essence of the diagnostic potential of MRI (Figure 5.14).

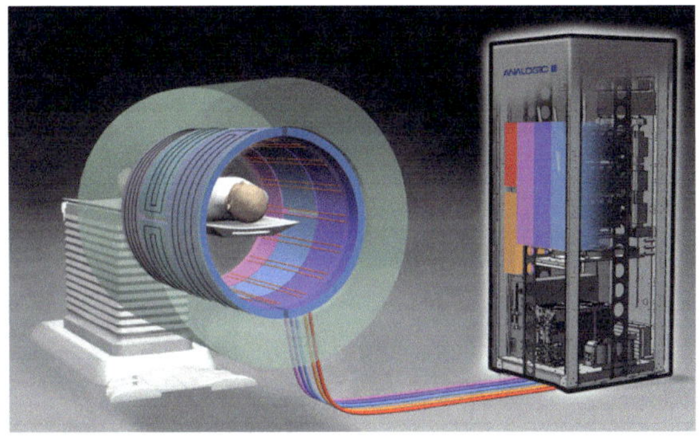

Figure 5.14. MRI gradient coil arrangement and their field effects.

Source: https://mriquestions.com/uploads/3/4/5/7/34572113/703508_orig.gif.

5.2.6. Software Used in MRI Image Reconstruction

Developments in magnetic resonance imaging (MRI) image reconstruction software have had a significant impact on the diagnostic imaging sector. These sophisticated algorithms, particularly those that leverage artificial intelligence and deep learning, improve image quality and reduce scanning times, thereby increasing efficiency in the hospital setting. For instance, accelerated imaging strategies and iterative reconstruction algorithms, such as those demonstrated in the investigation comparing AI-aided iterative methods to traditional fast spin-echo techniques, show significant improvements in signal-to-noise ratio (SNR) and subjective image quality ratings without compromising diagnostic performance (Liu et al., 2024). In addition, the development of convolutional neural network (CNN)-based reconstructions is an arena that is set to be an interesting avenue for optimizing under-sampled MRI data, as detailed in recent literature bridging such advanced computational methods with traditional multi-coil sensitivity encoding (SENSE) MRI scanners (Li et al., 2025). Such technologies identify the pioneering contribution of software advances in presenting high-fidelity images for effective clinical diagnosis (Figure 5.15).

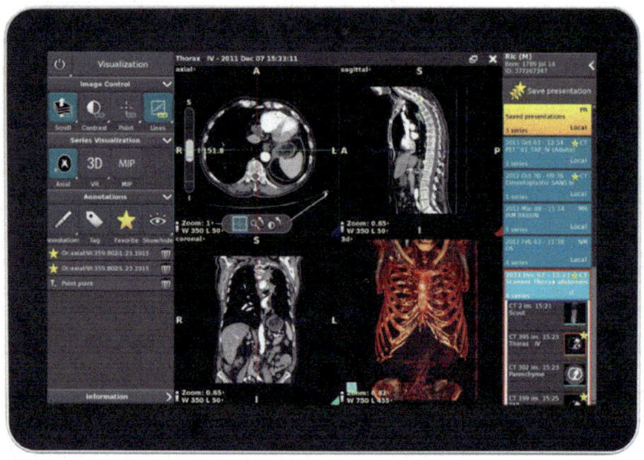

Figure 5.15. Interface of software used in MRI image reconstruction.

Source: https://media.springernature.com/lw685/springer-static/image/art%3A10.1007%2Fs13244-018-0620-7/MediaObjects/13244_2018_620_Fig5_HTML.gif.

5.2.7. Maintenance and Calibration of MRI Equipment

The smooth operation of MRI devices depends on stringent maintenance and calibration processes. MRI machines must be inspected at regular intervals and regulated, as any deviation in calibration will affect image quality and diagnostic accuracy. The establishment of a dynamic fault-repair knowledge base for MRI equipment has proven useful, providing systematized maintenance history tracking and access to technical guidance for efficient fault resolution (Chu et al., 2024). This user-friendly system not only facilitates the management of MRI equipment but also towards the larger goal of creating intelligent hospital environments. Regular calibration ensures that operation-critical parameters, namely magnet homogeneity and gradient integrity, are maintained within prescribed limits. Finally, an maintenance infrastructure not only prolongs the life of the equipment but also ensures patient safety and diagnostic reliability in a continuously evolving medical landscape (Figure 5.16).

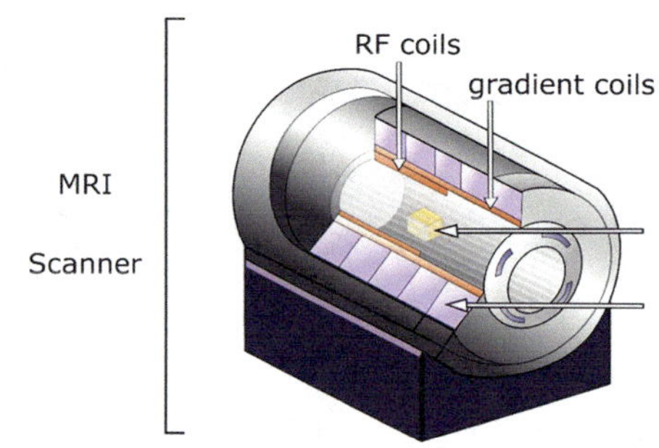

Figure 5.16. Calibration procedure using phantom in MRI scanner.

Source: https://media.springernature.com/full/springer-static/image/art%3A10.1038%2Fs41598-020-63581-9/MediaObjects/41598_2020_63581_Fig1_HTML.png.

5.2.8. Innovations in MRI Technology (e.g., 7T MRI)

As medical imaging technologies continue to advance, the introduction of ultra-high-field MRI systems, including the 7 Tesla (7T) MRI, represents a monumental leap in diagnostic capability. This innovation offers enhanced spatial resolution, thereby enabling clinicians to see anatomical structures with unprecedented resolution and clarity. The signal-to-noise ratio (SNR) gains from 7T MRI have not only maximized conventional imaging techniques but also enabled new clinical applications, such as functional MRI and brain connectivity mapping.

These advances have major implications for surgeries such as deep brain stimulation, whose success is greatly dependent on accurate surgical targeting. Specifically, ultra-high-field imaging helps reduce reliance on indirect landmarks commonly used during stereotactic neurosurgery, improving patient outcomes and reducing procedure risks (Lau et al., 2019; Tavaf et al., 2021). In accordance with this, the inclusion of 7T MRI in clinical practice points to its potential to revolutionize the levels of care in radiology (Figure 5.17).

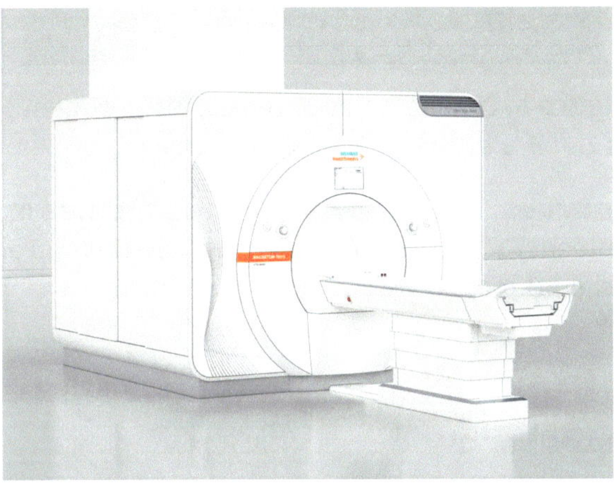

Figure 5.17. Illustration of ultra-high-field 7T MRI scanner.

Source: https://www.itnonline.com/sites/default/files/Siemens-Magnetom-Terra-7T-MRI.jpg.

5.2.9. Cost Considerations in MRI Technology

The evolution of MRI technology has been accompanied by drastic economic consequences that influence health facilities and patient access. Above all, the installation and maintenance of MRI machines are capital-intensive, with a proclivity to incur enormous upfront costs that can exceed a million dollars. The costs are complemented by the operational costs of having experienced technicians and radiologists to effectively decode complex imaging information. Additionally, despite newer MRI technologies such as 7 T MRI having higher diagnostic accuracy, they also pose cost problems because they are more expensive and require greater maintenance, making them difficult to use routinely in the clinic (Arachchige et al., 2024). Additionally, these costs can create disparities of access to MRI, leading to unequal outcomes among patients that tend to affect socioeconomically disadvantaged populations (Zhang, 2025) disproportionately. Hence, it is essential to understand and correct such cost determinants to enable equitable access to MRI technology in modern healthcare systems (Figure 5.18).

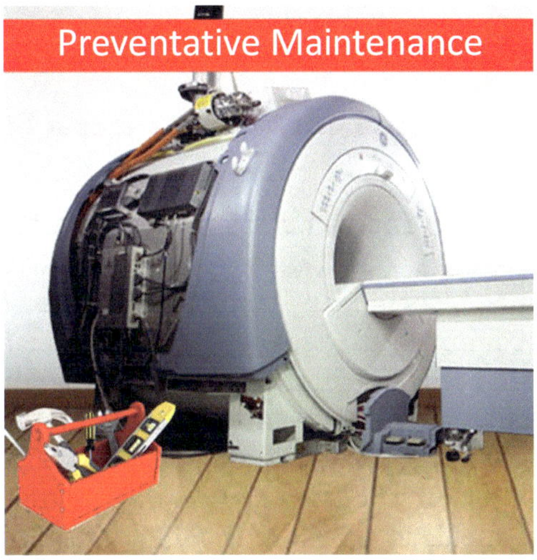

Figure 5.18. Maintenance of MRI systems.

Source: https://cdn2.hubspot.net/hubfs/180962/MRI_PM.jpg.

5.3. MRI Techniques and Protocols

Advancements in MRI have revolutionized diagnostic protocols and procedures, particularly for complex diseases such as cancer. Magnetic Resonance Fingerprinting and T2 mapping are some newer methods with higher potential for disease detection and quantification, which are highly crucial in oncology (Kutli et al., 2025). By optimizing protocols across field strengths of 3T and 1.5T, radiologists can deliver a diagnostic yield equivalent to 3 T while benefiting from higher signal-to-noise ratios, improved image quality, and reduced acquisition time. Aside from these advancements, standardized sequences remain essential, particularly in children, where protocols must be adhered to to avoid putting patients under anesthesia and contrast media (Jung, 2024). These developments not only enhance MRI's diagnostic accuracy but also underscore the need for tailored imaging methods that cater to a broad spectrum of patient populations, ultimately improving patient care and clinical outcomes in an ever-changing discipline.

5.3.1. Routine MRI Sequences (T1, T2, FLAIR)

Radiologists and clinicians must recognize the nuances of various MRI sequences while arriving at a diagnosis in many conditions. Three of the most commonly used sequences are T1-weighted, T2-weighted, and FLAIR sequences. All of these sequences provide varying contrasts that aid in identifying specific pathologies. T1-weighted scans yield excellent anatomical information and are particularly useful in showing fatty tissues. In contrast, T2-weighted scans detect structures that contain fluid and are thus highly useful in detecting edema and other abnormalities in brain tissue. Conversely, FLAIR sequences inhibit signals from cerebrospinal fluid (CSF) and, hence, lesions bordering on CSF spaces, that is, in hypoxic-ischemic encephalopathy, become more apparent as one would wish to identify them promptly (Kumar et al., 2025). Both sequences form a well-rounded toolkit for effective MRI interpretation (Şahap Törenek et al., 2024), with time being left for subtle decisions that can have a profound impact on patient management (Figure 5.19).

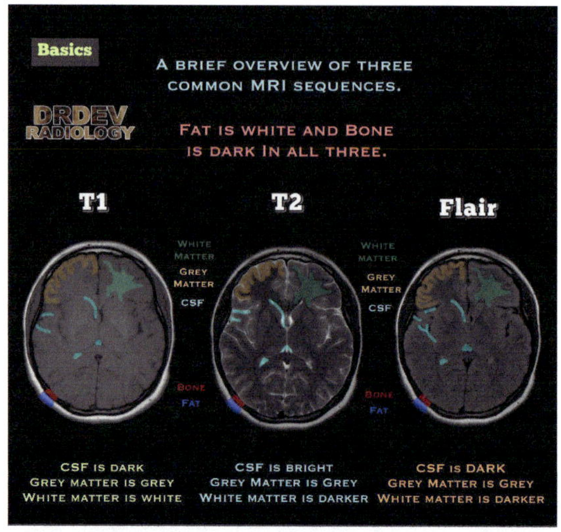

Figure 5.19. Examples of typical MRI sequences (T1, T2, FLAIR) of the brain.

Source: https://img.grepmed.com/uploads/13590/mri-brain-diagnosis-t2-clinical-original.jpeg.

5.3.2. Functional MRI (fMRI) and Its Applications

Visualization of brain activity in neuroscience has changed very dramatically with the advent of Functional Magnetic Resonance Imaging (fMRI). fMRI is not just an imaging method that measures brain activity as a function of the alterations in blood flow, but also tells us about the neural bases of cognition. By using principles of blood-oxygen-level-dependent contrast, fMRI allows scientists to identify specific brain regions engaged in tasks of varying difficulty, thereby linking function to structural anatomy. Developments in recent years have also made fMRI applications more advanced, such as resting-state functional connectivity analysis, which examines intrinsic networks of the brain in the absence of explicit stimuli. Such advances make it possible to understand brain organization and connectivity patterns better and confirm theories like the connectivity fingerprint, which categorizes brain areas based on their input and output connections as proposed by Passingham et al., thus making possible progress in basic and clinical neuroscience (Schaefer et al., 2017; Rogier et al., 2018) (Figure 5.20).

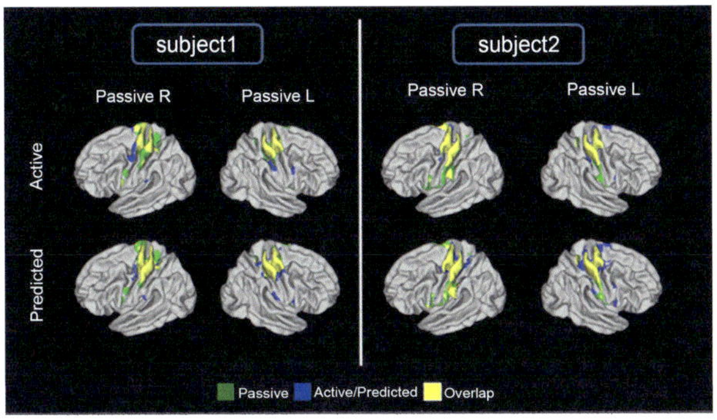

Figure 5.20. fMRI scan showing brain activation in motor task.

Source: https://media.springernature.com/lw685/springer-static/image/art%3A10.1007%2Fs11682-019-00239-9/MediaObjects/11682_2019_239_Fig6_HTML.png.

5.3.3. Diffusion-Weighted Imaging (DWI)

In contemporary medical imaging, the more advanced approaches such as diffusion-weighted imaging (DWI) have significantly enhanced diagnostic precision. DWI quantifies water molecule diffusion in tissues and provides useful data on cellular architecture and pathology, thereby facilitating the delineation of various conditions. For instance, studies have shown that DWI effectively differentiates perianal fistulas from other inflammatory processes, providing a non-invasive alternative to traditional contrast-enhanced imaging methods (Aggarwal et al., 2024). Moreover, the application of DWI is also seen in neuroimaging to differentiate between low-grade and high-grade meningiomas, thereby assisting in appropriate treatment planning (Mukku et al., 2024). These results highlight DWI's role as a crucial part of MRI protocols that can play an important role in providing valuable information to increase the specificity and sensitivity of clinical diagnoses. The inclusion of DWI in standard MRI practices, therefore, marks an important milestone in the advancement of medical imaging.

5.3.4. Contrast-Enhanced MRI Techniques

The addition of contrast-enhanced techniques to MRI has revolutionized the imaging diagnostic paradigm by making it possible to visualize tumorous tissue and discriminate between benign and malignant lesions. Dynamic contrast-enhanced MRI (DCE-MRI), for instance, provides critical details regarding hemodynamic features of lesions to enable more accurate diagnoses of tumor biology and physiology, as evidenced by studies on non-mass enhancement (NME) breast lesions demonstrating how features like heterogeneous enhancement correlate with malignancy risk (Bayoumi et al., 2024). Similarly, techniques such as dynamic susceptibility contrast MRI (DSC-MRI) further enrich the information by providing descriptions of perfusion dynamics, effectively bridging between structural and functional data (Tang et al., 2024). With the advent of these newer technologies, the usefulness of multiparametric approaches emerges, improving diagnostic performance and laying the groundwork for personalized therapeutic strategies. Generally, contrast-enhanced MRI techniques are an effective medical imaging breakthrough, both enhancing diagnostic precision and clinical outcomes.

5.3.5. MRI Angiography and Its Significance

The integration of advanced imaging technology into the clinical environment significantly enhances the ability to assess vascular disease via MRI angiography, a noninvasive technique that uses magnetic resonance imaging principles to visualize blood vessels. This modality is special in that it can provide high-resolution images of vascular structures without subjecting patients to the dangers of ionizing radiation, making it particularly valuable for the diagnosis and treatment of conditions such as aneurysms and arterial stenosis. Using specific pulse sequences and contrast modes, MRI angiography can distinguish normal and pathological vessels, helping with a range of surgical and therapeutic interventions, including pre-operative planning and post-operative assessment (Sabrina et al., 2024). Furthermore, the application of machine learning and artificial intelligence to MRI angiograms enhances their usability and diagnostic power, potentially revolutionizing the practice of vascular imaging in the clinical setting (Komenan, 2024). MRI angiography is thus a revolutionary technique in modern medicine, exemplifying the extensive implications of technology in healthcare outcomes.

5.3.6. Protocols for Specific Body Regions (Brain, Spine, Joints)

The diversity of MRI protocols necessitates a tailored strategy to different anatomical regions, including the brain, spine, and joints, each with its own individual diagnostic requirements. For brain imaging, protocols are biased toward T1- and T2-weighted images to render anatomy and identify pathologies such as tumors or ischemia in the best possible manner. By comparison, spinal imaging protocols can include specialized techniques such as diffusion tensor imaging to assess white matter integrity, as well as sequences designed to enhance visualization of neural structures and adjacent tissues. Imaging of joints, particularly the shoulder or knee, often uses fat-suppressed sequences to depict cartilage, ligaments, and other soft tissues, providing useful information on conditions such as tears or arthritis. These tailored procedures emphasize the importance of obtaining an understanding of specific imaging requirements to achieve optimal diagnostic precision and patient safety in MRI practice (Steven et al., 2021; Bryan et al., 2021).

5.3.7. Patient Preparation and Positioning in MRI

patient preparation and positioning are determinants of successful MRI outcomes, as they affect both the quality of the images produced and patients' comfort during the procedure. Before imaging, in-depth communication of the MRI procedure—such as the need for stillness—can reduce patient movement artifacts that negatively impact image quality. The role of proper positioning is further emphasized by statistics indicating that almost 98.78% of panoramic radiography errors result from patient positioning errors (Suparno et al., 2023). This relationship holds for MRI as well, where misalignment can mask anatomical features important for diagnosis. Furthermore, management of conditions such as claustrophobia and anxiety in patients via pre-scan reassurance, as well as the use of appropriate supports or cushions, has the potential to enhance compliance and comfort (Huang et al., 2024). Therefore, attention to the preparation protocol and positioning maximizes image integrity and improves the patient experience during MRI procedures.

5.3.8. Artifacts in MRI and How to Minimize Them

In MRI, numerous artifacts can severely degrade diagnostic precision and image quality, making it necessary to employ efficient minimization techniques. The most prevalent of these artifacts are motion artifacts, which are caused by patient movement during imaging and can be avoided by techniques such as breath-holding and faster imaging sequences. Also, susceptibility artifacts are produced by local magnetic field inhomogeneities, which are normally exacerbated by the presence of ferromagnetic material, to highlight the importance of maintaining a clear appreciation of an MRI environment to improve patient safety and image quality (Gaeta et al., 2024). Moreover, chemical shift artifacts can distort fat-water interfaces in images, but this can be corrected by applying fat-saturation techniques in pulse sequences (Mukherjee et al., 2025). Such techniques cumulatively enhance the integrity of MRI images and result in more accurate clinical assessments and improved patient outcomes.

5.3.9. Advanced Imaging Techniques (e.g., Spectroscopy)

The comingling of advanced imaging techniques and MRI is critical for enhancing diagnostic data and expanding applications in clinical usage. Among these techniques, magnetic resonance spectroscopy (MRS) stands out through its capacity to provide biochemical information about tissues, complementing the anatomical information afforded by conventional MRI. This new technique facilitates the study of metabolic processes by examining the chemical composition of tissues, allowing clinicians to detect abnormal states, such as tumors, using metabolic markers. Technology, including more effective magnetic field shimming, has developed enormously and hence improved the field homogeneity required for MRS, ultimately providing clearer and more precise spectral data and image quality (Shang et al., 2024). In addition, hyperspectral imaging and Raman spectroscopy are emerging as promising techniques that, when integrated with MRI, can reveal intricate biochemical and structural information about tissues and enable more precise evaluations in real-world clinical settings (Lan et al., 2024). Thus, the convergence of these advanced approaches with MRI is revolutionizing the diagnostic frontier.

5.4. Clinical Uses of MRI

The past decade has seen the clinical setting increasingly recognize MRI's pivotal role in diagnosing many medical conditions. Most visibly pronounced in neurological, musculoskeletal, and oncologic applications, MRI's ability to generate high-resolution images without the need for ionizing radiation has revolutionized patient management. For instance, its undisputed soft-tissue contrast is of great value for tumor identification and typing in the brain, enabling precise treatment planning and post-therapeutic follow-up evaluation of changes (Preetha et al., 2024). Moreover, developments in pulse sequences, such as ultrashort echo time (UTE) techniques, have enhanced MRI's performance in the imaging of mineralized tissues in dentistry, providing alternatives to traditional radiographic modalities based on the use of ionizing radiation (Vaddi et al., 2025). The use of deep learning techniques in MRI analysis has great promise in streamlining tumor detection and improving diagnostic accuracy, with a profound impact on clinical processes and patient outcomes in a wide range of medical specialties.

5.4.1. Neurological Applications of MRI

Magnetic Resonance Imaging (MRI) has transformed the diagnosis and treatment of neurological disorders with its advent. With its ability to provide unrivaled soft tissue contrast, MRI enables the detection of a wide range of neurological conditions, from tumors to trauma-related disorders. The application of techniques such as Diffusion Tensor Imaging (DTI) supplements standard imaging protocols by elucidating microscopic changes in brain tissue that are pivotal in conditions such as neonatal hypoxic-ischemic encephalopathy (HIE) (Onda et al., 2023). Furthermore, the application of advanced functionalities such as Functional MRI (fMRI) has allowed clinicians to explore patterns of brain activity, thereby improving therapeutic interventions and predictive assessments (Krish, 2024). The evolution of MRI in neurological applications underscores its pivotal role in both acute clinical care and long-term planning, making a significant leap toward improved patient outcomes in this intricate field of medicine.

5.4.2. MRI Musculoskeletal Imaging

The use of MRI has transformed the care of musculoskeletal disorders, enabling soft tissues and joints to be accurately imaged without exposing patients to ionizing radiation. This capability is most beneficial for assessing cartilage degeneration, ligament injury, and muscle diseases, where standard imaging devices are deficient. MRI provides high-contrast images using methods such as T1- and T2-weighted sequences, enhancing the delineation of different tissue types (N/A, 2011). Pulse sequence optimization, such as spin-echo and inversion recovery, plays a critical role in optimizing image quality for musculoskeletal applications. Additionally, by measuring fluid dynamics using diffusion and perfusion imaging, doctors can obtain valuable information about conditions such as osteoarthritis and tendon injury. As a result, MRI has emerged as a valuable tool in musculoskeletal imaging, allowing a non-invasive approach to the diagnosis and monitoring of complicated diseases (N/A, 1997).

5.4.3. Cardiovascular MRI techniques

The introduction of advanced imaging modalities into cardiovascular evaluation has revolutionized diagnostic procedures, particularly through MRI. The modality stands out because it provides information on multiple dimensions of both structural and functional heart details and has emerged as a gold standard for such assessments.

Among its many applications, cardiovascular MRI plays a pivotal role in assessing epicardial adipose tissue, a cornerstone for understanding nonischemic cardiovascular diseases, especially those related to type 2 diabetes (Kotha et al., 2024). MRI techniques such as T1 mapping are also crucial for elucidating pathologic mechanisms that affect cardiac tissues by investigating relaxation times influenced by tissue composition and disease states (Gaeta et al., 2024). Together, these methods not only enhance diagnostic precision but also facilitate the assessment of therapeutic responses, thus highlighting their role in modern cardiovascular practice.

5.4.4. Oncological Applications of MRI

In modern oncology, MRI's ability to provide high-fidelity anatomical and functional evaluation has made it a crucial tool for diagnosing and managing cancer. In particular, MRI is helpful in evaluating soft-tissue tumors, where its high contrast resolution is superior to that of conventional imaging techniques. Using advanced techniques such as diffusion-weighted imaging and dynamic contrast-enhanced MRI, physicians can assess tumor characteristics, including cellularity and perfusion, both of which are important for planning therapy. Also, with increasing applications of artificial intelligence (AI) in oncological imaging, the future for automating image analysis and enhancing diagnostic efficiency is promising. But there remain barriers in introducing AI tools into daily clinical use, with ongoing collaboration between clinicians and researchers still required (Masino et al., 2024). As MRI technology has improved, its use in designing personalized therapeutic schedules is bound to expand, only further making it a vital tool in the treatment of cancer (Paudyal et al., 2023).

5.4.5. Pediatric Applications of MRI

Over the past decade, the use of MRI in pediatrics has advanced significantly in diagnosing and treating a wide range of conditions in children. The flexibility of MRI technology enables it to serve as a non-invasive, radiation-free imaging modality, particularly important when dealing with the fragile anatomy and physiology of children. Pediatric MRI applications are more likely to include the assessment of neurological disorders, such as cerebral abnormalities or tumors, as well as musculoskeletal disorders arising from growth. Besides, MRI's ability to generate highly detailed images enhances the detection of developmental abnormalities, which can be invaluable for planning therapeutic intervention. Most of all, improvements in pulse sequence generation and image contrast mechanisms have further optimized pediatric imaging protocols, thereby enhancing diagnostic accuracy and minimizing patient stress (N/A, 1997; N/A, 2011). With a new methodology, MRI continues to improve the care context for pediatric patients, paving the way for improved health outcomes.

5.4.6. Planning MRI for Surgery

Preoperative imaging is a part of surgical planning, particularly in those surgeries where anatomical precision is critical. MRI has proven to be a valuable resource in this regard, providing high-quality images of the soft-tissue structures involved in surgical planning. Its ability to delineate significant features, e.g., tumor borders and local invasion, can go a long way towards aiding treatment plans. For instance, studies have shown that preoperative staging with diffusion-weighted imaging (DWI) improves cancer staging accuracy by providing important information on tumor aggressiveness, as evidenced by reduced apparent diffusion coefficient values associated with deep invasion and other prognostic factors (Gehad et al., 2024). Additionally, MRIs' function includes assessing intricate anatomical variations that can affect surgical techniques, for example, cochlear implantation surgeries, where imaging before surgery can accurately foretell surgical challenges (Jerosha et al., 2024). Such thorough imaging, in turn, yields better surgical outcomes.

5.4.7. Role of MRI in Treatment Response Monitoring

A key aspect of contemporary medical imaging is ongoing monitoring for treatment response; a field where MRI dominates. With its higher-quality contrast in soft tissues and its ability to provide dynamic visualization of tumors, MRI is at the forefront of realizing personalized therapeutic approaches for numerous cancers. For instance, MRI has helped monitor the responses of glioblastoma patients to therapy by using advanced analysis tools, such as clustering analysis of functional MRI data, to detect subtle changes in tumor characteristics (Simone et al., 2024). Furthermore, breakthroughs in deep learning enhanced MRI segmentation accuracy so that clinicians may make timely adjustments to treatment protocols based on quantified patient response to treatment (Liu et al., 2024). MRI thus not only provides disease status at the moment but also enables strategic planning of future interventions, increasing its value in the cancer treatment and monitoring continuum.

5.4.8. Limitations and Challenges in Clinical Applications

The clinical application of MRI is hampered by several significant limitations and difficulties that detract from its full value and potential in modern medicine. The inherent complexity of MRI technologies is one such limitation, which gives rise to variability in image quality and interpretation and is aggravated by factors such as patient movement and susceptibility artifacts. Also, the presence of certain substances, such as macromolecules and gadolinium-containing contrast media, can significantly alter T1 relaxation times, making diagnosis of pathologies without clear imaging signs problematic (Gaeta et al., 2024). In addition, despite technological advances in functional magnetic resonance imaging, there are challenges in its clinical application, particularly in mental illnesses such as schizophrenia, wherein issues of cost, availability, and realistic application of fMRI findings in clinical decision making persist (Voineskos et al., 2024). This must be resolved to optimize MRIs' contribution to patient outcomes and improve diagnostic accuracy.

5.4.9. Case Studies Demonstrating MRI Effectiveness

In considering the broad-based strengths of MRI, several case studies demonstrate its effectiveness in practice. For instance, a dynamic contrast-enhanced MRI (DCE-MRI) study demonstrated enhanced diagnostic benefit in distinguishing sinonasal lymphoma from sinonasal carcinoma, using varying imaging parameters to achieve an area under the curve of 0.945 when combining DCE-MRI and diffusion-weighted imaging data (Liu et al., 2024). A relevant study demonstrated the effect of guided imagery as an intervention to reduce levels of patient anxiety during MRI scans, demonstrating a significant reduction in anxiety scores post-intervention (Shojaie et al., 2024). Such case studies not only highlight MRI's versatility in a range of clinical conditions but also illustrate how adjunct therapies can enhance the overall patient experience and diagnostic yield. These findings support the growing importance of MRI in today's diagnostic imaging, affirming its essential role in patient care.

SUMMARY

Progress in MRI has transformed diagnostic imaging, providing unprecedented insight into soft tissue anatomy and improving patient care. As has been detailed throughout this essay, the unique capacity of MRIs to create high-contrast images and their varied pulse sequences and sophisticated hardware equipment enable clinicians to effectively diagnose a wide variety of conditions. The significance of safety protocols, including RF heating control and implant problems, cannot be overstated as these are vital in ensuring patient health during the imaging procedures. Moreover, studies into image contrast mechanisms and artifact minimization are further enhancing MRI technology, reflecting once again its dynamic nature in the healthcare industry. Lastly, as outlined in recent studies, for example, exploring ways of bowel preparation for MRI (Wang et al., 2024) and cardiovascular diseases evaluated through CMRI (Zareiamand et al., 2023), the potential of MRI in the future is vast for increasing diagnostic accuracy and patient outcomes.

The MRI examination encompasses a broad array of fundamental principles and technological aspects that enable it to be effective in medical diagnostics. The description goes as far as the most essential physics of nuclear magnetic resonance, such as coverages of spin and magnetic moment, Larmor frequency, and relaxation mechanisms that are the basis of MRI's operating principles. Further, key hardware components, including various magnets, gradient coils, and RF transmitters, are reviewed to determine their roles in image formation. More significantly, the spin-echo and gradient-echo sequences' pulse sequence design is discussed, and how these protocols influence the quality and contrast of images is explained. The physics of image contrast caused by T1 and T2 weighting and proton density are imperative for tissue discrimination. Finally, artifacts related to motion and susceptibility, as well as protection concerns in association with RF heating and ferromagnetic hazards, define the entire scope of MRI application in the clinical setting (Bonetti et al., 2016; Waseem et al., 2018).

The application of MRI in medicine has profoundly changed diagnostic methods and the delivery of care. First identified as a means to produce detailed pictures of soft tissue, MRI has also been developed to incorporate many advanced applications, including fMRI and diffusion tensor imaging (DTI), to yield information on brain activity and the integrity of nerve tracts, respectively. These developments enable clinicians to detect previously challenging-to-visualize pathologies, such as early tumors or slight alterations of the nervous system. In addition, artificial intelligence and machine learning are just beginning to interpret MRIs autonomously, advancing diagnostic validity and efficiency in the clinical setting. For instance, deep learning methods have been shown to produce promising results in diagnosing illnesses like Alzheimer's disease and to reflect the evolving role of MRI in facilitating timely intervention and customized treatment schedules (Tjoa et al., 2020; Jo et al., 2019). As MRI technology advances, its potential to enhance patient outcomes is increasingly realized.

CLOSER LOOK

MAGNETIC RESONANCE IMAGING IN MODERN MEDICINE: LIFELONG LEARNING, CLINICAL VALUE, AND ETHICAL CONSIDERATIONS

In a day and age when technology is improving at lightning speed, the role of continuing education in Magnetic Resonance Imaging (MRI) cannot be overstated. With the rapid development of technology, professionals must remain abreast of new methods and technological improvements that enhance diagnostic yields and protect patients. Continuing education ensures a deeper understanding of MRI physics, enabling radiologists and technicians to use sophisticated pulse sequences and optimize imaging protocols. Moreover, with the advent of artificial intelligence affecting medical imaging processes, an educated workforce is required to impart necessary skills to deal with the complexities associated with machine learning technology in MRI (Tjoa et al., 2020). Finally, professional education promotes technical skills required to address evolving challenges, as well as interpretive skills to evaluate and utilize advanced imaging modalities in the right context (Williams et al., 2018). Thus, the assurance of lifelong learning remains the foundation of professionalism in MRI. Magnetic Resonance Imaging (MRI) has radically changed patient management and outcomes across most medical specialties.

Its non-invasiveness allows for widespread imaging without the use of ionizing radiation, characteristic of other modalities, representing an important advance in pediatric therapy where radiation sensitivity is a factor. Evidence indicates that MRI plays a pivotal role in diagnosing conditions such as tumors, neurological disorders, and cardiovascular disease, leading to individualized treatment plans that enhance prognosis (Théo et al., 2021). Further, the ability to assess vascular organs and soft-tissue contrast provides vital information that can inform intraoperative decisions and thereby reduce the need for exploratory surgery and its attendant risks. As MRI becomes increasingly woven into routine practice within healthcare systems, its impact appears as enhanced diagnostic accuracy and optimized patient outcomes. As a result, the clinical advantages of MRI benefit not only from effective patient care but also from therapeutic strategy advancements (Young-Kim et al., 2020). Implementation of MRI in medical practice poses substantial ethical issues to be carefully addressed to promote patient well-being and informed decision-making.

As MRI technology advances, ethical considerations regarding incidental findings rise to the forefront. For instance, while MRI can identify abnormal results that may be of no clinical significance, revelation of such types of findings has the potential to cause anxiety and unjustified follow-up treatments for patients who were initially unaware of potential health issues (Sullivan et al., 2024). Furthermore, the existence of MRI technology creates health inequalities, where underprivileged patients may not receive an equal opportunity for screening (Lorenzo, 2025). In consequence, there should be a balance between the benefits of sophisticated imaging technology and the ethical need to provide equal access, transparency, and support to patients navigating the complexities of their healthcare information. With advancing medical imaging technology, the role of MRI technology is seen to be a prominent area of significance.MRIs' capacity to produce high-resolution images without ionizing radiation has revolutionized diagnostic imaging, particularly in neuroimaging and musculoskeletal assessment. Worth mentioning, its advantages extend beyond mere visual presentation; the technique enables unique contrast mechanisms that enhance tissue discrimination, aiding precise disease localization and characterization. Further, technologies such as fMRI and diffusion tensor imaging have expanded the application of MRIs to fields such as brain mapping and understanding neural pathways, a promising indicator of the future.(Wu et al., 2023) Despite challenges such as artifacts and safety procedures remaining, a shift in focus towards ongoing education and the improvement of technology is underway—MRI remains an essential piece of equipment that exemplifies the confluence of innovation and patient care in current medicine. (María et al., 2020)

REFERENCES

1. Abadi, E., Segars, W. P., Tsui, B. M. W., Kinahan, P. E., Bottenus, N., Frangi, A. F., Maidment, A., Lo, J., & Samei, E. (2020). Virtual clinical trials in medical imaging: a review. *Journal of Medical Imaging, 7*(04), 1. https://doi.org/10.1117/1.jmi.7.4.042805Aboitiz, A., Alexander, A., Andersson, A., Assaf, Y., Barazany, D., et al. (2016). Microstructural parameter estimation *in vivo* using diffusion MRI and structured prior information. https://core.ac.uk/download/29416144.pdf (accessed on 14th July 2025).
2. Abreu, M. T., Sandborn, W. J., Cataldi, F., D'Haens, G. R., Feagan, B. G., Hanauer, S. B., Jairath, V., et al. (2020). Defining endpoints and biomarkers in inflammatory bowel disease: Moving the needle through clinical trial design. *Gastroenterology, 159*, 2013–2018.e7. https://doi.org/10.1053/j.gastro.2020.07.064 (accessed on 14th July 2025).
3. Aggarwal, P., Malik, R., Sarawagi, R., & Kumar, A. (2024). Comparing the efficacy of a combination of diffusion-weighted imaging and T2-STIR (short tau inversion recovery) imaging with contrast-enhanced MRI in the evaluation of perianal fistula. *Cureus, 16*. https://www.semanticscholar.org/paper/e88e0e384d1ac66680eabb447eb890a6f29387e6 (accessed on 14th July 2025).
4. Akbarzadeh, A., Samiei, M., & Davaran, S. (2012). Magnetic nanoparticles: Preparation, physical properties, and applications in biomedicine. *Nanoscale Research Letters, 7*. https://doi.org/10.1186/1556-276x-7-144 (accessed on 14th July 2025).
5. Baltz, V., Manchon, A., Tsoi, M., Moriyama, T., Ono, T., & Tserkovnyak, Y. (2018). Antiferromagnetic spintronics. *Reviews of Modern Physics, 90*. https://doi.org/10.1103/revmodphys.90.015005 (accessed on 14th July 2025).
6. Bayoumi, D., Shokeir, F. A., Karam, R., & Elboghdady, A. (2024). Validity of dynamic contrast-enhanced magnetic resonance imaging of the breast versus diffusion-weighted imaging and magnetic resonance spectroscopy in predicting the malignant nature of non-mass enhancement lesions. *Egyptian Journal of Radiology and Nuclear Medicine*. https://www.semanticscholar.org/paper/6e6fa4b7c934cba7f2445925e43a702c734ffa74 (accessed on 14th July 2025).
7. Begley, S. L., McBriar, J., Pelcher, I., & Schulder, M. (2024). Intraoperative MRI: A review of applications across neurosurgical specialties. *Neurosurgery, 95*, 527–536. https://www.semanticscholar.org/paper/b258a8e6ec8bc5df94c0857984101c5a5f132770 (accessed on 14th July 2025).
8. Berry, D., Gordon, J. A., Adair, V., Frank, L. R., & Ward, S. R. (2024). From voxels to physiology: A review of diffusion magnetic resonance imaging applications in skeletal muscle. *Journal of Magnetic Resonance Imaging, 61*, 595–615. https://www.semanticscholar.org/paper/592b4b6da1f3a670c84af00a1fd5af6612cebab9 (accessed on 14th July 2025).
9. Bhuiyan, M. M. H., Gupta, K. D., Hossain, I., Islam, M., et al. (2023). Introduction of medical imaging modalities. http://arxiv.org/abs/2306.01022 (accessed on 14th July 2025).
10. Bian, W., Jang, A., & Liu, F. (2024). Multi-task magnetic resonance imaging reconstruction using meta-learning. *Magnetic Resonance Imaging*. https://www.semanticscholar.org/paper/b8a16fd8d823cfe683c19d58bec77a023b5bf1ef (accessed on 14th July 2025).
11. Bogart, L. K., Johansson, C., Kazakova, O., Pankhurst, Q. A., et al. (2017). Standardization of magnetic nanoparticles in liquid suspension. https://core.ac.uk/download/111037210.pdf (accessed on 14th July 2025).

12. Bonetti, S. (2016). X-ray imaging of spin currents and magnetization dynamics at the nanoscale. http://arxiv.org/abs/1611.07691 (accessed on 14th July 2025).
13. Borgheresi, A., De Muzio, F., Agostini, A., Ottaviani, L., Bruno, A., Granata, V., Fusco, R., et al. (2022). Lymph nodes evaluation in rectal cancer: Where do we stand and future perspective. *Journal of Clinical Medicine, 11*, 2599–2599. https://doi.org/10.3390/jcm11092599 (accessed on 14th July 2025).
14. Box, M. W., Marsh, L., Major, J., Puga, T. B., Poffenbarger, M., & Riehl, J. T. (2025). Safety and utility of magnetic resonance imaging of patients with external fixators: A systematic review. *OTA International, 8*. https://www.semanticscholar.org/paper/b55b0c2f4c31daca4a39ed46b509b8b9df905215 (accessed on 14th July 2025).
15. Brookes, M. J., Leggett, J., Rea, M., Hill, R. M., Holmes, N., Boto, E., & Bowtell, R. (2022). Magnetoencephalography with optically pumped magnetometers (OPM-MEG): The next generation of functional neuroimaging. *Trends in Neurosciences, 45*, 621–634. https://doi.org/10.1016/j.tins.2022.05.008 (accessed on 14th July 2025).
16. Cameron, D., Gatehouse, P. D., Prasad, S. K., Vassiliou, V., et al. (2018). Magnetic resonance imaging: Physics basics for the cardiologist. https://core.ac.uk/download/157862011.pdf (accessed on 14th July 2025).
17. Campbell, S. C., Uzzo, R. G., Karam, J. A., Chang, S. S., Clark, P. E., & Souter, L. (2021). Renal mass and localized renal cancer: Evaluation, management, and follow-up: AUA guideline: Part II. *The Journal of Urology, 206*, 209–218. https://doi.org/10.1097/ju.0000000000001912 (accessed on 14th July 2025).
18. Chu, C., Ji, Z., & Li, B. (2024). [Research on construction of knowledge base for MRI equipment maintenance based on knowledge graph]. *Zhongguo yi liao qi xie za zhi = Chinese Journal of Medical Instrumentation, 48*(5), 544–548. https://www.semanticscholar.org/paper/b26023e7ebfb4922d343a5c4b8d0231bfef633ba (accessed on 14th July 2025).
19. Cong, W., Durairaj, K., & Feng, P. (2013). Mathematical methods in biomedical imaging. *Computational and Mathematical Methods in Medicine, 2013*. https://www.semanticscholar.org/paper/c4e277be086f9294ac19a3c0a78c6ffce1359128 (accessed on 14th July 2025).
20. De Simone, M., Iaconetta, G., Palermo, G., Fiorindi, A., Schaller, K., & de Maria, L. (2024). Clustering functional magnetic resonance imaging time series in glioblastoma characterization: A review of the evolution, applications, and potentials. *Brain Sciences, 14*. https://www.semanticscholar.org/paper/a71557b6f019a8f7fdd0e0a3dbcbad1c308bb6ef (accessed on 14th July 2025).
21. Ding, Q. (2025). Advances in medical imaging equipment: A review of research progress and clinical applications. *Highlights in Science, Engineering and Technology*. https://www.semanticscholar.org/paper/0b6e1cf961cfae2ad3203a11c49a9fabcf8e5289 (accessed on 14th July 2025).
22. Farrant, J. P., Black, N., Yamagata, K., Soltani, F., Orsborne, C., Yan, C. K., Clark, D. J., et al. (2025). Comprehensive reference ranges for cardiovascular magnetic resonance: Time to move on from single center data? *The International Journal of Cardiovascular Imaging, 41*, 913–932. https://www.semanticscholar.org/paper/7e7bdb1c7a3904ea8950202fe065bb3865b43173 (accessed on 14th July 2025).

23. Gaeta, M., Galletta, K., Cavallaro, M., Mormina, E., Cannizzaro, M. T., Lanzafame, L. R. M., D'Angelo, T., et al. (2024). T1 relaxation: Chemo-physical fundamentals of magnetic resonance imaging and clinical applications. *Insights into Imaging, 15*. https://www.semanticscholar.org/paper/35c2a557a83fd535c60d4cf12b8971ec683590ca (accessed on 14th July 2025).

24. Gu, D., Shi, F., Hua, R., Wei, Y., Li, Y., Zhu, J., Zhang, W., et al. (2022). An artificial-intelligence-based age-specific template construction framework for brain structural analysis using magnetic resonance images. *Human Brain Mapping, 44*, 861–875. https://www.semanticscholar.org/paper/2b877f89d4ba3e999d43f990f9b96ebc649ce187 (accessed on 14th July 2025).

25. Harshe, G. U. (2024). *Magnetic Resonance Imaging in Evaluation of Endometriosis: Case-Based Pictorial Essay*. https://www.semanticscholar.org/paper/04ebd3e8a20f4dab57e042337083787ded99ef27 (accessed on 14th July 2025).

26. Heskamp, L., Birkbeck, M. G., Baxter-Beard, D., Hall, J., Schofield, I., Elameer, M., Whittaker, R. G., et al. (2024). Motor unit magnetic resonance imaging (MUMRI) in skeletal muscle. *Journal of Magnetic Resonance Imaging, 60*. https://www.semanticscholar.org/paper/b20fd02a9fc95935246b3ab336c887e82f94ae1b (accessed on 14th July 2025).

27. Huang, J., Wu, Y., Wang, F., Fang, Y., Nan, Y., Alkan, C., Abraham, D., et al. (2024). Data- and physics-driven deep learning-based reconstruction for fast MRI: Fundamentals and methodologies. *IEEE Reviews in Biomedical Engineering, 18*, 152–171. https://www.semanticscholar.org/paper/a381766b436d69949e38a8a3c4220fa622ec44b7 (accessed on 14th July 2025).

28. Huang, L. (2017). Nuclear magnetic resonance methods for characterization of mass transport in porous materials. https://core.ac.uk/download/132609283.pdf (accessed on 14th July 2025).

29. Hughes, S. J., & Ciulli, A. (2017). Molecular recognition of ternary complexes: A new dimension in the structure-guided design of chemical degraders. *Essays in Biochemistry, 61*, 505–516. https://doi.org/10.1042/ebc20170041 (accessed on 14th July 2025).

30. Jayaraman, M. (2008). Neurovascular imaging. *Topics in Magnetic Resonance Imaging: TMRI, 19*(5), 223. https://www.semanticscholar.org/paper/f9688bfea80fdfab9f3ab311585e1ce42f4e81fa (accessed on 14th July 2025).

31. Jerosha, S., Subramonian, S. G., Mohanakrishnan, A., Muralidharan, Y., & Natarajan, P. (2024). Preoperative assessment using CT and MRI scans of the temporal bone to determine the degree of difficulty in cochlear implant surgery. *Cureus, 16*. https://www.semanticscholar.org/paper/4eb07e97e39fff50fa1dafc3c2a3a023ac342e6c (accessed on 14th July 2025).

32. Jiang, Z., Zhang, M., Zhang, Q., & Xie, Y. (2024). A low-field magnetic resonance signal transmission and reception processing platform. *2024 7th International Conference on Information Communication and Signal Processing (ICICSP)*. https://www.semanticscholar.org/paper/3a712ae655dc0b2c4613f5c2beb8699ce8d7d396 (accessed on 14th July 2025).

33. Jo, T., Nho, K., & Saykin, A. J. (2019). Deep learning in Alzheimer's disease: Diagnostic classification and prognostic prediction using neuroimaging data. *Frontiers in Aging Neuroscience, 11*. https://doi.org/10.3389/fnagi.2019.00220 (accessed on 14th July 2025).

34. Jung, A. Y. (2024). Basics for pediatric brain tumor imaging: Techniques and protocol recommendations. *Brain Tumor Research and Treatment, 12*, 1–13. https://www.semanticscholar.org/paper/ab89d83c6cf356754a7fb8394c247b43514836f1 (accessed on 14th July 2025).

35. Kamel, R. J., Karim, S. N., Musa, M. M., Naeem, M., et al. (2024). Advancements in medical imaging technologies: Ultrasound, X-ray, and MRI. https://core.ac.uk/download/620857181.pdf (accessed on 14th July 2025).

36. Kelly, C., Karthikesalingam, A., Suleyman, M., Corrado, G. S., & King, D. (2019). Key challenges for delivering clinical impact with artificial intelligence. *BMC Medicine, 17*. https://doi.org/10.1186/s12916-019-1426-2 (accessed on 14th July 2025).

37. Kholmatov, J. A., Askarov, O. O., Pilania, H., & Kawale, K. V. (2023). Applications of physics in diagnostic imaging. *European Journal of Medical Genetics and Clinical Biology*. https://www.semanticscholar.org/paper/2a0cbb11533ae7eeea6c5fc94e274b3523533898 (accessed on 14th July 2025).

38. Kim, Y. H., Chen, S. A., Ernst, S., Guzmán, C., Han, S., Kalarus, Z., Labadet, C., et al. (2020). 2019 APHRS expert consensus statement on three-dimensional mapping systems for tachycardia developed in collaboration with HRS, EHRA, and LAHRS. *Journal of Arrhythmia, 36*, 215–270. https://doi.org/10.1002/joa3.12308 (accessed on 14th July 2025).

39. Komenan, Y. (2024). Beyond today's MRI: Machine learning and AI pioneering tomorrow's imaging landscape. *Current Journal of Applied Science and Technology*. https://www.semanticscholar.org/paper/9b9d85c11e70a40a7c5865fdd41f5fdf4d91a143 (accessed on 14th July 2025).

40. Kotha, S., Plein, S., Greenwood, J. P., & Levelt, E. (2024). Role of epicardial adipose tissue in diabetic cardiomyopathy through the lens of cardiovascular magnetic resonance imaging–A narrative review. *Therapeutic Advances in Endocrinology and Metabolism, 15*. https://www.semanticscholar.org/paper/19eb66621d13930a78c35e66d92c39f4023f11d5 (accessed on 14th July 2025).

41. Krish, A. H. (2024). Comparative analysis of traditional and modern imaging techniques in neurological disorders. *International Journal for Multidisciplinary Research*. https://www.semanticscholar.org/paper/4e51f03494dccbec769e279f352f3bc65a77572e (accessed on 14th July 2025).

42. Kui, X., Fan, Z., Ji, Z., Li, Q., Liu, C., Si, W., & Zou, B. (2025). A comprehensive survey on magnetic resonance image reconstruction. *ArXiv, abs/2503.07097*. https://www.semanticscholar.org/paper/c386ba84d843a019cf26a43be30310edc625f3c8 (accessed on 14th July 2025).

43. Kumar, G. S., Borah, P., Islam, A., & Kashyap, S. (2025). Patterns of magnetic resonance imaging and early detection via diffusion-weighted imaging of neonatal hypoxic brain injury: A cross-sectional study. *Indian Journal of Neonatal Medicine and Research*. https://www.semanticscholar.org/paper/7a3adb61edb72df31ea095e48861017121d7d08a (accessed on 14th July 2025).

44. Kutlić, G., & Dolić, K. (2025). Comparison of magnetic resonance imaging of the prostate 1.5T and 3T. *Radiološki vjesnik*. https://www.semanticscholar.org/paper/e3c8040d16b3720e2ba723bdded803525d88db57 (accessed on 14th July 2025).

45. Kwok, W. (2024). Radiofrequency interference in magnetic resonance imaging: Identification and rectification. *Journal of Clinical Imaging Science, 14*. https://www.semanticscholar.org/paper/2320ec0375628f9ce7dc247dbd0ec0ddbc05e7f6 (accessed on 14th July 2025).

46. Lan, W., Hui, X., Nicolaï, B., Verboven, P., Qin, J., Renard, C. M. G. C., Jaillais, B., et al. (2024). Visualizing the structural and chemical heterogeneity of fruit and vegetables using advanced

imaging techniques: Fundamentals, instrumental aspects, applications and future perspectives. *Critical Reviews in Food Science and Nutrition*. https://www.semanticscholar.org/paper/702b0372ae38bedd862b154c1f257eec200bc891 (accessed on 14th July 2025).

47. Lau, J. (2019). Ultra-high field magnetic resonance imaging for stereotactic neurosurgery. https://core.ac.uk/download/215393664.pdf (accessed on 14th July 2025).

48. Lee, G., Does, M., Avila, R., Kang, J., Harkins, K., Wu, Y., Banks, W. E., et al. (2023). Implantable, bioresorbable radio frequency resonant circuits for magnetic resonance imaging. *Advanced Science, 11*. https://www.semanticscholar.org/paper/08d63dde13fea3a3f9d278292b11c2095d151979 (accessed on 14th July 2025).

49. Li, K., Kc, P., Li, H., Myers, K. J., Anastasio, M. A., & Zeng, R. (2025). Estimating task-based performance bounds for accelerated MRI image reconstruction methods by use of learned-ideal observers. *ArXiv*. https://www.semanticscholar.org/paper/42d7f0d34caec7e9e3817425b2f92ad55fafcd85 (accessed on 14th July 2025).

50. Liebschner, D., Afonine, P. V., Baker, M. L., Bunkòczi, G., Chen, V. B., Croll, T. I., Hintze, B. J., et al. (2019). Macromolecular structure determination using X-rays, neutrons and electrons: Recent developments in *Phenix*. *Acta Crystallographica Section D Structural Biology, 75*, 861–877. https://doi.org/10.1107/s2059798319011471 (accessed on 14th July 2025).

51. Liu, C., Wang, Y., Zhang, D., Zhou, J., Wu, Y., Guo, Y., Liu, R., et al. (2024). Value of multiparametric magnetic resonance imaging in distinguishing sinonasal lymphoma from sinonasal carcinoma: A case control study. *BMC Medical Imaging, 24*. https://www.semanticscholar.org/paper/3ca4abdcac4f97d5d6b1535b2e5d24894a492612 (accessed on 14th July 2025).

52. Liu, H., Chen, Y., Zhang, M., Bu, H., Lin, F., Chen, J., Xiao, M., et al. (2024). Feasibility of knee magnetic resonance imaging protocol using artificial intelligence-assisted iterative algorithm protocols: Comparison with standard MRI protocols. *Frontiers in Medicine, 11*. https://www.semanticscholar.org/paper/77d9bd698c1d998361385f05d475899aca6472c4 (accessed on 14th July 2025).

53. Liu, Z., Kainth, K., Zhou, A., Deyer, T., Fayad, Z., Greenspan, H., & Mei, X. (2024). A review of self-supervised, generative, and few-shot deep learning methods for data-limited magnetic resonance imaging segmentation. *NMR in Biomedicine, 37*. https://www.semanticscholar.org/paper/a69c737b3d2a902a9aaa06effe01f991215520b8 (accessed on 14th July 2025).

54. Malandris, K., Katsoula, A., Liakos, A., Bekiari, E., Karagiannis, T., Theocharidou, E., Giouleme, O., et al. (2024). Accuracy of controlled attenuation parameter for liver steatosis in patients at risk for metabolic dysfunction-associated steatosis liver disease using magnetic resonance imaging: A systematic review and meta-analysis. *Annals of Gastroenterology, 37*, 579–587. https://www.semanticscholar.org/paper/8ebd83ad5cc86bc45dc9b50058d98c7f6e56497b (accessed on 14th July 2025).

55. Mars, R. B., Passingham, R. E., & Jbabdi, S. (2018). Connectivity fingerprints: From areal descriptions to abstract spaces. *Trends in Cognitive Sciences, 22*, 1026–1037. https://doi.org/10.1016/j.tics.2018.08.009 (accessed on 14th July 2025).

56. Masino, F., Eusebi, L., Montatore, M., Muscatella, G., Gifuni, R., Ferrara, V., Marcellini, M., et al. (2024). Fundamentals of dual energy CT and its emerging applications in bladder cancer. *Digital Diagnostics*. https://www.semanticscholar.org/paper/916a7aecddf44ea6eca3e3fe1648160204708a5e (accessed on 14th July 2025).

57. Mohamed, T., Ismail, K. I., Shawky, M., Abdel, I., Lebda, A., Abdel, A., Al-Sammak, A., et al. (2024). Crohn's disease imaging and possible role of magnetic resonance imaging: Review article. *The Egyptian Journal of Hospital Medicine*. https://www.semanticscholar.org/paper/97c6cba85fe02d2a5d9baac9f78a73a2d1653a70 (accessed on 14th July 2025).

58. Mukherjee, T., Mendiola, E. A., Fugate, E., Lindquist, D., Myers, K., Sadayappan, S., & Avazmohammadi, R. (2025). Augmented long-axis acquisition in cardiac magnetic resonance imaging improves cardiac strain accuracy. *2025 IEEE 22nd International Symposium on Biomedical Imaging (ISBI)*. https://www.semanticscholar.org/paper/6080b177a210f8e1c4b8082cb55e5d3f3c3d9666 (accessed on 14th July 2025).

59. Mukku, S. R., Malikireddy, P., & Karpur, S. (2024). Diagnostic accuracy of diffusion-weighted imaging and perfusion-weighted imaging with dynamic susceptibility contrast in differentiating World Health Organization Grade-I meningioma from high-grade meningioma with histopathology as gold standard. *MRIMS Journal of Health Sciences*. https://www.semanticscholar.org/paper/001446bd18dc103203d2b0ddc243d04c9e64a879 (accessed on 14th July 2025).

60. Nagawa, K., Inoue, K., Hara, Y., Shimizu, H., Tsuchihashi, S., Matsuura, K., Kozawa, E., et al. (2024). Three-dimensional magnetic resonance imaging-based statistical shape analysis and machine learning-based prediction of patellofemoral instability. *Scientific Reports, 14*. https://www.semanticscholar.org/paper/0079fba2fb08dcb2ff4ef56ac92b293a1c011249 (accessed on 14th July 2025).

61. Nanz, D., Pazahr, S., & Sutter, R. (2023). 7 T musculoskeletal MRI: Fundamentals and clinical implementation. https://core.ac.uk/download/611954256.pdf (accessed on 14th July 2025).

62. Nensa, F., Bamberg, F., Rischpler, C., Menezes, L., Poeppel, T., Fougère, C., Beitzke, D., et al. (2018). Hybrid cardiac imaging using PET/MRI: A joint position statement by the European Society of Cardiovascular Radiology (ESCR) and the European Association of Nuclear Medicine (EANM). *European Journal of Hybrid Imaging, 2*, 1–23. https://www.semanticscholar.org/paper/307aeed8993f4561660ca1d80d54440e63fb7ae6 (accessed on 14th July 2025).

63. Onda, K., Chavez-Valdez, R., Graham, E., Everett, A., Northington, F., & Oishi, K. (2023). Quantification of diffusion magnetic resonance imaging for prognostic prediction of neonatal hypoxic-ischemic encephalopathy. *Developmental Neuroscience, 46*, 55–68. https://www.semanticscholar.org/paper/2955d9be046e2dde9d869c76e244dccffc5dcbef (accessed on 14th July 2025).

64. Patra, J. K., Das, G., Fraceto, L. F., Campos, E. V. R., Rodriguez-Torres, M. P., Acosta-Torres, L. S., Díaz-Torres, L. A., et al. (2018). Nano based drug delivery systems: Recent developments and future prospects. *Journal of Nanobiotechnology, 16*. https://doi.org/10.1186/s12951-018-0392-8 (accessed on 14th July 2025).

65. Paudyal, R., Shah, A., Akin, O., Do, R. K. G., Konar, A., Hatzoglou, V., Mahmood, U., et al. (2023). Artificial intelligence in CT and MR imaging for oncological applications. *Cancers, 15*. https://www.semanticscholar.org/paper/bc6b56919568e1f2ed447bc24a93befa9f6bfee2 (accessed on 14th July 2025).

66. Perera Molligoda Arachchige, S., & Politi, L. (2024). Potential applications of 7 Tesla magnetic resonance imaging in pediatric neuroimaging: Feasibility and challenges. *World Journal of Clinical Pediatrics, 13*. https://www.semanticscholar.org/paper/2a2d3fc6a8cd4d5f414f9c8c3e1894b2d38159c9 (accessed on 14th July 2025).

67. Pezel, T., Silva, L. M., Bau, A. A., Teixiera, A., Jerosch-Herold, M., & Coelho-Filho, O. R. (2021). What is the clinical impact of stress CMR after the ISCHEMIA trial? *Frontiers in Cardiovascular Medicine, 8*. https://doi.org/10.3389/fcvm.2021.683434 (accessed on 14th July 2025).
68. Preetha, R., Jasmine, M., Priyadarsini, P., & Nisha, J. S. (2024). Automated brain tumor detection from magnetic resonance images using fine-tuned EfficientNet-B4 convolutional neural network. *IEEE Access, 12*, 112181–112195. https://www.semanticscholar.org/paper/7a84add39881dc4c6dd628e665d9fe7541da94e8 (accessed on 14th July 2025).
69. Rizzo, G., & Tonni, G. (2023). Advances in maternal–fetal imaging. *Journal of Clinical Ultrasound, 51*. https://www.semanticscholar.org/paper/6ffad020790043540c4efaad238f458931b50782 (accessed on 14th July 2025).
70. Rosin-Paumier, S., El Youssef, R., Abdallah, A., Perrin, J. C., & Leclerc, S. (2023). Characterizing water transfer in compacted soils in the context of energy storage: Contribution of magnetic resonance imaging (MRI). *Symposium on Energy Geotechnics 2023*. https://www.semanticscholar.org/paper/0f59473607f12862b7cb27b72447c3114075151e (accessed on 14th July 2025).
71. Rout, M., Lipfert, M., Lee, B. L., Berjanskii, M., Assempour, N., Fresno, R. V., Serra Cayuela, A., et al. (2023). MagMet: A fully automated web server for targeted nuclear magnetic resonance metabolomics of plasma and serum. *Magnetic Resonance in Chemistry: MRC*. https://www.semanticscholar.org/paper/eb7dd8a9ac9ef7d30bb7190107ae5e87449ee29a (accessed on 14th July 2025).
72. Runge, S. B., Precht, H., Jensen, I. E., Jensen, K., Johannesen, T. A., Pedersen, M., & Christensen, N. (2024). Children centered care: Child and parent perspectives on a multi-faceted concept for magnetic resonance imaging without anesthesia–A survey. *Pediatric Radiology, 55*, 334–346. https://www.semanticscholar.org/paper/daa559d1670ede80ff5be55df7c04bacf338d0a7 (accessed on 14th July 2025).
73. Saito, S., & Ueda, J. (2024). Preclinical magnetic resonance imaging and spectroscopy in the fields of radiological technology, medical physics, and radiology. *Radiological Physics and Technology, 17*, 47–59. https://www.semanticscholar.org/paper/6fd029088fa0ef8963098cc046744af326e3226e (accessed on 14th July 2025).
74. Saleh, G. A., Abdelrazek, R., Hassan, A., Hamdy, O., & Tantawy, M. S. I. (2024). Diagnostic utility of apparent diffusion coefficient in preoperative assessment of endometrial cancer: Are we ready for the 2023 FIGO staging? *BMC Medical Imaging, 24*. https://www.semanticscholar.org/paper/f657badd5b5e5f9c19820bf40b08895819149f8e (accessed on 14th July 2025).
75. Schaefer, A., Kong, R., Gordon, E. M., Laumann, T. O., Zuo, X. N., Holmes, A. J., Eickhoff, S. B., et al. (2017). Local-global parcellation of the human cerebral cortex from intrinsic functional connectivity MRI. *Cerebral Cortex, 28*, 3095–3114. https://doi.org/10.1093/cercor/bhx179 (accessed on 14th July 2025).
76. Schmidt, S. (2020). On the quantification of fluid mechanical properties by means of magnetic resonance imaging. https://core.ac.uk/download/323364012.pdf (accessed on 14th July 2025).
77. Schneider, B. J., Naidoo, J., Santomasso, B., Lacchetti, C., Adkins, S., Anadkat, M. J., Atkins, M. B., et al. (2021). Management of immune-related adverse events in patients treated with immune checkpoint inhibitor therapy: ASCO guideline update. *Journal of Clinical Oncology, 39*, 4073–4126. https://doi.org/10.1200/jco.21.01440 (accessed on 14th July 2025).

78. Segura, J., Fernández-Valle, M. E., Cruz-Díaz, K., Romero-de-Ávila, M. D., Castejón, D., Remiro, V., & Cambero, M. I. (2024). Magnetic resonance imaging (MRI) of Spanish sheep cheese: A study on the relationships between ripening times, geographical origins, textural parameters, and MRI parameters. *Foods, 13*. https://www.semanticscholar.org/paper/c501c2a2afd2f2f87a9159299b79f3ee1bc3f783 (accessed on 14th July 2025).

79. Sempere, L. F. (2025). Ethical considerations and implications of multi-cancer early detection screening: Reliability, access and cost to test and treat. *Cambridge Quarterly of Healthcare Ethics: CQ: The International Journal of Healthcare Ethics Committees*. https://www.semanticscholar.org/paper/e4ebafeb8d43c090e33d33683a53c39b865c4cde (accessed on 14th July 2025).

80. Seu, V., & Maliga, O. (2025). Evaluation of magnetic resonance imaging in the detection of lumbar disc herniations in relation to clinical signs. *Bulletin of the Academy of Sciences of Moldova. Medical Sciences*. https://www.semanticscholar.org/paper/19eb3465adcc9ba0a530e80f16727a8bb9ae6ddb (accessed on 14th July 2025).

81. Shang, Y., Simegn, G., Gillen, K., Yang, H. J., & Han, H. (2024). Advancements in MR hardware systems and magnetic field control: B0 shimming, RF coils, and gradient techniques for enhancing magnetic resonance imaging and spectroscopy. *Psychoradiology, 4*. https://www.semanticscholar.org/paper/31382d51c6f3a71fd57cf26a3f8117317b62570f (accessed on 14th July 2025).

82. Shen, D., Wu, G., & Suk, H. I. (2017). Deep learning in medical image analysis. *Annual Review of Biomedical Engineering, 19*, 221–248. https://doi.org/10.1146/annurev-bioeng-071516-044442 (accessed on 14th July 2025).

83. Shojaie, A., Amiri, H., Dehesh, T., & Bagherian, B. (2024). Anxiety of patients undergoing magnetic resonance imaging (MRI): The effectiveness of guided mental imagery. *Topics in Magnetic Resonance Imaging, 33*, e0314. https://www.semanticscholar.org/paper/de9c3d9619b7f56f7ae87940bfae3b71e0f6c9ed (accessed on 14th July 2025).

84. Stoltzfus, M. T., Capodarco, M. D., Anamika, F., Gupta, V., & Jain, R. (2024). Cardiac MRI: An overview of physical principles with highlights of clinical applications and technological advancements. *Cureus, 16*. https://www.semanticscholar.org/paper/088daa6f29ce882dae61062e4e26cf731d022282 (accessed on 14th July 2025).

85. Sullivan, G., Quigley, A., Choi, S., Teed, R., Blesa Cábez, M., Vaher, K., Corrigan, A., et al. (2024). Brain 3T magnetic resonance imaging in neonates: Features and incidental findings from a research cohort enriched for preterm birth. *Archives of Disease in Childhood. Fetal and Neonatal Edition, 110*. https://www.semanticscholar.org/paper/ab478e0fef07f9ceac2b6088ca1cf748baab4124 (accessed on 14th July 2025).

86. Suparno, N. R., Faizah, A., & Nafisah, A. N. (2023). Assessment of panoramic radiograph errors: An evaluation of patient preparation and positioning quality at Soelastri Dental and Oral Hospital. *The Open Dentistry Journal*. https://www.semanticscholar.org/paper/e4e57159f0ea2a95df11193837e0275f2f580e22 (accessed on 14th July 2025).

87. Tang, L., Wu, T., Hu, R., Gu, Q., Yang, X., & Mao, H. (2024). Hemodynamic property incorporated brain tumor segmentation by deep learning and density-based analysis of dynamic susceptibility contrast-enhanced magnetic resonance imaging (MRI). *Quantitative Imaging in Medicine and Surgery, 14*, 2774–2787. https://www.semanticscholar.org/paper/501065bf603c46b83bde3f71d3d43b7f28ebdaf5 (accessed on 14th July 2025).

88. Tavaf, N. (2021). Improving signal to noise ratio in ultra-high field magnetic resonance imaging. https://core.ac.uk/download/478871378.pdf (accessed on 14th July 2025).

89. Tjoa, E., & Guan, C. (2020). A survey on explainable artificial intelligence (XAI): Toward medical XAI. *IEEE Transactions on Neural Networks and Learning Systems, 32*, 4793–4813. https://doi.org/10.1109/tnnls.2020.3027314 (accessed on 14th July 2025).

90. Törenek, Ş., Bilgin, E. Y., Ünal, Ö., Batur, A., Topçu Çakır, B., Bükte, Y., & Önbaş, Ö. (2024). Magnetic resonance imaging findings in patients with multinodular vacuolating neuronal tumors. *Medical Science and Discovery*. https://www.semanticscholar.org/paper/f911a640f3cfebfbd875371ef3f85b4fc5ca1d73 (accessed on 14th July 2025).

91. Vaddi, P., Parasher, S., & Khurana, S. (2025). Beyond X-rays: Unveiling the future of dental diagnosis with dental magnetic resonance imaging. *Diagnostics, 15*. https://www.semanticscholar.org/paper/aeb28aad43f636aa034b5c4d7af887e6a2d2197b (accessed on 14th July 2025).

92. van Osch, M. V., Wåhlin, A., Scheyhing, P., Mossige, I., Hirschler, L., Eklund, A., Mogensen, K., et al. (2024). Human brain clearance imaging: Pathways taken by magnetic resonance imaging contrast agents after administration in cerebrospinal fluid and blood. *NMR in Biomedicine, 37*. https://www.semanticscholar.org/paper/9f30da6234a545704eace368644b26b082bc4d7d (accessed on 14th July 2025).

93. Vangijzegem, T., Lecomte, V., Ternad, I., Van Leuven, L., Müller, R. N., Stanicki, D., & Laurent, S. (2023). Superparamagnetic iron oxide nanoparticles (SPION): From fundamentals to state-of-the-art innovative applications for cancer therapy. *Pharmaceutics, 15*, 236–236. https://doi.org/10.3390/pharmaceutics15010236 (accessed on 14th July 2025).

94. Vu, J., Bhusal, B., Jiang, F., & Golestanirad, L. (2024). Comparative analysis of RF heating of cardiac implantable electronic devices (CIEDs) in conventional closed-bore vs. vertical open-bore MRI systems. *2024 46th Annual International Conference of the IEEE Engineering in Medicine and Biology Society (EMBC)*. https://www.semanticscholar.org/paper/b4264cb6fd1b7fef0f435782be3440d54dc3974a (accessed on 14th July 2025).

95. Wan, Q., Peng, H., Liu, F., Liu, X., Cheng, C., Tie, C., Deng, J., et al. (2024). Ability of dynamic gadoxetic acid–enhanced magnetic resonance imaging combined with water-specific T1 mapping to reflect inflammation in a rat model of early-stage nonalcoholic steatohepatitis. *Quantitative Imaging in Medicine and Surgery, 14*, 1591–1601. https://www.semanticscholar.org/paper/6697525d6bbef7481c0182c27db569c400e0e1b4 (accessed on 14th July 2025).

96. Wańczura, P., Aebisher, D., Leksa, D., Mytych, W., Dynarowicz, K., Myśliwiec, A., Leksa, N., et al. (2024). Photodynamic therapy of atherosclerotic plaque monitored by T1 and T2 relaxation times of magnetic resonance imaging. *International Journal of Translational Medicine*. https://www.semanticscholar.org/paper/c37d96e23fedff7dd4824841ed9c203245fcfb2a (accessed on 14th July 2025).

97. Wang, Y., Dai, M., Zheng, M., Jin, Y., Wen, Q., Cui, B., Zhang, Z., et al. (2024). Bowel preparation after mid-gut tubing enhanced the efficacy and compliance of magnetic resonance enterorrhaphy in Crohn's disease: A randomized controlled trial. *Therapeutic Advances in Gastroenterology, 17*. https://www.semanticscholar.org/paper/de9ec6d191fcea560f3b14347b1c5237ed8e755d (accessed on 14th July 2025).

98. Waseem, M. (2018). Collisional properties of Fermigases withp-wave interactions. https://core.ac.uk/download/186661780.pdf (accessed on 14th July 2025).

99. Williams, B., Mancia, G., Spiering, W., Agabiti Rosei, E., Azizi, M., Burnier, M., Clément, D., et al. (2018). 2018 ESC/ESH guidelines for the management of arterial hypertension. *Journal of Hypertension, 36*, 1953–2041. https://doi.org/10.1097/hjh.0000000000001940 (accessed on 14th July 2025).

100. Wu, D., Chen, Q., Chen, X., Han, F., Chen, Z., & Wang, Y. (2023). The blood–brain barrier: Structure, regulation and drug delivery. *Signal Transduction and Targeted Therapy, 8.* https://doi.org/10.1038/s41392-023-01481-w (accessed on 14th July 2025).

101. Yadav, P., Lokhande, A., Prasanna, B. L., & Thorat, G. (2024). Conceptual importance of imaging and signal processing in the medical science. *2024 International Conference on Healthcare Innovations, Software and Engineering Technologies (HISET).* https://www.semanticscholar.org/paper/58d2c820d6e4c4ac0ade0de4d21e05d6f78e13cf (accessed on 14th July 2025).

102. Zareiamand, H., Darroudi, A., Mohammadi, I., Moravvej, S. V., Danaei, S., & Alizadehsani, R. (2023). Cardiac magnetic resonance imaging (CMRI) applications in patients with chest pain in the emergency department: A narrative review. *Diagnostics, 13.* https://www.semanticscholar.org/paper/7dcda9e9186b047e95da8a829f3dae86eebd1c42 (accessed on 14th July 2025).

103. Zhang, Y. (2025). Enhancing rectal cancer liver metastasis prediction: Magnetic resonance imaging-based radiomics, bias mitigation, and regulatory considerations. *World Journal of Gastrointestinal Oncology, 17.* https://www.semanticscholar.org/paper/7fd4f92e462f214b01666d0e725a946ca9bd1dd2 (accessed on 14th July 2025)

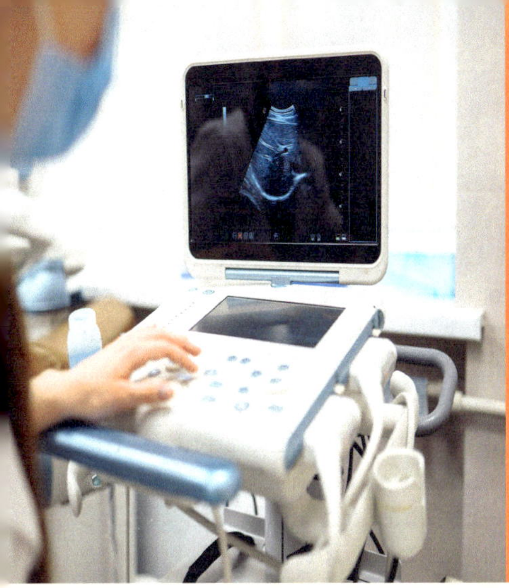

Chapter 6

ULTRASOUND PHYSICS AND INSTRUMENTATION

Contents

Introduction

Ultrasound is an excellent medical device that uses sound waves to create images of the body's interior. It works by creating high-frequency sound waves that bounce off tissues and organs. The bouncing sound waves are translated into images that doctors can see in real time. This non-invasive imaging technology is highly recognized for safety, versatility, and efficacy. Although traditionally associated with obstetrics, where it is used to monitor fetal development, ultrasound is now used in numerous medical specialties, including cardiology, radiology, and orthopedics. With advances in technology, combining ultrasound with sophisticated instruments yields greater precision and improved diagnostic value, thereby transforming clinical practice. Ultrasound knowledge entails not only an understanding of its operational principles but, more significantly, its growing significance in contemporary medicine and the related issues of its technological progress. Central to ultrasound application is its engagement with physical principles governing the behavior of sound waves in different tissues. Sound wave interaction with biological materials demands advanced understanding of acoustic properties such as impedance contrast, attenuation, and frequency-dependent scattering. The shift from a fundamental basis to practice demands technical precision in the design and calibration of equipment to achieve optimal image quality during tests. This is reflected in research studies, which focus on developments in instrumentation to meet the particular demands of diverse clinical cases. One such case is the testing of combined technologies, such as ultrasound-modulated optical tomography, where one can see the advantage of combining ultrasound with other modalities to enhance imaging capability and accuracy. These innovations constitute a commitment to the development of better ultrasound techniques and to addressing clinical needs emerging in the fluid healthcare environment, thereby finding application in the field of medical imaging (Arridge et al., 2015). Additionally, the hardware involved with ultrasound plays an integral role in the success of diagnostics, since innovation continues to redefine the boundaries and horizon of this technology. A critical review of the available equipment determines a scene that is mainly designed to deal with comprehensive clinical concerns, but finds certain challenges in certain applications. As shown in background studies, adjustments to instrumentation technology are typically required to accommodate unique situations, such as those encountered in spaceflight studies that focus on cardiovascular function under modified gravitational forces. The necessity for mission-specific instrumentation calls for the demand for priorities of future research and development, emphasizing the importance of sustained innovation in the field. With existing technology, users can effectively employ a range of ultrasound applications; however, addressing mission-specific demands remains an optimal field for future innovation (Ganiaris et al., 2025). This is to emphasize the need for further research to expand both the theoretical foundation and the clinical utility of ultrasound across various medical environments.

6.1. Principles of Ultrasound Physics

The underlying principles of ultrasound physics lie at the junction of wave physics and sound transmission, with critical applications in medicine and industry. Ultrasound uses sound waves with frequencies typically greater than 20 kHz, above the human hearing range. The generation of ultrasound waves normally uses piezoelectric transducers that transform electrical energy into mechanical movement to produce high-frequency acoustic waves. These waves travel through various media, such as tissues and fluids, and encounter boundaries, which result in reflection, refraction, and scattering. One needs to understand these interactions, since back-scattered echoes contain significant information about the structure and composition of the medium through which the ultrasound has passed. This foundation is central in offering the competence of ultrasound equipment in various applications. A significant topic in ultrasound physics is the examination of wave behavior as it propagates through different materials. Upon meeting media boundaries, the propagation of ultrasound waves is influenced by the acoustic characteristics of the materials in question, namely density and acoustic impedance. Reflection occurs whenever sound waves enter an interface with a dissimilar acoustic impedance, while refraction can bend the wave into a new medium. Other factors, such as internal pipe wall roughness, are also capable of introducing uncertainties that may degrade measurement quality, particularly in instances such as clamp-on ultrasonic flowmeters. In line with research findings, internal surface roughness can affect flow profiles, leading to substantial ultrasound scattering and, therefore, impacting the fidelity of the resulting flow data. Limiting these variability issues is essential to enhance the reliability of measurements and imaging systems derived from ultrasound (Cegla et al., 2018). Furthermore, the evolution of nondestructive evaluation (NDE) techniques demonstrates ultrasound's ability to extend beyond flaw detection to quantitative assessment of structural integrity. Novel NDE methods employ ultrasound to examine the mechanical properties of materials, such as tensile strength and ductility, as well as their microstructural properties. Although most of these new techniques are still undergoing validation and have not yet entered regular use, they promise to revolutionize how industries measure material properties non-destructively. By overcoming instrumentation constraints and achieving practical application, ultrasound promises to improve monitoring and maintenance operations across engineering fields significantly. With the development of this technology, the use of ultrasound in conjunction with advanced analysis software and more powerful equipment will enable better measurement of material properties, helping ensure that structural components meet high safety and performance standards (Klima et al., 2025).

6.1.1. Sound Wave Propagation and Characteristics

Sound wave transmission is generally described in terms of its ability to transfer energy through an intermediary, with the typical process being absorption, reflection, and refraction of acoustic waves. These play a vital role in describing ultrasound applications across its various uses, particularly in medical imaging. The velocity with which sound waves travel depends on the density and rigidity of the medium, resulting in different velocities for different materials. This measurable relation plays a vital role in the development of techniques maximizing sound wave propagation for accurate imaging and diagnostics. A detailed understanding of these principles is imperative, as ultrasonic devices can be designed to manipulate sound waves for effective imaging techniques in medical fields, thereby enabling non-destructive examination of internal body parts. Properties of a sound wave, like frequency, wavelength, and amplitude, are all-important in ultrasound technology, controlling image quality and diagnosticity (Figure 6.1).

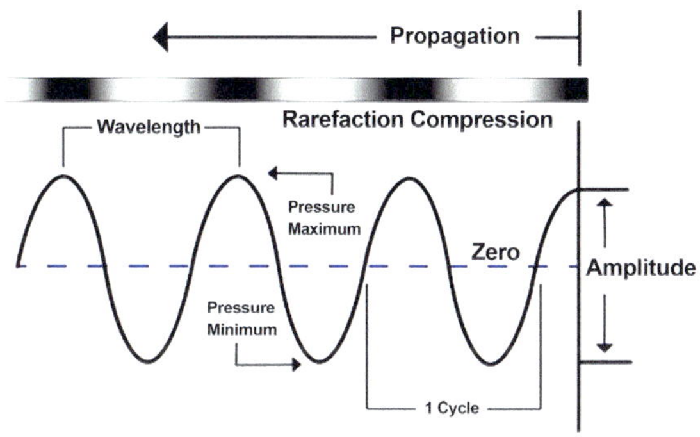

Figure 6.1. Diagram illustrating the fundamental principles of sound wave propagation in ultrasound.

Source: https://th.bing.com/th/id/OIP.8CMsxL0VnIGpIi3F2Q3erAAAAA?rs=1&pid=ImgDetMain.

Higher frequencies tend to offer higher resolution but with greater attenuation in tissues, while lower frequencies offer deeper penetration but with lower image detail. Such a trade-off between frequency and imaging depth is the dominant consideration in the design of ultrasound equipment and dictates specific applications in clinical environments. The relationship between acoustical parameters and resulting images underscores the importance of deriving sound wave parameters for optimal diagnostic effectiveness. As sound waves travel through biological tissues, tissue structure, density, and temperature also influence their behavior, so it is essential to have a clear understanding of these interactions to enhance imaging skills in ultrasound physics and instrumentation. Recent developments in acoustic methods have demonstrated strong potential to expand the application of ultrasound techniques, especially in opaque and complex systems. For instance, acoustic approaches to fluid mechanics have gained popularity, wherein multiphase flows, such as fluidized beds, which are important in medical and engineering sciences, can be described. Measurement of sound speed, attenuation, and frequency shifts is one of the measures employed, which is of significance in determining the fluid-particle interaction dynamics. These can greatly enhance our understanding of material behavior and properties. As tasked in recent studies, such developments in ultrasonic technology pave the way for improved monitoring and characterization methods, facilitating the shift towards deeper applications for diagnostics and therapeutic intervention, especially regarding real-time assessment of fluid dynamics in the human body, thus unifying the art of acoustics and medicine (Angeli et al., 2021; Klima et al., 2025).

6.1.2. Frequency and Wavelength of Ultrasound

The relationship between frequency and wavelength is fundamental to understanding ultrasound technology. Frequency, or the number of oscillations per second, is in hertz (Hz), while wavelength is the distance between consecutive peaks of a wave. The inverse relationship is given as $v = f\lambda$, where v is the velocity of sound in the medium, f is the frequency, and λ is the wavelength. In medical ultrasound, typical frequencies range from 1 to 10 MHz, which correspond to reasonably short wavelengths. Short wavelengths enhance resolution, enabling better imaging of superficial structures. Higher frequencies are attenuated faster in biological tissues this comes at the trade-off of reduced penetration and image quality. Therefore, frequency selection directly affects the diagnostic utility of ultrasound and underscores the need to understand this relationship in clinical use and in instrument design. The frequency selection in the use of ultrasound also determines the characteristics of sound waves as they travel through other media. Ultrasonic waves, while traveling through different materials, may experience velocity and wavelength changes based upon changes in the density and elasticity of such materials. For instance, the frequencies of ultrasonic surgical instruments are likely to be optimized to maximize cutting efficiency on mineralized tissues. This setting is of utmost significance, as instrument resonance, based on its length in terms of half-wavelengths, has significant implications for performance parameters. Optimized devices at specific frequencies, such as these devices, can efficiently carry out ablation of tissue while causing minimal damage to adjacent tissues. In addition, multi-frequency endoscopic devices have been proposed to improve surgical performance, but they can introduce nonlinear dynamic behaviors that complicate surgical outcomes. An understanding of frequency and wavelength enables optimization of advanced ultrasound use and its related equipment in surgery. Besides their impacts on imaging and surgical accuracy, frequency and wavelength cannot be downplayed as inputs for flow measurement technologies (Figure 6.2).

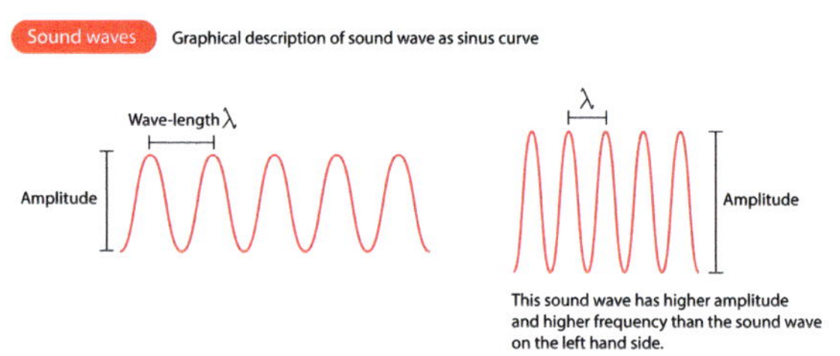

Figure 6.2. Graphical comparison of frequency and wavelength parameters in diagnostic ultrasound.

Source: Adapted from https://ecgwaves.com/wp-content/uploads/2019/10/ultrasound-sound-waves-wave-length-amplitude-1024x427.jpg.

Ultrasonic flowmeters use frequency and wavelength principles to calculate fluid velocity by measuring the time it takes sound waves to travel a set distance through a medium. Clamp-on ultrasonic flowmeters, though non-invasive, often suffer from uncertainties caused by internal pipe wall roughness, which can scatter ultrasonic waves and complicate measurement. The literature observes that moderate roughness alone leads to systematic errors in velocity measurement, underscoring the nuanced interaction between device technology and environmental factors. Therefore, a thorough understanding of the interdependence between wavelength and frequency in ultrasound not only contributes to healthcare delivery but also drives innovation in industrial flow-measuring technologies, enhancing overall efficacy and precision across diverse fields (Cegla et al., 2018; Cardoni et al., 2015).

6.1.3. Interaction of Ultrasound with Biological Tissues

Ultrasound behavior in biological tissues is complex and depends significantly on the acoustic properties of the materials being examined. As ultrasound waves pass through tissues, they encounter a variety of interfaces and structures that result in reflections, refractions, and scattering. The magnitude of the interactions relies to a large extent on the density and elasticity of the biological tissues, which determine the way in which ultrasound energy is absorbed and transmitted. Tissues such as muscle and fat have varying acoustic impedances, so a portion of the sound energy bounces back when it travels from one of these materials to another instead of passing through. This characteristic is fundamental throughout the imaging process because it serves to define the different types of tissue, hence enhancing the accuracy of the diagnosis (Figure 6.3).

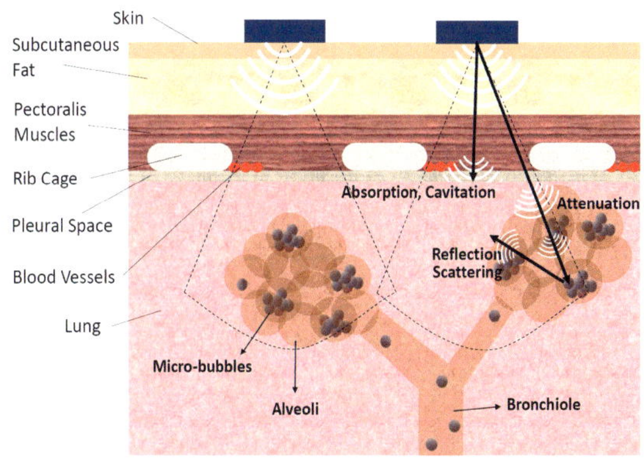

Figure 6.3. Schematic of ultrasound interaction mechanisms with various biological tissues.

Source: https://www.researchgate.net/publication/349491768/figure/fig2/AS:993851166687235@1613963991434/Diagram-representing-ultrasound-propagation-through-the-tissue-layers-reaching-the.png.

In addition to reflection and refraction, ultrasonic energy absorption by tissue is a critical phenomenon in its interaction with tissue. Tissues vary in their absorption coefficients, which determine the efficiency with which they convert acoustic energy to thermal energy. For example, soft tissues will absorb ultrasound at relatively lower rates compared to denser tissue like bone. This differential absorption has the advantage of targeting a specific site in the body and could potentially enable therapeutic application via focused ultrasound surgery. It is, however, challenging as high levels of absorption can create undesirable thermal tissue damage. The full appreciation of the specific interactions of ultrasound with various tissues thus becomes a requirement for optimizing both imaging diagnosis and treatment. Furthermore, advancements in mimicking materials for tissues have grown our knowledge of the interactions above, facilitating improved clinical practice as well as research. Such materials, specifically designed to mimic the acoustic features of human tissues, serve as phantoms for testing ultrasound equipment and methods. Recent research suggests that the creation of repeatable experimental platforms using such phantoms enables a detailed investigation of ultrasound behavior under varied conditions. By studying the electrical characteristics of various tissue substitutes, scientists can better tailor their methods to mimic natural biological reactions, improving the quality of diagnostic imaging. Furthermore, these advances not only enhance the accuracy of ultrasound equipment but also enable the identification of novel applications in biomedical engineering, underscoring the need for continued research and development in ultrasound physics and equipment (Bowen et al., 2004; Alquaydheb et al., 2018).

6.2. Transducer Technology

Transducer technology is the enabling technology for ultrasound physics and instrumentation, enabling the conversion of electrical energy into acoustic waves and vice versa. Transducers, the dominant piezoelectric devices, play a vital role in producing sound waves that can travel through biological tissue to facilitate the imaging of internal structures. The ability to understand the principles of operation of transducers, such as resonance frequency and bandwidth, allows practitioners to optimize image resolution and depth of penetration. The newer advances in transducer development, namely miniaturization and increased sensitivity, have revolutionized ultrasound imaging, enabling the imaging of smaller structures with greater clarity. In addition, the continuously evolving nature of the materials used for transducer design, such as polyvinylidene fluoride, further contributed to performance parameters, ultimately enabling more diagnostics. Transducer technology not only supports imaging but also makes a significant contribution to several non-invasive medical monitoring methods. For example, Doppler ultrasound methods are used to detect air embolism in astronauts performing extravehicular activities, illustrating the systems' flexibility in extreme conditions. Such a minimally invasive approach is pivotal, as it provides immediate feedback on cardiovascular performance with no risk associated with invasive techniques. The technology review referenced in Greene et al. (2025) refers to an extensive overview of the medical ultrasound market, with special focus given to the intricate interplay between advanced transducer designs and their corresponding applications. Such ability highlights the indispensable nature of robust transducer technology in both clinical settings and specialist applications, such as space, where traditional monitoring methods might prove restrictive. The advances in transducers also represent the necessity for interdisciplinary collaboration in ultrasound instrumentation. By merging the disciplines of engineering, physics, and medicine, it is possible to create highly specialized transducers. Encouraging the spirit of cooperation can lead to novel products tailored to cope with the diverse and demanding needs of medical imaging. The evaluation of equipment, as per Ganiaris et al. (2025), reveals that while underlying technologies exist, their adaptation for specific purposes, such as spaceflight or specific patient treatment contexts, entails ongoing research and development. As clinicians continue to look to ultrasound technologies, the role of transducers in enhancing diagnostic accuracy and therapeutic applications grows, reaffirming their significance in the new context of medical imaging.

6.2.1. Types of Ultrasound Transducers

In ultrasound physics and instrumentation, various types of ultrasound transducers play a pivotal role in diagnostic imaging and therapeutic applications. These transducers convert electrical energy into sound waves and vice versa, enabling visualization of the body's internal structures. The two primary categories of transducers are linear and convex transducers. Linear transducers, characterized by a rectangular, flat configuration, produce high-resolution images, particularly effective for superficial structures like vascular studies and musculoskeletal evaluations. In contrast, convex transducers feature a curved array, enabling broader tissue coverage and deeper penetration, making them suitable for abdominal and obstetric imaging. Both types highlight the adaptability of ultrasound technology in addressing diverse clinical needs, thereby enhancing patient diagnosis and treatment. Another significant classification of ultrasound transducers is the distinction between single-element and multi-element transducers. Single-element transducers use a singular crystal to emit and receive sound waves, predominantly found in simple applications where cost efficiency is paramount. Conversely, multi-element transducers comprise multiple individual crystals that work in tandem to produce enhanced images at higher frame rates and with better spatial resolution. This technology is particularly beneficial in scenarios requiring rapid imaging, such as in cardiac diagnostics, where real-time images can inform immediate clinical decisions. The evolution of multi-element technology has advanced ultrasound capabilities, empowering practitioners with the tools necessary for comprehensive diagnostic insights and effectively addressing the complexities of human anatomy. Additionally, the emergence of specialized ultrasound transducers, such as volumetric and needle-guidance transducers, exemplifies the innovation in ultrasound technology aimed at achieving precise, targeted outcomes. Volumetric transducers enable three-dimensional imaging, enhancing visualization of anatomical relationships and facilitating complex assessments, particularly in obstetric and gynecological examinations. Needle guidance transducers, on the other hand, assist clinicians in performing minimally invasive procedures with increased accuracy. By providing real-time imaging feedback, these transducers significantly improve the efficacy of interventions, such as biopsies or fluid aspirate procedures. The integration of these specialized transducers into clinical practice underscores the ongoing advancements in ultrasound instrumentation, enhancing the overall scope and effectiveness of ultrasound applications in medicine (Chan et al., 2009; Ganiaris et al., 2025) (Figure 6.4).

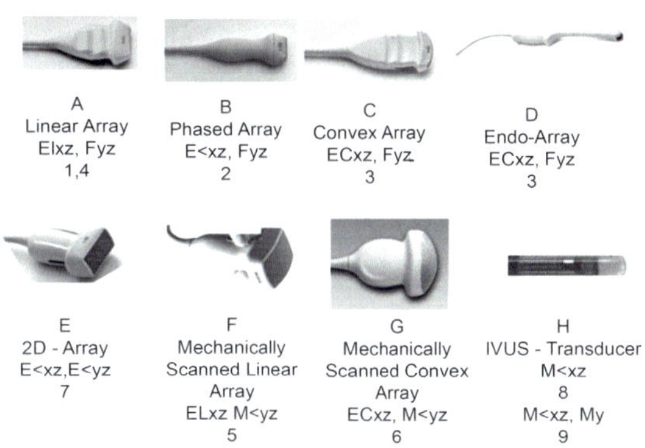

Figure 6.4. Overview of ultrasound transducer classifications by application type.

Source: https://onlinelibrary.wiley.com/cms/asset/09f799c1-8d62-416f-a911-eca2ef12ee2b/jum2013324573-fig-0004-m.jpg.

6.2.2. Piezoelectric Effect and Its Significance

The piezoelectric effect is a significant phenomenon behind most ultrasound physics and instrumentation applications. . The piezoelectric effect occurs when certain materials generate an electric charge in response to mechanical stress, making them ideally suited for acoustic wave-to-electronic signal and electronic signal-to-acoustic wave conversion. Transducers for ultrasound imaging utilize the piezoelectric effect to generate ultrasonic waves that reflect off organs and tissues, allowing image creation from the reflected echoes. Not only does this two-way feature of transducers permit imaging, but it also provides critical quantitative data, enhancing diagnostic capability across different clinical settings. (Figure 6.5).

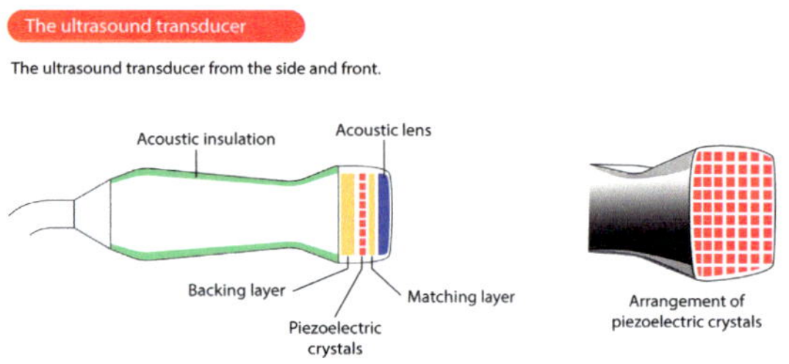

Figure 6.5. Visualization of the piezoelectric effect in ultrasound transducer crystals.

Source: https://ecgwaves.com/wp-content/uploads/2019/10/ultrasound-transducer-piezoelectric-crystals-effect-echocardiography.jpg.

Therefore, understanding the physics of the piezoelectric effect becomes essential for technological progress in ultrasound. One of the primary applications of the piezoelectric effect in ultrasound devices is improving the precision and effectiveness of measurements. The development of sophisticated ultrasonic instruments, such as segmental ultrasonic plethysmographs, reflects how piezoelectric sensors can enhance measurement reliability and minimize the effects of environmental influences. Research indicates that such devices yield more precise limb-volume readings, which are significant for assessing physiological states such as venous return during weightlessness. Furthermore, the instrument's ability to produce reliable results enables continuous assessments of orthostatic intolerance—a condition exacerbated by conditions such as weightlessness. By combining the piezoelectric effect with sophisticated algorithms, next-generation ultrasound devices can provide more detailed diagnostic information, essential to both ground- and space-flight medicine (Ganiaris et al., 2025; Bhagat et al., 2025). The significance of the piezoelectric effect does not stop at the diagnostic frontier but extends to therapeutic use as well. The ability to manipulate and control acoustic energy enables the development of several therapeutic ultrasound techniques, such as lithotripsy and high-intensity focused ultrasound (HIFU). Such methods employ focused ultrasonic waves to target and destroy diseased tissues, such as kidney stones or tumors, demonstrating the capabilities of piezoelectric materials in medical treatments. Research also further expands the boundaries of ultrasound application by developing enhanced piezoelectric materials and modifying their functional characteristics. This route underscores the importance of the piezoelectric effect in ultrasound instrumentation and physics as the foundation for future innovations intended to advance medicine's diagnostic and therapeutic objectives.

6.2.3. Transducer Design and Its Influence on Image Quality

Transducer design plays an important role in determining the quality of images developed in diagnostic imaging. Transducers convert electrical signals to mechanical vibrations and vice versa, and their efficiency determines the resolution and quality of the image. An efficient transducer ensures maximum frequency and bandwidth for accurate imaging of anatomical features. These include aperture size, element spacing, and the selection of appropriate piezoelectric materials, all of which contribute to image quality. For instance, larger apertures can yield more focused beams with lower side lobes and greater axial resolution. This precision is critical in uses such as High Intensity Focused Ultrasound (HIFU), where beam precision can have a profound influence on the effectiveness and safety of treatment, as evidenced by recent innovations aimed at overcoming beam defocusing due to tissue heterogeneity, highlighting the key role played by transducer design in clinical success (Constanciel et al., 2018) (Figure 6.6).

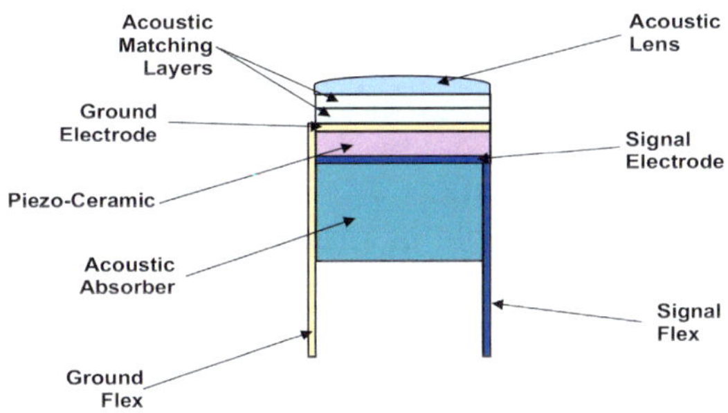

Figure 6.6. Cross-sectional design of a typical ultrasound transducer showing components and beam profile influence.

Source: https://www.researchgate.net/profile/Murtaza-Ali-2/publication/265425106/figure/fig1/AS:669430530977802@1536616084584/Ultrasound-Transducer-Cross-Sectional-View.png.

Aside from hardware issues, the computational methods employed alongside transducer technologies also impact image quality. Current state-of-the-art developments in signal processing techniques, including source encoding procedures alongside structured optimization algorithms like the regularized dual averaging (RDA) algorithm, reflect this synergy. These computational designs enable more sophisticated image reconstruction processes to handle complex data interactions, particularly in high-end imaging modalities such as Ultrasound Computed Tomography (USCT). By addressing diffraction effects and reducing noise at no cost to resolution, these algorithms enhance the interpretability of ultrasound images. Additionally, ongoing research aimed at optimizing these algorithms continues to improve, underscoring the need to marry transducer design with effective software applications to push the boundaries of diagnostic imaging, particularly for applications such as breast cancer screening (Anastasio et al., 2017). Furthermore, the future of transducer design is intricately linked to developments in ultrasound imaging modalities and technologies. With increasing imaging complexity, enhancements to transducer capabilities are critical to meet the challenge. Miniaturization, sensitivity, and the integration of multimodal capabilities are leading to higher-resolution, higher-definition imaging. Moreover, engineering-biophysics collaboration has led to the study of novel materials and shapes that would deliver dramatic improvements in beamforming and focusing performance. Integration of sophisticated transducer designs not only improves picture quality but also expands the potential applications of ultrasound in diagnostics and therapy, repeatedly reaffirming the merits of good transducer design as part of the overall scheme of ultrasound physics and engineering.

6.3. Imaging Techniques in Ultrasound

The discipline of ultrasound technology encompasses a variety of imaging modalities that improve diagnostic imaging capabilities in diverse medical applications. At the focal point of ultrasound imaging is the generation of sound waves, which are employed to irradiate the body's tissues by transducers. The sound waves reflect back to the transducer to form images through reconstruction that depict structures and functions of the body. There are various types of ultrasound, including A-mode, B-mode, and Doppler ultrasound, each intended for a specific use. A-mode (amplitude mode) provides one-dimensional information about the amplitude of an echo, while B-mode (brightness mode) produces two-dimensional images that reflect anatomical structures. Doppler ultrasound, on the other hand, measures blood flow, enabling doctors to gauge vascular status. As the discipline evolves, the integration of advanced imaging technologies continues to improve how experts view and analyze internal body functions, thereby enhancing clinical performance. The operation of ultrasound imaging depends on the understanding of the physics of waves and instruments. Ultrasound sound waves typically range from 1 to 20 MHz, allowing efficient penetration and resolution depending on use. Higher frequencies offer higher resolution but shallower penetration, while lower frequencies penetrate deeper but lose some detail. The selection of frequency depends on the specific diagnostic requirement, such as imaging shallow structures versus deep organs. Image quality also depends on factors such as the design of the transducers (e.g., size and shape) and the transmission medium for the sound waves. Effective utilization of these parameters is critical to delivering accurate and consistent imaging results; thus, education in ultrasound physics and instrumentation is a must for healthcare providers. Furthermore, technological advances in ultrasound imaging have enabled revolutionary applications, particularly in real-time and three-dimensional (3D) imaging.

Real-time ultrasound enables clinicians to visualize physiological processes in real time, allowing them to make informed decisions as they perform procedures such as biopsies or surgery. Progress in 3D ultrasound provides an overall visualization of anatomy, supplying volumetric data that enhances interpretative accuracy. By fusing numerous two-dimensional images, clinicians achieve a better representation of the region of interest. This capacity is of especial utility in obstetric and gynecologic imaging, where it can be utilized to enhance the assessment of fetal development, placental position, and other factors. With ever-advancing instrumentation technology, the use of advanced imaging techniques marks a revolutionary shift in diagnostic protocols, confirming the irreplaceable role of ultrasound in contemporary medicine (N/A, 2008; Ganiaris et al., 2025).

6.3.1. B-Mode Imaging and Applications

B-mode imaging, or brightness mode imaging, is a staple of ultrasound physics and instrumentation. It forms two-dimensional images by reflecting ultrasound waves off body interfaces, yielding varying echoes based on the density and acoustic properties of the tissues.

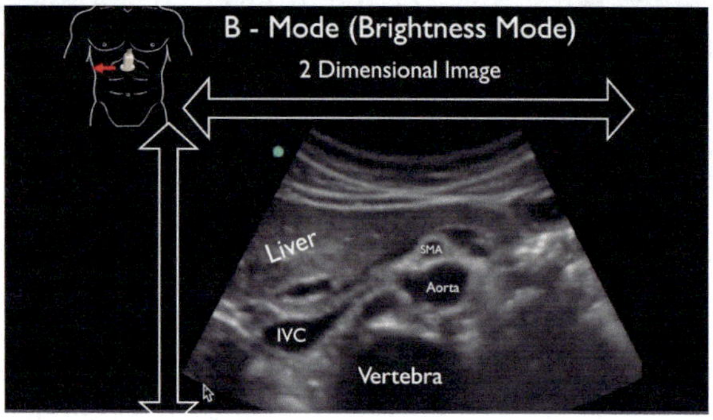

Figure 6.7. B-Mode imaging example highlighting structural details in abdominal scanning.

Source: https://i.ytimg.com/vi/qhCKDKy3LoY/maxresdefault.jpg.

The grayscale images thus formed are paramount for providing essential information during diagnostic workup, allowing clinicians to visualize anatomical structures in real time. This noninvasive technique is especially valuable in obstetrics, cardiology, and abdominal organ scanning, where accurate visualization can change patient diagnosis and treatment. As technology continues to improve, advances in transducer design and signal processing have enhanced spatial resolution and image quality, increasing diagnostic confidence across a broad spectrum of medical specialties. Besides, B-mode imaging has increasingly been combined with other imaging modalities to broaden its indications and provide multidimensional data. Its combination with Doppler ultrasound is an example that enables dynamic assessment of blood flow alongside the structural images obtained with B-mode techniques (Figure 6.7).This combined approach is central to determining cardiovascular status, particularly disease conditions such as stenosis or vascular malformations. In addition, advances in ultrasound technology, like the development of handheld machines, have enabled point-of-care application, which fosters immediate diagnosis in diverse environments from emergency medicine to rural care.

Through expediting clinical decision-making, these integrated uses underscore B-mode imaging's versatility and importance in contemporary medical practice and equipment. Continuing optimization of B-mode imaging is also observed in recent studies of its interaction with new-generation imaging technologies. Recent publications have demonstrated the potential of applying new technologies, such as photorefractive polymers, to enhance imaging through scattering media and improve diagnostic accuracy even further.

These innovations offer the potential to overcome certain disadvantages of traditional ultrasound techniques, including signal decay and depth-penetration limitations in complex tissues. As argued in discussing the merits of new methodologies for material characterization, seeking better imaging techniques remains a necessity. Each new method, created with a specific clinical or research purpose, brings potential benefits and the need for meticulous evaluation of its operational and cost-effectiveness relative to standard procedures. This reflects the need for ongoing refinement of ultrasound technology and the strategic integration of new technologies.

6.3.2. Doppler Ultrasound for Blood Flow Analysis

The application of Doppler ultrasound in blood flow analysis is a significant advancement in medical imaging, leveraging physics principles to measure hemodynamic parameters. The procedure is painless, using the principle of Doppler where frequency changes of ultrasound waves represent movement of blood cells in the circulatory system. By creating sound waves and measuring the resulting frequency changes as they reflect off moving red blood cells, doctors can obtain valuable information about blood velocity and flow patterns. Such systems are required not only for identifying vascular disease but also for continuous tracking of patients' cardiovascular status —an important intersection between technology and patient care in contemporary medicine. The uses of Doppler ultrasound extend beyond traditional domains, enabling cutting-edge applications, particularly in previously challenging environments. Notably, research has shown the importance of Doppler ultrasound for assessing cardiovascular function in astronauts during EVAs (Figure 6.8).

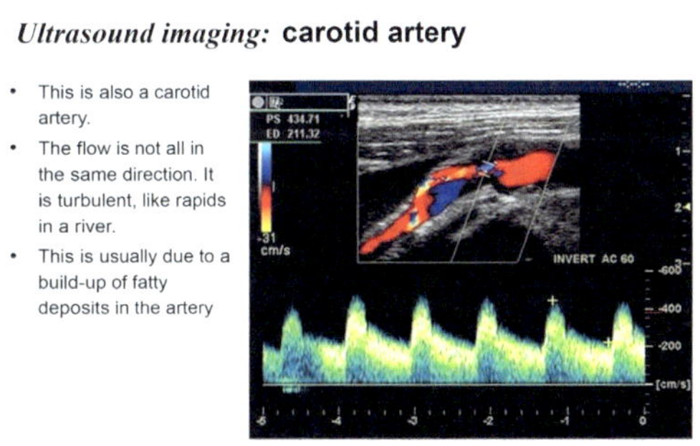

Figure 6.8. Doppler ultrasound image demonstrating blood flow in a major artery.

Source: https://th.bing.com/th/id/R.592907ec8cd13451cfe681576a153895?rik=5J0JYwX8GWqhkw&riu=http%3a%2f%2fslidetodoc.com%2fpresentation_image_h%2f1fdc5208b6b9c6859c1049a5c031af1b%2fimage-3.jpg&ehk=SkX%2b1OUGTvVIWlG4QYDKzGsJaDceFDFbACF7BGU8vo4%3d&risl=&pid=ImgRaw&r=0.

The technology enables continuous monitoring of blood flow, which is essential for understanding the physiological effects of microgravity. As outlined in recent studies, the incorporation of Doppler ultrasound into spaceflight missions reveals a general tendency toward greater readiness among astronauts to respond to various physiological demands (Greene et al., 2025). This achievement points to another aspect of Doppler ultrasound: not just accommodating Earth-based medical procedures but also necessary for ensuring astronauts' health amid the unique stresses of space travel. The development of Doppler ultrasound technologies also points to a radical shift in instrumentation procedures aimed at improving data reliability and accuracy. As a review of current technologies shows, the incorporation of state-of-the-art Doppler techniques has necessitated individualized accommodations to accommodate individual medical and environmental situations. Advances in sensor design and data processing algorithms have enabled equipment that meets exacting performance requirements and performs well even under extreme conditions encountered on space missions. This emphasis on technology assessment has been vital: familiarity with the cardiovascular measurement parameters that must be dealt with for special situations assures that the future of Doppler ultrasound will not only benefit routine medical diagnosis but also complex situations like space flight (Ganiaris et al., 2025).

6.3.3. Progress in 3D and 4D Ultrasound Imaging

The advancements in 3D and 4D ultrasound imaging have transformed obstetric and gynecologic practice and enabled unparalleled visualization of fetal anatomy and motion. The modalities facilitate comprehensive assessment of fetal growth, with early detection of abnormalities and improved patient care. Using 3D ultrasound, clinicians can obtain volumetric images of the fetus, enabling them to assess structures in 3D. It enhances diagnostic accuracy by providing detailed, realistic images of anatomical structures such as the heart and face, which are often difficult to interpret from conventional 2D images. In addition, 4D ultrasound brings in the time dimension, with real-time motion, allowing clinicians to understand better complex functions such as fetal breathing and cardiac rhythm, further refining prenatal assessment and offering expectant parents a more intimate relationship with their unborn baby (Figure 6.9).

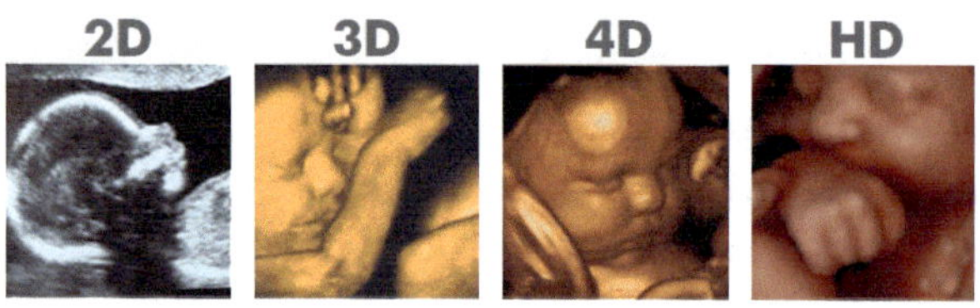

Figure 6.9. 3D and 4D ultrasound comparison in fetal imaging.

Source: https://www.onelikeme.com/wp-content/uploads/2d3d4d_animated_MASTER1.gif.

The use of advanced computer technologies has played a key role in enhancing the performance of 3D and 4D ultrasound imaging. Sophisticated image reconstruction and processing algorithms enable the creation of higher-resolution, more informative images. Such advances involve the creation of super phantoms, which provide new test materials that closely approximate physiological conditions. Super phantoms are designed to replicate the intricate anatomical and functional characteristics of human tissue, thereby enabling improved imaging modalities. As listed in recent literature, such phantoms are better than the traditional phantoms because they allow one to make incremental improvements in ultrasound technology prior to it being taken to the clinic, underpinning their relevance for technology validation and training in the clinical community (Anastasio et al., 2023; Anastasio et al., 2024). This technology paves the way for further progress, keeping 3D and 4D ultrasound imaging in the development stage by rigorous testing and use in practical conditions. In addition, the application of enhanced 3D and 4D ultrasound imaging is not confined to obstetrics but extends to other medical disciplines, such as cardiology and oncology. To illustrate, in cardiology, 3D echocardiography facilitates improved visualizations of cardiac structures, enabling more accurate diagnoses and treatment. Similarly, cancer imaging is enhanced by precise measurement of tumor vascularity and size using advanced ultrasound. Visualization of real-time physiological function enables clinicians to adjust treatment in response to feedback. As these imaging modalities continue to advance, they have the potential to unlock fundamental insights into disease pathology and to dictate the course of therapy. Overall, the combination of ultrasound physics and advanced instrumental innovations in imaging re-engineers clinical practice and enhances patient care significantly.

6.4. Ultrasound Instrumentation

The evolution and development of ultrasound machines have significantly advanced medical imaging, enabling non-invasive visualization of internal structures. Leading the technology is the use of transducers that can convert electrical energy to sound waves and vice versa. Upon encountering various tissues, the sound waves generate echoes that are processed to form images. The quality of such images is highly influenced by parameters such as frequency, wavelength, and degree of tissue interaction that can enhance or reduce the quality of the resulting visualization. It is essential to know the physics of the propagation of ultrasound waves and tissue interaction in this regard to obtain the best imaging outcomes. Thus, ongoing research in new transducer designs and upgrade technologies is of paramount importance in the continued advancement of ultrasound equipment, expanding its applications to diagnostics as well as therapeutic procedures. As ultrasound systems evolved, so did methods of signal processing that enhance image quality as well as diagnostic sensitivity. Today's ultrasound systems employ advanced algorithms to eliminate noise and improve image resolution, thereby optimizing the effectiveness of clinical assessments. One of the significant breakthroughs in this field is harmonic imaging, which exploits the nonlinear nature of sound waves to produce more detailed images at higher frequencies. This is supplemented by the addition of Doppler techniques to measure blood flow dynamics, rendering it a useful tool for both structural and functional assessment of cardiovascular status. There must be ongoing education and training for ultrasound professionals to become proficient with these modern machines, thereby enhancing patient outcomes. Beyond standard imaging, ultrasound use does not end with conventional imaging but extends to guided interventions and even specialist areas such as space medicine, where cardiovascular assessment becomes a critical parameter. The growing demand for portable, easy-to-use ultrasonics signals a paradigm shift in the discipline, enabling point-of-care diagnosis in any setting. Such flexibility is valuable in situations where rapid decision-making has to be done, like emergency care. However, to truly exploit the potential of such technologies, patient safety, ergonomics, and precision should also be considered when thinking about instrumentation. For instance, Ganiaris et al. (2025) bring to light the need to assess the appropriateness of instrumentation in new environments, as mission-based specifications at times demand modifications to existing technologies to address a range of clinical needs. Ongoing assessment and innovation of ultrasound instrumentation will indeed play a pivotal role in shaping the future of medical practice across specialties.

6.4.1. Components of An Ultrasound Machine

The fundamental components of an ultrasound machine serve as the backbone for its functionality, playing critical roles in the generation, transmission, and reception of sound waves. At the core of the ultrasound device is the transducer, which converts electrical energy into ultrasound waves and vice versa. This component relies on piezoelectric materials that vibrate to produce high-frequency sound waves when an electrical current is applied.

The efficient operation of the transducer is pivotal, as it directly influences the quality of the images produced. Furthermore, the transducer must be carefully synchronized with the imaging software to ensure accurate spatial representation of the tissues being examined. Without the transducer's precise function, diagnostic outputs would be severely compromised, underscoring its importance in the machine's architecture (Figure 6.10).

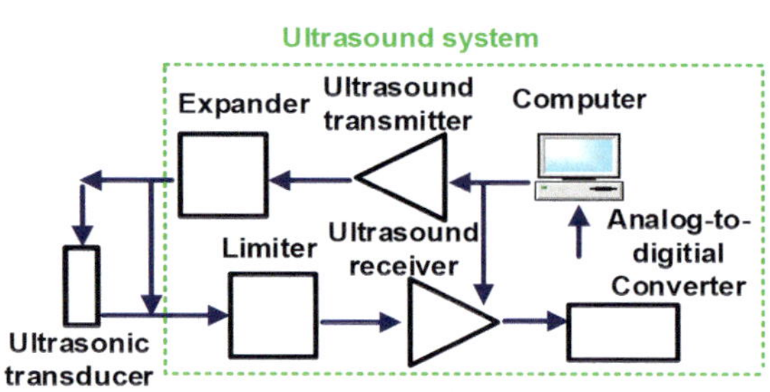

Figure 6.10. Block diagram of the main components within an ultrasound machine.

Source: https://www.researchgate.net/publication/358328698/figure/fig1/AS:1153498016165889@1652026766893/Block-diagram-of-the-ultrasound-system.jpg.

Apart from the transducer, ultrasound machines utilize electronic components that facilitate data processing and display. The pulser generates electronic pulses that energize the transducer, causing it to create sound waves. After transmission, the echoes return from tissue are transformed to electrical signals by the transducer and amplified by the receiver for improved imaging. Sophisticated digitization techniques process these signals, reducing them to a pattern that radiologists can visually recognize. This combination of components points to the advanced engineering that supports real-time imaging. The use of advanced software for image processing and noise filtering is another indicator of the role of electronics in ultrasound technology, making it a key diagnostic tool in contemporary medicine. Finally, the device's functionality extends beyond image creation to other developments such as Doppler imaging and elastography. These are expert techniques that utilize the device components to quantify blood flow and tissue stiffness, respectively. For example, Doppler ultrasound exploits the quantification of changes in the frequency of reflected sound waves from moving blood cells to enable clinicians to measure hemodynamics accurately. Besides, other futures involve integrating nanotechnology with ultrasound machines, such as systems composed of tiny robots communicating via ultrasonic waves, as studied in recent research (AIUM et al., 2012). All these have the potential to improve diagnostic efficiency, reflecting the evolving field of ultrasound physics and devices. This complex set of components not only indicates the technical prowess of ultrasound technology but also its quality contribution to patient care.

6.4.2. Signal Processing of Ultrasound System

The field of ultrasound systems relies heavily on sophisticated signal processing methods, which are key to transforming raw acoustic data into meaningful diagnostic information. With the help of advanced algorithms, ultrasound devices can improve image quality, enabling anatomical structures to be visualized with clarity. As such, signal processing methods such as time-gain compensation, filtering, and image reconstruction are essential in this regard.

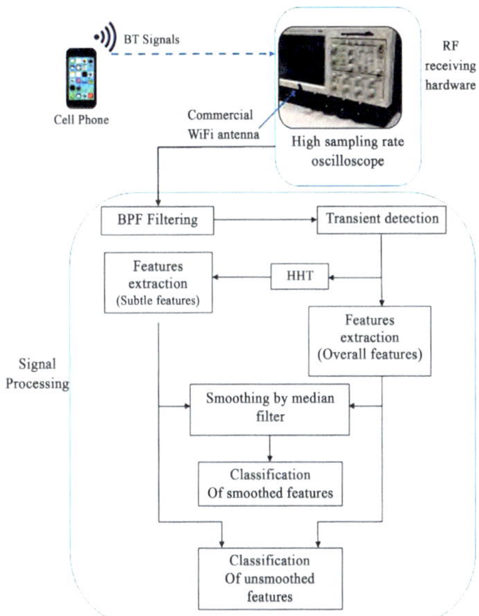

Figure 6.11. Signal processing flowchart for real-time ultrasound data acquisition.

Source: https://www.researchgate.net/profile/Ali-Kara-7/publication/332646590/figure/fig1/AS:751609667674116@1556209117350/Signal-acquisition-setup-and-flow-chart-of-signal-processing.png.

These methods minimize the effects of noise and attenuation, which will obscure the crispness of ultrasound images. With advancing technology, researchers continually advance these processes to provide better resolution and accuracy. Enhanced signal processing capabilities ultimately lead to improved diagnostic performance, and the necessity for ongoing development in ultrasound physics and instrumentation remains central to providing accurate medical evaluations. Besides, the use of computer technology in ultrasound equipment has revolutionized medical imaging. Digital signal processing (DSP) enables real-time manipulation and analysis of ultrasound signals, resulting in faster, more accurate diagnoses (Figure 6.11).

With DSP applied, systems can easily eliminate unwanted noise and artifacts, resulting in cleaner images and more reliable data interpretation. Adaptive techniques can also adjust processing parameters based on the nature of the received signals. This flexibility is crucial to various clinical conditions, particularly in dynamic situations like cardiology or obstetrics, where patients' care needs to be decided upon in a timely manner, impacting patients' care quite significantly. With the development of ultrasound technology, the role of signal processing also keeps on increasing, allowing the medical community to make the most of high-quality images for the evaluation of paramount significance. Though ultrasound scanners have seen tremendous improvements from advances in signal processing, calibration, and installation problems remain paramount. For instance, the accuracy of ultrasound measurements can be vastly affected by variables such as the acoustic properties of the medium and the geometrical properties of the measurement setup. Studies have established that variables such as internal pipe wall roughness must be accounted for, especially in clamp-on ultrasonic flowmeter applications subject to uncertainties arising from environmental conditions. Surface roughness-induced ultrasound scattering can introduce systematic errors in measurements; thus, proper calibration procedures are required. Therefore, ongoing research into understanding and minimizing such influences remains central to further refining the reliability and performance of ultrasound systems in practice, so that they continue to be sensitive to the needs of practitioners and patients, as emphasized in existing research on variability of performance in the applications of ultrasound (Cegla et al., 2018; Ganiaris et al., 2025).

6.4.3. Display Technologies Employed in Ultrasound Imaging

The evolution of display technology in ultrasonography has significantly transformed doctors' imaging practices. Former ultrasound equipment used cathode ray tube (CRT) technology, which, while effective, offered limited resolution and contrast—with advances in digital technology, modern-day ultrasound equipment embraced the use of liquid crystal displays (LCDs) and light-emitting diodes (LEDs), which supply higher image quality and visibility.

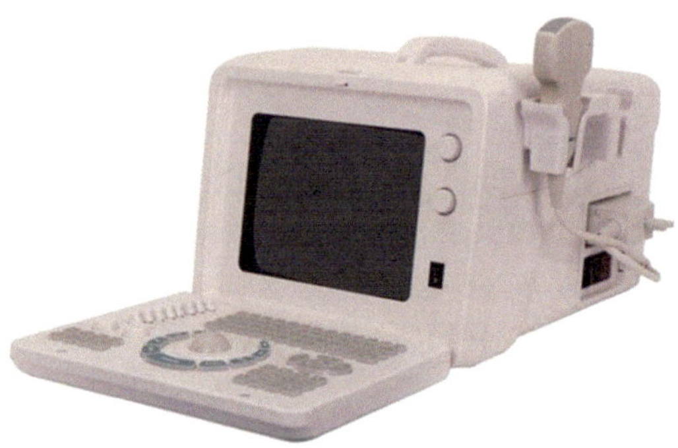

Figure 6.12. CRT display Bx-550 ultrasound machine.

Source: https://tiimg.tistatic.com/fp/1/001/837/crt-display-bx-550-ultrasound-machine-for-medical-use-211.jpg.

These new screens enable better visualization of anatomical and pathological features, resulting in accurate diagnoses. Such advances in display technology not only enhanced the aesthetic appeal of images but also improved the functionality of ultrasound machines, making real-time imaging crucial in many clinical settings. Interfacing color Doppler and spectral Doppler imaging technologies has continued to enhance ultrasound systems' visual capabilities. They enable the measurement of tissue motion and blood flow, providing crucial information for the evaluation of cardiac, vascular, and obstetric illnesses (Figure 6.12).

Color Doppler imaging uses a color overlay on the grayscale images to indicate blood flow direction and speed, making it easier for practitioners to interpret complex dynamics. Advances in display processing power also enable simultaneous visualization of multiple modalities, such as the combination of 2D and 3D imaging. Multimodality enables broader assessment during examinations, thereby enhancing the diagnostic capabilities of healthcare practitioners. Furthermore, the advent of high-definition and three-dimensional (3D) ultrasound imaging has redefined the norm of diagnostic imaging. High-definition monitors provide more advanced visualization of tissue structures, whereas 3D imaging generates volumetric data, offering unparalleled information about spatial relationships. They are particularly crucial for obstetric imaging, where exquisite detail of fetal anatomy is essential. By integrating 3D visualization techniques with emerging display technologies, clinicians can provide more accurate evaluations and improve patient outcomes. Continuous development in display technologies will definitely be at the forefront of the evolution of the discipline of ultrasound imaging and make it an inevitable resource in today's medicine, as seen from contemporary resources (N/A, 1985 and (N/A, 2011)

6.5. Safety and Bioeffects of Ultrasound

The safety and bioeffects of ultrasound imaging have been of concern in medical physics, particularly given its widespread use across a variety of clinical applications. Standard diagnostic ultrasound is safe in that it uses non-ionizing radiation, but recent research is raising concerns about potential adverse effects. An extensive study highlighted the neurotoxic impact of prenatal ultrasound scanning on developing fetuses, indicating that excessive exposure could result in changes in hematological indices, such as red blood cell count and hemoglobin levels, among newborns in animal models. These findings underscore the need for firm rules on exposure duration and intensity, with a particular requirement that even routine practices be periodically reevaluated in light of new science and evolving applications of ultrasound technology (Razak et al., 2013). New technology introduces the development of wearable ultrasound devices, which pose particular concerns regarding safety and bioeffects. Unlike standard systems that typically use acoustic energy for short periods, wearable ultrasound technology allows extended exposure. This aspect raises concerns about extended acoustic exposure, particularly potential thermal and mechanical bioeffects on tissues. These aspects have to be taken into account in order to ensure safety for patients who may benefit from continuous monitoring or treatment. Moreover, as wear time increases, issues related to skin health and comfort also need to be evaluated. Hence, comprehensive research is needed to address these potential risks and establish safety procedures that ensure maximum benefit of wearable ultrasound technology with minimal or no harm (Andre et al., 2024). The complexity of ultrasound safety and bioeffects requires interdisciplinary research among scientists, engineers, and clinicians. The use of multiple experts ensures a holistic understanding of the engineering principles underlying ultrasound devices and their clinical impact. Proper such collaboration is necessary to extend research on safety aspects and standardize protocols, considering diagnostic as well as therapeutic use. Keeping the focus on bioeffects, despite advancing technology, will enable practitioners to provide effective patient care with minimal risk. More studies of ultrasound bioeffects will eventually lead to a more informed and cautious application of ultrasound, particularly as novel technologies are forthcoming and its uses extend into other areas of clinical medicine (Razak et al., 2013; Andre et al., 2024).

6.5.1. Ultrasound Safety Regulatory Standards

There is a need to develop regulatory standards for ultrasound safety to ensure the continued efficiency and reliability of ultrasound technologies in research, clinical, and medical use. These guidelines are developed by regulatory bodies, like the Food and Drug Administration (FDA) in the United States, that govern the production, operation, and use of ultrasound devices. These guidelines encompass a set of safety criteria, including thermal and mechanical indices, to reduce potential risks to operators and patients. In practical terms, adhering to these guidelines not only protects patient welfare but also encourages confidence among health practitioners regarding the efficiency of ultrasound treatments. Technological advancements, such as the development of photoacoustic imaging (PAI), have prompted ongoing reviews of these regulatory frameworks to ensure they remain relevant to the rapidly evolving technologies in medical imaging (Assi et al., 2023) (Figure 6.13).

Furthermore, the lack of globally accepted standards can negatively impact the consistent application of ultrasound technologies. Specifically regarding biophotonic applications, such as PAI, the lack of standardized phantoms for technical verification impedes the use of reliable, reproducible results. The creation of appropriate tissue-mimicking phantoms can address regulatory requirements by providing standards against which new ultrasound technologies can be validated. The most recent research is now requiring increased collaboration between scientists, engineers, and regulatory agencies to close these standardization gaps. By developing standards for phantom design and testing, stakeholders can simplify the evaluation of ultrasound safety and efficacy (Bohndiek et al., 2022). This will make it easier to integrate new technology into clinical use while ensuring conformity with safety standards.

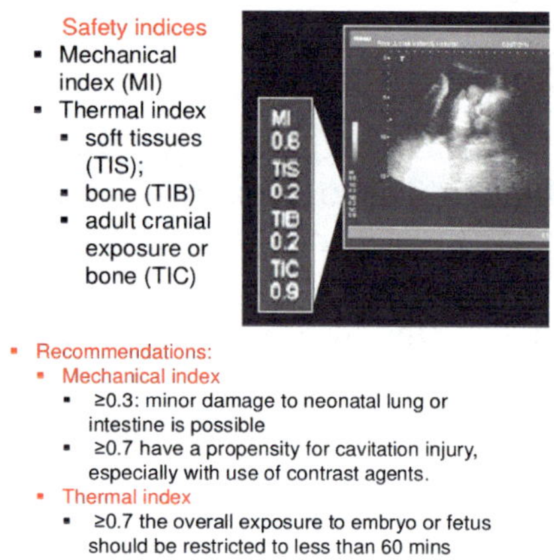

Figure 6.13. Infographic summarizing international regulatory safety limits for ultrasound exposure.

Source: https://futuremed-tr.com/documents/posts/5db7afeea5e53.jpg?1572319214.

Also, as the ultrasound technology landscape continues to evolve, regulatory bodies must continually revise their regulations to incorporate new advancements in imaging modalities and methods. The emergence of sophisticated ultrasound applications, such as elastography or contrast-enhanced ultrasound, brings with it further regulatory sophistication, where regulators' continuous exchange with physicians becomes inevitable. Fighting the novel threats in ultrasound safety regulation will require a proactive strategy founded on extensive education and training of concerned professionals handling such equipment. Creating watchfulness regarding non-compliance with safety standards can foster a safety culture in ultrasound practice, ultimately serving patients' interests and upholding confidence in this valuable imaging modality.

6.5.2. Tissue Bioeffects That Are Possible

The use of ultrasound in medical imaging has potential bioeffects on the tissues being imaged, which need to be closely examined. The amplitude and frequency of the acoustic energy used in ultrasound scanning can cause a range of physiological changes in biological tissues.

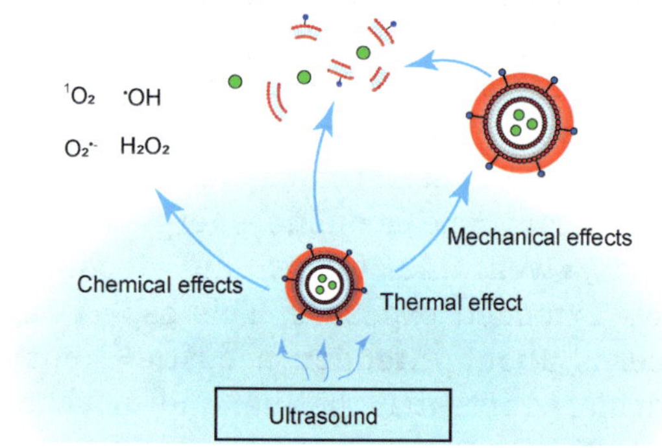

Figure 6.14. Illustration of potential thermal and mechanical effects of ultrasound on soft tissues.

Source: https://th.bing.com/th/id/OIP.Ul8iN-v1lwfvU6emluAgIQHaEr?rs=1&pid=ImgDetMain.

Notably, the research has demonstrated exposure to ultrasound can induce thermogenic effects, particularly in developing fetal tissue. For instance, an experiment using pregnant rabbits proved an association between exposure to ultrasound and drastic alterations of neonatal hematological parameters, such as a severe decrease in the number and hemoglobin level of the red blood cells. These findings highlight the need for rigorous guidelines and regulation of ultrasound examinations to minimize the risk of potential bioeffects, especially among sensitive groups such as fetuses, whose developmental stages are highly sensitive to environmental stimuli (Razak et al., 2013). Prolonged acoustic exposure from sophisticated ultrasound systems, such as wearable ultrasound devices, also increases the complexity of interpreting the impact of bioeffects on tissue. Such probes, which permit long-term monitoring by providing acoustic energy for longer durations than standard ultrasound machines, pose problems of cumulative exposure (Figure 6.14).

Increased exposure time could introduce a greater risk of thermal damage or mechanical strain in tissues if factors of safety are not adequately accounted for. With researchers and clinicians moving into the implications of wearable ultrasound, there is a requirement to consider both biological responses to acoustic energy and impact on skin well-being. Prudent balancing of benefits versus risks will ultimately decide the clinical usefulness of such novel technologies (Andre et al., 2024). Quantification of the bioeffects on tissue resulting from ultrasound exposure requires not only an understanding of ultrasound physics but also an interdisciplinary effort involving biological contributions. Continued research into the mechanisms underlying ultrasound-altered tissue changes is required to advance ultrasound technology safely for patients.

The union of engineering design and biological understanding may make it easier to create safer ultrasound, potentially leading to clearer standards in exposure limits as well as procedural perfection. With advancing imaging and monitoring technologies, these bioeffects will continue to be a crucial part of ultrasound physics and instrumentation to avoid overuse, optimize benefits, and maintain patient safety and health (Razak et al., 2013; Andre et al., 2024).

6.5.3. Safe Practice Guidelines for Ultrasound

Safe ultrasound practice is critical to patient safety and the success of ultrasound imaging. Training and competence on the part of the operator are emphasized in guidelines because the accuracy of ultrasound diagnosis is, to a large degree, dependent upon the experience and proficiency of the technician. Misinterpretation and unnecessary risk to the patient can result if training is insufficient. Moreover, operators need to stay updated with advancements in technology and techniques in ultrasound imaging.

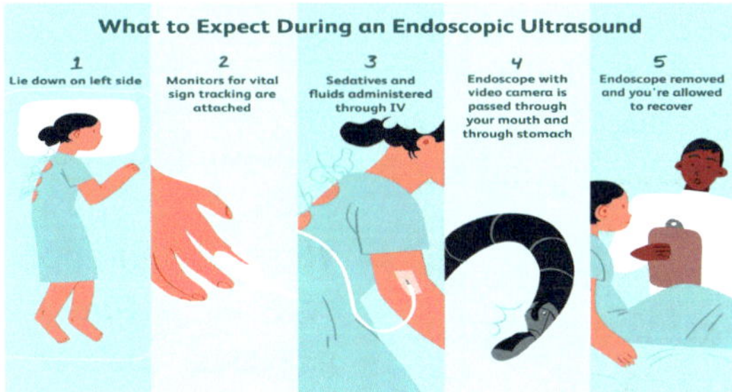

Figure 6.15. Summary chart of recommended practices for minimizing ultrasound risks during clinical use.

Source: https://www.verywellhealth.com/thmb/SFNipqkPTxXQ0H7Sy-6WPnxXaYY=/750x0/filters:no_upscale():max_bytes(150000):strip_icc()/endoscopic-ultrasound-uses-side-effects-procedure-results-4176265_color1-5c05a05e46e0fb00010588a2.png.

This encompasses familiarization with new devices and techniques, which is relevant given the field's rapid pace of change, including future techniques such as photoacoustic imaging. According to educational guidelines, practitioners can derive the maximum benefit from the application of ultrasound technology, prevent potential harm, and ultimately ensure quality patient care in accordance with the highest standards of practice. In addition to operator education, strict sterilization and disinfection protocols are essential for safe ultrasounds. As ultrasound transducers directly contact the patient's skin, equipment cleanliness is extremely important to prevent cross-contamination and infection (Figure 6.15).

Recommendations are to regularly clean and disinfect ultrasound probes before and after each use, especially in high-risk departments such as obstetrics and gynecology. The establishment of these hygienic standards is further enforced by clear procedures and guidelines that healthcare administrators must ensure. In addition, instances where the use of gel or other mediums is required should consider hypoallergenic mediums to minimize allergic reactions among hypersensitive patients. By implementing stringent disinfection protocols, healthcare professionals contribute to creating safe ultrasound environments and enhancing patient confidence. Standardizing ultrasound practice is critical to safety and patient outcomes. Innovations in simulation-based training and the use of flow phantoms can facilitate learning among ultrasound technicians significantly. In addition to recent advances, a Complex Flow Phantom model was created, which not only confirms the consistency of ultrasound machines but also provides further insight into fluid dynamics across imaging modalities. Through continuous assessment using tools such as Computational Fluid Dynamics (CFD) and validation methods, technicians can refine their skills before handling real patients. As noted, the ability to self-check methods ensures consistency and replicability, which are essential for achieving excellence in ultrasound physics and instrumentation. This adherence to standard methods ensures diagnostic reliability and fosters compliance with current guidelines on safe ultrasound practice, thereby enhancing overall patient safety standards (Assi et al., 2023; Ambrogio et al., 2019).

6.6. Clinical Applications of Ultrasound

Its medical applications have expanded dramatically in recent decades, from a mere diagnostic modality to an all-inclusive technology with the ability of responding to a myriad of various medical needs. Initially used primarily for obstetric scanning to monitor fetal development, ultrasound is now employed in many fields of medicine, including cardiology, urology, and emergency medicine. Its ability to provide real-time imaging renders it invaluable for guiding minimally invasive procedures such as biopsies and catheter placements.

Additionally, advancements in ultrasound technology, including Doppler and 3D imaging, have greatly enhanced its diagnostic capabilities, providing clinicians with robust information about blood flow and organ morphology. This versatility of application confirms ultrasound's role as a fundamental modality in clinical practice, further validating its applicability not only as a diagnostic tool but also as an integral component of therapeutic treatment protocols. Among ultrasound's applications is its use in cardiac assessments, where it helps evaluate cardiac structure and function. Echocardiography, utilizing ultrasonic waves, is used for non-invasive diagnosis of cardiac ailments such as valvular heart disease, heart failure, and congenital heart disease. By visualizing the movement of the heart walls and blood flow through the cardiac chambers, the technique enables physicians to diagnose and monitor a variety of heart diseases effectively. The ability to perform echocardiography at the bedside gives it an essential role in emergency and critical care settings, allowing rapid decision-making for potentially time-critical conditions. With the ongoing evolution of the medical environment, the integration of advanced ultrasound technology into core cardiac management remains to enhance patient outcomes and streamline clinical practice.

Further, ultrasound, which is outside the range of traditional imaging, significantly influences therapeutic intervention by enabling procedures such as ultrasound-guided interventions. Real-time visualization of anatomic structures has improved clinicians' ability to perform various procedures, particularly in musculoskeletal medicine and pain management. For instance, ultrasound guidance of corticosteroid injections ensures accurate placement, decreasing complications and maximizing therapeutic effect. This capability not only enhances patient safety but also increases the likelihood of successful outcomes, underscoring the significant impact ultrasound has on medical practice. As the practice evolves further, the use of ultrasound technology in numerous therapeutic settings will see further expansion, promoting improvements in the quality of patient care and increasing the precision of procedures in multiple medical settings (Figure 6.16).

6.6.1. Obstetric and Gynecological Ultrasound

The practice of maternal-fetal medicine and gynecology has been revolutionized by the application of obstetric and gynecologic ultrasound as a non-invasive imaging modality with accurate diagnostic precision. The application of such ultrasound modalities enables fetal growth monitoring, diagnosis of placental position, and diagnosis of congenital malformations during pregnancy. In gynecology, further, ultrasound remains an important modality for the assessment of disorders such as ovarian cysts, fibroids, and uterine bleeding. Real-time imaging enables clinicians to make timely, informed decisions, resulting in improved patient outcomes. The development of such practices demands an understanding of the physics of ultrasound technology, such as sound wave propagation, frequency selection, and the interaction between tissue and the ultrasound beam, to provide an approach for efficient diagnosis and management in clinical practice. Furthermore, advancements in ultrasound technology have enabled the development of portable devices, making obstetric and gynecological services highly accessible. Miniaturization has led to the development of miniature ultrasound devices, including pocket ultrasound devices, which are more convenient for practitioners, particularly for those in low-resource environments. Studies quantifying the performance of such hand-held units show that they can provide immense diagnostic capacity equal to that of standard ultrasound equipment, particularly for non-cardiologic populations (Santoro et al., 2010). The ability to perform complete examinations for peripheral or disadvantaged communities, hence, represents an immense milestone in maternal health, allowing for early detection of complications that can arise during pregnancy. With ongoing research and development, the use of these technologies in everyday clinical practice has the ability to greatly impact accessibility, enhancing maternal and fetal health results. In addition to technological advancement, ultrasound teaching and education are fundamental in making healthcare workers capable of using the advancements effectively. Proper training equips professionals with skills to interpret ultrasound scans appropriately, enhancing diagnosis. With the advancement of ultrasound technology and contributions from physics and medical imaging innovators like Ian Donald, there remains a need for ongoing professional training in this field (Johnston et al., 2006). This keeps practitioners current with new techniques, attuned to the nuances of ultrasound physics, and able to apply these skills to provide high-quality obstetric and gynecologic care. Ultimately, as demand for ultrasound services grows, investment in education and training will be required to sustain the high level of patient care characteristic of modern medical practice.

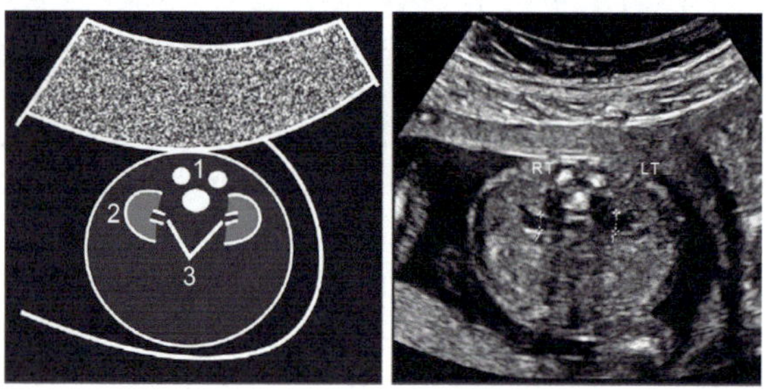

Figure 6.16. A pictorial guide for the second trimester ultrasound.

Source: https://onlinelibrary.wiley.com/cms/asset/0343ee49-796d-41ed-8ca0-118867d1486f/ajum00106-fig-0034-m.jpg.

6.6.2. Cardiac Ultrasound and Echocardiography

The field of echocardiography and ultrasound is a core discipline in the fields of ultrasound physics and instrumentation because it can display the structures and function of the heart in real time. It is an imaging technique that uses high-frequency sound waves to produce dynamic, two- and three-dimensional images of the heart noninvasively. The echocardiographic imaging mode offers diversity, with applications including transthoracic and transesophageal echocardiography, each suited to specific clinical scenarios and patient groups. By assessing chamber dimensions, wall motion, and valve function, echocardiography is a fundamental tool for diagnosing cardiovascular disease, planning therapeutic intervention, and monitoring treatment outcomes. The incorporation of Doppler ultrasound further enhances the ability to measure hemodynamics and provides vital information on blood flow patterns, which are imperative for successful cardiac evaluation. The technical advancements in the equipment utilized in echocardiography reflect broader advancements in the engineering and physical sciences (EPS), which are a principal driver of advances in the health and life sciences (HLS). A solid foundation in ultrasound technology, including transducer design and image-algorithm processes, underpins the accuracy and effectiveness of cardiac imaging (Figure 6.17).

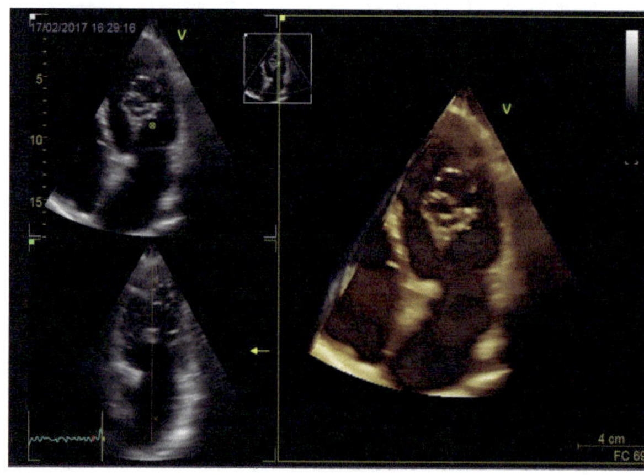

Figure 6.17. Echocardiographic image displaying heart valve function.

Source: https://www.researchgate.net/publication/320998361/figure/fig1/AS:654633995337729@1533088315598/Three-dimensional-transthoracic-echocardiographic-imaging-displaying-accessory-mitral.png.

In addition to basic B-mode imaging, more recent developments such as tissue Doppler imaging and strain imaging are now available to allow accurate assessment of myocardial function and tissue characterization. These advancements underscore the synergy between

EPS and HLS research, as advances in imaging technology are crucial to further developing the diagnostic capabilities of clinical cardiology. Thus, echocardiography is not only a superb illustration of the application of physical principles but also highlights how medical research and engineering fields must interact constantly to enable more efficient healthcare procedures (Smart et al., 2014). In terms of adapting cardiac ultrasound expectations, it is imperative to consider how technology affects diagnostic accuracy and patient outcomes. While echocardiographic instrumentation is generally accessible, its application in special situations—such as microgravity conditions on space missions—requires precise calibration and adjustment. Research into these accommodations shows both current technological capabilities and the need for continued development in instrumentation design (Ganiaris et al., 2025). This project not only adds to our understanding of cardiovascular physiology under varying conditions but also enhances the quality of patient care provided to patients on Earth. Furthermore, as echocardiography continues to advance, it is paramount for health professionals to maintain rigorous training and education in new technologies so they can effectively and dynamically utilize these advancements to improve patient management.

6.6.3. Musculoskeletal Ultrasound for Injury Evaluation

The use of musculoskeletal ultrasound (US) for injury assessment has gained popularity over the past several years in physical therapy and sports medicine. The imaging technique offers a non-invasive means to visualize soft tissues, joints, and other musculoskeletal structures, thereby aiding in the accurate diagnosis and management of injury. The ability to visualize real-time dynamics of musculoskeletal tissues during movement allows clinicians to quantify the extent of injury and guide rehabilitation protocols. Despite its advantages, the integration of the US into routine practice is challenged by barriers, one of the significant ones being a lack of comprehensive regulatory guidelines for physical therapists. These lacunae point to the need for stronger education models and competency-based training programs to develop practitioners with the competencies to properly utilize this technology in clinical settings (Bur Aía et al., 2019). As physical therapists increasingly integrate ultrasound, there is a growing need to identify its various applications (Figure 6.18).

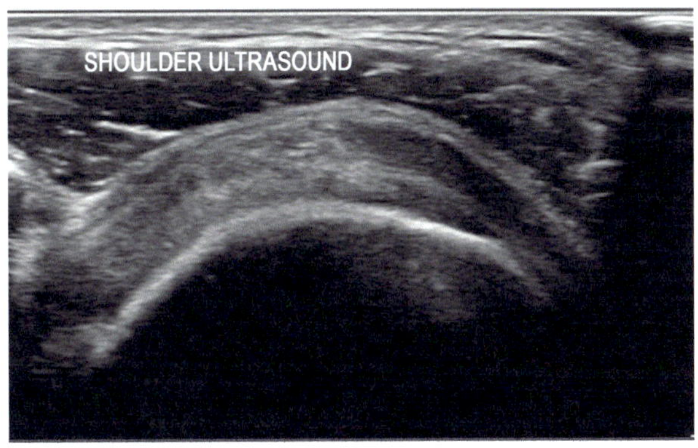

Figure 6.18. Musculoskeletal ultrasound scan identifying a partial tendon tear.

Source: https://ultrasoundscan.co.za/wp-content/uploads/2022/02/shoulder-600x365.jpg.

Musculoskeletal ultrasound is not only reserved for diagnostic purposes but also enables rehabilitation and intervention, with immediate feedback on treatment effectiveness. For instance, imaging of tendon healing can guide the determination to progress rehabilitation protocols or modify loading schemes. In this regard, an understanding of the depth and breadth of ultrasound use can facilitate high-value care in physical therapy. Such multidimensional injury assessment helps provide treatment plans tailored to patients' needs, thereby improving clinical outcomes and patient satisfaction. Its application in physical therapy can transform care delivery, and its role in the evolving rehabilitation landscape cannot be overemphasized (N/A, 2008). Furthermore, the future of musculoskeletal ultrasound in practice relies on enhancing learning opportunities for physical therapists. The current imbalance in training programs hinders the application of ultrasound technology in rehabilitation settings; thus, it is essential to develop a robust competency-based education model to address this gap. This model should emphasize theory and practical experience equally so that practitioners can successfully advance in ultrasound imaging and its clinical applications. These programs can include workshops, certification training courses, and collaborative studies that reinforce practice skills and evidence-based practice. With these educational standards met, the profession can ensure that physical therapists are not only competent in the use of ultrasound but can also make contributions to research and development in the field of musculoskeletal imaging (Bur Aía et al., 2019).

SUMMARY

In summarizing the broad scope of ultrasound physics and instrumentation, it is evident that the usage of such technology is extensive and very common in medical diagnosis and industrial applications. The non-invasive evaluation capabilities of ultrasound technologies enable doctors to draw appropriate conclusions from the resulting images. It is important to note that advances in instrumentation have enabled higher resolution and deeper penetration, crucial for exposing internal anatomical structures. As shown, maintaining such intricate systems requires continuous research and optimization of techniques to mitigate inaccuracies caused by various factors, such as internal pipe wall roughness when using ultrasonic flowmeters, as detailed in Cegla et al. (2018). Such stringent attention to detail not only validates the efficacy of ultrasound application but also emphasizes the importance of user training and operating expertise. Furthermore, exploring the horizon of future uses for ultrasound technology is a broad field of possibilities. The integration of new methods, such as Multiplexing Electric Field Sensors (MEFS), indicates a breakthrough revolution in non-invasive quality inspection techniques. Such developments address fundamental needs across diverse industries, including food quality and safety, underscoring the expanding potential of ultrasound technology beyond standard medical uses. Benefits of MEFS utilization demonstrate its potential in successfully detecting foreign objects and quantifying fat levels, indicative of its application in food quality monitoring systems, as illustrated in Capdeboscq et al. (2018). Beyond being cost-effective, ultrasound technology is also promising for its flexibility and non-destructiveness, indicative of a rosy future for ultrasound in the healthcare and food quality sectors. In short, the field of ultrasound physics and instrumentation continues to be dynamic with challenges and promising opportunities equally. The ability to reduce measurement uncertainties through more sophisticated methods directly enhances the credibility of ultrasound applications across various fields. As with the study of scattering effects in flow measuring instruments in (Cegla et al., 2018), further research is essential to minimize sources of potential inaccuracy and increase the reliability of ultrasonic assessments. Likewise, the encouraging advances in tools such as MEFS portend a new milestone in improving food security and quality surveillance systems. In the future, researchers and practitioners must collaborate to create ways of taking advantage of the full potential of ultrasound so that its applications are not only effective but also in compliance with the most up-to-date science and technology.

CLOSER LOOK

ULTRASOUND PHYSICS

Ultrasound physics is the study of the physical principles and properties that govern the generation, transmission, and reception of ultrasound waves in medical imaging. Ultrasound refers to sound waves with frequencies higher than the upper limit of human hearing, typically above 20,000 Hz. In medical imaging, most diagnostic ultrasound operates between 2 and 15 MHz. These high-frequency sound waves are produced by a transducer containing piezoelectric crystals, which convert electrical energy into mechanical vibrations. When activated, these crystals emit sound waves into the body. As these waves travel through tissues, they are reflected, refracted, scattered, or absorbed depending on the acoustic properties of the tissues they encounter. The returning echoes are captured by the same transducer, which then converts them back into electrical signals. The ultrasound machine processes these signals to create real-time images of internal body structures.A fundamental concept in ultrasound physics is the speed of sound in different media. In soft tissue, sound travels at an average speed of 1540 m/s. However, this speed can vary depending on the medium's density and elasticity. For example, sound travels faster through bone than through air. The difference in acoustic impedance—the product of tissue density and sound speed—between two adjacent tissues determines how much of the sound wave is reflected at their interface. Greater impedance differences produce stronger echoes, which appear brighter on the ultrasound image. This principle underlies ultrasound's ability to differentiate between structures such as organs, blood vessels, and abnormal masses.Another important concept is attenuation, the gradual loss of sound wave energy as it propagates through tissue. Attenuation occurs due to absorption, scattering, and reflection, and it increases with frequency. Higher-frequency ultrasound provides better resolution but is more rapidly attenuated, limiting its depth of penetration. Therefore, different transducer frequencies are used depending on the clinical application; for instance, high-frequency probes are suitable for superficial structures such as the thyroid, while low-frequency probes are better for imaging deeper organs such as the liver or uterus.Ultrasound imaging also relies heavily on the Doppler effect, which measures changes in the frequency of sound waves as they reflect off moving objects, such as red blood cells. This principle allows clinicians to assess blood flow in vessels, detect turbulence, and measure the velocity and direction of flow. Color Doppler, spectral Doppler, and power Doppler are techniques that enhance the evaluation of vascular structures and cardiac function.Overall, ultrasound physics provides the foundation for safe, non-invasive, and real-time imaging that is essential in many areas of medicine, including obstetrics, cardiology, emergency medicine, and musculoskeletal imaging. A thorough understanding of these principles helps ensure accurate image interpretation, optimal equipment use, and high-quality patient care.

REFERENCES

1. Abdul Razak, H. R., Ahmad Zaiki, F. W., Hassan, H. F., Md Dom, M., et al. (2013). Prenatal ultrasound heating impacts on fluctuations in hematological analysis of *Oryctolagus cuniculus*. https://core.ac.uk/download/300437974.pdf (accessed on 14th July 2025).
2. Hogg, T., Freitas, R. A., Jr, Hogg, T., & Freitas, R. A., Jr. (2012). Acoustic communication for medical nanorobots. *Nano Communication Networks*, *3*(2), 83–102. https://doi.org/10.1016/j.nancom.2012.02.002Alquaydheb, I. N., Eltawil, A. M., Khorshid, A. E., Kurdahi, F., et al. (2018). Physical multi-layer phantoms for intra-body communications. http://arxiv.org/abs/1806.04219 (accessed on 14th July 2025).
3. Ambrogio, S. (2019). Development of a complex flow phantom for diagnostic imaging. https://core.ac.uk/download/293755112.pdf (accessed on 14th July 2025).
4. Anastasio, M. A., Duric, N., Li, C., Matthews, T. P., et al. (2017). Regularized dual averaging image reconstruction for full-wave ultrasound computed tomography. http://arxiv.org/abs/1708.07221 (accessed on 14th July 2025).
5. Anastasio, M. A., Gupta, R., Maier-Hein, L., Manohar, S., et al. (2023). Imaging super phantoms. http://arxiv.org/abs/2308.12692 (accessed on 14th July 2025).
6. Anastasio, M. A., Gupta, R., Maier-Hein, L., Manohar, S., et al. (2024). Super phantoms: Advanced models for testing medical imaging technologies. https://core.ac.uk/download/621168560.pdf (accessed on 14th July 2025).
7. Andre, M., Chitnis, P., Croy, T., Sikdar, S., et al. (2024). Clinical, safety, and engineering perspectives on wearable ultrasound technology: A review. https://core.ac.uk/download/622191020.pdf (accessed on 14th July 2025).
8. Angeli, P., Hossein, F., Lettieri, P., Materazzi, M., et al. (2021). Application of acoustic techniques to fluid-particle systems–A review. https://core.ac.uk/download/480392622.pdf (accessed on 14th July 2025).
9. Arias Buría, J. L., Ellis, R., Fernández Carnero, S., Hides, J., et al. (2019). Imaging with ultrasound in physical therapy: What is the PT's scope of practice? A competency-based educational model and training recommendations. https://core.ac.uk/download/370420664.pdf (accessed on 14th July 2025).
10. Arridge, S. R., Leung, T. S., & Powell, S. (2015). Gradient-based quantitative image reconstruction in ultrasound-modulated optical tomography: First harmonic measurement type in a linearized diffusion formulation. https://core.ac.uk/download/79497083.pdf (accessed on 14th July 2025).
11. Assi, H., Bohndiek, S. E., Cao, R., Castelino, A., et al. (2023). A review of a strategic road mapping exercise to advance clinical translation of photoacoustic imaging: From current barriers to future adoption. https://core.ac.uk/download/580092264.pdf (accessed on 14th July 2025).
12. Bailey, M. R., Cleveland, R. O., Fineberg, N., Hartenbaum, S., et al. (2000). Design and characterization of a research electrohydraulic lithotripter patterned after the Dornier HM3. https://core.ac.uk/download/4870305.pdf (accessed on 14th July 2025).
13. Bhagat, P. K., & Kadaba, P. K. (2025). Development of limb volume measuring system. https://core.ac.uk/download/pdf/42848916.pdf (accessed on 14th July 2025).

14. Bohndiek, S. E., Hacker, L., Pfefer, T. J., Pifferi, A., Pogue, B. W., & Wabnitz, H. (2022). Criteria for the design of tissue-mimicking phantoms for the standardization of biophotonic instrumentation. https://core.ac.uk/download/554201238.pdf (accessed on 14th July 2025).
15. Bowen, J. W., Walker, G. C., Hadjiloucas, S., Berry, E., Chou, C. K., Brettle, D. S., Fitzgerald, A. J., Ghiglia, D. C., et al. (2004). Materials for phantoms for terahertz pulsed imaging. https://core.ac.uk/download/58598.pdf (accessed on 14th July 2025).
16. Capdeboscq, Y., Rittscher, A. E., Rittscher, J., Sulaimalebbe, A., et al. (2018). Foreign object detection and quantification of fat content using a novel multiplexing electric field sensor. http://arxiv.org/abs/1806.08596 (accessed on 14th July 2025).
17. Cardoni, A., Cerisola, N., Lucas, M., Mathieson, I., et al. (2015). Understanding nonlinear vibration behaviors in high-power ultrasonic surgical devices. https://core.ac.uk/download/42360528.pdf (accessed on 14th July 2025).
18. Cegla, F., & Gu, X. (2018). The effect of internal pipe wall roughness on the accuracy of clamp-on ultrasonic flow meters. https://core.ac.uk/download/157858824.pdf (accessed on 14th July 2025).
19. Chan, C. C., Dobie, G. I. I., Friedrich, M., Galbraith, H., et al. (2009). Miniature mobile sensor platforms for condition monitoring of structures. https://core.ac.uk/download/9558883.pdf (accessed on 14th July 2025).
20. Chougule, M. B., Dave, V. S., Haware, R. V., Shahin, A., et al. (2017). Emerging technologies for the non-invasive characterization of physical-mechanical properties of tablets. https://core.ac.uk/download/129153450.pdf (accessed on 14th July 2025).
21. Christie, D. A., & Tansey, E. M. (2006). Development of physics applied to medicine in the UK, 1945–90. https://core.ac.uk/download/30696186.pdf (accessed on 14th July 2025).
22. Constanciel, E., Drake, J. M., Hosseini, B., Mougenot, C., et al. (2018). A Bayesian approach for energy-based estimation of acoustic aberrations in high intensity focused ultrasound treatment. https://core.ac.uk/download/211387916.pdf (accessed on 14th July 2025).
23. Ganiaris, N. J., Polhemus, J. T., & Schappell, R. T. (2025). Cardiovascular instrumentation for spaceflight. https://core.ac.uk/download/pdf/42879383.pdf (accessed on 14th July 2025).
24. Greene, E. R., Nadeau, J. J., & Schulze, A. E. (2025). In-suit Doppler technology assessment. https://core.ac.uk/download/pdf/42809264.pdf (accessed on 14th July 2025).
25. Johnston, S. F. (2006). The physical tourist. *Physics in Glasgow: A heritage tour.* https://core.ac.uk/download/1393823.pdf (accessed on 14th July 2025).
26. Kippelen, B., Marder, S. R., Peyghambarian, N., Röckel, H., et al. (1998). Transillumination imaging through scattering media by use of photorefractive polymers. https://core.ac.uk/download/4871475.pdf (accessed on 14th July 2025).
27. Klima, S. J., & Vary, A. (2025). Nondestructive techniques for characterizing mechanical properties of structural materials: An overview. https://core.ac.uk/download/pdf/42842083.pdf (accessed on 14th July 2025).

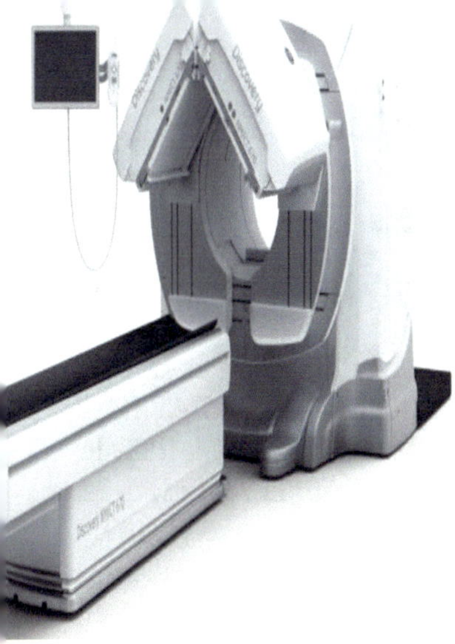

Chapter 7

NUCLEAR MEDICINE: GAMMA CAMERA AND SPECT

Contents

Introduction

Nuclear medicine is a significant intersection of imaging and therapeutic practice, revolutionizing the way physicians diagnose and treat certain ailments. The field utilizes radiopharmaceuticals that emit gamma rays, which are interpretable by specialized cameras to provide detailed descriptions of the body's physiological processes. Most notably, gamma cameras and Single Photon Emission Computed Tomography (SPECT) altered the imaging landscape, enabling high-resolution visualization of organ function and anatomy. Apart from making real-time diagnosis possible, these technologies not only follow treatment efficacy but also track therapy efficacy in a variety of diseases, most significantly in cardiology and oncology. Since it is a developing branch of medicine, nuclear medicine continues to grow and adopt new technologies that enhance imaging and improve patient care, underscoring its significant role in the broader scheme of modern medicine. Perhaps most critical to the success of nuclear medicine are radioisotope production and radiochemistry, which provide the foundation for radiopharmaceuticals. The two primary sources of such isotopes are generators and reactors, each with distinct advantages and implications for clinical practice. Radioisotopes generated by reactors are generally the preferred choice because of their high specific activity and accessibility; however, isotopes generated by generators offer logistical advantages, including ease of access and transport. The elaborate processes of radiolabeling such isotopes guarantee their specific binding of target tissues to enhance imaging specificity. Additionally, rigorous quality control measures must be implemented to verify the purity, potency, and safety of radiopharmaceuticals in accordance with regulatory standards and clinical practice guidelines. Thus, understanding these fundamental aspects is vital to improving imaging performance and protecting patients in nuclear medicine procedures. The gamma camera and SPECT system design and operation form the core of nuclear imaging advances. The image quality of acquired images is greatly influenced by factors such as the nature of the collimators, the properties of the scintillation crystals, and the arrangement of the photomultiplier array. The spatial resolution and sensitivity in imaging are, for example, predecided by the selection of collimators. Additionally, scintillation crystals that produce visible light after converting gamma photon energy are the center of camera detection. With technological innovations, detector design innovations such as the integration of cadmium-zinc telluride (CZT) into SPECT systems promise higher-quality images and more precise diagnoses. Combined, these technological advances not only optimize image resolution but also enable wider application of nuclear medicine procedures such as cardiac perfusion imaging and bone scintigraphy, thereby enhancing the field's clinical utility and impact on patient outcomes (Zuziak et al., 2023; Aleksa et al., 2025).

7.1. Principles of Gamma Cameras

The gamma camera design plays an essential role in the field of nuclear medicine, most critically in its ability to record and handle scintillation occurrences of gamma radiation. At its core is the collimator, which passively allows gamma photons to pass while maintaining spatial resolution, which is crucial to proper imaging. There are several types of collimators, such as parallel-hole, pinhole, and converging collimators, each with its own strengths and suited to specific imaging use. Camera imaging performance is directly affected by the use of the correct type of collimator, influencing sensitivity and resolution. Furthermore, collimator design and calibration must be aligned with the target imaging purposes to deliver optimal performance in detecting radioactive emissions from the body, as evidenced by the complexity of gamma camera design (Piwowarska-Bilska et al., 2019). Also of similar importance in gamma camera design is the scintillation crystal used to convert gamma photons into visible light. Common crystals used are sodium iodide thallium-activated (NaI(Tl) due to its high photon conversion efficiency and relatively good light output. The crystal properties, namely thickness and uniformity, have a decisive influence on the overall detection efficiency and imaging system resolution. When exposed to gamma rays, these crystals emit light pulses, which are then detected by photomultiplier tubes (PMTs) and amplified for analysis. Hence, the integration of high-quality scintillation crystals and an appropriate detection system provides the foundation for enhancing image quality and achieving accurate diagnostic results in nuclear medicine (Kane, 2002). Apart from fundamental design attributes, the imaging protocols used by gamma cameras also make a significant contribution to the attainment of high-quality diagnostic images. It involves defining the acquisition parameters, including image acquisition time, energy window values to reject lower energy scatter photons, and image corrections needed to minimize artifacts. Tuning such settings ensures clinicians obtain more precise images, which result in better diagnosis. For instance, parameters of the energy window are crucial in discriminating actual emission events from background noise, making the visual result more distinct. Further development of the sector, coupled with continuous improvements and optimizations in imaging protocols, will undoubtedly be instrumental for optimizing the clinical utility of gamma cameras in nuclear medicine (Piwowarska-Bilska et al., 2019).

7.1.1. Components of a Gamma Camera

The gamma camera is one of the principal imaging modalities in nuclear medicine, central to diagnostic image formation that images the body distribution of radiopharmaceuticals.

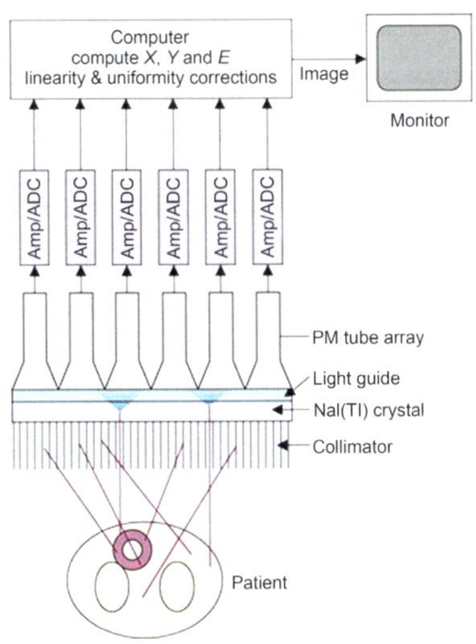

Figure 7.1. Schematic overview of a basic gamma camera system with labeled components.

Source: https://radiologykey.com/wp-content/uploads/2016/02/B9781416051985000137_f013-001-9781416051985.jpg.

Central to this system is the gamma camera collimator, which screens incoming gamma rays and allows only those from specific angles to pass through to the detector. Collimator design varies by type —parallel-hole, pinhole, or converging —and is selected based on imaging requirements and the body area of interest. Collimator efficiency directly affects image quality; an incorrect selection may result in decreased resolution or increased background noise, undermining diagnostic ability. A full appreciation of the collimator operation is necessary for the optimal use of the gamma camera and indirectly enhances patient care and diagnosis outcomes (Figure 7.1).

The heart of a gamma camera is the scintillation crystal, through which gamma radiation is transformed into visible light. The materials employed for this purpose are sodium iodide (NaI), which is used by preference because of its excellent scintillation properties. The thickness and material of the crystals decide the sensitivity and resolution of the camera; hence, proper care should be taken during the designing and calibration process. The scintillation events are then detected by photomultiplier tubes (PMTs), which multiply the light emitted by the crystal. Efficiency in light conversion and subsequent charge amplification are critical for the integrity of acquired images. With respect to the collimator, the nature of scintillation crystals is of vital significance to overall gamma camera performance, as they determine spatial resolution and detection sensitivity, both of which are critical for effective medical assessment. The photomultiplier array is the critical component that is paired with the scintillation crystal. The array consists of several PMTs that detect and enlarge the light emitted upon the interaction of gamma rays with the scintillation crystal. Tubes are carefully positioned in space to achieve optimal event detection and improve gamma camera localization accuracy. Each PMT converts the light of scintillation into electrical signals that are processed to determine the energy and position of the arriving gamma rays. This data enables the production of high-resolution images that doctors use to diagnose many diseases. Thus, ensuring the functional integrity of the photomultiplier array is vital, as its operation has immediate implications for image quality and diagnostic accuracy in nuclear medicine applications, thereby enhancing the gamma camera's value in clinical applications (Lamichhane et al., 2018; Andreas et al., 2020).

7.1.2. Functionality and Operation of Gamma Cameras

The function and operation of gamma cameras play a vital role in successful imaging in nuclear medicine. Central to the gamma camera's design is the employment of the scintillation crystal, which converts gamma radiation from radiopharmaceuticals into light. The most common substances employed in this purpose are sodium iodide doped with thallium (NaI(Tl), as it possesses high efficiency as well as good energy resolution. The emitted light is then detected by photomultiplier tubes (PMTs) and amplified to form images. The imaging relies heavily on the accurate placement of the collimator, which acts as a filter, permitting only gamma photons emitted in a specific direction to strike the crystal to increase spatial resolution and limit background noise, thereby improving the image quality needed for diagnostic purposes. Monitoring and optimizing gamma camera operating parameters are essential to achieving accurate imaging results. Acquisition parameters, energy window settings, and image corrections are critical parameters that require significant effort to optimize these systems. Acquisition parameters determine how data are acquired during imaging, with effects on image quality and patient safety. Energy window corrections are necessary to exclude low-energy photons not from the radiopharmaceutical of interest, ensuring that images are reliable and representative of the underlying physiology. Furthermore, various image correction techniques that account for scatter and detector nonuniformity are applied to enhance image resolution and diagnostic utility (Figure 7.2).

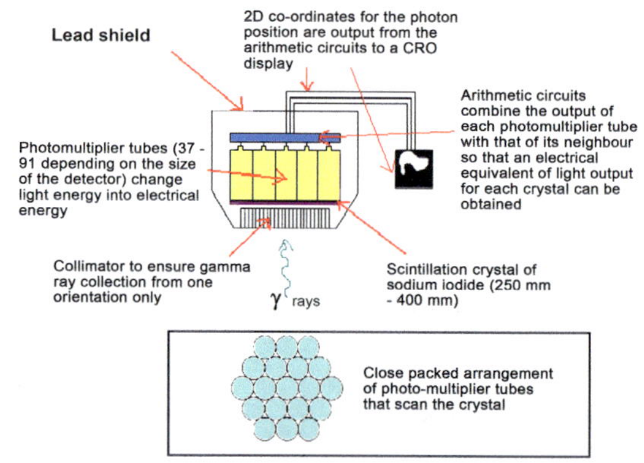

Figure 7.2. Flowchart illustrating the functionality and step-by-step operation of a gamma camera.

Source: https://www.researchgate.net/profile/Burak-Yalvac/publication/309536257/figure/fig1/AS:492845837623296@1494515012346/llustration-of-a-gamma-camera-7.png.

The interaction of these processes is important for getting the best quality outcome in imaging patients and the analysis that follows. Innovations in gamma camera technology over the recent past have led to hybrid imaging systems, including single-photon emission computed tomography (SPECT). SPECT has a superior ability to traditional gamma cameras through three-dimensional imaging via tomographic acquisition schemes. This allows enhanced visualization of the body's functional processes, thereby promoting more precise diagnoses and treatment planning. Reconstruction algorithms play a crucial role in transforming data from detectors into interpretable images, while attenuation correction procedures compensate for signal loss due to tissue absorption. The future of gamma camera technology, as indicated by advances in medical imaging informatics and integration with artificial intelligence, promises to enhance the precision of diagnostics and expand the clinical use of nuclear imaging modalities, as indicated by discussions in Andreas et al. (2020) and Sarrut et al. (2021) .

7.1.3. Applications in Clinical Settings

In medical practice, the development of nuclear medicine, particularly using gamma camera and SPECT (Single Photon Emission Computed Tomography) technologies, has transformed diagnostic imaging. Perhaps the most valuable application is in cardiac perfusion imaging, in which the assessment of myocardial blood flow is of paramount importance for the diagnosis and treatment of cardiovascular disease. Gating in SPECT imaging allows evaluation of function and perfusion, and hence an overall estimate of cardiac health. This feature is most pertinent in regions like the Caribbean and Latin America, where cardiovascular diseases have been seen to be highly prevalent. Moreover, the introduction of innovative technologies, such as cadmium-zinc-telluride (CZT) cameras, has enhanced image quality and diagnostic accuracy, enabling clinicians to select more optimal therapies (Pandey, 2024). Apart from its use in cardiology, SPECT also performs critical roles in other clinical practices, including in bone scintigraphy (Figure 7.3).

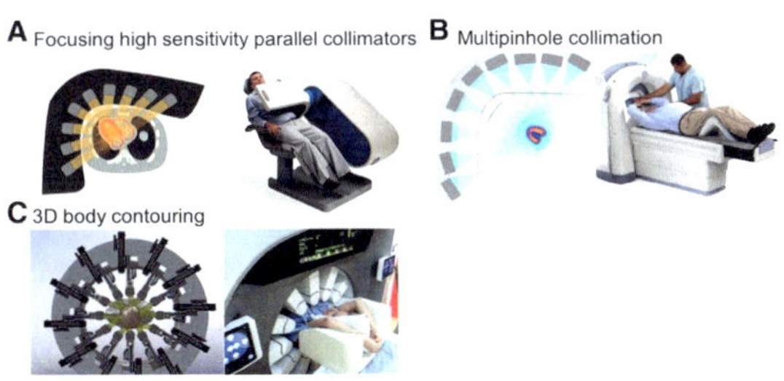

Figure 7.3. Example of gamma camera scans in clinical applications.

Source: https://jnm.snmjournals.org/content/jnumed/60/9/1194/F1.large.jpg.

This imaging modality is essential for identifying bone-metabolism disorders, including metastatic disease, infections, and inflammatory disease. By injecting radioisotopes, gamma cameras can obtain images that reflect the distribution of tracers in the skeletal system, leading to timely and accurate diagnoses. Furthermore, technical improvements in image correction protocols and reconstruction algorithms enhance the specificity and sensitivity of bone imaging, overcoming pitfalls posed by overlapping structures or patterns of radiopharmaceutical biodistribution. Real-time visualization of dynamic physiological processes has significant contributions to understanding various orthopedic diseases, thereby impacting patient management and the availability of treatment (Pandey, 2024).

Renal function studies also employ SPECT to obtain valuable information about kidney health. Quantitative assessment of renal perfusion and function is vital for diagnosing renal disease, including chronic kidney disease, and for assessing transplant viability. Gamma cameras enable measurement of parameters such as glomerular filtration rate (GFR) and effective renal plasma flow, which are crucial for assessing renal pathologies. With the evolution of sophisticated imaging protocols and quality-assurance programs, including uniformity and linearity testing, renal imaging accuracy continues to evolve. Practitioners appreciate this accurate information, facilitating easier prognostic assessment and tailored treatment planning. With the advancement of nuclear medicine, SPECT's adaptability in clinical practice remains essential for enhancing patient outcomes and care across a range of medical specialties (Peix et al., 2022).

7.2. Principles of SPECT Imaging

Among nuclear medicine procedures, Single Photon Emission Computed Tomography (SPECT) is an innovative imaging technique that produces three-dimensional images of body physiology in most tissues. SPECT imaging is based on the principles of gamma-ray detection and the sophisticated design of modern gamma cameras. This process exploits radiopharmaceuticals that emit one-photon radiation, which can be detected by the camera, enabling biological functions such as blood flow, metabolism, and receptor binding to be imaged. As imaging technology advances, innovations such as full-ring cadmium-zinc-telluride (CZT) detectors improve spatial resolution and sensitivity, enhancing diagnostic accuracy in clinical use. Rigorous inspection of imaging protocols, such as acquisition parameters and energy window settings, ensures the precision of acquired data, which is paramount for interpreting resulting images and decision-making in clinical practice (Aleksa et al., 2025).

Tomographic acquisition, one of the central processes in SPECT, enables cross-sectional image reconstruction that indicates the functional status of organs or tissues. Here, various reconstruction algorithms are used to optimize image quality and legibility, to the point that it is possible to visualize how radiotracers are distributed throughout the body. Finally, attenuation correction is an important step that reverses the scattering of gamma rays as they travel through tissues. Such a change is important for achieving accurate quantification of tracer uptake, which may be critical when assessing conditions such as coronary artery disease or cancer. By improving image sharpness and resolution, these advances advance SPECT imaging into an extremely useful application for clinicians to determine treatment strategies and maximize patient outcomes (Pawar et al., 2024). Quality assurance standards form the cornerstone in maintaining high standards necessary in SPECT imaging. Some of these are tests for linearity and uniformity, spatial resolution, and checks on system sensitivity. These quality assurance measures ensure that the imaging devices operate at their best and in a predictable manner, and give results that are dependable and can be trusted by clinicians. Given the hazards of misdiagnosis, the implementation of a robust quality assurance program in SPECT centers is non-negotiable. By regularly testing SPECT systems' hardware and software, medical specialists can mitigate risks and ensure that patient images accurately reflect physiological conditions. Ultimately, the complementarity of technological progress and strict quality control procedures ensures SPECT's role as a solid pillar in nuclear medicine diagnostics (Aleksa et al., 2025).

7.2.1. Definition and Significance of SPECT

The definition of Single Photon Emission Computed Tomography (SPECT) highlights its role as a key imaging modality in nuclear medicine practice. SPECT constitutes the detection of gamma radiation emitted from radiopharmaceuticals injected into a patient to image physiological functions in real time. SPECT differs from traditional planar imaging techniques in that it produces three-dimensional reconstructions of organ function, thereby increasing diagnostic potential for many clinical disorders. This capability is particularly useful for assessing blood flow and metabolic function in organs, notably the brain and heart. By integrating spatial and temporal information, SPECT significantly improves the accuracy of clinical diagnosis and treatment planning (Figure 7.4).

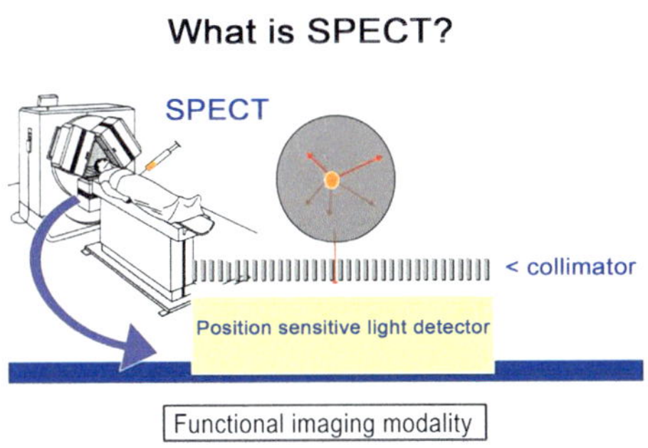

Figure 7.4. Conceptual diagram defining SPECT.

Source: Introductory texts on nuclear imaging techniques.

The benefit of SPECT is not only its advanced imaging capabilities but also its clinical applications across multiple specialties. According to recent studies, SPECT has emerged as a fundamental tool in myocardial perfusion imaging for the detection and management of coronary artery disease. Its ability to reveal functional impairments prior to structural alterations makes SPECT invaluable in early intervention strategies. Moreover, advances in SPECT technology, particularly the introduction of full-ring solid-state detectors, have enhanced image quality and diagnostic accuracy, the parameters necessary for good patient care. SPECT correlations with coronary angiography further fortify its role as a reliable non-invasive imaging tool in cardiology, thus minimizing the need for invasive procedures. Apart from cardiology, the versatility of SPECT extends to other clinical fields, such as oncology and neurology, where it is important for detecting cancer and evaluating neurodegenerative disorders. For example, SPECT imaging has been used to assess conditions such as Alzheimer's disease, where it can identify changes in cerebral blood flow associated with disease progression. The ongoing improvement of acquisition protocols and image reconstruction techniques, including attenuation correction, further raises SPECT's value in contemporary medical practice. Inconsistencies in quality control protocols between hospitals reinforce the need to standardize protocols, as reflected in ongoing benchmarking studies (Ramkishore et al., 2024). By addressing such variations and enhancing the quality assurance systems, SPECT can continue to provide accurate and reproducible diagnostic data necessary for inpatient management.

7.2.2. Comparison Between SPECT and Traditional Imaging Techniques

In a comparison of SPECT and traditional imaging modalities in terms of relative effectiveness, one sees that technological developments in SPECT confer a significant advantage in diagnostic capability and clinical application. Conventional imaging modalities, such as X-rays and traditional CTs, are primarily anatomical structure-based but generally too poorly functional. In contrast, SPECT not only images anatomical structures but also assesses physiological functions by measuring gamma rays emitted by radiopharmaceuticals (Figure 7.5).

This function-based imaging capacity is particularly valuable for diagnosing and monitoring disease, including cardiac and neurological conditions, where quantifying metabolic activity is essential for accurate medical evaluation and decision-making. SPECT's positioning at the interface of anatomy and physiology equates to its increased role in contemporary nuclear medicine. The technological innovations associated with SPECT, including high-tech signal amplifying machines and sophisticated reconstruction algorithms, are key to distinguishing it from traditional imaging. Notably, the transition away from massive photomultiplier tubes (PMTs) to more sophisticated detector technologies, such as position-sensitive PMTs and avalanche photodiodes, has improved spatial resolution and energy efficiency, thereby enhancing the overall quality of images produced. Besides, newer SPECT systems, such as those with collimators made of specialized materials and semiconductor material CdZnTe, enable faster scanning times and improved patient comfort.

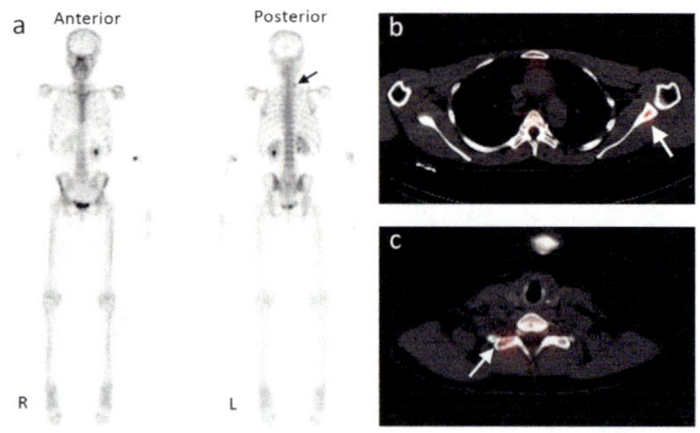

Figure 7.5. Planar bone scan versus SPECT. Images from a planar bone scan (a) and views from a single-photon emission computerized tomography (SPECT) through the thoracic (b) and cervical (c) spine in a 56-year-old woman with breast cancer. Subtle abnormal tracer accumulation is present at the root of the left neck on the planar bone scan (black arrow) with normal accumulation within the urinary tract and at the injection site (a). SPECT-CT demonstrates corresponding uptake in right transverse process of C7 (c white arrow) but additional uptake in the left scapula (b white arrow) not visible on the planar images alone.

Source: https://www.researchgate.net/publication/342225828/figure/fig1/AS:905714021187584@1592950458516/Planar-bone-scan-versus-SPECT-Images-from-a-planar-bone-scan-a-and-views-from-a.png.

These advancements not only make the imaging process more efficient but also improve diagnostic accuracy and precision in treatment planning, showing how SPECTs development continues to revolutionize clinical radiology procedures, particularly in specialized centers (AlSaadi et al., 2024). Furthermore, integrating quantitative analysis into SPECT imaging makes it twice as rewarding as with traditional modalities. Camera-specific modeling attempts to make SPECT and SPECT/CT reliable quantitative tools, providing clinicians with precise measurements of the metabolic function of tissues. This aspect is valuable for evaluating disease progression and treatment response, thus equipping healthcare providers with useful information with which to make informed, individualized treatment plans. SPECT's evolving role thus signifies not only technological capability but also its capacity to respond to complex clinical contexts across oncology, neurology, and cardiology. With conventional imaging modalities increasingly being replaced by multimodal imaging technologies, SPECT stands alone in providing combined information that significantly improves patient care outcomes and extends to broader applications in molecular imaging (Chatziioannou et al., 2004).

7.2.3. Advantages of SPECT in Diagnostic Procedures

The use of Single Photon Emission Computed Tomography (SPECT) in diagnostic imaging has a wide range of benefits, primarily its ability to furnish extensive functional imaging of organs. A key advantage is the improvement in spatial resolution compared to conventional imaging techniques. Such an improvement enables the visualization of minute abnormalities, especially in small organs like the brain and heart. The technology enables practitioners to visualize physiological processes in real time and, in so doing, to provide information on tissue metabolism and blood flow that is critical to accurate diagnoses. Moreover, the nearness of detectors to the organ target significantly improves sensitivity and image quality and supersedes the abilities of traditional imaging systems (Baviera et al., 2018) (Figure 7.6).

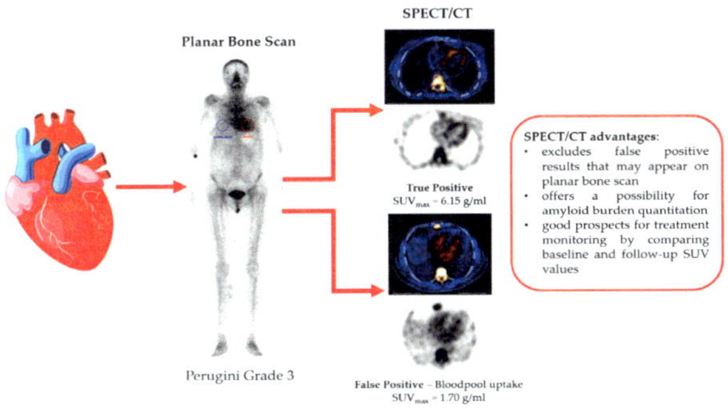

Figure 7.6. Summary of diagnostic advantages offered by SPECT imaging.

Source: Evidence-based studies in nuclear diagnostics.

This is particularly effective in clinical applications that require precise localizations of lesions or functional impairment, which are essential in the planning of suitable treatments. SPECT is also helpful because it is highly versatile across many clinical applications, including cardiac perfusion imaging, bone scintigraphy, and renal function testing. The modality is better at evaluating cardiac conditions and provides essential information regarding blood flow and myocardial viability, critical to patient management and intervention planning. In oncology, SPECT plays a valuable role in diagnosing metastatic bone disease and provides timely, accurate diagnoses that improve patient outcomes. Its capacity to non-invasively assess anatomical and functional parameters renders SPECT a valuable imaging modality that complements other imaging modalities to enrich the entire diagnostic armamentarium offered to medical practitioners (Armstrong et al., 2023). With the integration of SPECT into daily clinical practice, practitioners can achieve a more holistic understanding of patient trajectories, ultimately leading to better outcomes through evidence-based decision-making. In addition, technological advancements in SPECT have greatly expanded its utility, particularly for quantitative imaging. As such, quantification of radiotracer uptake facilitates precise dosimetry in therapeutic applications, particularly in the emerging field of theranostics. Such capabilities are vital for personalizing treatment regimens and longitudinally monitoring therapeutic impact. Standards set by credible institutions, such as the European Association of Nuclear Medicine, recognize the importance of standardized procedures to ensure quality and reliability in SPECT imaging (Armstrong et al., 2023). Respect for quality assurance ensures that SPECT remains a dynamic and responsive tool that aligns with clinical demands, making it a progressively potent and effective modality in the diagnostic toolkit of nuclear medicine. The integration of technological progress and medical application is set to solidify SPECTs position as a pillar of modern healthcare diagnosis.

7.3. Radiopharmaceuticals in Nuclear Medicine

The application of nuclear medicine with radiopharmaceuticals is crucial for enhancing diagnostic capability, particularly with the implementation of single-photon emission computed tomography (SPECT) technology. Radiopharmaceuticals are radioactive isotopes bound to pharmaceutical agents and can be directed to deliver within the human body. Gamma emitters used in such compositions are part of what makes them work in that they enable imaging of functional processes in organs via gamma cameras. Remarkably, around 85% of clinical radiopharmaceuticals can be used with SPECT, demonstrating their immense usefulness in the diagnosis of infectious and malignant disorders. As depicted in recent publications, these compounds have significantly improved imaging diagnostics for diseases ranging from cancer to cardiac diseases, justifying their dominance in contemporary nuclear medicine practice (Imran et al., 2020). Radiopharmaceutical production can be supplied by generator or reactor sources, a reality that has implications for the availability and purity of these valuable compounds. Isotopes from reactors are typically produced by neutron activation, while those from generators exploit a more readily accessible decay process and are consequently well suited to the clinical environment, where turnover is high. Besides, the choice of radiolabeling techniques is important to ensure the radioactive components are stable and retain their efficacy and biodistribution characteristics. Quality control is most important in such a scenario, encompassing radiochemical purity, specific activity, and sterility tests. Such procedures ensure that medicines are safe and effective for patient use, thereby improving the consistency of nuclear medicine diagnostic tests and enhancing patient care (Mishra, 2024). Technological advancements also call for ongoing optimization of quality control protocols in radiopharmaceutical manufacturing and application.

The intricate dependence of gamma camera design on operational characteristics of radiopharmaceuticals is at the heart of their operation. As required by various research studies, this involves calibrating image equipment to accommodate a range of radiopharmaceuticals and achieve maximum image quality and diagnostic performance. Each imaging modality, including SPECT, relies on a high-level understanding of the chemistry between radiopharmaceuticals and gamma camera technology. Inventions such as the application of artificial intelligence to imaging protocols have the potential to enhance scintigraphic data interpretation, yielding increasingly more profound insights into biological processes. Overall, such innovations illustrate the pivotal role of radiopharmaceuticals in contemporary nuclear medicine, enhancing diagnosis and therapeutic capabilities (Imran et al., 2020).

7.3.1. Types of Radiopharmaceuticals Used in Gamma Cameras and SPECT

Among the broad range of radiopharmaceuticals employed by gamma cameras and SPECT (Single Photon Emission Computed Tomography), technetium-99m (Tc-99m) is the most prevalent isotope. This is largely attributed to its optimal physical and chemical properties, including a half-life of around six hours, which facilitate adequate imaging without exposing patients to substantial radiation for long periods. Tc-99m can be incorporated into a wide variety of molecular compounds, enabling the selective imaging of many physiological and biological processes. For instance, Tc-99m-labeled compounds are used in myocardial perfusion imaging, where the relative distribution of blood to cardiac tissue is being quantified. The role of Tc-99m is central to the enhancement of nuclear medicine diagnosis and to its position as the basis for gamma camera applications. In addition to Tc-99m, iodine-123 (I-123) and indium-111 (In-111) are significant radionuclides used in certain clinical applications. I-123, with its favorable imaging characteristics, is widely used in thyroid scanning to assess function and detect abnormalities, such as nodules or cancers. Its 13-hour half-life allows for optimal imaging while minimizing the patient's radiation dose. On the other hand, In-111 is typically used for tumor imaging and infection labeling of monoclonal antibodies, capitalizing on its ability to bind to specific cancer cells or agents responsible. Both isotopes highlight the flexibility of radiopharmaceuticals that have been designed to counter specific diagnostic issues in various clinical areas, such as in oncological and endocrine assessment. The quality control of these radiopharmaceuticals is paramount to ensure their efficacy and safety when used clinically. Careful protocols are strictly adhered to to verify radiochemical purity, specific activity, and freedom from contaminants that could compromise diagnostic efficacy (Figure 7.7).

Gamma-emitting targeted agents with labelled radiotracers	Type of Cancer
Bombestine	• Endocrine organ tumor
Pentadecapeptide Technetium-99m	• Breast cancer • Prostate cancer • Gastro-entero-pancreatic tumors • Lunch cancer
Oxdronate-99mTc	• Bone diseases
Tilmanocept technetium-99m	• Breast cancer • Melanoma • Oral cavity cancer
Pertechnetate technetium-99m	• Urinary thyroid cancer • Bladder thyroid cancer
Iodinated bombesin I-125	• Endocrine cancer - with cell growth in the endocrine organ: > breast > prostate ovaries > testes
Bombesine rhenium-188	• Prostate tumor
FDG-F-18	• Soft tissue cancer • Prostate cancer
Oxdronate-99mTc	• Bone diseases

Figure 7.7. Commonly used radiopharmaceuticals in gamma cameras and SPECT.

Source: https://www.escopharma.com/images/upload/nuclear-medicine-radiopharmacy-unit-tables-10-min.jpg.

Techniques used for quality control include thin-layer chromatography and high-performance liquid chromatography to measure radiochemical purity. Moreover, handling and storage procedures are strictly controlled to prevent degradation of the radiopharmaceuticals. Such emphasis on quality control has a direct impact on the reliability of gamma cameras and SPECT imaging, as any fluctuation in radiopharmaceuticals would result in false positives or false negatives, adversely affecting patient care and treatment planning in such complex cases as with breast cancer and neuroendocrine tumors (Akram et al., 2017; Sundin et al., 2017).

7.3.2. Mechanism of Action of Radiopharmaceuticals

The mechanism of action of radiopharmaceuticals is fundamentally based on their ability to emit radiation detectable by imaging devices, thereby providing valuable information on physiological processes. Radiopharmaceuticals consist of radioisotopes that are either linked to targeting molecules or incorporated into systems that selectively interact with biological structures such as cells or tissues. The specific application enhances the dose to the target site while minimizing exposure to overlying normal tissue. Upon decay, the radioisotope emits gamma photons or beta particles, which gamma cameras or SPECT systems can image. Through this process, clinicians can view and assess several pathological conditions, such as tumors or cardiac dysfunction, with a level of specificity that other imaging devices cannot offer, as discussed in the context of technological innovation in molecular imaging in nuclear medicine (Witney et al., 2021). Radiation-induced necrosis is one example of a targeted therapeutic application of radiopharmaceuticals, including in Yttrium-90 radioembolization (Y90-RE). In this technique, Y90-marked microspheres are infused through the arterial vessels supplying the tumors, delivering radiation in a localized fashion (Figure 7.8).

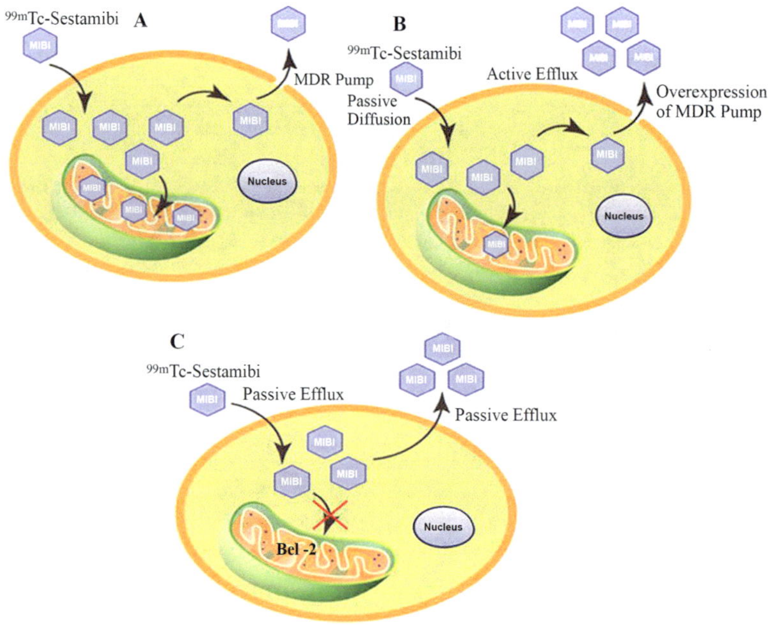

Figure 7.8. Illustration of the biochemical mechanism of action of radiopharmaceuticals at the cellular level.

Source: https://api.intechopen.com/media/chapter/73661/media/F2.png.

Upon administration, Y90 undergoes β-decay, emitting high-energy beta particles that induce cell damage via radiation-induced necrosis. Ionizing radiation destroys tumor tissue to a great extent, sparing adjacent healthy tissues, making use of the physical properties of the radioisotope to gain optimum therapeutic advantage. Furthermore, the released radiation from Y90 also generates Cherenkov light, which not only has the potential to enhance imaging but also enables real-time imaging during procedures, ultimately enriching therapeutic and diagnostic paradigms (Villalobos et al., 2020). At the end of the day, thinking about the action mechanisms of radiopharmaceuticals is not merely about imaging; it is also about therapeutic applications that capitalize on the inherent nature of radioisotopes. With ongoing developments in radiochemistry and imaging technology, the production of new radiopharmaceuticals targeted to specific molecular targets becomes increasingly critical for personalized medicine. This shift not only increases the specificity of diagnostic imaging but also concurs with the increased focus on individualized treatments in oncology and other fields. The synergy between radiopharmaceutical pharmacology and current imaging modalities showcases a paradigm change in nuclear medicine, underscoring the importance of ongoing research and development to meet evolving clinical demands (Witney et al., 2021).

7.3.3. Safety and Regulatory Considerations

Safety and regulatory matters have the highest priority in nuclear medicine, particularly for gamma cameras and SPECT. Regulatory agencies, such as the United States Nuclear Regulatory Commission (NRC), have stringent standards to ensure the safe management of radioactive substances used in diagnostic imaging. These standards involve training personnel, shielding the sources of radiation, and measuring exposure rates. Adherence to regulations not only ensures the health of healthcare professionals but also that of patients undergoing imaging examinations. It is necessary for nuclear medicine departments to stay informed about such regulations, as a lack of them may lead to severe legal ramifications and patient compromise. Thus, safety guidelines need to be incorporated into practice regularly to maintain the integrity of nuclear medicine. Quality assurance is vital to gamma camera and SPECT practice safety. The use of a systematic quality control process ensures that imaging devices work efficiently and effectively, thus minimizing unnecessary radiation exposure to patients (Figure 7.9).

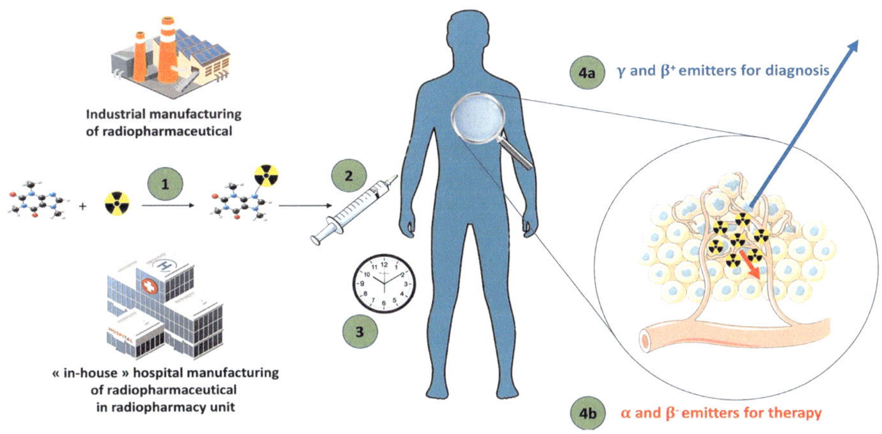

Figur 7.9. Chart outlining international safety and regulatory protocols for radiopharmaceutical use.

Source: IAEA and FDA regulatory documents.

Regular equipment maintenance and calibration, like uniformity, linearity, and system sensitivity test checks, play a vital role in achieving reproducible image results. Quantitative SPECT-CT, for instance, has advanced, necessitating stringent quality assurance methodologies to ensure imaging findings are accurate and safe, particularly in complex applications such as dosimetry and theranostics (Armstrong et al., 2023). All the protocols must be comprehensively inspected and authorized to ensure that safety standards are met, and trust between the patients and the clinicians is maintained. All parties must work together to establish and maintain effective safety and regulatory procedures in nuclear medicine. The European Association of Nuclear Medicine (EANM) provides guidelines to establish quantitative SPECT-CT services while ensuring compliance with safety standards (Nienhuis et al., 2023). By integrating experts from fields such as physics, dosimetry, and oncology, these guidelines provide extensive guidance on the safe use of nuclear medicine. Furthermore, ongoing education among healthcare providers on new technologies and regulations is critical to maintaining high levels of patient safety and quality care. Finally, devotion to ongoing safety and regulatory adherence not only makes nuclear imaging modalities more trustworthy but also encourages the broader growth of the discipline.

7.4. Image Acquisition and Processing

Image acquisition and processing in nuclear medicine are critical for accurate diagnostics and effective treatment planning. This stage encompasses the initial acquisition of images using gamma cameras, and determining the acquisition parameters is crucial. Acquisition time, energy window settings, and collimator selection are some of the parameters that can significantly affect the quality of the acquired images. The energy window, for example, is essential for differentiating genuine signals from background noise because it determines the gamma photon energy spectrum to be measured. It is necessary to employ optimal parameters so that artifacts are minimized and the anatomical and functional details within the images are enhanced in definition, a sign of the need for rigorous calibration and standardization of image acquisition procedures. Following the initial buyout, advanced processing techniques are employed to enhance image quality from gamma cameras and SPECT systems. Filtering and image correction are applied to remove various forms of distortion, such as scatter and attenuation, which can degrade precision and diagnostic value. Gaussian filters, for instance, improve image texture and reduce noise without drastically altering the desired signal. Furthermore, reconstruction algorithms are fundamental for reprocessing raw data into interpretable, meaningful images that facilitate the easy visualization of points of interest. Selection and tuning of such algorithms must be adequately tailored, as evidenced in studies that have developed impressive improvements in image quality using reconstruction parameter optimization, including iterations and filter types (Aleksa et al., 2025). These advances not only enhance diagnostic accuracy but also extend the clinical applications of nuclear medicine. Technological innovations such as full-ring SPECT systems are typical of the movement to improve imaging modalities with better spatial resolution and sensitivity. All these advances are at the core of multifaceted diagnoses, particularly in cardiology, where precise measurements of myocardial perfusion are crucial in managing coronary artery disease. As documented in comparative clinical evaluations of several systems, newer technologies have made remarkable progress in detecting pathologies and correlating results with invasive methods such as coronary angiography (Ghaneh et al., 2024). In total, these advances in image acquisition and processing represent a crucial step forward for nuclear medicine, laying the foundation for a future dedicated to enhanced diagnostic performance and better patient outcomes.

7.4.1. SPECT Image Acquisition Techniques

Within the Single Photon Emission Computed Tomography (SPECT) field, imaging acquisition protocols play a focal role in obtaining qualitative data that inform diagnostic outcomes. SPECT uses a rotating gamma camera to detect gamma rays emitted by radiotracers administered to patients. Tomographic acquisition generates high-resolution three-dimensional images by combining multiple two-dimensional images acquired at various angles around the patient. The process enhances contrast and spatial resolution over traditional planar imaging methods. By optimizing acquisition parameters such as number of projections, scan time, and patient position, clinicians can significantly improve image acutance, thus enhancing diagnostic stability and enabling better clinical decision-making. The efficacy of SPECT imaging also resides not just in its acquisition techniques but in very sophisticated reconstruction algorithms that convert raw data into understandable images. These techniques, including some filtered back-projection and iterative reconstruction algorithms, play a crucial role in mitigating problems such as photon scattering and attenuation, which can degrade image quality (Figure 7.10).

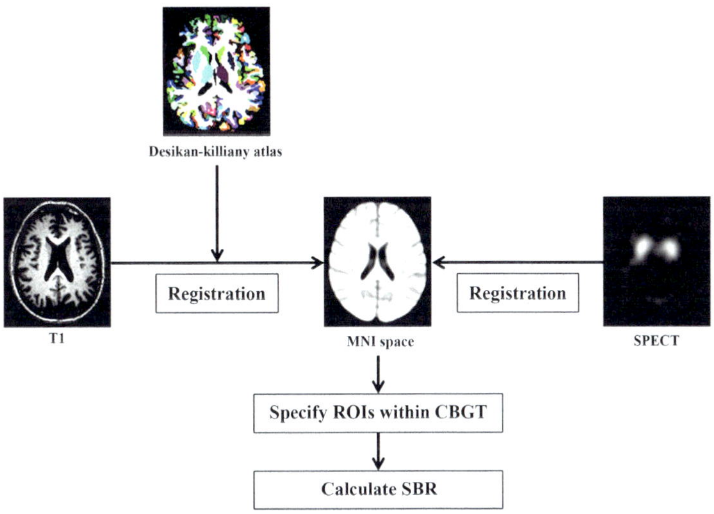

Figure 7.10. Overall image processing procedures of SPECT. The processing of SPECT image was similar to that of the DTI processing. The images were co-registered to common space (MNI space) to define the ROIs within the CBGT circuit. The mean intensity of each ROI was used to compute the regional SBR.

Source: https://www.researchgate.net/publication/311246309/figure/fig6/AS:669034769027080@1536521727388/Overall-image-processing-procedures-of-SPECT-The-processing-of-SPECT-image-was-similar.jpg.

Advanced iterative techniques are highly effective in reducing image noise and enhancing spatial resolution. The use of machine learning and artificial intelligence algorithms in image reconstruction is also further revolutionizing SPECT by enabling more efficient, faster data processing. Such technologies have the potential to improve diagnostic reliability by incorporating better visualization of physiological and anatomical structures vital for patient assessment. Quality control is an essential component of maintaining the accuracy of SPECT imaging technologies, hence keeping diagnostic programs valid. Linearity and uniformity tests, undertaken on a routine basis, ensure that imaging equipment operates at its maximum potential, enabling clinicians to make informed decisions in patient care. Continuous system sensitivity and spatial resolution monitoring through standardized protocols also plays a critical role in minimizing variability of results, as per guidelines laid out by organizations such as the European Association of Nuclear Medicine. The ongoing emphasis on high-quality acquisition techniques not only ensures standardization of practice but also enhances clinical utility across a range of diagnostic applications, such as cardiac perfusion imaging and bone scintigraphy, thereby reinforcing the significance of SPECT in modern medicine (Van et al., 2016; Andreas et al., 2020).

7.4.2. Image Reconstruction Techniques

In nuclear medicine, image reconstruction methods play a critical role in the quality and interpretation of diagnostic images generated by gamma cameras and Single Photon Emission Computed Tomography (SPECT) since raw data obtained from emitted gamma rays are converted into highly detailed pictorial representations using various mathematical methods.

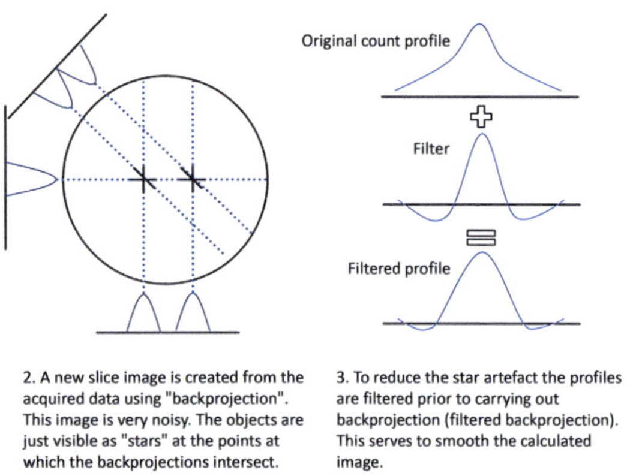

Figure 7.11. Diagrams of filtered back projection techniques used in SPECT.

Source: https://www.radiologycafe.com/wp-content/uploads/2021/04/nm-spect-backp2.png.

Among popular algorithms, Ordered Subsets Expectation Maximization (OSEM) became popular because it provided high-resolution images with a considerable reduction in reconstruction time. OSEM maximizes the use of projection data by iteratively updating image estimates to progressively higher levels, thereby improving the sharpness of anatomical and functional information central to clinical decision-making. Additionally, advances in algorithm complexity, including the inclusion of prior knowledge about the imaging equipment, further enhance the accuracy of the image reconstructions, hence strengthening the diagnostic capabilities in nuclear medicine. The reconstruction algorithm chosen determines explicitly the quality of information that can be recovered with SPECT imaging (Figure 7.11).

The development of algorithms such as the Maximum Likelihood Expectation Maximization (MLEM) has highlighted the importance of statistical methods in image reconstruction. MLEM uses a probabilistic model to reconstruct maximum-likelihood images from the true distribution of radioisotopes in the organs under imaging. Research indicates that combining advanced collimation techniques, including rotating-slat collimators, with MLEM produces notable improvements in image quality, with higher contrast-to-noise ratios for hot and cold lesions. More specifically, the improved photon collection efficiency of these collimators results in less noisy data and, therefore, better images that allow for accurate disease diagnosis and treatment (Staelens et al., 2011). small animal imaging with integrated modalities, such as SPECT and micro-CT, further advances in image reconstruction methods are evident. Two integrated imaging modalities are useful for a complete assessment of the functional and structural aspects of biological systems. For instance, the use of a standard gamma camera with a pinhole collimator facilitates the acquisition of high-resolution SPECT images that can be fused with the micro-CT images. These techniques enable scientists to obtain exact measurements of physiological parameters, such as pulmonary blood flow, with a high degree of accuracy (Clough et al., 2003).

Ongoing refinement of reconstruction fidelity, as evidenced by numerical simulations with nearly zero measurement error, underscores the potential of these methods to advance our understanding of biological processes and to optimize therapeutic strategies in preclinical and clinical contexts.

7.4.3. Quality Control of Image Processing

In nuclear medicine, Gamma Camera and SPECT imaging, proper image processing quality control is crucial for accurate diagnosis and improved patient safety. The process of acquiring images begins with accurate calibration of the imaging equipment, during which uniformity and linearity are evaluated.

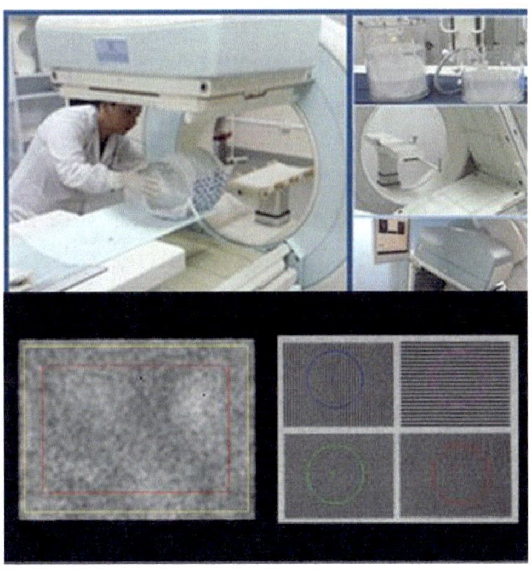

Figure 7.12. Checklist for quality control measures during SPECT image processing.

Source: Standard operating procedures from nuclear medicine departments.

These tests are crucial as they directly impact the image integrity of the images produced. If calibration is not tightly performed, slight deviations can lead to considerable errors in radiopharmaceutical distribution interpretation and, consequently, influence clinical decision-making. As illustrated in experimental research utilizing SPECT/micro-CT imaging to study angiogenesis, accurate image processing is paramount in the achievement of reliable information about biological processes, demonstrating the importance of quality control in ensuring the integrity of medical imaging modalities (Clough et al., 2008) (Figure 7.12).

Moreover, understanding the subtleties of image quality measures, such as spatial resolution and system sensitivity, is crucial to accurate quality assurance in SPECT imaging. Spatial resolution specifies the ability of the system to distinguish between two objects placed very close together, while sensitivity indicates the ability of the system to detect infinitesimal quantities of radioactive tracers. Periodic measurement and calibration of these parameters improve not only image quality but also diagnostic reliability. When creating new radiotracers, scientists must ensure that small-animal imaging systems are well established and capable of producing high-quality images. Such meticulous attention to detail helps ensure ongoing improvement in therapy and enables accurate evaluation of the treatment's efficacy (Bankstahl et al., 2015). Properly conducted quality control procedures thus ensure imaging modalities can cope with ever-increasing complexity in clinical practice. Finally, the use of advanced software packages for image processing is an important area in nuclear medicine quality control. While hardware devices like collimators and scintillation crystals are at the heart of initial image acquisition, sophisticated algorithms and software are crucial for subsequent processing and analysis. Precision in applying image corrections for scatter, attenuation, and motion must be maintained to obtain meaningful clinical information from the raw, unprocessed data. Moreover, such algorithms require regular updates and verification to keep up with the speed of technological developments and changing clinical requirements. Thus, an exclusive focus on quality control in every facet of image processing not only ensures the accuracy of SPECT imaging but also enhances its application in various clinical scenarios, from cardiac imaging to cancer evaluation. Overall, high standards of quality in quality control ensure effective implementation of nuclear medicine technologies and ultimately result in improved patient outcomes.

7.5. Clinical A pplications of Gamma Cameras and SPECT

The clinical application of gamma cameras and Single Photon Emission Computed Tomography (SPECT) is at its finest in cardiac perfusion imaging, which has transformed the face of cardiovascular diagnostics. This imaging modality evaluates myocardial blood flow, identifies areas of ischemia, and thus enables the clinician to make informed decisions about patient management. SPECT, particularly with newer technologies such as cadmium-zinc-telluride (CZT) detectors, provides superior resolution images with enhanced visualization of perfusion defects. Cardiovascular diseases, ranking among the leading causes of death worldwide, point towards the importance of such non-invasive diagnostic tests. The capability for gated-SPECT imaging enables precise measurements of cardiac function, detecting dilated cardiomyopathy and providing valuable information on therapy outcomes and prognosis. The history of cardiac imaging reflects ongoing efforts to maximize patient benefits through new nuclear medicine modalities (Pandey, 2024). Outside cardiology, gamma cameras and SPECT find vital applications in cancer, particularly in bone scintigraphy. This modality utilizes radiopharmaceuticals that bind to regions of increased bone activity, typically seen in the setting of metastasis, infection, or trauma.

The ability of SPECT to provide three-dimensional imaging allows for localization and quantification of disease processes in the skeleton, which is critical for planning treatment and follow-up. For instance, in breast or prostate cancer patients, early identification of bone metastases in the course of the disease may have significant implications for therapy, and therefore the role of nuclear imaging in the care of these patients. Furthermore, improvements in imaging technologies have upgraded the sensitivity and specificity of these techniques to offer more accurate staging and treatment response evaluation ultimately. Practitioners are increasingly utilizing these devices to customize the treatment protocol, which confirms the unreplaceable position of gamma cameras and SPECT in contemporary cancer practice (Peix et al., 2022). Besides, SPECT and gamma cameras are essential to renal function evaluation, which is an integral part of patient management in various kidney diseases. With techniques such as dynamic renal scintigraphy, both modalities quantify glomerular filtration rates and detect obstructions and other pathologies that influence renal function. With the aid of specific radiotracers, doctors can visualize renal blood flow and tubular function, helping them better understand the organ's current status. Renal scintigraphy is particularly valuable in pediatrics, where noninvasive assessment is of utmost importance. Nuclear medicine tests, such as renal scans, allow the monitoring to be accomplished safely without invasive procedures like renal biopsies. Thus, gamma cameras and SPECT are versatile tools for assessing renal health, not only aiding clinicians in making early interventions but also underscoring the increasing focus on patient-centered care practices in nephrology (Pandey, 2024).

7.5.1. Oncology Contribution to Tumor Identification

In cancer, the role of nuclear medicine, particularly with gamma cameras and SPECT, has greatly expanded the ability to detect tumors. The ability of these modalities to image metabolic activity within tissues means that the clinician can identify malignancies which are not apparent on anatomical imaging. Among the most important advantages of radioisotope application is their selectivity for targeting specific molecules in tumors, thus enabling early diagnosis and potentially better treatment. For example, the use of targeted radiotracers can significantly contribute to preoperative staging of tumor extent, leading to more precise surgery and individualized treatment plans. Furthermore, the integration of molecular imaging with anatomic imaging, such as CT scans, facilitates comprehensive tumor assessment and provides real-time information essential to effective clinical decision-making (Charles et al., 2024). Advances in gamma camera technology and image acquisition techniques have further optimized tumor detection in the clinic. SPECT imaging, characterized by visualization in three dimensions, augments detection of functional impairments related to various forms of tumors (Figure 7.13).

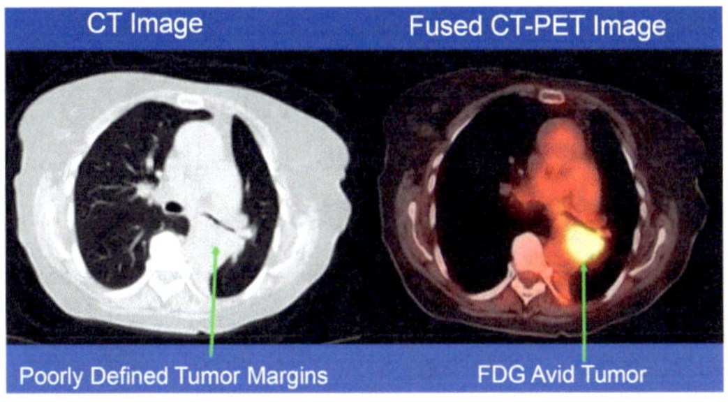

Figure 7.13. Gamma camera scan highlighting tumor detection in oncology cases.

Source: Oncology case studies in nuclear medicine.

The incorporation of high-technology image reconstruction algorithms and attenuation correction increases sensitivity and specificity. This is particularly evident in breast cancer diagnosis, where high-tech gamma camera scintimammography has been promising. With sensitivities of 89% to 95% reported across tumor types, this modality underscores the importance of nuclear medicine in identifying cancers undetectable with routine imaging. The integration of such technologically advanced imaging modalities into oncology practice is thus a paradigm shift towards more effective and personalized patient management (Popova et al., 2023). The integration of nuclear medicine in the procedures of oncology needs rigorous quality control procedures to determine diagnostic effectiveness and patient safety. Quality control procedures, such as uniformity and linearity tests, spatial resolution measurements, and system sensitivity testing, need to be performed to maintain the integrity of SPECT imaging. Such quality assurance methods are vital in order to avoid errors that would impact cancer diagnosis and treatment planning. Furthermore, the interdisciplinary collaboration between nuclear medicine and other disciplines, as emphasized in some cancer treatment protocols, increases the accuracy in identifying tumor markers and measuring response to treatment. By using radiopharmaceuticals that bind to specific molecular targets associated with cancer, oncologists can accurately track disease progression and treatment effectiveness. Therefore, nuclear medicine has served as a cornerstone in the ongoing search for optimizing tumor detection methods, which eventually led to improved patient outcomes in oncology (Charles et al., 2024).

7.5.2. Use in Cardiology to Evaluate Heart Disease

Nuclear medicine plays a central role in the assessment of heart disease in cardiology, particularly through the use of myocardial perfusion imaging (MPI). This technique allows precise evaluation of myocardial blood supply, important to CAD diagnosis. Using gamma cameras, doctors can create images that report the functional state of heart tissue at rest and after stress testing. Functionality is essential because ischemic regions might be occult in the absence of such imaging. Device innovation, such as in the Discovery CZT 530c, enhances diagnostic accuracy by highlighting myocardial perfusion abnormalities, particularly in high-risk patients, such as those with diabetes. Evidence indicates that nuclear medicine can effectively identify early coronary artery issues, hence facilitating proper intervention and leading to improved outcomes for patients (Lacko et al., 2024). Efforts to maximize the efficiency of SPECT systems have driven technological and methodological advances, significantly impacting cardiology practices. Recent surveys report myocardial perfusion scintigraphy as the dominant modality in nuclear cardiology, a testament to its status as the most frequently performed scintigraphic test (Figure 7.14).

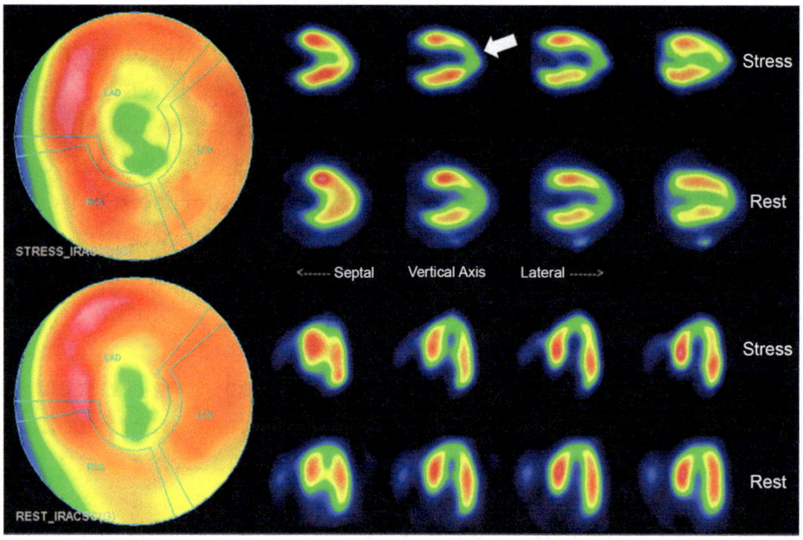

Figure 7.14. SPECT scan showing myocardial perfusion analysis for cardiac assessment.

Source: https://th.bing.com/th/id/OIP.E1RNImgECQa0IgyrhVs_PwHaEx?rs=1&pid=ImgDetMain.

During the years 2019–2021, the widespread application of SPECT equipment, such as cardiocentric cameras, revealed the pivotal role of cutting-edge imaging technologies in diagnostics. In addition to improving image quality through increased spatial resolution, these technologies facilitate the detection of microvascular disease, which is often overlooked during traditional evaluation. Their incorporation into routine clinical practice results in a comprehensive diagnostic strategy that is especially beneficial for patients with unusual symptoms or diabetes (Teresińska et al., 2023). Additionally, the incorporation of advanced algorithms into SPECT imaging offers significant benefits for evaluating cardiac viability. With the incorporation of attenuation correction and reconstruction algorithms, SPECT can produce more accurate images of myocardial perfusion, distinguishing viable from nonviable heart tissue. This diagnostic specificity is crucial in the management of patients with ischemic heart disease, where the decision for revascularization versus medical therapy is based on the characterization of myocardial ischemia and viability. Additionally, continued radiopharmaceutical development ensures the imaging procedure maintains radiation exposure at a minimum, thereby maintaining patient safety while providing optimal diagnostic return. Hence, nuclear medicine, in the form of SPECT imaging, remains a central component of contemporary cardiology, thereby improving the clinical management of cardiac disease (Lacko et al., 2024).

7.5.3. Applications in Neurology for Brain Disorders

In neurology, nuclear medicine uses advanced imaging technologies, such as Single Photon Emission Computed Tomography (SPECT), to investigate brain disorders with precision. SPECT's capability to quantify regional cerebral blood flow has tremendous insights into disorders such as Alzheimer's disease, Parkinson's disease, and other neurodegenerative illnesses. By visualizing dopaminergic circuits in the brain, SPECT enables doctors to differentiate between parkinsonian syndromes and other movement disorders, providing critical diagnostic information that enables successful treatment. Furthermore, the use of artificial intelligence in SPECT image processing holds the potential to enhance diagnostic accuracy, as such new techniques can lead to improved classification and segmentation of brain disease (Andreas et al., 2020). As SPECT technology advances, its neurological applications are expected to grow, enabling more specific patient treatment. The use of radiopharmaceuticals for SPECT in neurological applications underscores the need for quality control programs to ensure that diagnostic procedures are both safe and effective. Standardization and production of the agents are critical, especially as radiolabeling techniques advance, enabling the development of new tracers targeting specific neurotransmitter systems. For example, breakthroughs in imaging of the dopamine transporter have established guidelines that better diagnose disorders like Parkinson's disease, allowing for a more advanced understanding of dopaminergic function in the brain (Figure 7.15).

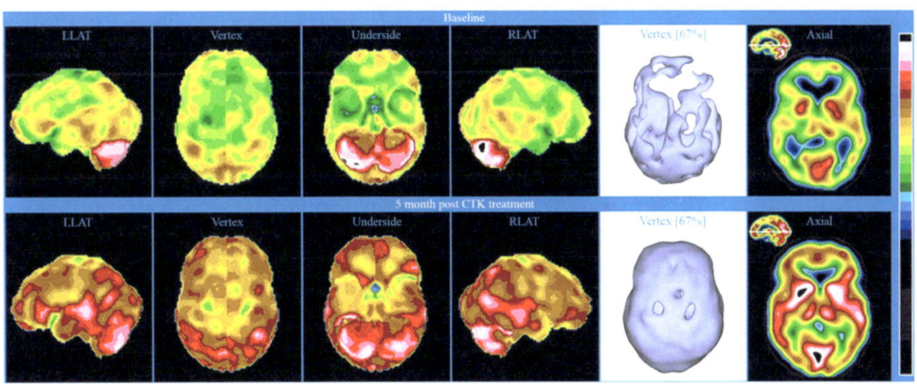

Figure 7.15. Functional brain scan using SPECT in the evaluation of neurological disorders.

Source: https://th.bing.com/th/id/OIP.5D8OMua0SbWyu9I-lQKt7gAAAA?rs=1&pid=ImgDetMain.

These recommendations highlight the clinical value of SPECT and its use in discrimination between various forms of Parkinsonism, and thereby on therapeutic management (Morbelli et al., 2020). Moreover, with ongoing research findings of new pathophysiological markers of cerebral disorders, development in radiopharmaceuticals will further increase the diagnostic role of nuclear medicine. Apart from its application in the diagnosis and differentiation of brain disease, SPECT imaging plays an important role in monitoring treatment response and disease progression in neurological patients. Repeated examination of cerebral blood flow and receptor activity over time is essential for assessing therapeutic efficacy. For instance, patients who are treated with dopaminergic therapy for Parkinsons disease can be monitored through SPECT imaging to measure alterations in the function of neurotransmitters, hence informing clinical practice in terms of medication titration. Moreover, new 3D reconstruction and visualization methodologies facilitate the ease of studying complex brain structures associated with various disorders, and hence, thorough investigations of neurological illnesses can be carried out (Andreas et al., 2020). As imaging devices and algorithms are increasingly refined, SPECT's role in the neurology field will grow, providing invaluable tools for diagnosis and the emerging dynamics of treatment in brain disease.

7.6. Challenges and Limitations

In nuclear medicine, gamma cameras and single-photon emission computed tomography (SPECT) have several limitations, making it difficult to use these imaging tools efficiently. One of the biggest challenges is in their production and availability as radioisotopes, from which radiopharmaceuticals are produced. The type of isotopic decay, coupled with their shorter half-lives, becomes an organizational burden in clinical practice where availability is time-sensitive. For instance, the need for isotopes with faster decay rates to produce high-quality images while maintaining low patient radiation exposure significantly constrains choice. In addition, the application of advanced radiolabeling techniques yet again inhibits the preparation of high-quality radiopharmaceuticals since errors in labeling compromise image quality or initiate inaccurate diagnostic findings, making quality control an important factor in nuclear medicine procedures (Volpe et al., 2021). The second significant shortcoming in nuclear medicine is related to imaging equipment sensitivity and resolution. While SPECT provides valuable three-dimensional data regarding the distribution of radioactive tracers in the body, the inherent sensitivity of the systems is typically inferior to that of certain other devices such as positron emission tomography (PET).

This limitation demands longer acquisition times or the use of larger quantities of radioactive sources to yield high-quality images, thereby posing problems of patient exposure and discomfort. Moreover, variations in collimator geometry and scintillation crystal properties can affect spatial resolution and contrast, leading to less precise diagnostics. Technological innovation and imaging reconstruction algorithms are ongoing activities but standardization across systems remains an issue, leading to inconsistent clinical outcomes (Andreas et al., 2020). Additionally, the application of artificial intelligence and machine learning in the field remains challenging since the massive volume of data generated during the imaging procedure is problematic. The reliance on sophisticated algorithms in image analysis and interpretation poses challenges in itself, including the need for significant computing power and a mechanism for handling large datasets. Beyond technical considerations, there are ethical and privacy concerns with using patient information to train algorithms and increase diagnostic sensitivity. While adding artificial intelligence has the potential to improve informatics in imaging for disease segmentation and classification, current systems must be carefully validated to be safe and reliable for clinical use (Andreas et al., 2020; Volpe et al., 2021). Therefore, while there is potential for improvement in nuclear medicine, significant hurdles must be overcome before these improvements can be effectively realized.

7.6.1. Technical Limitations of Gamma Cameras and SPECT

The technological limitations of gamma cameras and SPECT imaging systems are central to understanding their actual applications and effectiveness in the clinical setting. The spatial resolution of gamma cameras is a principal limitation, inherently constrained by the physics of photon detection and collimation. Though better collimator designs, such as pinhole and converging collimators, do enhance spatial resolution, they are not able to match the greater resolution of CT or MRI technology. For critical situations in which there are small lesions or intricate anatomical details, where the inferior resolution will be deceptive or lead to a missed diagnosis, this is particularly crucial.

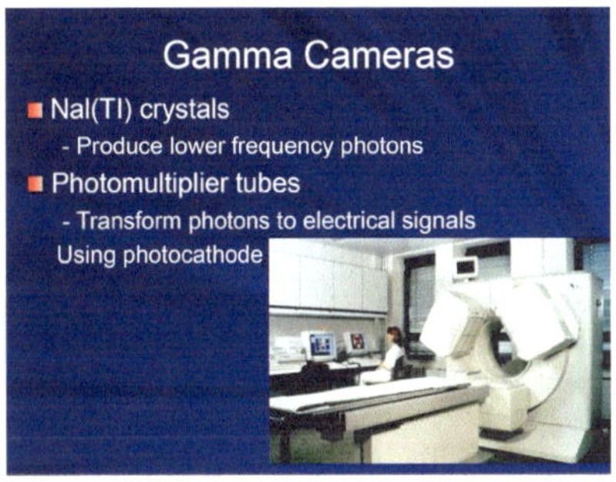

Figure 7.16. Technical diagram detailing the limitations of current gamma camera hardware.

Source: https://image2.slideserve.com/4083230/gamma-cameras1-n.jpg.

In addition, non-uniformity in the response of the scintillation crystals can further degrade image quality, calling for continuous calibration and quality assurance testing to confirm diagnostic integrity. Except for spatial resolution, gamma camera sensitivity is also problematic in regions of high activity or when measuring states of low absorption. SPECT imaging, while advanced in three-dimensional image reconstruction, is plagued by a trade-off between temporal resolution and sensitivity. Higher sensitivity typically comes with longer acquisition times, which are more prone to inducing motion artifacts and decrease patient comfort, especially for dynamic imaging like cardiac perfusion imaging. In addition, lower sensitivity can impair the ability to visualize minor changes in tracer distribution and thereby lead to a tendency towards poor clinical performance (Figure 7.16).

The reliance on energy window optimization also increases its analysis complexity, since improper settings can lead to incorrect data interpretation, reducing the technique's general applicability in certain cases. Attenuation correction is another critical technical challenge that faces SPECT imaging. Even with sophisticated reconstruction algorithms, accurately compensating for gamma-ray attenuation from nearby tissues can be difficult. This issue is further complicated in the case of highly obese patients or in heterogeneously dense tissues, in which photon scatter can taint results. In line with the issues discussed above, a lack of standardization between calibration methods and image processing algorithms contributes yet another variable among systems that could affect the reproducibility of results. Consequently, SPECT study analysis often requires skilled personnel to circumvent these inbuilt constraints, again sustaining the need for ongoing research and technological advancement to make gamma camera and SPECT imaging more accurate and reliable (Van et al., 2016; Camilleri et al., 2016).

7.6.2. Patient Safety and Radiation Exposure

In nuclear medicine, particularly with techniques such as Single Photon Emission Computed Tomography (SPECT), patient safety is paramount because of ionizing radiation exposure. While ionizing radiation plays a major role in diagnostic imaging, it can pose risks that require stringent safety measures. SPECT imaging techniques use radiopharmaceuticals that emit gamma radiation. When carrying out these procedures, healthcare providers need to understand the nuances of radiation safety procedures to prevent exposure to both patients and healthcare workers. For instance, maintaining appropriate distance from the patient can effectively reduce occupational exposure. Studies emphasize that when healthcare workers hold more than a meter away from patients following injection of radiopharmaceuticals, their exposure to radiation is significantly minimized, underscoring the importance of spatial awareness at clinical facilities (Hasan et al., 2025). In addition, the formulation and implementation of National Diagnostic Reference Levels (NDRLs) would be extremely important for improving patient safety in nuclear medicine (Figure 7.17).

Procedure		Approximate effective radiation dose	Comparable to natural background radiation for
ABDOMINAL REGION	Computed Tomography (CT) - Abdomen and Pelvis	10 mSv	3 years
	Computed Tomography (CT) - Abdomen and Pelvis, repeated with and without contrast material	20 mSv	7 years
	Computed Tomography (CT) - Colonography	6 mSv	2 years
	Intravenous Pyelogram (IVP)	3 mSv	1 year
	Radiography (X-ray) - Lower GI Tract	8 mSv	3 years
	Radiography (X-ray) - Upper GI Tract	6 mSv	2 years
BONE	Radiography (X-ray) - Spine	1.5 mSv	6 months
	Radiography (X-ray) - Extremity	0.001 mSv	3 hours
CENTRAL NERVOUS SYSTEM	Computed Tomography (CT) - Head	2 mSv	8 months
	Computed Tomography (CT) Head, repeated with and without contrast material	4 mSv	16 months
	Computed Tomography (CT) - Spine	6 mSv	2 years
CHEST	Computed Tomography (CT) - Chest	7 mSv	2 years
	Computed Tomography (CT) - Lung Cancer Screening	1.5 mSv	6 months
	Radiography - Chest	0.1 mSv	10 days
DENTAL	Intraoral X-ray	0.005 mSv	1 day
HEART	Coronary Computed Tomography Angiography (CTA)	12 mSv	4 years
	Cardiac CT for Calcium Scoring	3 mSv	1 year
MEN'S IMAGING	Bone Densitometry (DEXA)	0.001 mSv	3 hours
NUCLEAR MEDICINE	Positron Emission Tomography - Computed Tomography (PET/CT)	25 mSv	8 years
WOMEN'S IMAGING	Bone Densitometry (DEXA)	0.001 mSv	3 hours
	Mammography	0.4 mSv	7 weeks

Figure 7.17. Radiation dose chart.

Source: https://i0.wp.com/theradiologictechnologist.com/wp-content/uploads/2020/04/Untitled-design-60.png?w=560&ssl=1.

These levels not only serve as criteria for radiation doses administered during various procedures but also assist health centers in limiting unnecessary radiation exposure during diagnostic imaging. A national dose survey of adult patients found that NDRLs effectively support compliance with safety standards across hospitals (Skovorodko et al., 2022). By establishing these reference levels, radiologists can be confident that the doses given are within safety limits while still being effectively diagnostic. With technological advances in the imaging field, it will be necessary from time to time to review and revise these levels to keep up with the evolution of SPECT practice and advances in radiopharmaceuticals. Lastly, the use of advanced monitoring and quality assurance procedures has further safeguarded patients in nuclear medicine. These individuals have established mechanisms to continually test and improve the accuracy and precision of diagnostic images while protecting against unwanted exposure to radiation. Routine tests and adherence to safety standards rigorously can minimize risks associated with SPECT procedures. Performing uniformity, linearity, and spatial resolution tests, for example, ensures that gamma cameras and imaging devices used are capable of detecting and transmitting crucial patient data without sacrificing safety. Hence, an integrative method that combines the latest technological advancements with stringent safety protocols must be implemented to ensure patient comfort in nuclear medicine (Hasan et al., 2025).

7.6.3. Future Challenges in Nuclear Medicine Technology

Technological developments in nuclear medicine, particularly in gamma camera and SPECT technology, are subject to many future challenges that could slow them down. Among the largest challenges is the need for higher sensitivity and specificity in imaging methods. The present imaging modalities, as useful as they are, are prone to image artifacts and spatial resolution limitations. The use of newer digital signal processing technologies, along with machine learning algorithms, can solve the problem; however, transitioning from existing to newer technologies requires significant capital expenditure and training. Again, there is a constant need to ensure the safe manufacturing and quality assurance of radiopharmaceuticals in accordance with good manufacturing practices. By resolving these issues, the capability to provide more accurate and up-to-date diagnoses in the clinic can be significantly improved, enhancing the overall discipline of nuclear medicine (Volpe et al., 2021) (Figure 7.18).

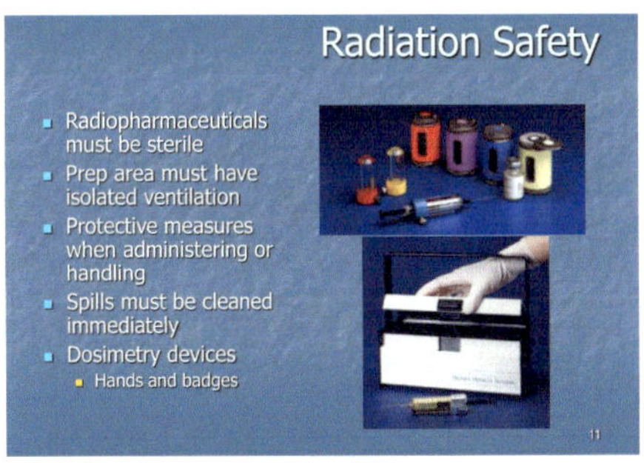

Figure 7.18. Infographic summarizing patient safety practices in nuclear medicine.

Source: https://image1.slideserve.com/3037668/radiation-safety-l.jpg.

In alignment with this is the administration of the complexity in radioisotope production and supply. The more radioisotopes that are required, the more the existing supply chain must adjust and be efficient in meeting those requirements. The process not only encompasses producing isotopes from reactors and generators but ensuring that they are transported adequately without compromising their integrity and losing much wastage. The reliance on aging nuclear facilities can contribute to this need for innovation. Domestic production facilities for the required radioisotopes can help overcome these problems and enhance the availability of health centers. Besides, the regulatory landscape for nuclear materials is changing every day; hence, nuclear medicine practitioners must be experts in keeping pace with such developments to embrace safe and compliant practices (Andreas et al., 2020). Lastly, the introduction of artificial intelligence (AI) into nuclear medicine technology is both a challenge and an opportunity. AI has the potential to transform image interpretation and processing, but its introduction requires careful consideration of ethics, patient confidentiality, and data management. When huge volumes of data are captured in medical imaging, the challenge becomes maximizing data analysis to yield actionable information that enhances patient care. The need for robust medical data governance policies also comes to the forefront to effectively manage the amount of digital data coming from diverse imaging modalities. A framework that is interoperable and harmonizes AI solutions with clinical workflows would enhance the accuracy and effectiveness of nuclear medicine procedures, along with resolving the ethical and logistical problems associated with this integration (Volpe et al., 2021).

SUMMARY

In this chapter on nuclear medicine, with the focus laid on gamma camera technology and single photon emission computed tomography (SPECT), several salient themes emerge. The chapter understandably addresses radioisotope production and chemistry to support image procedures. It contrasts reactor- and generator-based sources, focusing on the dynamics of radiolabeling techniques and the supreme importance of quality control in radiopharmaceuticals for safety and efficacy. This foundation of knowledge is essential for clinicians to master the uses of various isotopes in medical imaging to perfection. Understanding these basics lays the foundation for the safe and effective use of nuclear medicine as a diagnostic tool in all branches of medicine, ultimately to the advantage of patient care. A large majority of the chapter discusses gamma cameras' design and operation. It sheds light on collimator selection and types, the properties of the scintillation crystal important for gamma photon detection, and the functions of the photomultiplier array for converting scintillation into electrical signals. All these elements are instrumental to the quality of the imaging output. Further, the thorough examination of planar imaging protocols also highlights acquisition parameters, energy window settings, and image corrections to be made, enabling medical practitioners to promptly and competently interpret diagnostic images. This technical expertise not only enhances gamma camera capabilities but also underscores the intricacy of producing high-quality diagnostic images. The chapter concludes by examining SPECT technology, emphasizing its tomographic capability, reconstruction algorithms, and attenuation correction algorithms. These are important for improving the spatial resolution and overall accuracy of nuclear imaging. Quality assurance processes are highlighted, including tests for uniformity and linearity, spatial resolution checks, and measurement of system sensitivity, to maintain the integrity of images. Finally, let's examine the diverse clinical applications of SPECT, such as cardiac perfusion imaging, bone scintigraphy, and renal function imaging, thus lending emphasis on the utilitarian role of the above technologies in real-world health care. The comprehensive discussion highlights the development and challenges of nuclear medicine as a constantly evolving science (Wilson et al., 2021; Skotland et al., 2022).

CLOSER LOOK

THE EVOLVING ROLE OF GAMMA CAMERAS AND SPECT IN PRECISION MEDICINE

The development of gamma cameras and single-photon emission computed tomography (SPECT) has revolutionized healthcare, particularly diagnostic imaging. They have dramatically enhanced clinicians' ability to image and assess various medical conditions more accurately and precisely. The role of gamma cameras in imaging protocols, and their design features regarding collimator choice and scintillation crystal properties, contribute significantly to overall diagnostic image quality. The ability to non-invasively evaluate physiological functions in organs, for example, myocardial perfusion during cardiac investigations, underscores their role in influencing treatment planning and patient outcomes. This diagnostic specificity not only facilitates early treatment but also contributes to the broader aims of precision medicine by maximizing treatment strategies for the unique needs of individual patients. In addition to their diagnostic function, gamma cameras and SPECT have facilitated advances in clinical application that intersect a variety of medical specialties. For instance, in the diagnosis of neurological disorders, dopaminergic SPECT imaging has become a mainstay diagnostic tool for Parkinsonian syndromes, as recently emphasized by procedural guidelines formulated by the European Association of Nuclear Medicine and the Society of Nuclear Medicine and Molecular Imaging (Morbelli et al., 2020). These recommendations emphasize the need for harmonization and semi-quantification in reading imaging data, and hence fostering homogenized practice by healthcare centers. The integration of new tracers and newer imaging technologies also considerably enhances diagnostic capability, making it possible to better differentiate diagnoses and treatment options for the patient, ultimately leading to improved clinical outcomes. With the evolving technology of nuclear medicine, the potential for incorporating artificial intelligence and advanced algorithms into the imaging procedure cannot be overstated. Emerging deep learning architectures have the potential to revolutionize the processing and review of gamma camera and SPECT data (Andreas et al., 2020). The integration of these innovations may lead to greater accuracy in disease diagnosis and organ delineation, thereby improving the general performance of the imaging informatics environment. Facilitating real-time data analysis and decision-making, these innovations have the potential to dramatically transform patient care, enabling healthcare practitioners to deliver more effective diagnostics and treatment plans that are harmonized with each patient's individualized biological context. In this context, the current research into gamma cameras and SPECT has significant implications for future healthcare provision.

REFERENCES

1. Akram, M., Iqbal, M., Daniyal, M., & Khan, A. U. (2017). Awareness and current knowledge of breast cancer. *Biological Research, 50*(1), 33. https://doi.org/10.1186/s40659-017-0140-9Aleksa, G., Jarusevicius, P., Pacaitytė, A., & Vajauskas, D. (2025). Comparative analysis of cardiac SPECT myocardial perfusion imaging: Full-ring solid-state detectors versus dedicated cardiac fixed-angle gamma camera. *Medicina, 61*. https://www.semanticscholar.org/paper/24e90044d313a62ab39361504e2aca871a6a1259 (accessed on 14th July 2025).
2. AlSaadi, A., Jain, A., Al-Jabri, A., Delanerolle, G., Zabah, J., Shi, J. Q., Phiri, P., et al. (2024). Technological advances in SPECT and SPECT/CT imaging. https://core.ac.uk/download/613741130.pdf (accessed on 14th July 2025).
3. Armstrong, I. S., de Geus-Oei, L. F., Denis-Bacelar, A. M., Dickson, J., et al. (2023). EANM practice guideline for quantitative SPECT-CT. https://core.ac.uk/download/604657624.pdf (accessed on 14th July 2025).
4. Bankstahl, J., Belcari, N., Krämer, S., Vandenberghe, S., et al. (2015). Accurate molecular imaging of small animals taking into account animal models, handling, anesthesia, quality control and imaging system performance. https://core.ac.uk/download/55743381.pdf (accessed on 14th July 2025).
5. Benlloch Baviera, J. M., González Martínez, A. J., & Sánchez, F. (2018). Organ-dedicated molecular imaging systems. https://riunet.upv.es/bitstream/handle/10251/154033/Gonz%c3%a1lez%3bS%c3%a1nchez%3bBenlloch%20-%20Organ-Dedicated%20Molecular%20Imaging%20Systems.pdf?sequence=7&isAllowed=y (accessed on 14th July 2025).
6. Camilleri, M., & Linden, D. R. (2016). Measurement of gastrointestinal and colonic motor functions in humans and animals. *Cellular and Molecular Gastroenterology and Hepatology, 2*, 412–428. https://doi.org/10.1016/j.jcmgh.2016.04.003 (accessed on 14th July 2025).
7. Chatziioannou, A. F., Kirov, A. S., Assié, K., Behrens, H., Berger, L., Bielajew, A. F., Hirayama, H., Nelson, W. R., Rogers, D. W. O., et al. (2004). GATE: A simulation toolkit for PET and SPECT. https://core.ac.uk/download/34921078.pdf (accessed on 14th July 2025).
8. Clough, A. V., Dawson, C. A., Haworth, S. T., Molthen, R. C., et al. (2004). Quantification of bronchial circulation perfusion in rats. https://core.ac.uk/download/213084485.pdf (accessed on 14th July 2025).
9. Clough, A. V., Dawson, C. A., Johnson, R. H., Molthen, R. C., et al. (2003). SPECT imaging of pulmonary blood flow in a rat. https://core.ac.uk/download/213084483.pdf (accessed on 14th July 2025).
10. Clough, A. V., Gordon, J. B., Haworth, S. T., Molthen, R. C., et al. (2008). Bronchial circulation angiogenesis in the rat quantified with SPECT and micro-CT. https://core.ac.uk/download/213086433.pdf (accessed on 14th July 2025).
11. Ghaneh, M., Nasseri, S., Sadeghi, R., Zakavi, S., Vosoughi, H., & Mommennezhad, M. (2024). Optimization of image quality in pelvis lymphoscintigraphy SPECT/CT using Discovery NM/CT 670. *World Journal of Nuclear Medicine, 24*, 20–30. https://www.semanticscholar.org/paper/e93d8e95a02ba13e0d34600573b85cce59a61cdc (accessed on 14th July 2025).
12. Hasan, B., Chowdhury, M. S. A., Mahmud, S., Zerin, F., Akter, Y., Hossain, N., Hossain, F., et al. (2025). Radiation dose assessment around patients in single photon emission computed

tomography units during bone scintigraphy and DTPA renogram. *Bangladesh Journal of Nuclear Medicine.* https://www.semanticscholar.org/paper/43e0fa5fa3d6540c524e1b6a4e225b9c53da12b5 (accessed on 14th July 2025).

13. Hitchcock, C. L., Chapman, G., Mojzisik, C., Mueller, J. K., & Martin, E. W. (2024). A concept for preoperative and intraoperative molecular imaging and detection for assessing extent of disease of solid tumors. *Oncology Reviews, 18.* https://www.semanticscholar.org/paper/ed218a8b784a5298fbd5262af50b700564b5d085 (accessed on 14th July 2025).
14. Imran, M. B., & Naqvi, S. A. R. (2020). Single-photon emission computed tomography (SPECT) radiopharmaceuticals. https://core.ac.uk/download/335288469.pdf (accessed on 14th July 2025).
15. Kane, S. (2002). Introduction to physics in modern medicine. https://www.semanticscholar.org/paper/73e6cda683edcb60d6295e9fa42e67e5769151e7 (accessed on 14th July 2025).
16. Kusmirek, J., Magnusson, J. D., & Perlman, S. (2020). Current applications for nuclear medicine imaging in pulmonary disease. *Current Pulmonology Reports, 9*, 82–95. https://www.semanticscholar.org/paper/803c920d86fff9fcbb092aea35cd292f2ba7d2f2 (accessed on 14th July 2025).
17. Lacko, A., Straka, J., Hrubon, A., Babečka, J., & Lacko, L. (2024). Myocardial perfusion scintigraphy in diagnostic of coronary heart disease. *American Journal of Internal Medicine.* https://www.semanticscholar.org/paper/98f5f744f0dc543abf9385787c0b1ffda37ddad1 (accessed on 14th July 2025).
18. Lamichhane, N., Udayakumar, T. S., D'Souza, W., Simone, C. B., Raghavan, S. R., Polf, J., & Mahmood, J. (2018). Liposomes: Clinical applications and potential for image-guided drug delivery. *Molecules, 23*, 288. https://doi.org/10.3390/molecules23020288 (accessed on 14th July 2025).
19. MacRitchie, N., Frleta-Gilchrist, M., Sugiyama, A., Lawton, T., McInnes, I. B., & Maffia, P. (2020). Molecular imaging of inflammation–Current and emerging technologies for diagnosis and treatment. *Pharmacology & Therapeutics, 211*, 107550. https://doi.org/10.1016/j.pharmthera.2020.107550 (accessed on 14th July 2025).
20. Mishra, A. (2024). Gamma cameras: Exploring the technology, applications, and future prospects. https://core.ac.uk/download/617006397.pdf (accessed on 14th July 2025).
21. Morbelli, S., Esposito, G., Arbizu, J., Barthel, H., Boellaard, R., Bohnen, N., Brooks, D. J., et al. (2020). EANM practice guideline/SNMMI procedure standard for dopaminergic imaging in Parkinsonian syndromes 1.0. *European Journal of Nuclear Medicine and Molecular Imaging, 47*, 1885–1912. https://doi.org/10.1007/s00259-020-04817-8 (accessed on 14th July 2025).
22. Nienhuis, H. L. A., Pastoor, E. M., Slart, R. H. J. A., Tingen, M. H. N., et al. (2023). Correction to: Positron emission tomography in the diagnosis and follow-up of transthyretin amyloid cardiomyopathy patients: A systematic review. https://core.ac.uk/download/604657630.pdf (accessed on 14th July 2025).
23. Oelschlegel, A. M., & Goldschmidt, J. (2020). Functional neuroimaging in rodents using cerebral blood flow SPECT. *Frontiers in Physics, 8.* https://doi.org/10.3389/fphy.2020.00152 (accessed on 14th July 2025).
24. Panayides, A. S., Amini, A. A., Filipović, N., Sharma, A., Tsaftaris, S. A., Young, A. A., Foran, D. J., et al. (2020). AI in medical imaging informatics: Current challenges and future directions.

IEEE Journal of Biomedical and Health Informatics, 24, 1837–1857. https://doi.org/10.1109/jbhi.2020.2991043 (accessed on 14th July 2025).

25. Pandey, A. (2024). An introduction to the physics of nuclear medicine. *Journal of Medical Physics, 49*, 133–134. https://doi.org/10.4103/jmp.jmp_1_24 (accessed on 14th July 2025).
26. Pawar, Y. P., Shimpi, H., Shrivastav, A., Awasare, S. U., Rakshit, S., Karpe, M., Damle, A. A., et al. (2024). Role of advance nuclear medicine imaging techniques in preclinical drug development and three R's in animal research. *Journal of Laboratory Animal Science.* https://www.semanticscholar.org/paper/872cfab68fb460e6cccc2938a232921c5865a79c (accessed on 14th July 2025).
27. Peix, A., Mesquita, C. T., Gutiérrez, C., Puente, A., Dueñas-C, K. A., Massardo, T., Berrocal, I., et al. (2022). Current status of nuclear cardiology practice in Latin America and the Caribbean, in the era of multimodality cardiac imaging approach: 2022 update. *Nuclear Medicine Communications, 43*, 1163–1170. https://doi.org/10.1097/mnm.0000000000001630 (accessed on 14th July 2025).
28. Piwowarska-Bilska, H., Supińska, A., Iwanowski, J., Tyczyńska, A., & Birkenfeld, B. (2019). PET–advanced nuclear imaging technology for medicine. *Pomeranian Journal of Life Sciences, 65*, 45–53. https://www.semanticscholar.org/paper/71a3bff61c6dd1e9944398a9c59376f193e4c668 (accessed on 14th July 2025).
29. Popova, N. S., Krzhivitskiy, P., Novikov, S., Danilov, V., Valitova, A., Bryantseva, Z. V., Chernaya, A., et al. (2023). Radionuclide imaging of breast cancer: Experience of FSBI "N.N. Petrov National Medical Research Centre of Oncology" of the Ministry of Healthcare of Russian Federation. *Medical Visualization.* https://www.semanticscholar.org/paper/6ead186f297d9fd981cb20091b3e85590656df93 (accessed on 14th July 2025).
30. Ramkishore, N., Crocker, J., Martin, R., Yap, K. S., & Brady, Z. (2024). A survey of gamma camera and SPECT/CT quality control programs across a sample of public hospitals in Australia. *Physical and Engineering Sciences in Medicine.* https://www.semanticscholar.org/paper/727657e0acd3ea279afec0c479aa03931ccf4aae (accessed on 14th July 2025).
31. Sarrut, D., Bała, M., Bardiès, M., Bert, J., Chauvin, M., Chatzipapas, K., Dupont, M., et al. (2021). Advanced Monte Carlo simulations of emission tomography imaging systems with GATE. *Physics in Medicine and Biology, 66*, 10TR03. https://doi.org/10.1088/1361-6560/abf276 (accessed on 14th July 2025).
32. Sergieva, S., Mangaldgiev, R., Dimcheva, M., Nedev, K., Zahariev, Z., & Robev, B. (2021). SPECT-CT imaging with [99mTc]PSMA-T4 in patients with recurrent prostate cancer. *Nuclear Medicine Review. Central & Eastern Europe, 24*(2), 70–81. https://www.semanticscholar.org/paper/0a32cb1f9031cbbc8441e3951cbd15d808885606 (accessed on 14th July 2025).
33. Skotland, T., Iversen, T.-G., Llorente, A., & Sandvig, K. (2022). Biodistribution, pharmacokinetics and excretion studies of intravenously injected nanoparticles and extracellular vesicles: Possibilities and challenges. *Advanced Drug Delivery Reviews, 186*, 114326. https://doi.org/10.1016/j.addr.2022.114326 (accessed on 14th July 2025).
34. Skovorodko, K., Komiagienė, R., Maciusovic, M., Gilys, L., Vajauskas, D., Grigonienė, V., Žiliukas, J., et al. (2022). Nationwide survey on radiation doses received by patients in nuclear medicine imaging procedures. *Journal of Radiological Protection, 42.* https://www.semanticscholar.org/paper/1f81c5d1d8aac89c436d5f6f1a537013cf35bca5 (accessed on 14th July 2025).

35. Staelens, S., Van Holen, R., & Vandenberghe, S. (2011). Tomographic image quality of rotating slat versus parallel hole-collimated SPECT. https://core.ac.uk/download/55809080.pdf (accessed on 14th July 2025).

36. Sundin, A., Arnold, R., Baudin, É., Ćwikła, J. B., Eriksson, B., Fanti, S., Fazio, N., et al. (2017). ENETS consensus guidelines for the standards of care in neuroendocrine tumors: Radiological, nuclear medicine and hybrid imaging. *Neuroendocrinology, 105*, 212–244. https://doi.org/10.1159/000471879 (accessed on 14th July 2025).

37. Teresińska, A., & Królicki, L. (2023). Registry of nuclear medicine procedures in cardiology in Poland in 2019–2021. *Nuclear Medicine Review. Central & Eastern Europe, 26*(0), 158–164. https://www.semanticscholar.org/paper/1fcdead6231186b4642db38aef2e5dc56ad9b8f0 (accessed on 14th July 2025).

38. Van den Wyngaert, T., Strobel, K., Kampen, W. U., Kuwert, T., van der Bruggen, W., Mohan, H., Gnanasegaran, G., et al. (2016). The EANM practice guidelines for bone scintigraphy. *European Journal of Nuclear Medicine and Molecular Imaging, 43*, 1723–1738. https://doi.org/10.1007/s00259-016-3415-4 (accessed on 14th July 2025).

39. Villalobos, A., Soliman, M., Majdalany, B., Schuster, D., Galt, J., Bercu, Z., & Kokabi, N. (2020). Yttrium-90 radioembolization dosimetry: What trainees need to know. *Seminars in Interventional Radiology, 37*, 543–554. https://www.semanticscholar.org/paper/ea6788823898126eca5eca669f35a7f431186b3c (accessed on 14th July 2025).

40. Volpe, A., Pillarsetty, N., Lewis, J. S., & Ponomarev, V. (2021). Applications of nuclear-based imaging in gene and cell therapy: Probe considerations. *Molecular Therapy–Oncolytics, 20*, 447–458. https://doi.org/10.1016/j.omto.2021.01.017 (accessed on 14th July 2025).

41. Wilson, C., Aarons, L., Augustijns, P., Brouwers, J., Darwich, A. S., de Waal, T., Garbacz, G., et al. (2021). Integration of advanced methods and models to study drug absorption and related processes: An UNGAP perspective. *European Journal of Pharmaceutical Sciences, 172*, 106100. https://doi.org/10.1016/j.ejps.2021.106100 (accessed on 14th July 2025).

42. Witney, T., & Blower, P. (2021). The chemical tool-kit for molecular imaging with radionuclides in the age of targeted and immune therapy. *Cancer Imaging, 21*. https://www.semanticscholar.org/paper/5ad767b5ba0d26dcf71594c9155fd4b35bacfbd5 (accessed on 14th July 2025).

43. Woźniak, M., Płoska, A., Siekierzycka, A., Dobrucki, L. W., Kalinowski, L., & Dobrucki, I. T. (2022). Molecular imaging and nanotechnology—Emerging tools in diagnostics and therapy. *International Journal of Molecular Sciences, 23*, 2658. https://doi.org/10.3390/ijms23052658 (accessed on 14th July 2025).

44. Yitbarek, D., & Dagnaw, G. G. (2022). Application of advanced imaging modalities in veterinary medicine: A review. *Veterinary Medicine Research and Reports, 13*, 117–130. https://doi.org/10.2147/vmrr.s367040 (accessed on 14th July 2025).

45. Zuziak, P., Ilnicka, N., Matyja, D., Sadlik, M., & Abod, L. (2023). Application of nuclear medicine techniques in sports medicine. *Journal of Education, Health and Sport.* https://www.semanticscholar.org/paper/2628fe825c40c71d012f0b10d30575f27562242c (accessed on 14th July 2025).

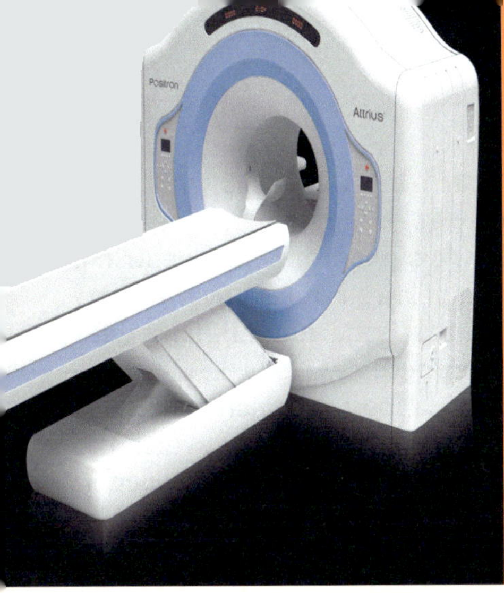

Chapter 8

POSITRON EMISSION TOMOGRAPHY (PET) BASICS

Contents

Introduction

The underlying physics of positron emission tomography (PET) is rooted in the β^+ decay process. In this process, a proton in a nucleus is converted into a neutron by the emission of a positron, the antimatter counterpart of an electron. Once emitted, the positron travels a short distance before annihilating an electron with a resultant pair emission of two 511 keV photons traveling in opposite directions. Annihilation is the central mechanism of PET imaging because coincidence photon detection enables localizing the original positron emission. Coincidence detection is therefore a fundamental aspect of building PET systems to achieve proper spatial imaging of the metabolism of biological tissues. Ultimately, a thorough understanding of these fundamental principles forms a solid ground for the extended applications of PET technology in medicine. Extended PET technology developments also arise from the complexities of PET scanner components, namely the detector materials employed in the systems. Familiar materials such as Lutetium Oxyorthosilicate (LSO) and Bismuth Germanate (BGO) possess excellent properties, including high stopping power and rapid decay times, which are valuable for the effective detection of annihilation photons. Moreover, the inclusion of the Time-of-Flight (ToF) feature enhances the spatial resolution of PET imaging by exploiting differences in photon detection times and facilitates improved three-dimensional localization of radiopharmaceutical uptake. The combination of scintillators with photomultiplier tubes (PMTs) is yet another vital aspect that maximizes the signal quality obtained from photons that are detected. As these are fabricated and improved, the overall performance of PET systems improves as well, significantly affecting diagnostic accuracy and patient outcomes in clinical applications. Quantitative PET imaging relies heavily on accurate data acquisition and reconstruction to support valuable biological inferences. List-mode or frame-mode acquisition directly influences temporal and spatial resolution, essentially determining the quality of the final image. In addition, application of analytic and iterative reconstruction algorithms improves positron emission precision by minimizing artifacts, scatter, and random events that obscure accurate signals. These methods are critical for achieving the Standardized Uptake Value (SUV), a standard measure of radiopharmaceutical uptake in targeted tissues. Novel kinetic modeling and partial-volume corrections will be needed to further improve the accuracy of quantitative results, enabling reasonable interpretations of metabolic function and disease follow-up studies, for example, in oncology and cardiology. The symbiotic blend of these elements accounts for the sophisticated nature of PET as a viable imaging technique in modern-day medical diagnostics.

8.1. Principles of PET Imaging

In positron emission tomography (PET), understanding the mechanisms of β^+ decay underlies most applications of the imaging modality. The β^+ decay mechanisms are essential because they occur when a nucleus with more protons than neutrons changes a proton into a neutron by emitting a positron and a neutrino. When the emitted positron travels over a short distance in biological tissue, it annihilates with an electron and produces two 511 keV gamma photons emitted in opposite directions. These are the principles of PET imaging, in which the detection of these photons allows reconstruction of the original positron emission event, a process termed coincidence detection. The ability to accurately identify these events allows for the mapping of tissue metabolic activity and the acquisition of valuable information concerning numerous physiological and pathological processes, including cancer and cardiovascular disease. PET scanners comprise components that directly affect the efficacy and effectiveness of image outcomes. Among these components, detector materials such as bismuth germanate (BGO) and lutetium oxyorthosilicate (LSO) play an important role in so far as they are sensitivity and resolution determinants of the scans. While BGO is defined by high density and efficient gamma-ray absorption, LSO is defined by lower response times as well as improved energy resolution. Besides, time-of-flight (TOF) capability provides better localization accuracy by measuring the time taken by the annihilation photons to reach the detectors. The process significantly reduces image noise and optimizes image quality. Furthermore, scintillator-photomultiplier tube (PMT) coupling is also important since it determines the conversion efficiency from scintillation light to an electric signal for imaging. All these elements combined ensure that PET technology delivers timely and accurate diagnostic data. Quantitative PET imaging is a significant advancement in this regard, enabling exact physiological data to be derived from images. The Standardized Uptake Value or SUV is an important measure in this regard, as it standardizes measured radioactivity in an area of interest relative to the patient's body weight to enable the detection of metabolic abnormalities. Kinetic modeling also allows for better characterization of the underlying physiological mechanisms of radiopharmaceutical uptake, particularly in oncology. As noted, [18F] FDG is the most widely used radiotracer in clinical PET, particularly in oncology, because it can target regions of increased glucose metabolism within tumors. Nonetheless, consideration of effects such as partial-volume correction should be made to enhance image quantification, particularly when assessing small lesions. Thus, technical advances in quantitative methods continue to enhance the clinical utility of PET imaging and provide additional information on patient status and responses to interventions.

8.1.1. Basic Physics of Positron Emission

The physics of positron emission is based on β^+ decay, a process in which a proton in a nucleus is transformed into a neutron, accompanied by the emission of a positron and a neutrino. This is about some radionuclides commonly used in positron emission tomography (PET). For instance, fluorine-18, a typical radiotracer, emits β^+ decay and later emits positrons that interact with nearby electrons. Particle-antiparticle annihilation produces two gamma photons that travel in nearly opposite directions. Explaining these decay modes is important, since they provide the background information required for the production of radiopharmaceuticals and their application in PET imaging, with precision in the detection and reading of such emissions being critical for correct diagnosis and therapeutic evaluation (Rosa et al., 2015). The annihilation process releases photons, which are critical for PET imaging. When the positron that is emitted by the radionuclide is met by an electron, they annihilate one another and form two 511 keV gamma photons that are emitted from the interaction point. The detection of these annihilation photons is of utmost importance for creating an image of the tracer distribution within the body. By applying a coincidence detection process, PET scanners identify these photons in coincidence, enabling localization of the annihilation process through triangulation of data from several detectors. This sophisticated detection process is crucial for enhancing spatial resolution as well as specificity within imaging and, as such, the overall efficiency of PET for clinical use (Eckardt et al., 2003). Coincidence detection not only helps identify the precise location of the radiotracer but also reduces background noise and improves the signal-to-noise ratio. During a PET scan, temporal detection of photons becomes important; thus, detector synchronization is required to identify photons from the same annihilation event. This strategy makes it more precise to determine the physiological processes in the body, and that is of prime importance for diagnosing disorders like tumors and coronary artery disease. Advances in coincidence detection technology, as well as the physics of positron emission, have gone a long way toward advancing the field of nuclear medicine, ultimately leading to improved patient outcomes through precise imaging and targeted treatment (Rosa et al., 2015) (Figure 8.1).

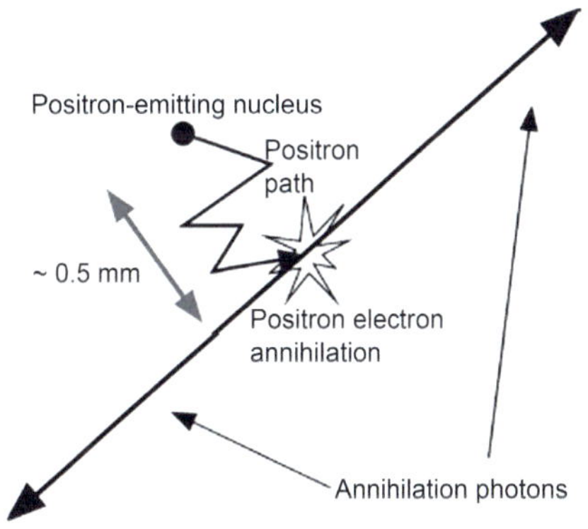

Figure 8.1. Diagram illustrating the basic physics of positron emission and annihilation.

Source: https://radiologykey.com/wp-content/uploads/2016/09/9781604061543_c001_f001.jpg.

8.1.2. Mechanism of Radiotracer Uptake

In Positron Emission Tomography (PET), radiotracer uptake is the primary mechanism for effective imaging and diagnosis. Radiotracers usually consist of agent molecules that are copies of naturally occurring molecules within the body, tagged with a radioisotope that emits positrons. The phospholipid bilayer of the cell membrane restricts the diffusion of such compounds, thereby determining their uptake in target tissues. Parameters such as blood flow, tissue perfusion, and metabolism may significantly affect this uptake, thereby enhancing the imaging of physiological and disease processes. As PET imaging has evolved, so has the understanding of these processes, which led to the development of more sophisticated tracers that allow for unique information of tumor metabolism, neuroinflammation, and other major biological processes, ultimately leading to enhanced diagnosis and therapy (Beyer et al., 2010).

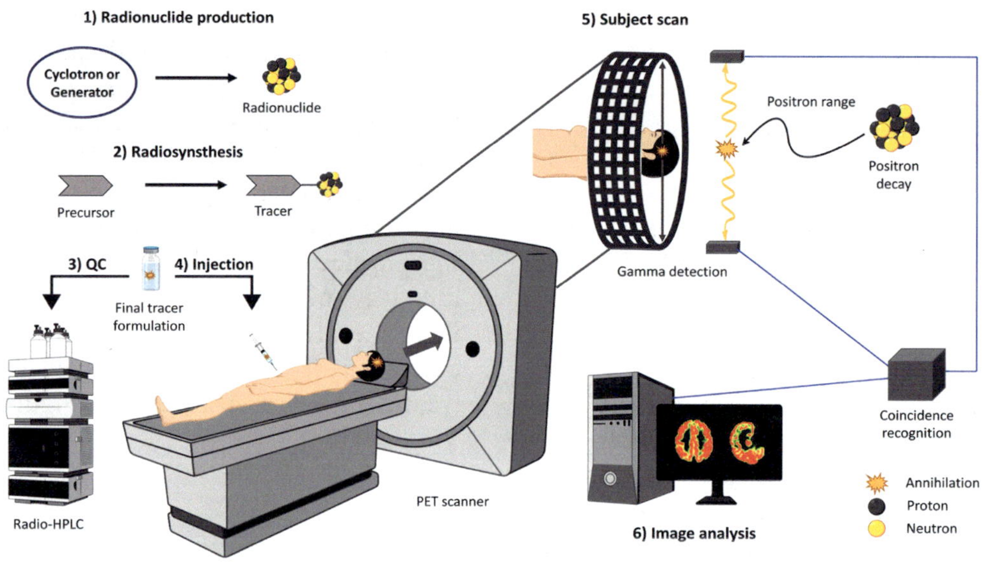

Figure 8.2. Schematic of a radiotracer molecule used in PET imaging.

Source: https://media.springernature.com/full/springer-static/image/art%3A10.1038%2Fs41467-023-36377-4/MediaObjects/41467_2023_36377_Fig1_HTML.png.

Technological advances have also promoted advancements in the accuracy of radiotracer uptake quantitation with quantitative PET imaging. The Standardized Uptake Value (SUV) has been commonly employed to allow comparison across studies and patients and to measure the extent of tracer deposition in multiple tissues. Such a measure demands accurate calibration of the imaging apparatuses, emphasizing the achievement of good kinetic modeling of tracer kinetics. Variables affecting SUV are radiotracer dose, timing of image acquisition, and factors related to the patient such as body mass index and hydration status. A full understanding of these variables enables the clinician to better interpret PET imaging results, thereby leading to proper management of conditions such as cancer and cardiovascular disease (Kaprelyan et al., 2015). In addition, recent advances in PET technology have led to the development of new radiopharmaceuticals designed to image targeted biological activity at the molecular level. Radiotracers such as [^18F]-FDG are now standard due to their application in imaging tumor glucose metabolism. Similarly, new biomarker-targeting tracers enable visualization of disease-related pathways and offer enhanced diagnostic capability. Continued studies on the production and quality control aspects of these radiotracers are necessary to ensure their safety and effectiveness. This constantly evolving profile of PET radiopharmaceuticals not only demonstrates the interplay between imaging science and medicine but also reveals new applications, including personalized medicine strategies and the evaluation of therapeutic responses (Beyer et al., 2010) (Figure 8.2).

8.1.3. Detection of Gamma Rays in PET

Gamma detection is an important component of Positron Emission Tomography (PET) that enables visualization of metabolic activity in the body. Upon positron emission, a beta-plus decay occurs, in which a positron emitted by a radiotracer annihilates an electron, resulting in mutual destruction. This destruction results in the emission of two gamma photons at opposite directions at an angle of 180°. The concurrent detection of such photons forms the basis of coincidence detection, enabling accurate localization of the radiotracer in a patient's body. Detection is based on advanced scintillator materials that convert the gamma rays into measurable light signals, which are thereafter processed to produce accurate images of physiological processes. Precise detection accuracy underlies the need to enhance diagnostic accuracy across various clinical applications. Detection of gamma rays in PET is dominated by the choice of detector material. Common materials such as Bismuth Germinate (BGO) and Lutetium Oxyorthosilicate (LSO) exhibit good scintillation properties. They can efficiently convert gamma-ray interactions into scintillation light, a necessity for photomultiplier tubes (PMTs) or avalanche photodiodes to detect it. Emerging technologies have enabled the creation of scintillator-optical fiber systems capable of delivering improved spatial resolution and enhanced gamma-ray localization using intersecting fibers. For instance, the use of primary scintillating fibers and secondary fibers at non-zero angles enables the detection system not only to recognize the site of gamma-ray incidence but also to determine their incidence path, thereby enhancing overall PET imaging capacity (Anderson et al., 1994).

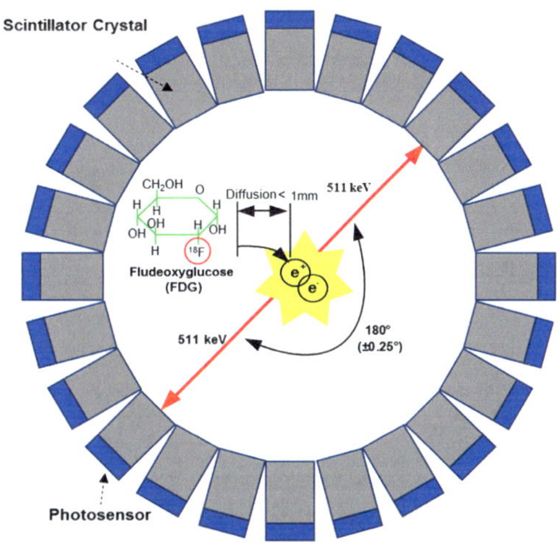

Figure 8.3. PET scanner detector ring showing the arrangement of scintillation crystals.

Source: https://www.researchgate.net/publication/337325700/figure/fig1/AS:11431281390734114@1745285857206/The-basic-principle-of-a-positron-emission-tomography-PET-system-A-PET-detector-ring.tif.

Moreover, PET's improvements in data-acquisition systems affect how gamma rays are detected and processed. Its two prominent modes, list-mode and frame-mode, offer versatility in data acquisition across a range of temporal resolutions. List-mode acquisition permits the registration of every coincidence event as it is continuously detected, thereby enabling more advanced analysis and iterative reconstruction techniques, which are important for achieving optimal image quality. Frame mode might group events into predefined time bins, which could simplify data handling but sacrifice resolution in dynamic exams. The effective combination of scatter and random correction algorithms further enhances gamma ray detection precision by minimizing spurious event noise. In these many-splendored ways, gamma ray detection in PET improves, leading to better and more informative imaging necessary for modern diagnostic radiology (Adenilson et al., 2008) (Figure 8.3).

8.2. Radiotracers Used in PET

The use of radiotracers in Positron Emission Tomography (PET) is paramount, as these agents are the fundamental imaging tools for the mapping of physiological events within the body. The most common radiotracer used is [^18F]-fluorodeoxyglucose (FDG), a glucose analogue that helps visualize tissue metabolic activity. This is particularly useful in oncological purposes, where it is noted that cancerous cells have elevated glucose metabolism. Moreover, FDG enables differentiation between malignant and benign lesions, which is critical for precise diagnosis and treatment planning. Other promising radiotracers include new agents like those that bind to prostate-specific membrane antigen (PSMA) for imaging prostate cancer. The development of these tracers has significantly impacted clinical decision-making and patient outcomes by providing greater diagnostic specificity than conventional imaging techniques (Davis et al., 2018). Beyond [^18F]-FDG, advancements have led to the development of new radiotracers that are specific to particular diseases. Tracers in this category include F-18 fluciclovine and carbon-11 choline, which are increasingly used to detect recurrent prostate cancer, especially for monitoring serum prostate-specific antigen (PSA) levels. Researchers have shown that gallium-68/PSMA PET imaging can detect recurrence in 51.5% of patients presenting with low PSA levels, underscoring its clinical utility. The advanced method facilitates detection at earlier stages, and thereby, timely therapeutic intervention could improve patient prognosis (Davis et al., 2018). Consequently, radiotracer development not only enhances PET imaging accuracy but also is amenable to tailored patient care strategies. Quality control processes are essential in providing dependable and safe radiotracers for use in PET. Synthesis and manufacture of radiopharmaceuticals involve rigorous protocols to minimize impurities and ensure radioisotope stability, both pivotal to achieving accurate imaging data.

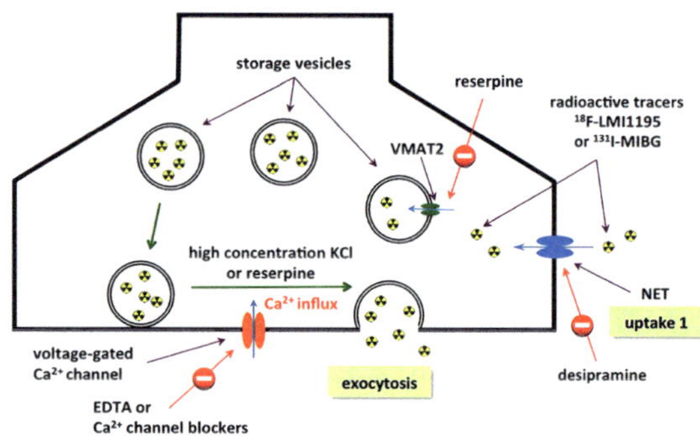

Figure 8.4. Illustration of the mechanism of radiotracer uptake in cells.

Source: https://www.researchgate.net/publication/322967521/figure/fig6/AS:963417703739407@1606708088942/Illustration-of-radiotracer-uptake-storage-and-release-mechanisms-in-PC12-cells-In.gif.

In addition, there are standardized procedures for the handling and storage of radiotracers that must be followed to maintain their efficacy and patient safety. Quality control, when incorporated into the clinical process, enhances the reproducibility and reliability of PET imaging results, which is paramount for both therapy and diagnosis. As quality assurance measures and radiotracer technology become more advanced, PET continues to be an important tool in modern medicine, contributing to both diagnostic capabilities and patient outcomes (Figure 8.4).

8.2.1. Commonly Used Radiotracers and Their Applications

PET technology has undergone significant advancements, with the development of numerous radiotracers that enhance diagnostic capabilities. The most common tracer is [^18F]-fluorodeoxyglucose (FDG), and its advantage is that it allows observation of metabolic activity in tissues. The tracer is able to do this by mimicking glucose so that the metabolic functions can be studied in conditions such as cancer, where cell function exceeds the normal level. The scope of FDG applications extends beyond oncology; it is also particularly important in neurological and cardiovascular disease. Studies indicate that measuring glucose uptake with FDG can reveal areas of increased metabolic activity, which is a highly valuable biomarker for distinguishing between malignant and benign lesions (Collins et al., 2018). Over the last few years, new tracer molecules have been synthesized, greatly expanding the range of PET imaging modalities. Among these, PSMA tracers have been noted for their potential to image prostate cancer, provide information regarding tumor burden, and be applied in treatment planning. Tracers that target amyloid have also revolutionized the diagnosis of Alzheimer's disease by enabling the visualization of amyloid plaques in the brain. The increasing diversity of radiotracers gives rise to the demand for novel approaches to manufacturing and validating them. The latest advancements in automated radio synthesizers have made the synthesis process more efficient, thereby improving the production of multiple tracers without compromising quality (Collins et al., 2018). Not only does this address increasing demands for various imaging agents, but it also facilitates timely delivery for clinical use. The indication for PET imaging is not limited to classical oncological applications; it now extends to neurodegenerative conditions and other complex diseases. For instance, in amyotrophic lateral sclerosis (ALS), PET can measure cerebral blood flow and metabolism to provide critical information about disease evolution. Such uses emphasize the importance of selecting a radiotracer based on clinical needs and the pathology being studied. With the inclusion of various radiotracers within the clinic, physicians can better understand disease dynamics and plan therapy accordingly. With evolving PET imaging, clinicians and scientists must understand the use and impact of widely accepted radiotracers to advance the field (Figure 8.5).

PET Radiotracer	Physical Half-Life ($t_{1/2}$)/Minutes	Physiological Process or Function	Clinical Application	Production Method
[^{13}N]Ammonia	9.8	Blood perfusion	Myocardial perfusion	Cyclotron
[^{15}O]Water	2.1	Blood perfusion	Brain activation studies	Cyclotron
2-Deoxy-2-[^{18}F]fluoro-*D*-glucose (FDG)	109.8	Glucose metabolism	Oncology, Cardiology, Neuropsychiatry	Cyclotron
[^{11}C]Raclopride	20.3	D_2 receptor agonist	Movement disorders	Cyclotron
[^{11}C]Methionine	20.3	Protein synthesis	Oncology	Cyclotron
[^{11}C]Flumazenil	20.3	Benzodiazepine receptor antagonist	Epilepsy	Cyclotron
[^{15}O]Carbon dioxide	2.1	Blood perfusion	Brain activation studies	Cyclotron
[^{18}F]Fluoromizonidazole	109.8	Hypoxia	Oncology-response to radiotherapy	Cyclotron

Figure 8.5. Comparison chart of different PET radiotracers and their clinical uses.

Source: Journal of Nuclear Medicine.

8.2.2. Production Methods for Radiotracers

Synthesis of radiotracers for positron emission tomography (PET) involves sophisticated methodologies aimed at both efficiency and quality of the synthetic methods. Traditional approaches typically consisted of discrete, custom-configured radio synthesizers for individual tracers, and consequently, problems arose when clinical situations required the use of diverse tracers. However, recent advances have led to modular radio synthesizers with disposable cassettes and kits, allowing operators to produce a variety of tracers from a single platform. This revolution simplifies the whole process with minimal need for dramatic hardware alteration for individual tracers, optimizing flexibility and productivity in radiopharmaceutical manufacturing (Collins et al., 2018). These innovations represent a significant leap in tracer synthesis, providing greater accessibility to institutions that seek to introduce PET imaging into a variety of research and clinical applications (Figure 8.6).

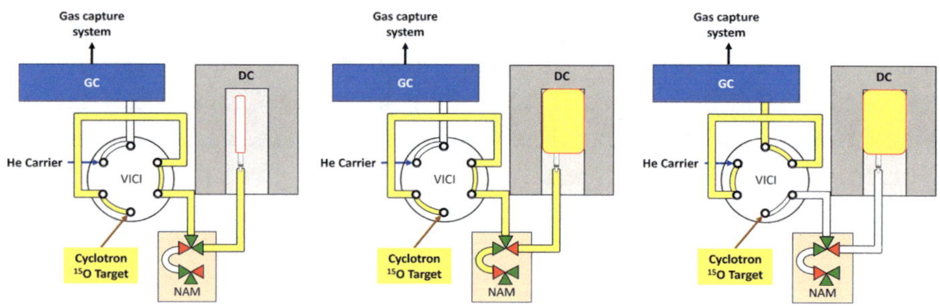

Figure 8.6. Cyclotron facility used for production of PET radiotracers.

Source: https://www.mdpi.com/diagnostics/diagnostics-14-00902/article_deploy/html/images/diagnostics-14-00902-g001.png.

Synthesis automation is another essential innovation that seeks to minimize the burden on hand radiochemistry. The existing protocols indicate that automated synthesis of new PET tracers can be systematically facilitated using a radio-synthesizer such as the ELIXYS, which features user-friendly software and robust radiochemistry. This automation involves translating the complex hand synthesis protocols into straightforward unit operations, which can be programmed with a simple graphical interface. Using a streamlined procedure, operators develop synthesis programs with the assurance of maximum yield and purity, which ultimately yield clinical-grade tracers (Collins et al., 2018). By breaking complex synthesis processes into manageable steps, this automation not only enhances productivity but could also improve the reproducibility and reliability of PET tracers. Moreover, the addition of simplified chemical and biological methods to the synthesis of PET radiotracers reflects a broader transition toward speeding research translation from the academy to the clinic. New modular concepts in synthetic methodology and bioconjugation enable researchers to make better use of available infrastructure. This flexibility addresses the imperative need to increase the pace of development of imaging agents, while minimizing radiosynthesis burden and increasing PET imaging availability to researchers. These new methods are not only crucial to the development of higher-tracer productivity but also hold the potential for new applications, such as gene-expression imaging and macromolecular delivery systems, that could significantly reshape the field of PET imaging across many biomedical fields (Figure 8.7).

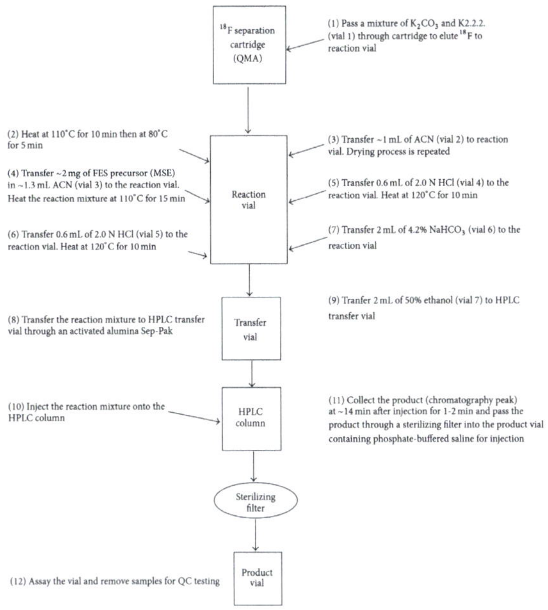

Figure 8.7. Flowchart of radiotracer synthesis process.

Source: https://www.researchgate.net/figure/Schematic-flow-chart-of-the-process-for-radiosynthesis-of-FFES_fig7_237817148.

8.2.3. Safety and Regulatory Considerations for Radiotracers

Safety and regulatory considerations for the use of radiotracers in Positron Emission Tomography (PET) are critical to patient health and effective imaging outcomes. Radiopharmaceuticals such as [^18F]-FDG are subject to strict regulations on manufacturing, quality control, and use in the clinical setting. This is regulated by good manufacturing practices (GMP), which demand comprehensive validation processes for each radiotracer. These regulations help minimize the risks associated with differential pharmacokinetics and biodistribution of radiotracers, as improper handling can lead to excess radiation exposure or diagnostic errors. Moreover, the generation of novel tracers should consider not only their therapeutic efficacy but also safety, which calls for thorough investigation and consensus among parties to harmonize approaches and align with clinical needs, ensuring that clinical uses are both safe and effective (Aloj et al., 2025) (Figure 8.8).

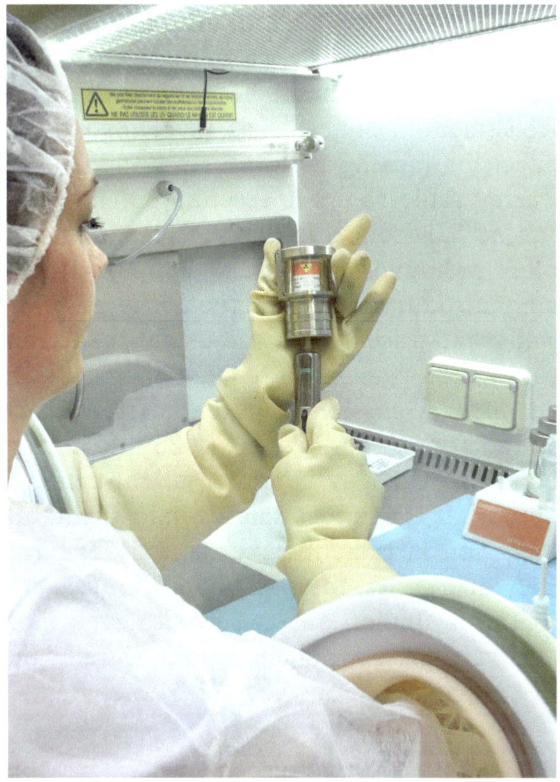

Figure 8.8. Safety protocols in handling radiotracers in a nuclear medicine lab.

Source: https://www.lemerpax.com/web/wp-content/uploads/2024/10/shielded_hotcell_for_manipulating_radioisotopes.jpg.

Recognition of molar activity (Am) in PET radiopharmaceutical production is essential from a regulatory perspective. Am is vital in effective imaging, especially in receptor-targeted studies. Thus, removing contamination with stable isotopes is important, as exemplified by studies showing that fluorinated tubing can inadvertently introduce stable fluorine during the synthesis of [^18F]-fluoride (Sarja et al., 2019). Regulatory frameworks require strong quality control measures that account for all possible sources of contamination, which can affect diagnostic accuracy. Safety assessments must also include comprehensive dosimetry studies to analyze the biological effects of radiotracers, further supporting the need to adhere to set safety standards throughout the lifecycle of the radiopharmaceutical. In the context of PET imaging more broadly, regulatory and safety issues are relevant to the ethical side of patient involvement in clinical trials. Involving patients in decision-making about the risks and benefits of using radiotracers is essential for informed consent, particularly in the emerging landscape of PET radiopharmaceuticals, with new tracers being introduced to the market. Whereas older established tracers have well-established safety profiles, new agents will require closer scrutiny and open discussion of potential side effects and radiation risk (Aloj et al., 2025). Regulatory bodies increasingly support patient-centered approaches that stress safety while facilitating innovation in radiotracer design. By ensuring safety and ethics, the transition from research to clinical applications can be achieved more effectively, thereby enhancing the overall value of PET imaging in oncology and other fields.

8.3. PET Imaging Procedure

The PET imaging process begins with the intravenous injection of a radiopharmaceutical —a molecule labeled with a radioactive isotope that serves as a tracer in the body. The most common radiopharmaceutical is [^18F]-FDG, which targets glucose metabolism and is highly valuable in oncologic imaging. The tracer accumulates in tissues with higher metabolic activity, allowing tumors and other disease states to be visualized through imaging. Following injection, the patient is imaged with a PET scanner, which detects annihilation photons produced when positrons from the radiotracer combine with electrons in the body, creating gamma rays that can be localized to map the tracer's distribution in tissues. The use of newer detector materials, such as Bismuth Germanium Oxide (BGO) and LSO, improves imaging performance by providing greater resolution and sensitivity in detection.

The data has to be reconstructed after scanning to generate useful images from raw detector information. Data can be processed with list-mode or frame-mode acquisition techniques, which affect the form of the data before reconstruction. Analytic and iterative methods, such as filtered back projection and iterative reconstruction, are two of the most popular methods to use for this; iterative reconstruction typically yields better image quality and noise performance. To further improve image accuracy, adjustments for randoms and scatter corrections are needed. These adjustments compensate for potential interference in the imaging data caused by photons that do not result from the targeted positron annihilations, providing a more precise reflection of the inherent physiology. Quantitative PET imaging analysis has been enabled by various metrics that allow interpretation of tracer uptake and its relationship to physiological status. Among the most frequently employed parameters is the Standardized Uptake Value (SUV), which provides a normalized measure of radioactivity in an area of interest relative to the dose injected and the patient's body weight. This parameter is essential for discriminating between benign and malignant lesions and for measuring treatment response. Kinetic modeling is also used to estimate more advanced tracer-kinetic parameters and assess metabolic rates in tissues. Techniques such as partial-volume correction are also essential to account for the limited resolution of PET imaging, which can lead to underestimation of uptake in small lesions. The use of these quantitative methods in the PET imaging process helps clinicians make informed decisions regarding patient management and treatment protocols, as substantiated by studies using PET imaging in the evaluation of the therapeutic efficacy and disease course of malignancies (Adenilson et al., 2008; Dehdashti et al., 2017) (Figure 8.9).

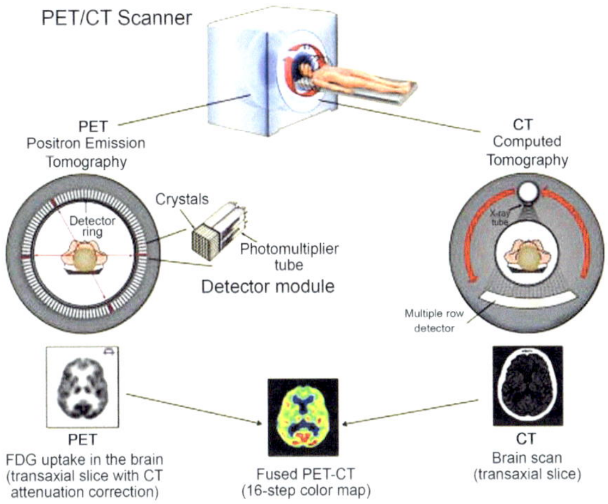

Figure 8.9. PET/CT scanner showing combined functional and anatomical imaging.

Source: Siemens Healthineers.

8.3.1. Patient Preparation for a PET Scan

Preparation for a positron emission tomography (PET) scan involves following protocols to ensure optimal image quality and patient safety. First and foremost, patients must fast for at least six hours before the procedure. Fasting reduces interference from food and glucose metabolism and can improve visualization of radiopharmaceutical uptake. Furthermore, patients should disclose any medications they are on, especially those that affect glucose metabolism or act as sedatives, as these can affect the outcome of the scans. In addition, individuals with diabetes need to consult with their physician about adjusting their insulin and diet prior to the scan to obtain accurate imaging results. These steps enhance the quality and interpretability of the PET scan, enabling precise diagnosis when needed in modern clinical practice (Deandreis et al., 2016). Psychological preparation for the process is also important, as anxiety has the potential to affect physiological status and could distort the result. Relief exercises, such as imagery or deep breathing, are advised for the patients for at least a couple of hours before the test. Informing patients about the procedure steps and what sensations they will experience can also alleviate fear and anxiety, making the process easier.

Health care providers must establish a permissive communication climate in which patients can express their concerns and fears about the PET scanning process. By resolving these affective issues, health care providers can foster a positive attitude among patients, thereby enhancing cooperation during imaging. Subsequently, such preparation is core not only for comfort and safety but also for the production of high-quality imaging information vital for proper clinical assessment (Bird et al., 2025). On reaching the imaging center, patients will undergo a brief registration process and then be escorted to the PET scanning room. To start, a radiopharmaceutical, typically [^18F]-FDG, will be administered intravenously. Following the injection, patients need to remain still for approximately 30 to 60 minutes to allow sufficient absorption of the radiotracer into the tissues. During this waiting period, it is critical for patients to restrict movement to ensure maximum accumulation of the radiotracer, which will provide better images during scanning. Also, it is preferable that patients are not spoken to or engaged in stimulating activities, as these can alter metabolic rates and thus impact the quality of the scan. Hence, this overall preparation encompasses dietary and emotional considerations, all of which are important for achieving accurate and reliable PET imaging results (Deandreis et al., 2016).

8.3.2. Step-by-Step Procedure of a PET Scan

Positron emission tomography (PET) scanning is an exact imaging exam that begins with intravenous administration of a radiopharmaceutical, most often [^18F]-fluorodeoxyglucose ([^18F]-FDG). The radiotracer is administered intravenously to allow it to distribute throughout the body. [^18F]-FDG is taken up very intensely in metabolically active tissues, such as tumors, because they metabolize more glucose than normal tissues. Subsequent to injection, the patients typically wait from 30 minutes to 90 minutes to allow the radiotracer to accumulate in the target tissue for optimal imaging results. The waiting period provides time for distinguishing cancer cells from normal cells based on their metabolism, as cancer cells have a greater affinity for glucose, resulting in improved visual demarcation on the scan. Thus, the initial stages of the PET process set the required basis for later imaging accuracy and diagnostic effectiveness (N/A, 2022). Once the uptake period is complete, patients are positioned in the PET scanner, a device that measures gamma rays emitted by the radioactive tracer. The scanner employs multiple detector rings around the patient to achieve full-body coverage and obtain three-dimensional images. The patient will need to remain stationary while scanning, typically between 20 and 40 minutes, to prevent motion artifacts in the photos that can impair their quality.

In doing this, the detectors capture the annihilation photons released when the radiotracer's positrons interact with body electrons, and the gamma rays move in varying directions. These are essential signals used for building accurate tomographic images, reflecting areas of abnormal metabolic activity and identifying suspected pathological conditions (N/A, 2022). Once the data is obtained, the next essential step is image reconstruction. This process can use either list-mode or frame-mode acquisition techniques; both are versatile and advanced tools for sensitive data collection. Advanced reconstruction algorithms, analytic algorithms, and iterative algorithms are utilized to convert raw data into interpretable images. Scatter corrections and random coincidences are also corrected for in order to enhance image precision to make the output an accurate representation of actual physiological states. The result is a high-resolution image that can be quantitatively assessed in measurements such as the Standardized Uptake Value (SUV) and that assists in determining the metabolic behavior of tissues. This painstaking step-by-step procedure culminates in the production of a diagnostic agent of prime importance in oncological diagnosis and management of diseases in general (Czuczejko et al., 2017).

8.3.3. Post-Scan Protocols and Patient Care

After a Positron Emission Tomography (PET) scan, the following post-scan procedures should be implemented to enhance patient safety and the accuracy of the ensuing diagnosis. Patients may be instructed to remain at the facility for several hours after the scan, as radiopharmaceutical administration is likely to cause temporary side effects, such as allergic reactions or discomfort. Moreover, monitoring vital signs may be necessary, particularly in individuals with known sensitivities to injected tracers. Such a measure enables one to promptly identify any unwanted reactions and resolve them, therefore minimizing the risks associated with post-scan interventions. Further, proper communication of what occurs during this phase assists in lowering anxiety, thus transforming the overall experience into a more positive one. Patient care does not end in the immediate aftermath of the PET scan. Instead, it is also responsible for complete follow-up instructions. Health care providers are highly important when explaining any post-scan activity suggestions, including hydration to help eliminate radiopharmaceuticals from the body. The patients also need to be informed of potential symptoms requiring immediate medical attention, including ongoing fatigue or unusual reactions.

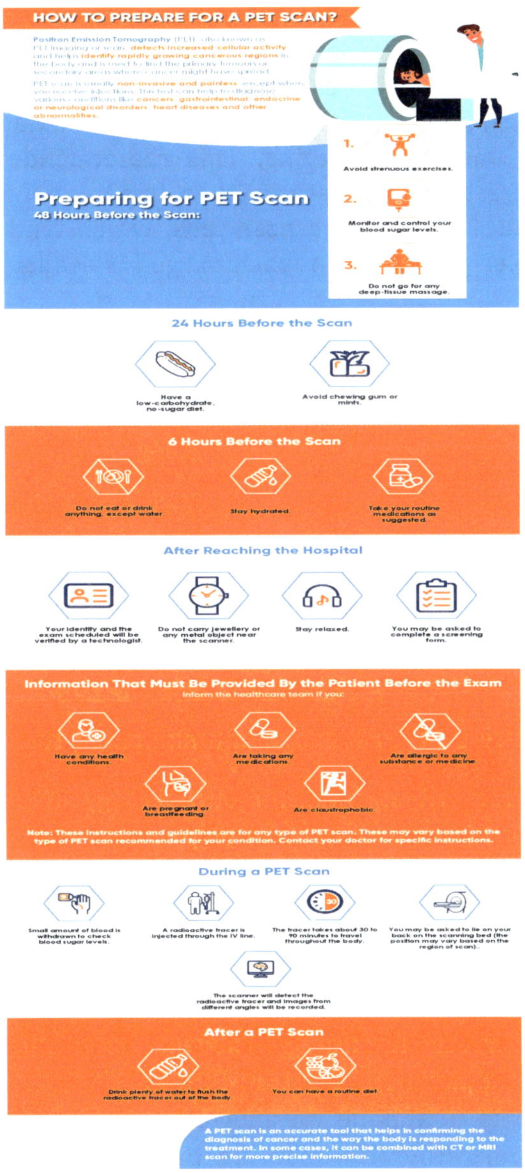

Figure 8.10. Post-scan care instructions for patients following a PET scan.

Source: American Cancer Society.

Well-educated patients are better equipped to manage their own care, leading to improved health outcomes. Empowering patients through education is most important, as this provides a sense of control in their healthcare process, which is best practice in patient-led care. Except for immediate post-scan care, systematic interpretation of PET scan results is needed in the long term to manage patients. Radiologists and medical practitioners should use standardized uptake values (SUVs) to facilitate objective assessment and comparison across multiple patient scans (Wilson et al., 2011). The numerical value permits differentiation between malignant and benign tissue, enhancing the reliability of diagnosis and further decision-making regarding treatment. The blending of newer imaging technologies, such as hybrid PET/CT and PET/MRI, also allows for a more informed assessment of complex clinical cases. These advances underscore the imperative of continuous professional development for health workers to keep pace with evolving protocols, thereby maximizing patient outcomes through more accurate diagnoses and tailored treatment modalities (Figure 8.10).

8.4. Applications of PET in Medicine

The clinical uses of Positron Emission Tomography (PET) are diverse and vital, particularly in cancer. Staging and cancer detection are one of the most important applications of PET. The radiopharmaceutical [^18F]-FDG, a glucose analog, is commonly used due to its ability to selectively accumulate in metabolically active neoplastic cells, thereby highlighting primary tumors and metastases with extremely high sensitivity. Studies have indicated that [^18F]-FDG PET has higher sensitivity for detecting oral neoplasms' margin delineations, particularly in the highly vascular areas such as the lingual and laryngeal regions. Furthermore, the technique shows high sensitivity for detecting lymph node metastasis, but variability in specificity has been noted in some studies. Thus, PET integration into oncological assessment will significantly enhance patient treatment and prognosis (Culp et al., 2019). Apart from oncology, PET also has a pivotal role in assessing inflammatory illnesses and other conditions. Not only is the tracer [^18F]-FDG superior in oncology, but it has also proven effective in the diagnosis of inflammatory illnesses, such as periodontitis and dental implant infections, proving the tracer's use beyond tumor imaging. Additionally, the second tracer, [^18F]-NaF, is highly useful for the evaluation of bone disorders, including metastatic disease and temporomandibular joint disorders.

Experiments in humans have indicated a satisfactory correlation between [^18F]-NaF scans and clinical symptomatology, citing the tracer's ability to quantify the effects of treatment. The increasing use of PET across various medical fields, including inflammation assessment and pain therapy, underscores its growing importance in modern medicine (Culp et al., 2019). Another major development in PET applications is the integration of hybrid PET/CT and PET/MRI modalities. Hybrid imaging modalities combine metabolic information from PET with anatomical data from CT or MRI, resulting in enhanced diagnostic accuracy and a streamlined clinical workflow. The fusion enables accurate attenuation correction using attenuation mapping and multimodality registration of anatomical and functional data. Aside from that, the advances have also led to an optimized clinical workflow, which facilitates quicker and more effective diagnosis and treatment planning. As hospitals and clinics increasingly adopt hybrid imaging technologies, the impact of PET on personalized medicine will become increasingly profound, ultimately leading to better patient outcomes and more efficient resource utilization within healthcare environments.

8.4.1. Role of PET in Oncology

The use of positron emission tomography (PET) in cancer is closely linked to the use of radiopharmaceuticals, in particular [^18F]-FDG, which has established itself as a gold standard for oncologic imaging. This radionuclide is characteristically attracted to hypermetabolic tissues, primarily cancer cells, which tend to prefer glucose even when oxygen is available.

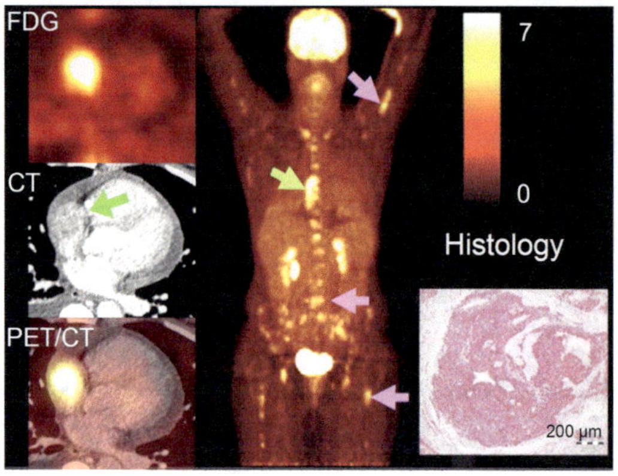

Figure 8.11. PET image of a malignant tumor.

Source: https://jnm.snmjournals.org/content/jnumed/53/6/856/F5.large.jpg.

This metabolic reprogramming enables PET to effectively define tumor boundaries and assess tumor viability, thereby qualifying it as a pivotal resource in oncology diagnostics and treatment strategy. The complex synthesis and application of [^18F]-FDG in PET imaging aim to illuminate the metabolic landscape of tumors, thereby enabling better diagnostic accuracy and patient management strategies, as demonstrated in most clinical applications (Rosa et al., 2015). Understanding the biochemical actions of these radiotracers enables clinicians to maximize PET's potential for cancer diagnosis and therapy monitoring. Advances in hybrid imaging technologies, such as PET/CT and PET/MRI, have further consolidated PET's place in oncology (Figure 8.11).

By integrating PET functional imaging with anatomical precision from computed tomography (CT) or magnetic resonance imaging (MRI), clinicians can overcome the limitations of conventional imaging modalities. Multimodality brings better tumor localization, staging, and assessment of therapy response, providing comprehensive information that supports individualized medicine in oncology. In addition, multimodality registration and attenuation correction procedures improve overall image quality, enabling more accurate clinical interpretations in clinical workflows (Rosa et al., 2015).

Consequently, the incorporation of advanced technologies into oncology practice underscores the added significance of PET in enabling optimal patient outcomes through customized therapeutic interventions. With the evolving situation in oncology in mind, the quantitative potential of PET imaging cannot be overstressed. Parameters such as the standardized uptake value (SUV) and kinetic modeling promote a more advanced strategy to tumor characterization and assessment of treatment response.

The SUV provides a quantifiable metric for assessing tumor metabolic activity, useful for treatment planning and prognostication. Furthermore, with the development of partial-volume correction techniques, PET image quality has been significantly enhanced, leading to improved discrimination between benign and malignant lesions. While oncologists strive to navigate the complexities of cancer treatment, the sophisticated imaging capabilities of PET establish its pivotal role in advancing the field, enabling optimal interventions tailored to each patient's unique malignancy profile (Czuczejko et al., 2017).

8.4.2. Use of PET in Neurology

The application of Positron Emission Tomography (PET) in neurology has radically improved the examination and treatment of many neurological disorders. By facilitating visualization of cerebral metabolic processes, PET is a vital adjunct to the diagnosis and monitoring of diseases like Alzheimer's disease, epilepsy, and brain tumors. The most commonly used radiopharmaceutical in this area is [^18F]-FDG, which labels areas of altered glucose utilization, enabling neurologists to measure functional changes in the brain associated with neurodegenerative disease. The dynamic nature of PET scanning, which indicates alterations in physiology rather than structure alone, provides a unique perspective on the course of disease and response to therapy, making it irreplaceable in the clinical environment (Mishra A, 2024). Furthermore, combining PET with anatomic imaging modalities such as CT and MRI further enhances its diagnostic utility. Hybrid imaging approaches such as PET/CT and PET/MRI provide complementary information to the respective sensitivities of PET, PET, and high-resolution anatomy from CT or MRI. This complementarity leads to a more detailed assessment of brain lesions, enabling improved discrimination among tumor types and better treatment planning. At the research level, improvements in PET technology, such as the addition of Time-of-Flight (ToF) capability, further improve image resolution and reduce scan times, rendering the process more comfortable and efficient for patients (Rosa et al., 2015). All such improvements serve further to increase the general utility of PET in clinical neurology, securing it as a foundation stone in modern-day diagnosis (Figure 8.12).

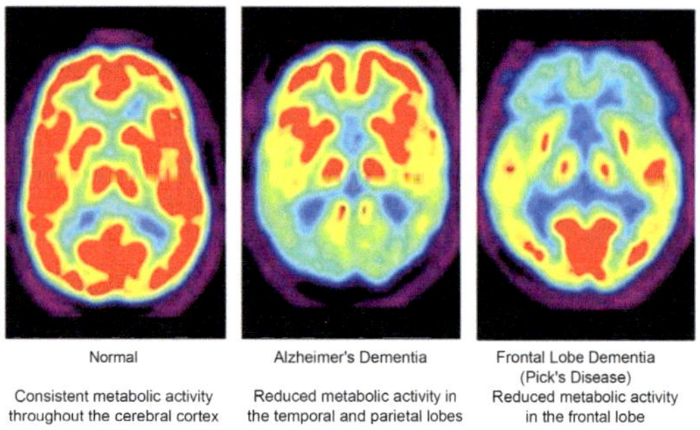

Figure 8.12. PET brain scan in neurology.

Source: https://akumin.com/wp-content/uploads/Brain-Scan.jpeg.

The continued development of new tracers targeting individual neurobiological processes is further expanding the role of PET in neurology. As an illustration, amyloid plaque-bound tracers provide essential information about the pathology of Alzheimer's disease, which facilitates early diagnosis and therapy. Similarly, neurotransmitter system-targeting radiopharmaceuticals show great potential in the exploration of psychiatric disorders and their neurochemical substrate. With additional uses outlined by research, PET is poised to make a significant impact not only in diagnostics but also in the development of personalized therapy techniques. The synergistic benefits of newer imaging techniques and innovative tracers highlight the revolutionary potential of PET for the comprehension and treatment of neurological diseases (Mishra, 2024).

8.4.3. Uses in Cardiology

In cardiology, PET has been a breakthrough imaging modality, enabling the assessment of a wide array of cardiovascular diseases. PET is more effective than other imaging techniques in evaluating myocardial perfusion and metabolism, allowing physicians to determine the viability of cardiac tissues, particularly in patients with coronary artery disease. Using radiopharmaceuticals such as [^18F]-FDG, PET allows visualization of glucose metabolism, which is essential for detecting areas of myocardial ischemia or infarction. It has been critiqued that the clinical application of PET extends beyond diagnosis and plays a significant role in treatment planning and patient management in cardiac practice (Lowin et al., 2025). Its ability to provide accurate information about the heart's metabolic status helps guide therapeutic decisions, especially when conventional imaging techniques are inadequate, thereby enhancing overall patient outcomes in cardiology. Going on to expand its applications, PET is also an important tool for evaluating heart failure by assessing cardiac function and determining the disease's etiology. By combining it with other imaging modalities, such as CT, performing integrated assessments enhances diagnostic accuracy. Multimodality imaging exploits attenuation correction and anatomical information from CT and adds the requisite functional imaging from PET. It is beneficial in heart failure when traditional methods do not yield specific results. Furthermore, consensus opinion demands standardized reporting in nuclear cardiology with precise imaging outcome descriptions, thereby improving communication among caregivers and ensuring optimal treatment planning (Agostini et al., 2017). This integration eventually leads to tailored therapies according to the specific needs of individual patients, offering the key to optimal clinical management. In addition to myocardial perfusion and function, PET is vital in the detection and quantification of the progression of coronary artery disease and response to treatment. The use of new tracers and kinetic modeling enhances the accuracy of PET imaging for the quantification of coronary blood flow and the assessment of revascularization therapies. With the progression of PET technology, its use in cardiology will also grow, ultimately adopting more advanced techniques such as artificial intelligence for image analysis and interpretation. The literature also identifies the potential of PET for cardiovascular risk stratification, enabling more accurate prediction of adverse events. As clinicians continue to advance the tremendous potential of PET imaging in cardiology, its capacity to provide crucial information on cardiac well-being will certainly inform contemporary cardiac care strategies (Lowin et al., 2025) (Figure 8.13).

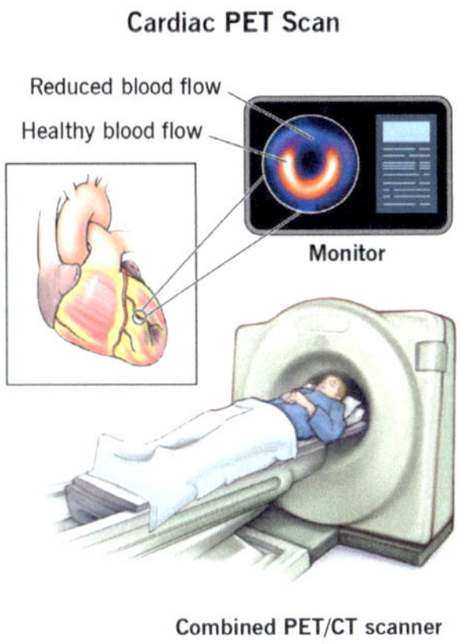

Figure 8.13. Cardiac PET image.

Source: https://my.clevelandclinic.org/-/scassets/images/org/health/articles/17376-cardiac-pet-scan.

8.5. Advantages of PET Imaging

The advantages of Positron Emission Tomography (PET) imaging are tremendous, particularly in clinical diagnostics. A advantage of PET imaging is its ability to provide accurate information on metabolic activity and, hence, to permit diseases to be identified at much earlier stages than traditional imaging techniques. For instance, PET's ability to detect cancer cells with elevated glucose metabolism enables early diagnosis and treatment. Early treatment can significantly improve patient outcomes because it can be administered before the disease progresses. Besides, PET imaging is noninvasive and provides detailed information about physiological processes, thereby being widely used in oncologic and neurological assessments, where early detection enables improved patient management and survival (Rosa et al., 2015). PET imaging also has the advantage of quantification, which is important for monitoring patient response to therapy. The Standardized Uptake Value (SUV), a numeric value on a PET scan, allows doctors to accurately estimate the uptake of radiopharmaceutical agents and, therefore, the metabolic activity of tissues. Quantification is also important for assessing treatment success, as SUV changes indicate whether a treatment is effective or whether other options should be pursued. Furthermore, kinetic modeling in PET imaging enables more precise calculation of tracer kinetics, again enhancing the possibility of creating individualized treatment plans. The inclusion of these quantitative parameters in the clinical process significantly improves the decision-making process as well as encourages personalized medicine (Chatziioannou et al., 2004). Also, the introduction of hybrid imaging modalities such as PET/CT and PET/MRI has extended the clinical utility of PET imaging by combining the functional imaging benefit of PET with the high spatial resolution anatomical detail provided by CT and MRI scans. This multimodality imaging modality not only allows for improved attenuation correction but also more accurate tumor localization. Such integration not only enhances image quality but also optimizes clinical processes, enabling better patient management and more accurate prediction of treatment outcome. Integration of anatomical and functional information provides healthcare practitioners with a comprehensive understanding of the patient's condition, maximizing diagnostic efficiency and therapeutic decision-making. With ongoing advancements in molecular imaging, the advantages of PET will continue to expand, underscoring its pivotal role in contemporary medicine (Rosa et al., 2015) (Figure 8.14).

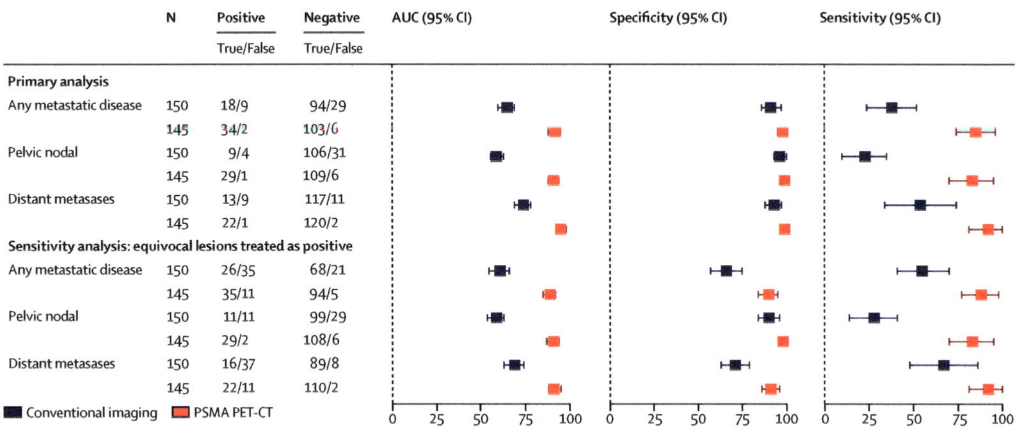

Figure 8.14. Comparing sensitivity and specificity of PET versus other imaging modalities.

Source: https://www.researchgate.net/profile/Michael-Hofman/publication/340093589/figure/fig1/AS:1003358911488000@1616230814710/Accuracy-sensitivity-and-specificity-of-conventional-imaging-compared-with-PSMA-PET-CT.png.

8.5.1. High Sensitivity and Specificity

In medical imaging, the sensitivity and specificity of positron emission tomography (PET) are most important for treatment and diagnosis. Sensitivity refers to a test's capacity to correctly identify the disease in patients, whereas specificity refers to an ability to exclude those without the disease. For instance, in PET/CT assessment for the detection of colorectal lesions, sensitivity was 36%, which increased significantly to 85% for lesions 11 mm or larger, with a clear correlation between lesion size and detectability (Halpern et al., 2018). Such detection of larger tumors with greater accuracy demonstrates the importance of size for the clinical usefulness of PET, particularly in oncology. The implications of these results favor the use of PET as a valuable agent for early cancer diagnosis, thereby enhancing patient prognosis through earlier intervention. The combination of high sensitivity and specificity can be particularly helpful in distinguishing malignant from benign lesions, especially in detecting bladder cancer. Traditional imaging techniques, despite their utility, are insensitive to specific tumor types or grades. For example, cystoscopy is commonly performed as an initial-line diagnostic but cannot effectively detect carcinoma *in situ* (CIS) or differentiate benign and malignant masses (Halpern et al., 2018). In such scenarios, PET/CT emerges as a valuable adjunct for the precise evaluation of suspicious lesions missed by other modalities. Furthermore, PET/MRI has been shown to better distinguish normal from disease tissue than PET/CT, potentially enhancing diagnostic accuracy and specificity in bladder cancer evaluation. Therefore, the integration of these advanced imaging modalities can have a considerable effect on the patient management strategies for patients diagnosed with bladder cancer. While PET imaging is not without its drawbacks, it does possess several advantages. The vulnerability to false-negative findings, particularly for small lesions, highlights the importance of proper interpretation of PET findings. In the case of colorectal cancer, lesions below a diameter of 10 mm are typically at high risk of being false-negative, highlighting a problem with sensitivity (Katagiri et al., 2011). Hence, while high specificity implies that PET correctly excludes non-diseased subjects, published sensitivity should be carefully considered when

PET is being used for screening. As researchers continue to develop new tracers and imaging methods, efforts are underway to improve PET sensitivity and thereby enhance its value across a range of clinical applications. Ultimately, further development of PET technology is expected to address these limitations, with the hope that high sensitivity and specificity will be available to increase detection rates at each stage and type of cancer (Figure 8.15).

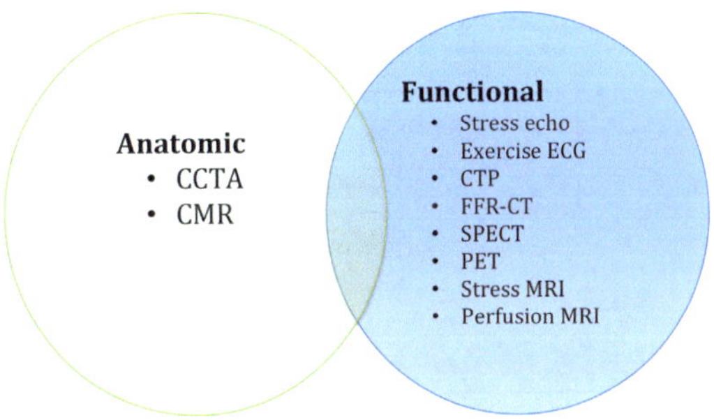

Figure 8.15. Visual representation of functional versus anatomical imaging differences.

Source: https://www.researchgate.net/publication/316080874/figure/fig5/AS:668320839761929@1536351513620/Cardiac-studies-divided-by-anatomical-and-functional-imaging-Color-version-of-figure-is.png.

8.5.2. Non-Invasive Nature of the Procedure

The non-invasive technique of Positron Emission Tomography (PET) virtually optimizes its value as a diagnostic tool in modern medicine. In contrast to other image-based modalities that may be invasive via surgical interventions or the application of ionizing radiation, PET relies on the detection of gamma rays emitted by positron annihilation reactions and thereby enables precise visualization of metabolic processes within the body. This technological superiority is responsible for the early diagnosis of diseases, especially in oncology, where early intervention has a significant influence on the recovery of patients. PET has been shown to play an essential role in cancer treatment by providing an *in vivo* quantitative assessment of physiological and biological processes (Marinis D et al., 2008). This unintrusive method not only reduces patient discomfort but also limits the risk of complications from invasive procedures, making PET increasingly popular as a diagnostic imaging tool. The fact that PET is unintrusive further enhances patient compliance and access, considerations that are important to healthcare professionals when planning diagnostic procedures. The process is typically performed by intravenous administration of a radiotracer, which mimics biological functions within the body and is therefore practical and comfortable for the patient. Following injection of patients must undergo the imaging session in a specially modified scanner that produces high-resolution images based on the tracer's distribution. This cost-effective process, without the need for anesthesia or lengthy recovery, expands the patient population eligible for diagnostic imaging.

This standard of acceptability further demonstrates the non-invasive nature of PET, which improves clinical workflow in healthcare centers and underscores its significance in facilitating health diagnostics. Furthermore, the application of PET in investigating non-obstructive coronary artery disease is a demonstration of the advancements in non-invasive imaging technologies. By using PET as a channel for assessing coronary microvascular dysfunction, cardiac health can be better assessed with greater accuracy, without the risks of invasive coronary angiography. Present studies are investigating the therapeutic potential of drugs, such as ticagrelor, on coronary flow reserve using PET imaging, thereby opening the way for new treatments tailored to this condition (Puvalowski et al., 2019). This new approach emphasizes the importance of PET not only for diagnosis but also for monitoring treatment efficacy over time in a non-invasive manner. These applications demonstrate greater adoption of PET as an essential component of the continuum of care, with a focus on diagnostic capability rather than patient comfort and safety (Figure 8.16).

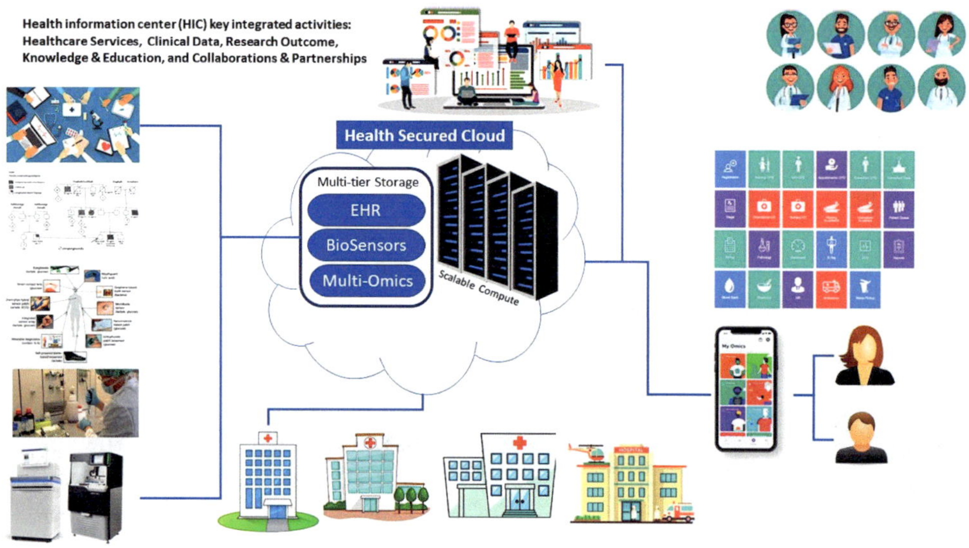

Figure 8.16. Non-invasive procedure of PET serves to improve clinical workflow in various healthcare settings.

Source: https://pub.mdpi-res.com/processes/processes-11-00939/article_deploy/html/images/processes-11-00939-ag.png?1679387548.

8.5.3. Ability to Provide Functional Information

In medical imaging, the ability to provide functional information with Positron Emission Tomography (PET) is crucial for both diagnostic and therapeutic use. PET imaging captures the biochemical function of the body by detecting annihilation photons from positron-electron collisions. PEt spatial and temporal resolution allow for a detailed representation of metabolic function, making it incredibly beneficial in oncology, cardiology, and neurology. For example, using the radiopharmaceutical [^18F]-FDG, physicians can visualize glucose metabolism and obtain information on tumor viability and brain function. By combining quantitative ability with imaging, a non-invasive means for assessment of disease progression and response to treatment is achieved, and in so doing, underscores PET's fundamental role in modern medical diagnostics and its promise in overcoming functional versus anatomical imaging incompatibilities. PET scanner technology has advanced significantly, enhancing its ability to provide functional information accurately. Substances such as Bismuth Germanate (BGO) and Lutetium Oxyorthosilicate (LSO) play a significant role in detecting photons and energy resolution. Moreover, recent developments, such as Time-of-Flight (TOF) capability, improve the accuracy of positron emission localization, significantly enhancing the functional images produced. Besides, the scintillator materials and photomultiplier tubes (PMTs) are combined to allow the system to have maximum sensitivity as well as temporal response. Maximization of these systems renders PET not only a diagnostic tool but also a technology with the potential to deliver fine-grained information about functional abnormalities in biological systems, reflecting its inevitable role in personalized medicine. Quantitative aspects of PET imaging quite remarkably enhance its potential to provide functional data, particularly in the area of kinetic modeling and standardized uptake values (SUV). Through methods such as regional tracer uptake analysis, clinicians can derive meaningful quantitative measures that delineate disease burden. Methods such as partial-volume correction are necessary to enhance the precision of such measures, especially in small anatomical regions. In addition, refinement of correction algorithms for scatter and random events renders images clearer and quantitative data more accurate. The ability to integrate functional imaging data with clinical parameters enables predictive modeling that guides treatment planning. Ongoing refinement of these quantitative methods makes PET the premier functional imaging modality, poised to provide valuable insights in research and clinical settings.

8.6. PET Challenges and Limitations

The constraints and challenges facing Positron Emission Tomography (PET) are multifactorial and can compromise its diagnostic sensitivity and clinical utility. One of the biggest challenges is the intrinsic difficulty of accurately quantifying radiotracer uptake due to physiological factors, such as increased background activity from normal tissues. This effect is most pronounced in heterogeneously diseased conditions, such as non-small cell lung cancer (NSCLC), where tumor characteristics can have a significant influence on imaging results. Besides, as mentioned in current studies, the application of radiomics attempts to extract substantial amounts of data from medical imaging, but at the same time also introduces data complexity in terms of management and analysis, as clinicians will need to rely on advanced computational methods to interpret meaningfully (Benedict et al., 2018). The subtleties of tissue differentiation require high-resolution imaging modalities that PET alone may not provide, further complicating patient evaluation and care. Another consideration to be balanced is the cost-effectiveness of PET as a diagnostic tool. Advanced imaging technologies have the potential to improve patient surgical planning and outcomes, but whether incremental value exists beyond routine diagnosis remains uncertain.

A study noted the lack of randomized controlled trials that unequivocally demonstrate the usefulness of PETs in clinical decision-making and questioned their cost-effectiveness (Chang et al., 2020). At the cost level, the high expense of radiotracer production, maintenance of sophisticated imaging equipment, and retention of expert personnel may limit access, particularly in institutions plagued by shortages. It is thus essential that a cost-benefit analysis is carried out to ensure that the use of PEt is implemented in line with the overall health care objectives of efficiency and patient-centered care. Lastly, merging PET with other imaging modalities, such as CT or MRI, as functional as it is, contributes to the challenges. Hybrid approaches offer the advantage of providing complete anatomical and functional data; however, multimodal imaging can complicate imaging protocols and clinical procedures. To illustrate, variations in image-acquisition settings and reconstruction protocols can lead to inconsistent interpretation, with consequences that may include delayed correct diagnosis (Chang et al., 2020). Thus, training and standardization requirements in multimodality registration are of utmost importance. As PET continues to evolve in the field of medical imaging, these pitfalls should be continually worked to enhance its practical application within clinical settings further and optimize patient care (Figure 8.17).

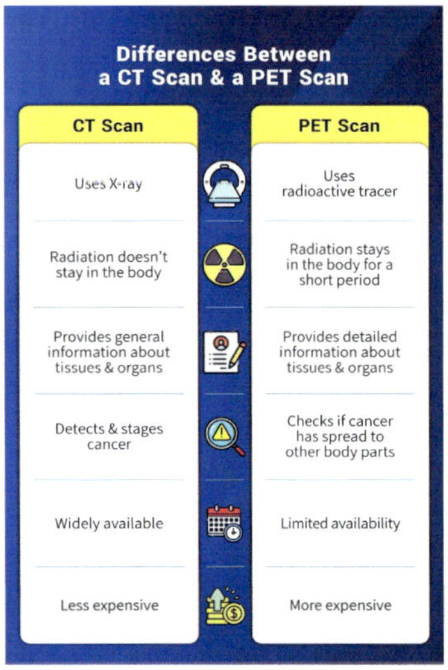

Figure 8.17. Functional vs anatomical imaging.

Source: https://actchealth.com/images/5-ways-a-ct-scan-is-different-from-a-pet-scan/02.webp.

8.6.1. Cost and Accessibility Issues

The advent of Positron Emission Tomography (PET) has immensely enhanced diagnostic capabilities but also raised drastic cost and accessibility issues. The technology is extremely costly in terms of equipment, training, and maintenance, and it can place a drastic financial burden on healthcare facilities, particularly those that are underfunded. This disparity in resources even manifests itself in unequal PET scan access, with patients in more advanced regions having access to the most advanced imaging, while patients in poorer regions receive diagnostic services as a luxury. More expensive PETs, dominated by the complexity of acquiring radiopharmaceuticals and operating sophisticated imaging equipment, even further fuel such imbalances. Having imaging guidelines and policies available to standardize utilization could help buffer costs; however, the initial investment required still deters most healthcare centers from adopting PET technology. One of the most significant contributors to PET technology accessibility is the rising demand for imaging services, often outpacing the growth of available equipment. As evidenced, the ratio of exams to scanners has increased in most countries, reflecting a trend in which the number of patients requiring PET scans has risen without a corresponding increase in diagnostic machines to meet that demand (Gianino et al., 2023). Thus, the efficiency of PET imaging practices is brought into focus, as an overreliance on available machines minimizes wait times and improves patient satisfaction (Figure 8.18).

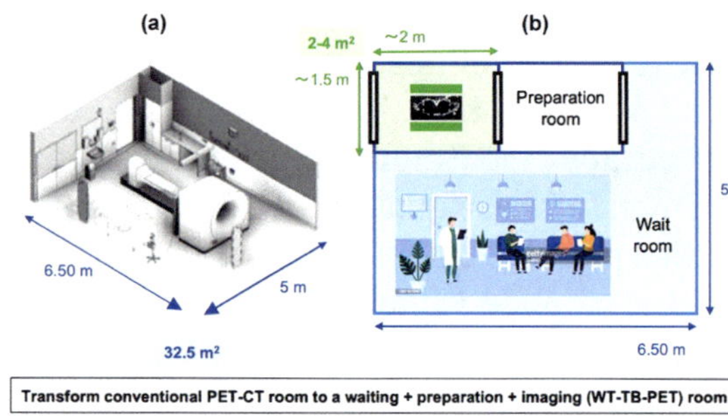

Figure 8.18. PET scanner space.

Source: https://www.researchgate.net/publication/372466539/figure/fig4/AS:11431281195418374@1696384250386/a-Large-installation-space-needed-for-conventional-PET-CT-scanner-b-Compact.png.

In addition, such limitations can cause delays in timely diagnosis, which unduly burden populations dependent on overextended public health systems. Redressing the balance between healthcare demand and affordable operating costs is instrumental in furthering the accessibility of PET technology while providing timely and effective patient care. Further, the development of novel radiopharmaceuticals and imaging modalities holds tremendous promise to make PET scans more effective and efficient, as well as to introduce new cost drivers. As PET imaging progresses, advances in the synthesis of tracers, such as those from prostate-specific membrane antigen (PSMA) ligands, have the potential to improve the precision of diagnostic tests vastly (Yogesh et al., 2023). However, the incorporation of these newer imaging technologies typically requires additional financial and logistical commitments for their production and distribution. The challenge is to balance proper access to these newer technologies so that advances do not become a new source of inequality in the healthcare system. By applying artificial intelligence and other optimization platforms, healthcare systems can potentially rationalize PET use, reduce costs, and facilitate a more equitable system of patient care in advanced imaging.

8.6.2. Limitations in Spatial Resolution

One of the principal spatial resolution constraints in Positron Emission Tomography (PET) is intrinsically a function of the physical properties of the emitted positrons and consequent annihilation photons. Positrons from radioactive tracers meet electrons within the body and annihilate to produce two 511 keV photons. The positron range and energy are significant factors since higher positron energy leads to a correspondingly broader range of annihilation points detected, resulting in lower spatial resolution images. The design of the detector and the intrinsic limiting resolution of scintillator materials also have a role to play in this regard. For example, choices of detector materials like BGO or LSO can significantly impact the localization accuracy and image quality of reconstructed PET scan images. Incorporating future directions of overcoming the limitation in spatial resolution with the addition of current reconstruction algorithms is also available, but these have their own limitations as well. Techniques such as iterative reconstruction, while helpful for improving image resolution, are time-consuming to compute and can introduce artifacts unless properly calibrated. The incorporation of Time-of-Flight (TOF) technology in current PET machines has improved resolution by exploiting the timing differences of the photons that are sensed. However, disparities in spatial resolution among different isotopes, such as Fluorine-18, Gallium-68, and Yttrium-90, reflect the constant pursuit of having similar quality in all applications in the clinic. Ga-68, for instance, has higher spatial resolution than F-18, posing challenges for the precise localization of tumors in imaging (D'Asseler et al., 2019). The limitations of spatial resolution significantly affect PET imaging's diagnostic capabilities, particularly in oncology and neurology. Compromised resolution can lead to inaccuracies in the estimation of standardized uptake values (SUVs), which play a vital role in evaluating treatment response and disease progression. As spatial resolution impacts the estimates of metabolic tumor volume as well as visual image quality, it is of utmost importance to utilize advanced hybrid imaging systems, such as PET/MRI, in order to achieve better attenuation mapping. By incorporating visualization-augmenting technologies alongside selective radiopharmaceutical selection, certain spatial limitations can be avoided, enabling improved clinical outcomes. Regularized iterative reconstruction techniques have been shown to improve image quality and thus become a potential direction for enhancing PET imaging protocols (Behr et al., 2017).

8.6.3. Challenges in Radiotracer Development

The design of new radiotracers for positron emission tomography (PET) imaging poses a series of formidable challenges that must be carefully considered and addressed innovatively. One of the primary challenges is the physics of positron emission and the design of tracers to localize target tissues effectively. As recognized, the intrinsic resolution-noise trade-offs have significant implications on quantitative precision, posing challenges in clinical and research use in oncology, cardiology, and neurology (Kinahan et al., 2015). With growing demand for high-resolution imaging, innovations in the production and synthesis of radiotracers must catch up to ensure reliable performance under the strict safety regulations imposed by clinical use. Thus, the continuous innovation in PET imaging technologies must address these issues to facilitate broader use and implementation of PET in real clinical practice. Compounding such matters is the fast expansion of new PET tracers that span many of the major biological processes. While such breakthroughs offer promising opportunities for improved diagnostic imaging, they also pose logistical hurdles for operational schemes in radio pharmacy. Traditional synthesis of each tracer is performed with specialized apparatus and intricate protocols, thereby wasting time and resources (Collins et al., 2018). Adoption of a model that employs commercial radio synthesizers allows for the effective production of multiple tracers on one system, thus addressing problems of operational efficiency and scalability. However, such a strategy requires expertise to adapt existing protocols for automated systems, ensuring that each tracer produced is of clinical-grade quality rather than compromising either throughput or quality in radiotracer production. Finally, quality control protocols in the development and manufacture of PET radiopharmaceuticals are critical in overcoming intrinsic limitations in this rapidly evolving field. Ensuring that tracers attain the desired purity, yield, and stability is important when releasing them for clinical use. Specifically, the validation procedures that establish the safety and efficacy of each tracer should remain rigorous to ensure patient safety and the effectiveness of treatment (Collins et al., 2018). Furthermore, compatibility with hybrid imaging modalities such as PET/CT and PET/MRI underscores the need to ensure that all radiotracers function flawlessly across multiple imaging platforms. As technology and techniques of PET imaging continue to evolve, continuous improvement in quality control processes will be required to ensure effective, high-performance imaging solutions across multiple clinical specialties, ultimately allowing for improved diagnostic capacity of PET (Figure 8.19).

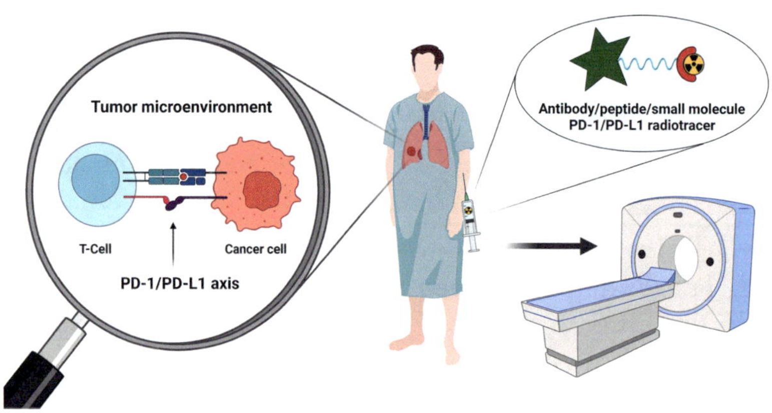

Figure 8.19. Emerging radiotracer molecules under development for advanced PET imaging.

Source: https://pub.mdpi-res.com/pharmaceuticals/pharmaceuticals-15-00747/article_deploy/html/images/pharmaceuticals-15-00747-ag.png?1655704960.

SUMMARY

Briefly, Positron Emission Tomography (PET) is a core nuclear medicine imaging modality owing principally to its promise of measuring metabolic processes in the living organism. A principal aspect of PET imaging is the physics of positron decay, in which positrons annihilate with electrons, yielding detectable photons for image reconstruction. This process utilizes advanced techniques, such as coincidence detection, to enhance precision in spatial localization within the body. Various detector materials like Bismuth Germanate (BGO) and Lutetium Oxyorthosilicate (LSO) are employed and this makes PET scanners effective and efficient. These developments are necessary to provide high-quality imaging because they directly influence the ability to detect subtle physiological changes, thereby enabling proper diagnosis and treatment planning (Eckardt et al., 2003). Equally critical is the acquisition and reconstruction protocol used in PET imaging. Whether one uses list-mode or frame-mode acquisition affects the final data processing and image quality. Central to this process are the analytic and iterative reconstruction techniques, both of which have associated strengths and weaknesses dependent on the clinical application. Additional requirements include scatter and random-event corrections to enable image accuracy optimization. Recent advancements exploit Monte Carlo simulations, which provide a robust framework for optimizing imaging protocols and improving reconstruction precision, particularly under realistic acquisition conditions. These developments do not only increase the reliability of PET imaging but also equip clinicians with improved diagnostic tools to measure disease (Chatziioannou et al., 2004) accurately. Furthermore, quantitative PET imaging, which operates on scales such as the Standardized Uptake Value (SUV), provides profound insight into metabolic activity. This quantification is valuable for interpreting therapeutic response and tumor behavior using kinetic modeling and partial-volume correction techniques. PET radiopharmaceuticals, especially [^18F]-FDG, have become standard in the diagnosis of numerous conditions, such as neurological and cancer illnesses, due to their sensitivity and specificity. Research into novel tracers, such as for PSMA or amyloid plaques, shows the rapid development in imaging technology in these disciplines. The combination of hybrid modalities such as PET/CT and PET/MRI enhances imaging accuracy through more sophisticated attenuation correction and multimodality registration, thereby streamlining clinical workflow and ultimately improving patient outcomes (Eckardt et al., 2003).

CLOSER LOOK

NEXT-GENERATION PET: ENHANCING RESOLUTION, SENSITIVITY, AND PRECISION MEDICINE

Advances in Positron Emission Tomography (PET) technology will revolutionize medical imaging and diagnostics. Much of the future work will focus on enhancing imaging resolution and sensitivity by incorporating new detector materials and sophisticated signal-processing techniques. New scintillator technologies, such as those based on lutetium-containing compounds, promise to deliver greater light output and energy resolution, resulting in higher-quality images. Furthermore, TOF PET technology will be enhanced to improve the detection of annihilation events as well as increase spatial resolution. All of these advances will not only enable earlier diagnoses of a wide range of diseases but also support treatment planning and monitoring and, ultimately, assist personalized medicine strategies in oncology and elsewhere. In addition to its imaging performance, the future of PET modality is in the development of new radiopharmaceuticals that image specific biological pathways. Improvements in imaging agent design, such as radiolabeled compounds targeting prostate-specific membrane antigen (PSMA) and amyloid plaques, are paving the way for more accurate estimates of tumor burden and neurodegenerative disease burden, respectively. These new tracers herald a move towards more individualized patient therapy, enabling targeted interventions for specific physiological and disease states. Accordingly, the simultaneous application of these new radiopharmaceuticals with existing PET technology will offer much-improved detection and monitoring of many diseases, thereby improving clinical outcomes and management strategies. Lastly, the combination of hybrid imaging modalities, such as PET/MRI, will provide new paradigms in imaging diagnosis. The combined benefits of PET and MRI enable comprehensive physiological and anatomical assessment, maximizing disease detection and therapy monitoring. These advancements will enable more robust attenuation mapping and multimodality registration, thereby improving the precise localization of pathologies. In tandem with these developments, future advances in artificial intelligence and machine learning algorithms are poised to optimize image reconstruction and analysis, further solidifying the role of PETs in clinical practice. As has been evident in literature, these technologies, when coupled with effective clinical workflow integration, will continue to transform the practice of medical diagnostics, positioning PET technology as a valuable solution to personalized medicine (Mishra, 2024; Carsrud et al., 2024).

REFERENCES

1. Schelhaas, S., Heinzmann, K., Bollineni, V. R., Kramer, G. M., Liu, Y., Waterton, J. C., Aboagye, E. O., Shields, A. F., Soloviev, D., & Jacobs, A. H. (2016). Preclinical applications of 3'-Deoxy-3'-[18F] fluoro-thymidine in oncology - A systematic review. *Theranostics*, *7*(1), 40–50. https://doi.org/10.7150/thno.16676Agostini, D., Delgado, V., et al. (2017). Reporting nuclear cardiology: A joint position paper by the European Association of Nuclear Medicine (EANM) and the European Association of Cardiovascular Imaging (EACVI). https://core.ac.uk/download/85210963.pdf (accessed on 14th July 2025).
2. Aloj, L., Barnes, A., Blower, P. J., Braun, M., et al. (2025). Translation of PET radiotracers for cancer imaging: Recommendations from the National Cancer Imaging Translational Accelerator (NCITA) consensus meeting. https://core.ac.uk/download/637013116.pdf (accessed on 14th July 2025).
3. Anderson, J. A., & Antich, P. P. (1994). Position sensitive radiation detector. https://core.ac.uk/download/211337499.pdf (accessed on 14th July 2025).
4. Badawi, R. D., Cherry, S. R., Qi, J., Shi, H., et al. (2020). Sub second total-body imaging using ultrasensitive positron emission tomography. https://core.ac.uk/download/305124759.pdf (accessed on 14th July 2025).
5. Ballon, J., Barbier, G., Barnoux, C., Berger, M., et al. (2005). Experimental study of a liquid Xenon PET prototype module. https://core.ac.uk/download/47313556.pdf (accessed on 14th July 2025).
6. Behr, S. C., Flavell, R. R., Hawkins, R. A., Mollard, P., et al. (2017). Effect of time-of-flight and regularized reconstructions on quantitative measurements and qualitative assessments in newly diagnosed prostate cancer with 18F-fluorocholine dual time point PET/MRI. https://core.ac.uk/download/323074353.pdf (accessed on 14th July 2025).
7. Benedict, S., He, Y., Qiu, J., Rong, X., et al. (2018). Radiomics for response and outcome assessment for non-small cell lung cancer. https://core.ac.uk/download/323070464.pdf (accessed on 14th July 2025).
8. Chaminade, T., & Stout, D. (2007). The evolutionary neuroscience of tool making. https://core.ac.uk/download/1671036.pdf (accessed on 14th July 2025).
9. Chang, E. F., Jetté, N., & Kwon, C. S. (2020). Cost-effectiveness of advanced imaging technologies in the presurgical workup of epilepsy. https://core.ac.uk/download/323063036.pdf (accessed on 14th July 2025).
10. Chatziioannou, A. F., Kirov, A. S., Assié, K., Behrens, H., et al. (2004). GATE: A simulation toolkit for PET and SPECT. https://core.ac.uk/download/34921078.pdf (accessed on 14th July 2025).
11. Cistaro, A., Cuccurullo, V., Mansi, L., Pagani, M., et al. (2014). Role of PET and SPECT in the study of amyotrophic lateral sclerosis. https://core.ac.uk/download/pdf/37835281.pdf (accessed on 14th July 2025).
12. Collins, J., Drake, C., Schopf, E., Slavik, R., et al. (2018). Automation of a positron-emission tomography (PET) radiotracer synthesis protocol for clinical production. https://core.ac.uk/download/323076375.pdf (accessed on 14th July 2025).

13. Culp, W. T. N., Spriet, M., & Willcox, J. L. (2019). Role of positron emission tomography in imaging of non-neurologic disorders of the head, neck, and teeth in veterinary medicine. https://core.ac.uk/download/323070037.pdf (accessed on 14th July 2025).

14. Czuczejko, J., Małkowski, B., Piskorska, E., Waśniowski, T., et al. (2017). Synthesis and application of (18F) fluorodeoxyglucose in oncology diagnosis. https://core.ac.uk/download/214942004.pdf (accessed on 14th July 2025).

15. D'Asseler, Y., De Vasconcelos Caribé, P. R. R., Deller, T. W., Koole, M., et al. (2019). NEMA NU 2-2007 performance characteristics of GE Signa integrated PET/MR for different PET isotopes. https://core.ac.uk/download/222452323.pdf (accessed on 14th July 2025).

16. Davis, B. J., Evans, J. D., Jethwa, K. R., Kwon, E. D., et al. (2018). Prostate cancer-specific PET radiotracers: A review on the clinical utility in recurrent disease. https://core.ac.uk/download/334787380.pdf (accessed on 14th July 2025).

17. de Souza da Fonseca, A., Bernardo-Filho, M., Beutel, M. E., Bouchelouche, K., Chaffanjon, P. C., Choe, W., Dennerstein, L., et al. (2008). Nuclear medicine procedures and the evaluation of male sexual organs: A short review. https://core.ac.uk/download/82923336.pdf (accessed on 14th July 2025).

18. Dehdashti, F., Freimark, B. D., Frye, J., Frye, S., Luehmann, H., Sultan, D., Shan, J. S., et al. (2017). First-in-man evaluation of 124I-PGN650: A PET tracer for detecting phosphatidylserine as a biomarker of the solid tumor microenvironment. https://core.ac.uk/download/129070165.pdf (accessed on 14th July 2025).

19. Eckardt, J. (2003). Effects of patient motion on absolute quantification of glucose metabolism in cardiac positron emission tomography (PET). https://miami.uni-muenster.de/Record/0f57b30a-a8bf-45a6-8c48-5510b07c40dd (accessed on 14th July 2025).

20. Gajos, A., Kacprzak, K., Korcyl, G., Krzemien, W., et al. (2020). J-PET framework: Software platform for PET tomography data reconstruction and analysis. https://core.ac.uk/download/344434920.pdf (accessed on 14th July 2025).

21. Gianino, M. M., Lenzi, J., & Martella, M. (2023). Diagnostic technology: Trends of use and availability in a 10-year period (2011–2020) among sixteen OECD countries. https://core.ac.uk/download/590239148.pdf (accessed on 14th July 2025).

22. Halpern, E. J., Kim, S., Salmanoglu, E., Thakur, M. L., et al. (2018). A glance at imaging bladder cancer. https://core.ac.uk/download/227055407.pdf (accessed on 14th July 2025).

23. Hooker, J. M. (2014). Modular strategies for PET imaging agents. https://core.ac.uk/download/28947967.pdf (accessed on 14th July 2025).

24. Jadhav, Y. R., Katkar, A. R., Choudhary, A. L., Misal, S. S., & Patange, A. (2023). Advancements in prostate cancer imaging: Implications for diagnosis and treatment. https://core.ac.uk/download/596247503.pdfijritcc.org (accessed on 14th July 2025).

25. Katagiri, A., Levin, B., Weston, B. R., Johnson, C. D., et al. (2011). Detectability of colorectal neoplasia with fluorine-18-2-fluoro-2-deoxy-D-glucose positron emission tomography and computed tomography (FDG-PET/CT). https://core.ac.uk/download/12551212.pdf (accessed on 14th July 2025).

26. Kinahan, P., & Vaquero López, J. J. (2015). Positron emission tomography: Current challenges and opportunities for technological advances in clinical and preclinical imaging systems. https://core.ac.uk/download/44311157.pdf (accessed on 14th July 2025).

27. La Rosa, F. (2015). Studies on ToF-PET using Cherenkov radiation. https://core.ac.uk/download/31158972.pdf (accessed on 14th July 2025).

28. Lowin, A., Pollicino, C., Fulham, M., Haywood, P., & Viney, R. (2025). Review of positron emission tomography at Royal Prince Alfred Hospital, CHERE Project Report No. 18. https://core.ac.uk/download/pdf/7070877.pdf (accessed on 14th July 2025).

29. N/A (2022). Computed-Tomography (CT) scan. https://core.ac.uk/download/534899146.pdf (accessed on 14th July 2025).

30. Qi, J., & Wang, G. (2013). Direct estimation of kinetic parametric images for dynamic PET. https://core.ac.uk/download/323070765.pdf (accessed on 14th July 2025).

31. Sarja, N. (2019). [18F] Fluoride: Molar activity and utility in radiosynthesis and in biological applications. https://core.ac.uk/download/198018378.pdf (accessed on 14th July 2025).

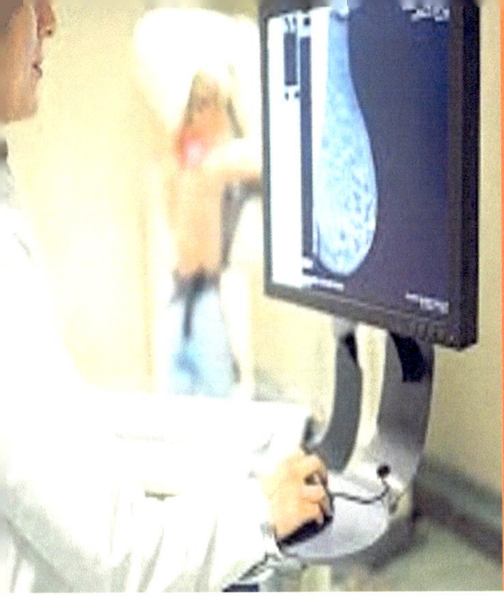

Chapter 9

CONTRAST MEDIA IN IMAGING: TYPES, ADMINISTRATION, AND SAFETY

Contents

Introduction

Contrast media used in contemporary diagnostic imaging play an essential role in rendering the inner structures visible so that they may be evaluated and diagnosed accordingly. Agents can be classified by class into iodinated contrast agents, gadolinium-based contrast agents, and ultrasound contrast agents. All these agents share the role of distinguishing soft tissue and vascular structures across various imaging modalities, including X-ray, MRI, and ultrasound. The evolution of contrast media has been marked by dramatic advances in composition and formulation, with improved safety profiles and patient tolerability. Despite all these advances, administration of contrast agents is complex due to economic considerations, ethical issues, and the need for rigorous patient selection. Radiologists need to balance the efficacy of the agents they employ with their potential risks, thereby achieving optimal diagnostic effectiveness and professionalism/cost-effectiveness (Cartocci et al., 2017). Increased application of contrast media demands thorough knowledge of their types and related safety protocols. Iodinated contrast agents are noted for their anti-allergic action, but they can cause adverse reactions, ranging from mere discomfort to severe anaphylactic reactions. With imaging technology evolving and the profile of patients undergoing these procedures changing, it is important that medical professionals are well aware of these risks. The pharmacovigilance profile of gadolinium-based drugs, with their relaxivity characteristics being non-uniform, also calls for serious evaluation, particularly concerning potential nephrogenic damage from their use in patients with underlying renal ailments. Sophistication supports robust safety measures and enlightened patient management policies across pre- and post-procedure phases (Bose et al., 2019). Information regarding contrast media administration involves not only selecting appropriate agents but also adhering to safety protocols.

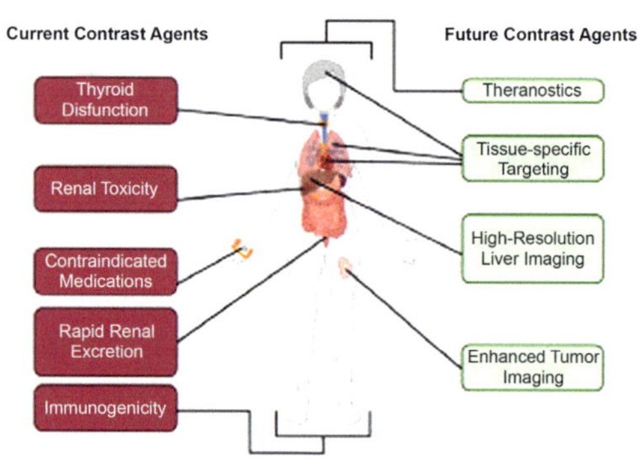

Figure 9.1. Overview of contrast media usage in diagnostic imaging.

Source: https://ars.els-cdn.com/content/image/1-s2.0-S1742706123005664-ga1.jpg.

There should be rigorous patient preparation, monitoring, and follow-up procedures to minimize the incidence of adverse reactions. Additionally, practitioners should be knowledgeable about hydration methods and medication adjustments based on the patient's profile. Learning to handle and respond to complications effectively can significantly improve patient outcomes and enhance the overall safety of imaging studies. Current best practices also emphasize the importance of honest patient communication informing patientsabout potential hazards and the necessity of immediate reporting of any out-of-the-ordinary symptoms. While the diagnostic imaging landscape evolves, the continuous review and improvement of safety guidelines continue to be important (Cartocci et al., 2017) (Figure 9.1).

9.1. Types of Contrast Media

The applications of contrast media in medical imaging are divided mainly based on their composition and the imaging methodologies which they enable. Iodinated contrast media are primarily utilized in fluoroscopy and CT due to their high radiopacity. This class of contrast media includes ionic and non-ionic types, each with subcategories with distinct physicochemical properties and safety profiles. Ionic agents, although conventionally employed, are associated with an increased incidence of side effects because they are more osmotically active. On the other hand, non-ionic preparations are less osmolal, have fewer side effects, and are thus preferred in contemporary imaging practice. These differences must be acknowledged by radiologists and medical practitioners when deciding on a proper contrast agent, particularly in terms of patient needs, including safety and susceptibility to side effects during procedures (Bose et al., 2019). A second general category of contrast media involves agents involving gadolinium, which is most frequently utilized in magnetic resonance imaging (MRI). They can be divided into macrocyclic and linear chelates, with the former having a more stable structure and thus lower risk of gadolinium release in the body. Relaxivity properties, which are required to achieve signal intensity increases in MRI, vary among gadolinium agents and influence their efficacy depending on the application. Also, special care should be taken in evaluating nephrogenic risks since patients with pre-existing renal disease can be at risk of nephrogenic systemic fibrosis, a profound side effect associated with gadolinium use. Thus, careful patient history and evaluation are also necessary in clinical practice for the correct application of gadolinium-containing contrast media for diagnostic imaging applications (Chui et al., 2014). Ultrasound contrast agents, which are usually based on microbubble technology, represent a third class of contrast media that enhance the acoustic properties of ultrasound imaging. Microbubbles consist of gas-filled capsules with a lipid or polymer shell, which are designed to backscatter ultrasound waves and thereby enhance contrast in circulation imaging and organ contours. The ultrasonic imaging setting's mechanical index is crucial to the functionality of microbubble contrast agents, as erroneous settings can lead to bubble destruction and insufficient imaging output. The safety profile of the agents has been carefully evaluated to determine them to be mostly safe for use with very limited minimal adverse reactions, yet there remains a need to acknowledge their potential limitations and patient-specific contraindications for a successful application in practice. With continued technological innovation in ultrasound contrast, their use in optimizing diagnostic accuracy is now more valued (Bose et al., 2019).

9.1.1. Iodine-Based Contrast Agents

Iodine imaging contrast agents, when it comes to medical imaging, have an imperative role of optimizing the quality and accuracy of the diagnostic images. These agents can be classified into two broad categories: ionic and non-ionic. Ionic contrast agents, which are osmolal to a high degree, are reported to have an increased rate of adverse effects in patients. Non-ionic preparations, with reduced osmolality, are reported to possess enhanced tolerance as well as safety profiles. This variation in terms is critical for radiologists to consider when selecting appropriate contrast media for patients with varying susceptibility to potential side effects. Above all, the development of non-ionic agents has greatly reduced the overall risk of complications in imaging procedures, thereby enhancing patient safety without compromising diagnostic effectiveness (Cartocci et al., 2017). In the evaluation of iodine-based contrast media, osmolality is a paramount determinant of their safety and efficacy. Osmolar contrast media are linked with increased risk for untoward effects, particularly in patient populations with pre-existing renal impairment or prior history of allergic reaction (Figure 9.2).

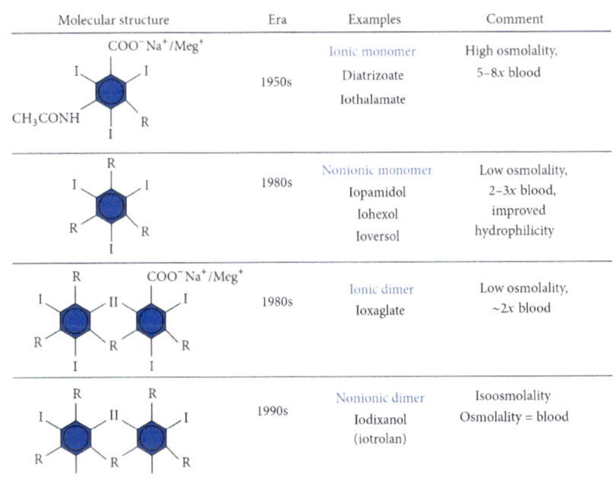

Figure 9.2. Chemical structure of an iodine-based contrast agent.

Source: https://www.researchgate.net/publication/260449277/figure/fig5/AS:1088953247629323@1636638094597/The-structure-of-iodinated-contrast-media-High-osmolality-contrast-media-HOCM-have-an.jpg.

On the other hand, low-osmolar contrast media were well tolerated, with reduced complications and greater patient comfort. Contrast medium selection is thus not only based on imaging characteristics but also on osmolality and its potential impact on patient safety. By employing low-osmolar non-ionic agents, clinicians can obtain the best patient outcomes and minimize the risk of side effects in imaging studies (Bose et al., 2019). Accurate dose calculation is of paramount importance when using iodine-based contrast media to achieve optimal imaging quality and patient safety.

The recommended dose depends on the patient's body weight, the type of imaging to be performed, and the type of contrast agent used. For instance, an appropriate dose must be accurately calibrated for maximum augmentation in vascular tissues or organs, considering the efficacy and, more importantly, the safety profile of the agent of choice. Furthermore, patient-specific factors, such as renal function, must also be considered to avoid nephrotoxicity, a known risk associated with the agents. By effectively balancing these parameters, radiologists can enhance diagnostic image quality while ensuring patients' health (Cartocci et al., 2017).

9.1.2. Barium Sulfate for Gastrointestinal Imaging

In GI imaging, barium sulfate is a critical radiopaque contrast medium that facilitates visualization of the GI tract. Barium sulfate, due to its characteristic X-ray absorption, is particularly well positioned to increase image contrast in fluoroscopy and radiography. Oral or rectal administration of barium sulfate coats the inside of the gastrointestinal tract. This coating effect provides radiologists with crisp delineations of the esophagus, stomach, and intestines, with abnormalities such as tumors, lesions, or structural defects standing out. In a curious twist, the physical state of barium sulfate — powder that forms a suspension upon mixing with water —facilitates easy application across imaging modalities. As a result, barium sulfate remains a mainstay in diagnostic imaging for a wide variety of gastrointestinal conditions. Barium sulfate administration must be carried out within certain guidelines to get the most out of it and minimize risk. The majority of patients drink barium in a liquid form, and the dosage may vary with the specific test being conducted (Figure 9.3).

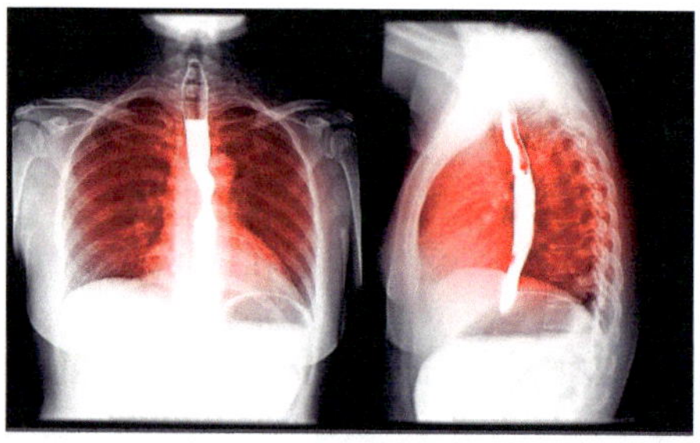

Figure 9.3. Radiograph showing barium sulfate contrast in a barium swallow test.

Source: https://www.carygastro.com/uploads/_1200x720_crop_center-center_100_none/Barium-Swallow.jpg.

For instance, a barium swallow would be of smaller volume than a barium enema. Before administration, health providers have a duty to make thorough evaluations of patients, including making a judgment that contraindications, such as suspected perforation or bowel obstruction, are taken into account. In addition, effective communication about the procedure's expectations can reassure anxious patients. As with all contrast agents, monitoring the patient before and after the procedure is essential to detect any adverse effects or procedural complications associated with barium sulfate injection.

These guidelines optimize the safety and efficacy of gastrointestinal imaging exams. While barium sulfate has advantages, it also poses risks. Complications that occur in the gastrointestinal tract, though not frequent, can occur, including constipation or fecal impaction, particularly in patients with existing bowel abnormalities. Besides, allergic reactions to the compound are uncommon but require readiness and protocols for immediate action. In clinical practice, the safety profile of barium sulfate must be continuously reviewed in accordance with guidelines to prevent adverse events during imaging. Practitioners must recognize the potential side effects and follow-up treatment needed after administration. For patients, awareness of the benefits and risks of barium sulfate can be helpful when preparing them for imaging tests. Both the handling of barium sulfate with care in gastrointestinal imaging and work to emphasize the importance of contrast media safety reinforce its implication in successful clinical diagnostics (Naeem et al., 2021; Catania et al., 2022).

9.1.3. Gadolinium-Based Agents for MRI

In magnetic resonance imaging (MRI), gadolinium-containing contrast agents have played a key role in enhancing image resolution and diagnostic accuracy. Gadolinium is a rare earth element with paramagnetic properties suitable for effective signal enhancement in MRI scans. Such agents are generally chelated to reduce toxicity while maximizing stability. Surprisingly, two disparate classes of gadolinium-containing contrast agents exist: linear and macrocyclic chelates. Macrocyclic agents are also known to have an outstanding safety profile due to greater chelation, thereby reducing the likelihood of gadolinium release into the body (Cartocci et al., 2017).

Given the varying conditions of patients and examination protocols, selecting the appropriate gadolinium-based agent is critical to optimizing diagnostic results without compromising patient safety. The relaxivity properties of these agents are particularly relevant to their effectiveness during MRI procedures. Relaxivity, or the degree to which a contrast medium enhances the magnetic resonance signal, depends on the chemical structure of the gadolinium complex. Macrocyclic agents generally have higher relaxivity because their more rigid and stable molecules are better suited to provide more explicit images of soft tissues. Research has also shown that gadobenate dimeglumine, for instance, has the highest r1 relaxivity among the clinically applied gadolinium-based contrast media, that is, best in breast MRI diagnosis (Kirchin et al., 2015) (Figure 9.4).

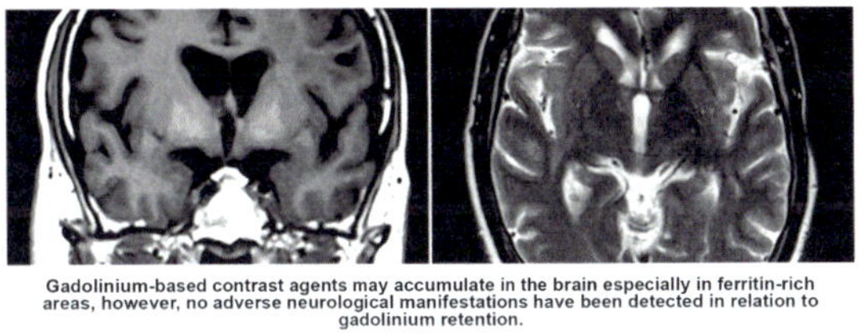

Figure 9.4. MRI scan using gadolinium contrast, highlighting brain enhancement.

Source: https://media.springernature.com/lw685/springer-static/image/art%3A10.1186%2Fs13244-024-01763-z/MediaObjects/13244_2024_1763_Figa_HTML.png?as=webp.

This variable enables radiologists to effectively choose the agent that yields high-quality images for specific exams, thereby enhancing overall diagnostic accuracy and patient care in the clinic. Although gadolinium-based contrast agents offer many benefits, there is a crucial consideration regarding nephrogenic systemic fibrosis (NSF), particularly among patients with compromised renal function. NSF is a severe condition that can occur in patients with renal impairment following gadolinium exposure, causing tissue fibrosis and systemic manifestations. Renal function screening before the administration of gadolinium is thus required to avoid associated risks. The doctors should adhere to the routine pre-procedure protocols, including hydration protocols to enhance renal function and potentially circumvent side effects (Cartocci et al., 2017). Lastly, understanding the balance between the diagnostic advantages of gadolinium-based agents and their risks underscores the importance of proper administration and regular monitoring in imaging protocols to ensure patient safety above all else.

9.2. Mechanisms of Action

When explaining contrast media's mechanism of action, it is essential to reflect on the specific properties that enable these drugs to enhance diagnostic imaging. Iodinated contrast dyes, for example, work essentially by absorbing X-rays. The chemical composition of such dyes enables strong differential attenuation between the tissues surrounding them and the region of interest, thereby increasing contrast and visibility in imaging procedures. Ionic compositions, which are quite effective, are more osmotically active than non-ionic compositions. This osmolality increase can lead to side effects, so non-ionic products are preferred in clinical applications because they offer a safety margin and a lower risk of complications. By reducing side effects and maximizing image quality, the mechanisms of iodinated agents simplify diagnosis, ultimately leading to better patient outcomes. Similarly, gadolinium-based contrast agents contain unique mechanisms that are vital for their use in magnetic resonance imaging (MRI). These agents act through a process known as relaxivity, which enhances the relaxation times of neighboring hydrogen protons in tissues. Relaxivity properties vary significantly between macrocyclic and linear chelates, with macrocyclic compounds typically exhibiting greater stability and fewer opportunities for gadolinium retention. This aspect matters particularly when considering the nephrogenic systemic fibrosis risk for patients with compromised renal function. The mechanisms that govern relaxivity and agent stability are essential for enhancing signal in the body's tissues with minimal potential to provoke side effects, thereby allowing a safer imaging experience among difficult patient populations. Consequently, understanding these processes enables clinicians to select appropriate contrast agents for individual patients' needs. Ultrasound contrast agents primarily consist of microbubbles, and they use distinct mechanisms of action with varying acoustic properties for improved imaging. Microbubbles vibrate when exposed to ultrasound frequencies, producing strong reflections that improve the resolution of ultrasound images. This process is mediated by a range of factors, including mechanical index settings during the procedure, which are used to optimize bubble behavior. Their biocompatibility and relatively low incidence of adverse effects enhance the safety profile of these contrast agents and qualify them as a desirable option for specific diagnostic applications. Though they possess a good but moderately confined history of security problems, due regard should still be given to physiological interactions between microbubbles and body systems to prevent potential complications. By providing greater insight into these mechanisms, clinicians can facilitate their navigation of ultrasound contrast agents to maximize diagnostic effectiveness while ensuring patient well-being.

9.2.1. How Contrast Media Enhance Imaging

In medical imaging, the role of contrast media is crucial to the diagnostic capacity of imaging modalities. Contrast media enhance the visibility of structures that are otherwise undetectable and enable radiologists to make accurate diagnoses. For instance, iodinated contrast agents are applied predominantly in computed tomography (CT) and fluoroscopy, where vascular dynamics, organ anatomy, and pathologies can be delineated by the contrast in attenuation among tissues. Whether an ionic or non-ionic formulation is employed may actually determine the efficacy and safety of imaging interventions, as shown by more recent studies that have reported increased patient tolerance for non-ionic agents (Cartocci et al., 2017) (Figure 9.5).

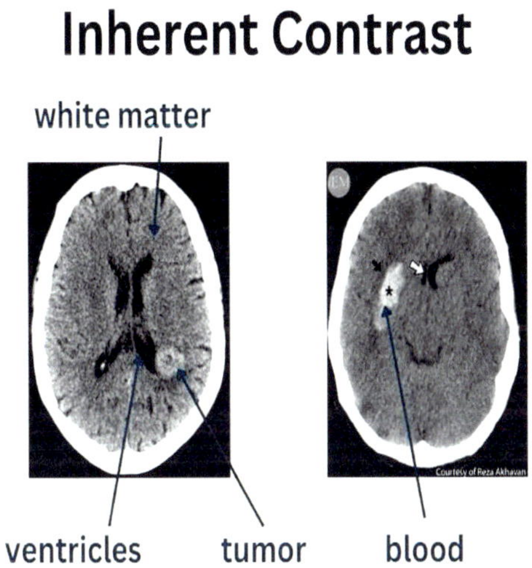

Figure 9.5. Diagram showing how contrast agents enhance tissue visibility.

Source: https://cdn.shortpixel.ai/spai/w_1005+q_lossy+ret_img+to_webp/howradiologyworks.com/wp-content/uploads/2023/12/15.jpg.

Thus, familiarity with the nuances of various contrast media formulations is essential to achieve maximal diagnostic yield while avoiding potential adverse effects. GBCAs are particularly vital in MRI, enabling better visualization of soft tissue and vascular structures. The relative properties of GBCAs, such as their relaxivity, will determine their ability to improve image contrast. Gadobenate dimeglumine, for instance, has been shown to have the highest r1 relaxivity of all available GBCAs and is therefore particularly suited to applications such as breast MRI, where sensitivity to cancer detection is of primary concern (Kirchin et al., 2015). By enhancing discrimination between malignant and benign lesions, gadolinium agents facilitate better clinical decision-making and individualized patient management plans. The selection of the most appropriate GBCA must therefore take into account its specific properties to ensure optimal diagnostic performance. Ultrasound contrast agents, typically composed of microbubbles, offer a new approach to enhancing imaging capability in echocardiography and vascular studies. Unlike traditional imaging technologies, ultrasound contrast agents amplify the ultrasound signal, enabling more definitive visualization of blood flow and tissue perfusion. The procedural mechanical index levels are key to optimizing the performance of these microbubbles and enabling their safe application with improved image quality. Safety profiles have shown lower risks of adverse reactions than those of iodinated or gadolinium agents, making it a promising alternative in certain clinical circumstances. The evolution of ultrasound contrast agents continually holds the potential for enhanced diagnostic accuracy, affirming the pivotal role of such agents in a multidisciplinary imaging approach (Cartocci et al., 2017). The simultaneous application of various classes of contrast media thus not only improves imaging precision but also facilitates clinicians in offering effective patient care.

9.2.2. Interacting with X-rays and Magnetic Fields

The interaction of contrast media with X-rays is key to making anatomical structures visible during imaging procedures. X-rays, being ionizing radiation, interact differently with contrast media depending on the chemical nature and density of the agents. Specifically, iodinated contrast agents have high atomic numbers that effectively absorb X-rays, thereby increasing contrast resolution. This interaction facilitates better visualization of blood vessels and soft tissues, aiding the detection of abnormalities such as tumors or vascular blockages. Further, there is a need for progress in knowledge of dosimetry to optimize the use of these agents, ensuring the minimum effective dose with the maximum diagnostic yield. This precision is necessary to balance the benefits of greater imaging with the risks of radiation exposure and the administration of contrast media. In magnetic resonance imaging (MRI), gadolinium-based contrast media are used to alter tissue magnetic susceptibility, thereby improving image clarity (Figure 9.6).

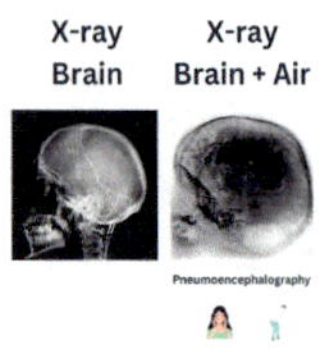

Figure 9.6. X-ray attenuation differences with and without contrast agent.

Source: https://cdn.shortpixel.ai/spai/w_1005+q_lossy+ret_img+to_webp/howradiologyworks.com/wp-content/uploads/2023/12/10.jpg t.

The interaction of the agents with the static magnetic field and radiofrequency pulses in MRI defines the quality of the image formed. For instance, linear gadolinium agents exhibit high uptake and rapid tissue washout, while macrocyclic agents are stable and less nephrotoxic. It is essential to understand the relaxivity properties of these agents, as variations can affect contrast enhancement and diagnostic insight. Besides, the introduction of gadolinium-based nanoparticles has opened promising avenues for therapeutic applications beyond imaging, suggesting a dual-modality approach with the potential to transform patient care through targeted therapy and enhanced imaging outcomes (Bianchi et al., 2015). Coupling nanotechnology with radiotherapy offers new avenues to enhance patient outcomes in radiation oncology. Nanotechnology advancements not only improve the effectiveness of contrast media but also have significant applications in precision medicine, enabling targeted delivery to malignant cells without harming surrounding normal tissues. For instance, work is underway to develop nanoparticles that can serve as radiosensitizers to improve the effectiveness of radiation therapy by amplifying cell damage inside the tumor region with minimal exposure to surrounding normal tissues (Butterworth et al., 2017). Such Imaging-Tx synergy remains at the basis of the growing trend toward personalized medicine, where imaging guided by advanced contrast agents may be able to determine the course of treatment. Such an evolving environment requires rigorous research and interdisciplinary cooperation between academic and clinical practitioners to harness to the maximum extent the therapeutic possibilities contained within these technological developments.

9.2.3. Role in Differentiating Tissues

The function of contrast media in distinguishing tissues is critical in current imaging methods, enormously improving diagnostic specificity and clinical decision-making. Contrast agents, such as iodinated substances and gadolinium-containing agents, increase the visibility of targeted tissues by altering their physical properties during imaging. For instance, the presence of iodine in contrast agents increases X-ray attenuation and thereby demarcates vascular tissues from surrounding tissues, which is critical for identifying abnormalities such as tumors or vascular disease. The agents assist radiologists in discriminating delicate structures in both acute and chronic disease, thereby contributing to timely interventions. Besides, newer technological developments in molecular imaging technologies, which make use of contrast agents for targeting particular cellular functions, provide a depth of understanding of pathological processes, including tumor biology and tissue inflammation, thus further increasing the usefulness of imaging beyond anatomical representation (Bose et al., 2019) (Figure 9.7).

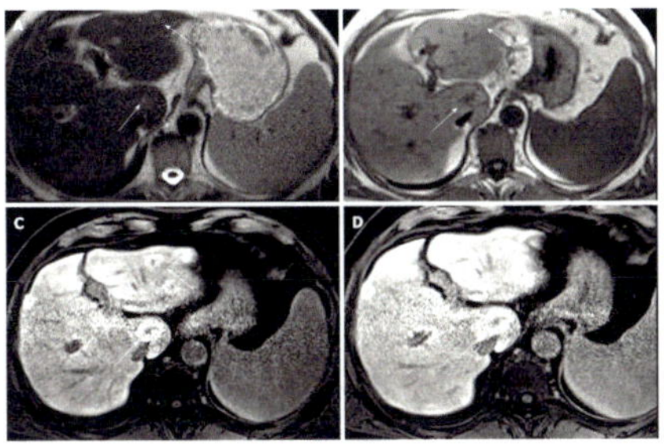

Figure 9.7. MRI signal intensity changes before and after gadolinium injection.

Source: https://www.researchgate.net/publication/51184937/figure/fig1/AS:339645121482752@1457989115137/Magnetic-resonance-images-before-and-after-gadolinium-injection-Half-fourier-acquisition.png.

Ultrasound contrast agents, which predominantly comprise microbubbles, are also helpful for discriminating tissues based on their specific echogenicity. Increased parenchymal-to-blood-flow contrast is achieved when microbubbles are injected intravenously, improving visualization of vascular and perfusion patterns. The uses are particularly beneficial in cardiac imaging and liver lesion analysis, in which discrimination between malignant and benign tissue is paramount. The mechanical index settings, which influence the destruction of microbubbles by ultrasound, also optimally improve imaging performance, enabling dynamic tissue perfusion evaluation. By using ultrasound contrast agents, medical professionals are better able to discern various pathologies more precisely and, thereby, enhance patient management (Janes et al., 2015). Last but not least, the safety profile of contrast agents cannot be overlooked in tissue discrimination. Awareness of potential adverse effects is essential to achieving optimal patient outcomes during imaging procedures. While most contrast media are well tolerated, there is potential nephrotoxicity with certain agents, particularly iodinated agents, in vulnerable populations. Thus, pre- and postprocedural recommendations, such as assessment of renal function and appropriate hydration status, become essential to avoid this risk. Close observation of these parameters not only ensures patient safety but also maximizes the diagnostic potential of imaging studies. The synergy between safety measures and advanced imaging modalities underscores the need for an integrated strategy for the use of contrast media in tissue differentiation and effective medical diagnosis (Bose et al., 2019).

9.3. Administrative Methods

The method of administration of contrast media plays a crucial role in determining the safety and effectiveness of diagnostic imaging protocols. Proven administration depends on several factors, including the contrast agent used and patient-related factors. In the case of iodinated contrast agents, for instance, the physician has to choose between ionic and non-ionic agents, which may significantly influence patient tolerance and success. Non-ionic agents are generally preferred due to their lower osmolality, fewer side effects, and improved patient comfort. In addition to the agent itself, calculating the dose is crucial; toxic doses may lead to complications such as nephrotoxicity. Radiologists must therefore be adept at determining the appropriate dose based on patient weight and specific imaging requirements to balance diagnostic yield and patient safety (Cartocci et al., 2017). Intravenous administration of gadolinium-containing substances requires a fine appreciation of the formulation—that is, between linear and macrocyclic chelates. Macrocyclic agents are used in the clinical environment due to their enhanced stability, reducing the potential for gadolinium dissociation and the resulting mobilization and adverse effects. Relaxivity of the agents also influences image quality; hence, screening involves examining how these properties affect visualization in magnetic resonance imaging. Producers also have to take account of nephrogenic gadolinium-based agent risks, especially in the context of patients with pre-existing renal dysfunction. This involves judicious patient assessment before administration based on guidelines that direct timing and technique of contrast medium delivery (Bose et al., 2019). Ultrasound contrast media, and particularly microbubbles, introduce new methods of administration that differentiate them from other contrast agents. These microbubbles increase echogenicity but require specific mechanical index settings during ultrasound scans to be best visualized in blood pools. Intravenous injection is the standard form of administration, and knowledge of its safety profile is crucial for successful application. For example, although microbubbles generally have a good safety profile, medical professionals need to be cautious about potential adverse effects and prepared to act immediately if required. Also crucial is the establishment of pre- and post-procedure protocols, such as hydration to support renal function and continuous monitoring for side effects, to prevent patient injury and optimize overall diagnostic outcomes (Cartocci et al., 2017).

9.3.1. Intravenous Administration Methods

In the context of contrast media administration, the intravenous (IV) technique of administration is essential in achieving rapid and effective distribution of imaging agents in the body. The IV route of administration is favored primarily because it can ensure immediate action, which is required in emergency imaging situations, such as acute strokes. Intravenous iodinated contrast media, for example, are widely used in computed tomography (CT) to enable vascular visualization and improve diagnostic performance. Intraprocedural intravenous administration of iodinated contrast during procedures such as CT angiography has been postulated to be unlikely to significantly increase the risk of symptomatic intracranial hemorrhage in patients undergoing thrombolytic therapy, suggesting procedural safety of this route (Teasdale et al., 2011). Therefore, education about appropriate IV administration methods and their clinical consequences can increase the overall effectiveness of imaging techniques (Figure 9.8).

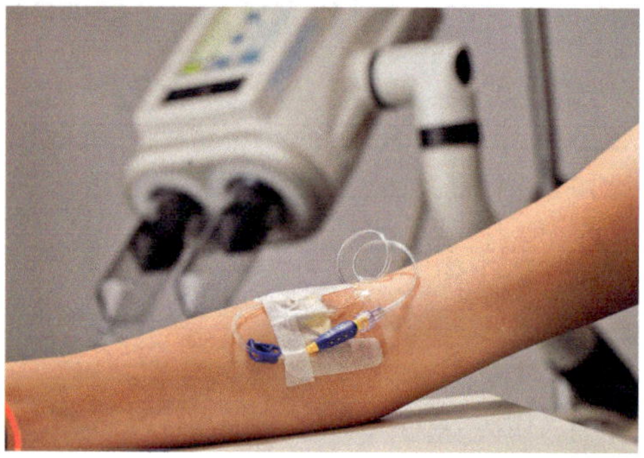

Figure 9.8. Intravenous (IV) setup for contrast media delivery.

Source: https://i.ytimg.com/vi/kJqMhxVpyU0/maxresdefault.jpg.

The safety and efficacy of IV administration methods also depend on the choice of the contrast agent preparation. Two significant iodinated contrast medium preparations are non-ionic and ionic. Non-ionic agents are predominantly used in clinical practice due to their lower osmolality, thereby reducing the risk of adverse effects such as nephrotoxicity and allergic reactions. Moreover, the volume of administration, which is normally between 50 and 150 mL, needs to be carefully calculated to achieve optimal imaging outcomes with a lower risk (Teasdale et al., 2011). Such meticulous deliberation underscores the importance of medical practitioners being well-versed in the unique characteristics of various contrast agents, as formulation type can play a vital role in determining patient outcomes during imaging studies. Also, appropriate pre- and post-procedure procedures are crucial to optimize the safety of intravenous contrast infusion. Appropriate hydration is necessary for all patients receiving iodinated contrast media to minimize renal injury, especially those with pre-existing renal impairment. Moreover, meticulous observation before and after the procedure can help significantly to reduce the incidence of adverse effects. For instance, patients should be observed following mild to moderate reactions and potential acute anaphylactoid effects following intravenous administration of contrast media. Establishing a comprehensive follow-up protocol with patient education on recognizing signs after the procedure can significantly enhance overall safety. As such, adherence to good pre- and post-procedure practices is required for effective patient care during imaging procedures involving intravenous contrast media.

9.3.2. Oral Administration Via the Gastrointestinal Tract

In gastrointestinal research, oral administration of contrast media is a fundamental technique used to enhance image quality and diagnostic accuracy. By ingesting contrast agents prepared to improve visibility of internal structures during imaging tests such as computed tomography (CT) scans and magnetic resonance imaging (MRI), this is accomplished. The principal focus is usually on specific formulations for the gastrointestinal tract that allow improved visualization of anatomical structures. For example, iodinated contrast media have been of interest due to their effectiveness in improving the radiographic visibility of the gastrointestinal system and allowing safe passage through the digestive tract. With these agents, clinicians can obtain better images, enabling more accurate diagnosis and treatment recommendations for patients with various gastrointestinal ailments (Figure 9.9).

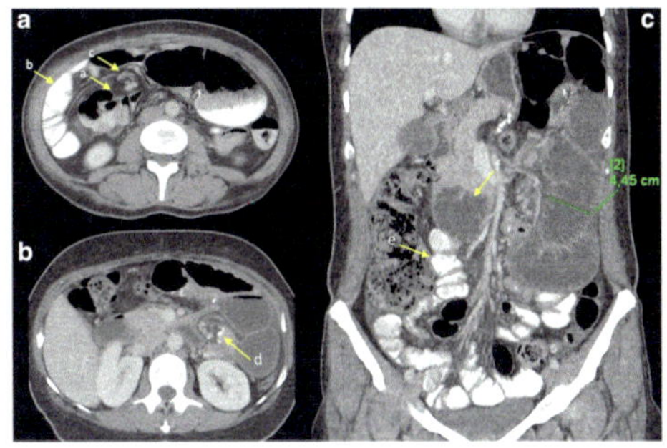

Figure 9.9. Oral administration of contrast medium for abdominal CT.

Source: https://www.researchgate.net/publication/325872892/figure/fig3/AS:962654323621889@1606526084702/A-Axial-abdominal-CT-image-after-oral-contrast-medium-administration-Medialization-of.png.

The safety profile of oral contrast media is of the highest priority, necessitating strict patient evaluation before use. Oral contrast media, particularly non-ionic low-osmolar ones, are well tolerated. However, they do carry a risk of adverse effects to some degree, albeit significantly less than with intravenous administration. Practice and clinical guidelines state that individuals with a history of contrast media reaction should undergo stringent screening to prevent potential risks. In particular, procedures such as premedication have been largely abandoned in favor of oral contrast administration, with the focus on alternative agents when required. The rare incidence of hypersensitivity reactions to oral contrast media, as indicated by clinical data, makes their standard inclusion in imaging protocols alongside safe and effective gastrointestinal studies (van de Ven et al., 2024). Along with safety, the pharmacokinetics of oral contrast media are essential to their efficacy in gastrointestinal imaging. Upon ingestion, the contrast media should pass through the gastrointestinal tract efficiently to achieve optimal visualization. Research studies involving animal models have analyzed the plasma and tissue disposition of different contrast media, which have provided vital information about their pharmacokinetic characteristics (Bascal et al., 2017). Optimal contrast media are needed to achieve a balance between luminal opacification and low systemic absorption. Furthermore, gastrointestinal motility, dosage, and formulation can also play a crucial role in influencing outcomes. The interplay of these will enable imaging specialists to optimize the use of oral contrast agents, consequently optimizing the diagnostic benefit of imaging studies for the assessment of gastrointestinal health and disease.

9.3.3. Intra-Arterial Administration for Specific Procedures

Intra-arterial contrast media injection is a key element in several imaging examinations, particularly angiographic and perfusion imaging studies. The procedure offers more targeted delivery of contrast material directly into blood vessels, facilitating enhanced visualization of vascular structures and disease. The precision of intra-arterial injection can significantly improve diagnostic quality and therapeutic procedures in the acute phase, for example, in cases requiring rapid assessment of stroke or tumor blood supply. The technique does carry inherent risks, for example, potential for thromboembolic events or contrast nephropathy. With selective patient selection and careful use of proven protocols, the benefits of intra-arterial contrast administration often outweigh the risks, provided clinical precautions are followed. The most serious concern in intra-arterial contrast delivery pertains to the risk of acute kidney injury (AKI). Despite advances in imaging techniques, the risk of AKI remains a critical concern that practitioners must avoid when administering iodinated contrast media (Figure 9.10).

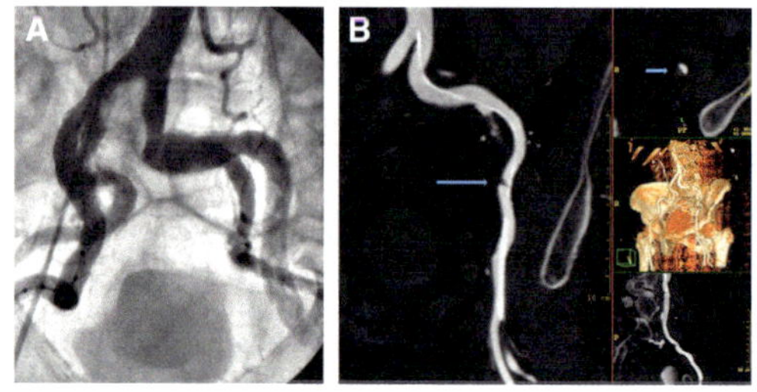

Figure 9.10. Arterial Dissection (A) Conventional angiogram. (B) Curved multiplanar reformatted images of an intra-arterial computed tomography angiogram revealing extensive dissection of the right iliac and femoral arteries. The intimal flap (red arrows) and its association with the catheter (blue arrows) are visible. (The dissection is likely to have been iatrogenic as part of the diagnostic cardiac catheterization and had no clinical sequelae).

Source: https://www.sciencedirect.com/science/article/pii/S1936878X09006913.

The literature evidence for the occurrence of contrast-associated AKI is mixed, with initial trials indicating a high risk and more contemporary trials identifying potential confounding by confounders that overestimated the rates. Nonetheless, however, underlying adverse effects on kidney function necessitate prevention, especially in those at high risk, because of the potential of AKI to produce worse clinical outcomes. Hence, hydration guidelines and careful monitoring are significant precautions to prevent this risk during and following intra-arterial procedures (Hoste et al., 2019). Furthermore, intra-arterial contrast administration must be well planned and executed to achieve optimal clinical benefit. Pre- and post-procedure guidelines are important for ensuring patient safety, particularly regarding hydration and renal function. Preprocedural routine renal function monitoring can provide important clues to potential risks. Procedural dosing within acceptable levels for patient-specific factors can enhance imaging quality while reducing side effects during the procedure. Post-procedure implementation of follow-up is important to assess for late complications. Proper education and preparation of the patients and the clinical team can enhance overall efficacy and safety outcomes when intra-arterial contrast media are used (Teasaddle et al., 2011).

9.4. Indications for Use

Requirements for contrast media application during imaging are key to optimizing diagnostic performance while ensuring patient safety. The primary objective of providing contrast agents, whether iodinated or gadolinium-containing, is to enhance visualization of internal structures and abnormalities during imaging. For instance, iodinated contrast agents are frequently employed in computed tomography (CT) because they improve the ability to define vascular systems and solid organs, thereby making it easier to detect tumors or vessel occlusions. It is critical that radiologists pay close attention to agent selection, tailored to the specific imaging modality, based on the patient's medical history, renal function, and potential for an allergic reaction. Radiologists must balance the efficacy of the contrast material against its safety profile, while accounting for economic considerations that also play a pivotal role in prudent decision-making regarding resource use and patient care (Cartocci et al., 2017). In pediatric imaging, the administration of contrast media must be even more cautious due to the characteristic physiological phenomena and developmental issues of children. Contrast media use in children is typically reserved for complex congenital defects, inflammation, or malignancies in which high-resolution imaging is required for optimal management. However, as the radiosensitivity of children and toxicity of chemical agents are greater than in adults, adherence to the principle of as low as reasonably achievable (ALARA) is mandatory. This principle extends to radiation dose during the imaging procedure as well as to judicious choice and administration of contrast media. Individually tailored protocols that adhere to established pediatric guidelines are essential to avoid complications while maximizing diagnostic potential (Nievelstein et al., 2010). For this purpose, careful assessment of contrast appropriateness is critical in safeguarding children undergoing imaging. Moreover, continued technological advancement in imaging necessitates a deeper understanding of the indications for contrast media in clinical use. With the advent of multidetector CT (MDCT) and magnetic resonance imaging (MRI), high-resolution imaging capability has significantly increased. Thus, indications for contrast enhancement must be reevaluated periodically as these technological advances unfold. Radiologists are tasked with weighing both the clinical presentation presented and the imaging modalities' capabilities available at hand while deciding on the necessity for contrast agents. Knowledge of each agent's characteristics—whether iodinated or gadolinium-based—is imperative to fostering wise and informed use. Therefore, continued education of healthcare professionals on the latest contrast media practice guidelines and current best practices remains vital to deliver safe and effective patient outcomes (Cartocci et al., 2017).

9.4.1. Diagnostic Imaging in Oncology

Diagnostic imaging plays a crucial role in the diagnosis, detection, and management of cancer. Diagnostic imaging encompasses numerous methods, a few of which are computed tomography (CT), magnetic resonance imaging (MRI), and positron emission tomography (PET), all of which rely on contrast media for enhanced image quality. Iodinated contrast agents used in CT scans are particularly significant because they make vascular tissues and tumors more visible, thereby enabling more consistent measurements of cancer progression or treatment response.

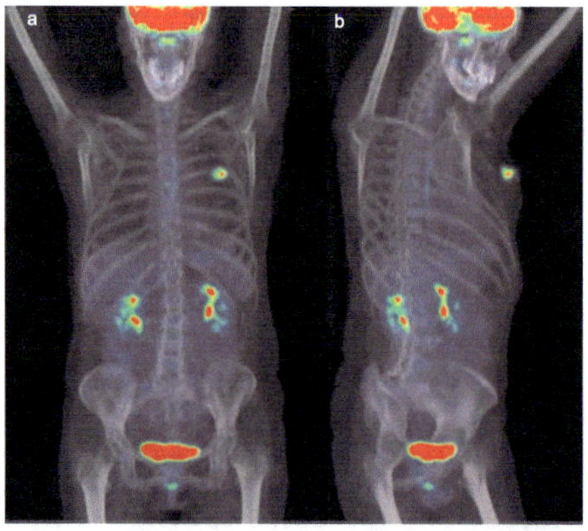

Figure 9.11. PET/CT scan of a patient with breast cancer. A trace amount of radiolabeled glucose (18 F-Fluorodeoxyglucose) was injected intravenously 1 h before the scan. The CT scan enables the visualization of the anatomical structures, such as the bone, in grayscale. The color-coded image represents the distribution of the molecular tracer in the body. The radiolabeled glucose shows normal uptake in the brain and elimination via the kidneys into the bladder. At the level of the left breast, there is an intense signal signifying the presence of hypermetabolic cells in the breast cancer. On the left (a) is the anterior view, and on the right (b) is the right oblique view of a 3D reconstructed image.

Source: https://www.researchgate.net/figure/PET-CT-scan-of-a-patient-with-breast-cancer-A-trace-amount-of-radiolabeled-glucose-18_fig1_233918959.

Moreover, understanding the character of ionic versus non-ionic preparations is essential in order to optimize imaging outcomes and minimize side effects. For instance, non-ionic agents are preferred due to their lower osmolality and reduced complications, underscoring the need for careful selection and administration of contrast media in oncology. The most frequently used agents in MRI for oncology imaging are gadolinium-based, due to their specific relaxivity properties, with a view to optimizing image contrast. When searching for tumors, the choice of macrocyclic or linear chelates is important, as macrocyclic chelates are more stable and reduce the rate of gadolinium leakage into tissue. Physicians also need to exercise caution with nephrogenic systemic fibrosis, a condition that occurs in rare but severe situations with gadolinium exposure in renal-impaired patients (Figure 9.11).

Identifying high-risk patient groups is important, enabling medical practitioners to apply appropriate preventive interventions, such as renal function screening prior to administration and other imaging modalities, where applicable. These represent an example of the ongoing process of ensuring optimal diagnostic imaging while ensuring patient safety. Pre-procedure and post-procedure guidelines also emphasize the role of patient safety in oncology imaging procedures. Before intravenous contrast media administration, clinicians should first confirm that the patient is properly hydrated to augment renal function and reduce acute kidney injury.

Post-procedure monitoring is also essential, particularly for detecting and managing potential side effects. These include the detection of mild to moderate reactions, which may escalate to more severe outcomes like acute anaphylactoid events. Patient counseling about likely symptoms and open communication channels can help early detection and control of complications during and after imaging procedures. In conclusion, an integrated approach to pre- and post-procedure care emphasizes the importance of safety in the proper use of contrast media in oncology diagnostic imaging.

9.4.2. Evaluation of Vascular Conditions

In the comprehensive evaluation of vascular disease, the use of contrast media in imaging cannot be overstated, particularly for assessing vascular pathology and anatomy. Iodinated contrast media is most commonly used in computed tomography (CT) and angiography, significantly enhancing visualization of blood vessels. By facilitating differentiation between vascular structures and the surrounding tissue, the agents allow not only unambiguous assessment of occlusions, stenoses, and aneurysms of the vessels but also play a crucial role in guiding interventional procedures. The decision between the ionic and non-ionic forms of iodinated contrast agents is a matter of choice, given that the non-ionic agents have the advantage of causing lower osmotic effects, thus helping reduce the frequency of adverse events. Therefore, understanding of these formulations and their relative uses is crucial in imaging vascular diseases with imaging modalities. Gadolinium-containing contrast agents are another essential class of contrast agents, predominantly utilized within magnetic resonance imaging (MRI) for vascular evaluations. Linear and macrocyclic chelates exhibit distinct stability profiles in this regard, influencing their safety and effectiveness in patients with established renal impairment. As greater focus is now being placed on nephrogenic systemic fibrosis, evaluation of the risk of gadolinium toxicity in individuals with compromised renal function has been of particular interest. Relaxivity is also a determinant of imaging quality; thus, careful selection based on patient-specific parameters is crucial. Assessment of vascular disease, especially in patients at risk for nephrogenic injury, requires familiarity with the biochemical actions of these agents and their effects on kidney function and general patient safety. In addition to the type of contrast agent used, strict pre- and post-procedure protocols are essential for reducing risks when vascular imaging is performed.

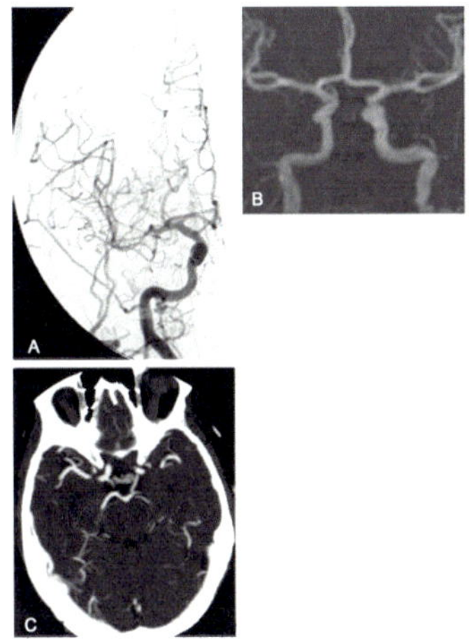

Figure 9.12. (A) During digital subtraction angiography (DSA), intra-arterial contrast is injected at a high rate and multiple images are acquired in rapid succession. Early images, before the arrival of the contrast, are used as masks to subtract bony structures; only vascular opacification remains. (B) Multiple axial magnetic resonance (MR) images constitute the basis of MR angiography. Moving protons, such as those of intravascular water, appear bright on conventional MR angiographic sequences. Stationary protons, such as those of the remainder of the brain parenchyma, appear dark. When stacked together, the axial images can be viewed in a fashion similar to conventional DSA. (C) Computed tomographic (CT) angiographic images include not only opacified vascular structures but also the osseous and soft tissue components of the brain. CT angiographic images are stacked together in groups of multiplanar volume reconstruction images and viewed in all three planes. The axial source images may need to be reviewed to clarify details. Three-dimensional (3D) surface-rendering techniques are available, but further development is needed before 3D-CT angiographic images become routinely useful.

Source: https://www.barrowneuro.org/for-physicians-researchers/education/grand-rounds-publications-media/barrow-quarterly/volume-17-no-3-2001/ct-angiography-and-stroke/.

Proper hydration is important for facilitating renal excretion of contrast material, particularly in the patient with baseline renal impairment. Medication manipulation, particularly those affecting renal perfusion and hemostasis, must be considered during patient preparation for vascular imaging studies. Proper post-procedure monitoring must also be instituted to early detect and treat any reaction. Side effects, while generally rare, can include allergic reactions or nephrotoxicity, and it is therefore key to an effective management strategy. Its application in clinical practice will enhance patient outcomes and improve the efficacy and safety of vascular condition evaluation (Cametti et al., 2015) (Figure 9.12).

9.4.3. Assessment of Gastrointestinal Disorders

Imaging modalities are critically involved in the evaluation and treatment of gastrointestinal disorders. Radiologic techniques with the use of contrast media make visualization of the GI tract better, facilitating accurate identification of abnormalities. Precautions should be taken when using iodinated contrast media, with the patient's renal status in mind, particularly in patients with pre-existing kidney disease, as these agents have the potential to induce contrast-induced nephropathy. Also, the new ultrasound technology, including the use of microbubbles as contrast agents, provides information on the vascular and structural characteristics of the GI tract.

The techniques endorsed by the Gastrointestinal Ultrasound (GIUS) task force aim to provide a comprehensive evaluation, integrating both normative anatomical data and pathological findings to enhance clinical outcomes in gastrointestinal imaging, according to EFSUMB recommendations (Calabrese et al., 2016). Further explanation of these advances, an understanding of the types of contrast agents is fundamental in the context of gastrointestinal evaluation. The distinction between ionic and non-ionic preparations becomes significant, especially regarding their osmolality, its impact on patient tolerance, and the likelihood of adverse reactions. Non-ionic agents, being of lower osmolality, have been found to cause fewer side effects, which increases patient comfort during imaging. As practitioners strive to strike a balance between minimizing risk and maximizing diagnostic efficacy, careful consideration must be given to the best contrast medium for optimal visualization and, thereby, proper diagnosis of GI pathology.

Additionally, adjunct procedures such as hydration status and pre-procedure screening enter into the picture to assist in the preservation of renal function, again emphasizing the significance of detailed pre- and post-procedure protocols to meet best-practice standards (Larauche et al., 2011). Because imaging plays a vital role in the diagnosis of gastrointestinal disorders, methods for managing adverse reactions to contrast media are invaluable. The reactions can vary in severity, requiring careful monitoring of patients during the imaging process. The application of preventive strategies, such as premedication in vulnerable patients, is still essential in avoiding the development of acute anaphylactoid reactions. Also, adherence to radiation protection protocols in radiopharmaceutical-based procedures is vital to patient safety as well as the prevention of unjustified exposure. Ongoing review and development of these protocols in light of emerging evidence are necessary to improve safety profiles in gastrointestinal imaging. These activities not only enhance the quality of patient care but also build confidence in the application of high-level imaging modalities as part of a diagnostic plan in the gastrointestinal sector (Calabrese et al., 2016) (Figure 9.13).

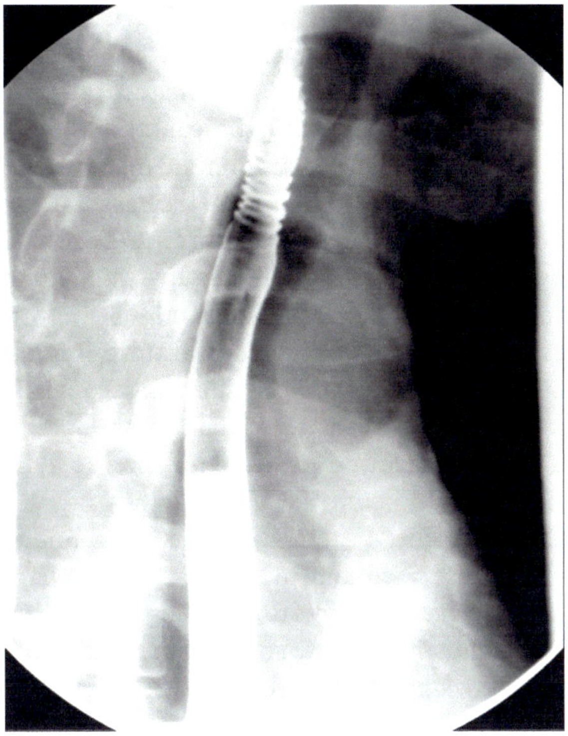

Figure 9.13. Fluoroscopic image of the gastrointestinal tract using contrast.

Source: https://radiologykey.com/wp-content/uploads/2021/06/f02-09-9780323680615.jpg.

9.5. Potential Risks and Side Effects

The use of contrast agents during imaging examinations can, while primarily necessary to enhance diagnostic accuracy, never be free of risks and side effects that require careful evaluation. The adverse events have primarily been categorized as mild, moderate, and severe reactions, the first one tending to present with acute anaphylactoid reactions. The latter, with symptoms of urticaria, edema, and in some cases, anaphylaxis, demand immediate clinical supervision. The likelihood of such events is dictated by a range of parameters, from the type of contrast used to patient demographics and comorbidities. In the context of the modern development of medical imaging, physicians have to be vigilant for such risks while tipping the balance in favor of the benefit from improved imaging against the risk of injury, a parameter that calls for consent and proper pre-procedure assessment on the part of healthcare practitioners (Cartocci et al., 2017). Over the last few decades, the safety record of contrast media has improved substantially due to innovations in formulation and routes of administration. Despite the advances, some risk must still be present, particularly in those patients with renal insufficiency or a history of adverse effects to the contrast media. Some gadolinium-based compounds have specifically been associated with nephrogenic systemic fibrosis (NSF), a serious but rare disease in patients with diminished renal function. Such problems necessitate careful pre-screening assessment and renal function studies before contrast administration. Second, the use of alternative imaging modalities, such as contrast-enhanced ultrasound (CEUS), is an excellent option, especially in children, because it minimizes exposure to iodinated agents and radiation, demonstrating a shift towards greater safety without sacrificing diagnostic efficiency (Cantisani et al., 2016). To offset contrast medium hazards, several preventive steps are increasingly implemented in clinical practice environments. These include rigorous pre-procedure protocols like scrutiny of patients' medical histories, prescribed medication, and established sensitivities. Proper hydration is also stressed as a pre- and post-procedure step to enhance renal clearance and offset nephrotoxicity risk. Anticipating potential side effects is also necessary; therefore, medical professionals are trained to recognize and manage such incidents effectively. Having strict monitoring and follow-up procedures in place also contribute to patient safety, in accordance with overall aims of optimizing imaging outcomes while ensuring minimal risk to patient health (Cartocci et al., 2017).

9.5.1. Allergic Reactions to Contrast Media

The application of the contrast media in imaging procedures, though required for diagnosis, is of concern due to allergic reactions. The reactions range from mild, like urticaria and pruritus, to the severe, including anaphylactic shock. The pathophysiology of allergic reactions is not well understood but is believed to involve a hypersensitivity reaction to contrast dyes, especially iodinated agents. These allergic reactions require close monitoring by medical practitioners, as they can occur immediately after injection. Surprisingly, such patients are at increased risk if they have had any history of allergic reactions to other drugs, a fact which confirms the importance of careful patient history before contrast medium administration. Furthermore, the pharmacological character and formulation—ionic or non-ionic—can influence the likelihood and severity of allergic reactions. Thus selection of formulation becomes a critical aspect of patient safety (Figure 9.14).

Allergic-like reactions to contrast

MILD	MODERATE	SEVERE
• limited urticaria • limited pruritus • limited cutaneous edema • limited "itchy"/"scratchy" throat • nasal congestion • sneezing • conjunctivitis • rhinorrhea	• diffuse urticaria • diffuse pruritus • diffuse erythema with stable vital signs • facial edema without dyspnea • throat tightness without dyspnea • hoarseness without dyspnea • wheezing/bronchospasm with mild or no hypoxia	• diffuse edema • facial edema with dyspnea • diffuse erythema with hypotension • wheezing/bronchospasm with significant hypoxemia • anaphylaxis • cardiopulmonary arrest* • pulmonary edema* *may be allergic-like or physiologic

Figure 9.14. Infographic showing symptoms of allergic reaction to contrast media.

Source: https://pbs.twimg.com/media/EG1I5dqWkAAQxcg.jpg:large.

Contrast media-induced allergic reactions should be handled proactively and reactively. For instance, premedication with antihistamines and corticosteroids can reduce the incidence of allergic reactions to a great extent in susceptible individuals. Recognition of individuals who are likely to have an acute anaphylactoid reaction, particularly in the case of a history of prior sensitivity or allergy, is significant. In mild and moderate reactions, symptomatic management itself is sufficient to minimize distress without compromising the imaging procedure. Acute severe reactions, though, require immediate medical intervention and might involve resuscitative measures. Furthermore, regular training for health care providers in recognizing and managing such reactions would enhance patient safety and confidence in receiving imaging with contrast media. New studies have highlighted adverse effects of iodinated contrast use, including intracranial hemorrhage, but the risk appears to be weighed against the diagnostic benefit. For instance, the use of iodinated contrast in CT scans has been criticized for potential associations with increased complications, but extensive evaluations have found that, when used appropriately, the risk is low. Surprisingly, intravenous iodinated contrast administered at typical diagnostic doses does not add considerably to the risk of symptomatic intracranial hemorrhage in patients receiving thrombolytic therapy. The findings highlight the need for ongoing research, with other evidence suggesting potential risks from gadolinium deposition in patients, to inform decision-making in imaging practice (Burke et al., 2016; Teasdale et al., 2011).

9.5.2. Nephrotoxicity and Its Consequences

Imaging with contrast media significantly enhances diagnostic yield but is not without risk, and one of its attendant risks is nephrotoxicity. Contrast-induced acute kidney injury (CA-AKI) is an endemic phenomenon, particularly in patients with baseline renal impairment. Intravenous administration of iodinated contrast media has been linked to negative alterations in renal function, primarily through effects on renal perfusion and tubular function. The underlying physiopathology of nephrotoxicity is ischemic injury to renal tissue, typically precipitated by renal vasoconstriction and alterations in glomerular filtration rate (GFR). Both iodinated and gadolinium-based contrast media have been found to induce these pathologic responses, so patient selection and pre-administration screening must be undertaken with caution to prevent the risk of adverse events (Maes et al., 2012) (Figure 9.15).

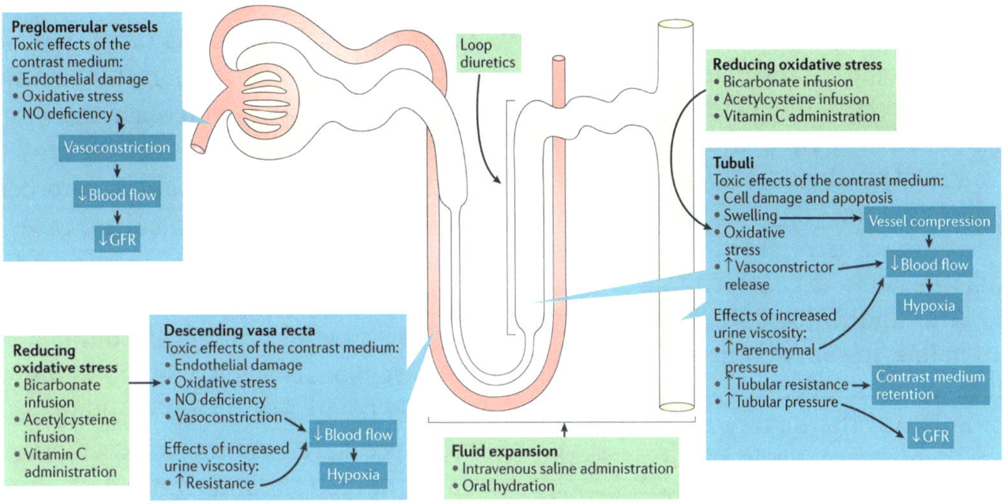

Figure 9.15. Diagram of nephrotoxicity pathway from iodine-based agents.

Source: https://media.springernature.com/lw685/springer-static/image/art%3A10.1038%2Fnrneph.2016.196/MediaObjects/41581_2017_Article_BFnrneph2016196_Fig3_HTML.jpg.

The impacts of nephrotoxicity are not restricted to acute renal damage alone. The long-term implications may include aggravation of chronic kidney disease (CKD) and enhanced susceptibility to subsequent nephrotoxic insults. For instance, among individuals receiving gadolinium-based contrast, it has been shown that even mild elevations in serum creatinine can signal covert tubular damage (Maes et al., 2012). Understanding the inter-relationship between the nature of the contrast media and risk will help to develop effective preventive measures. Established CKD, diabetes, and volume depletion are susceptible factors for which there are patient management interventions, like hydration protocols and pre-imaging adjustment of medications, that need to be instituted in order to prevent renal impairment. As the use of contrast media increases, advances have been made in identifying safer alternatives and protocols to effectively address nephrotoxicity risks. Recent studies show that some of these types, such as macrocyclic gadolinium agents, have less nephrotoxicity risk than linear agents, as evidenced by their safe track records among high-risk individuals, including CKD patients (Drews et al., 2024). Moreover, ongoing research is necessary to optimize imaging methods, such as monitoring serum creatinine levels before and after the procedure and implementing efficient follow-up mechanisms. By ensuring patient safety and using evidence-based practice, clinicians can minimize contrast media nephrotoxicity so that the benefit of enhanced imaging does not overtake renal injury.

9.5.3. Other Common Side Effects

Of the contrast media employed in diagnostic imaging, several mild to moderate side effects have manifested as common occurrences after administration. Symptoms such as headache, dizziness, and a sense of warmth are most commonly reported by patients, particularly with iodinated contrast media. These are typically short-lived and perhaps indicative of the body's normal physiological reaction to the introduction of a foreign substance. Though not dangerous, they can cause distress and discomfort to the patient undergoing imaging. Knowledge of this continuum of effects is relevant to healthcare professionals because it can facilitate a more compassionate and informed approach to patient care in imaging environments. Moreover, , reasonable control over these minor side effects can enhance the quality of the patient experience, thereby positively influencing the outcome of the diagnostic procedure (Cartocci et al., 2017). Among the major side effects of contrast media administration, skin reactions include rashes or urticaria (Figure 9.16).

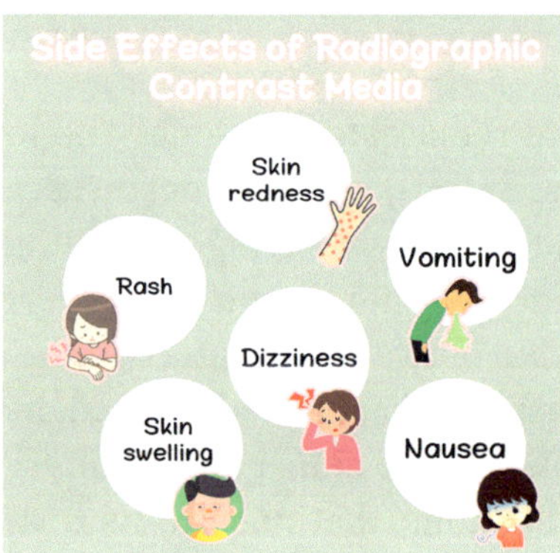

Figure 9.16. Common minor side effects of contrast agents (e.g., nausea, rash).

Source: https://pbs.twimg.com/media/E8NtGKSWUAAE-_m.jpg:large.

These cutaneous dermatologic reactions may be evoked by the immunogenicity of the contrast media, especially in susceptible patients. Most skin reactions are self-limiting and mild, but may anticipate more severe allergic reactions in some instances, warranting careful observation and reporting by healthcare personnel. Cutaneous effects should be communicated to radiologists and technologists so that timely awareness and intervention can be implemented where necessary. Additionally, the psychological impact of such reactions on patients must not be underestimated as fear of what might be an adverse reaction can increase their stress level. Continuous education regarding the side effects is crucial to optimize patient interactions and care (Ali et al., 2019). In severe cases, contrast media can trigger acute anaphylactoid reactions, although rare, which are serious enough to require careful discussion among providers. Such responses may include symptoms such as breathlessness, throat swelling, or a drop in blood pressure, resulting in a medical emergency. Early detection and control of such severe adverse reactions are essential because they can also affect patient safety during imaging. Prevention programs, such as rigorous screening for a history of allergy and pre-medication routines if required, can effectively reduce the risk of anaphylactoid reactions. An awareness of the full spectrum of potential side effects enables healthcare professionals to create a safer imaging room and, in turn, ensure that the benefits of diagnostic imaging outweigh the risks (Ali et al., 2019).

9.6. Safety Procedures and Policies

In the complex setting of medical imaging, adherence to safety rules and procedures when using contrast media is imperative. They ensure that the risk of potential adverse events with contrast injection is minimized while the diagnostic performance is optimized and patient safety is maintained. Radiologists have the duty to thoroughly review all patients' medical history and risks prior to the introduction of contrast agents. They must consider individual responses to these agents, especially in light of the evolving knowledge surrounding nephrogenic systemic fibrosis associated with gadolinium-based agents and allergies to iodinated contrast agents. Therefore, utilization of a systematic approach of safety steps is required, like pre-screening questions and establishing baseline renal function to ensure personalized patient care and optimal contrast agent use to augment diagnostic performance at the cost of patient safety (Cartocci et al., 2017). In addition to pre-procedure testing, post-procedure monitoring is also a significant component of the safety mechanism for the administration of contrast media. Following the administration of contrast media, patients should be observed for early signs of severe adverse effects, ranging from mild, self-limited reaction to anaphylactoid severe response.

An aggressive follow-up regimen, like hydration following the procedure, is critical in minimizing nephrotoxicity, particularly in patients with underlying renal impairment. Radiologists need to inform patients clearly about potential symptoms and provide definitive instructions on what to do next to obtain further medical treatment. The establishment of a systematic process of follow-up care addresses the need for patient education along with their active participation in their care, generating a culture of co-operation that leads to enhanced outcomes (Baio et al., 2016). Besides, continuing education and training for health professionals are integral to the proper implementation of safety protocols for contrast media. With advancements in imaging technology and changing guidelines, continuing professional education allows radiologists and technologists to stay abreast with best practices and new safety standards. This involves familiarity with the various characteristics of contrast agents, potential side effects, and recent studies on how to avoid risks associated with their use. Besides, multidisciplinary teamwork in healthcare ensures a collaborative approach to care, drawing on multiple perspectives and skills. Finally, prioritization of safety by intensive training and adherence to established guidelines not only protects the patient but also enhances the overall quality of imaging services (Cartocci et al., 2017).

9.6.1. Pre-Screening Patients for Allergies

In contrast agent imaging tests, pre-screening patients for allergic reactions is an essential step to ensure patient health. Before the administration of iodinated or gadolinium-based contrast agents, medical staff must carefully examine patient histories for any previous sign of an allergic reaction to contrast agents. This assessment is necessary because responses range from mild manifestations such as urticaria to their respective severe, life-threatening anaphylactoid reactions.

A successful pre-screening procedure would typically involve the administration of a comprehensive questionnaire that queries prior experience with contrast agents, food allergies, and other medical histories that might predispose patients to allergic reactions. Implementing these measures not only enhances patient safety but also enables the development of protocols to minimize the risk associated with contrast media use in diagnostic imaging procedures. Moreover, the need for appropriate patient screening is highlighted by the recognition that variations in patients' responses to contrast media are observed. Studies indicate that 40 million MRI scans are performed annually in the United States, underscoring the need for doctors to adhere to rigorous safety protocols during these procedures (Aran et al., 2023). By screening patients, clinicians can also identify those who may require additional precautions, such as pre-medication with corticosteroids or antihistamines, particularly in patients with a history of allergy (Figure 9.17).

Iodinated contrast media risk self-assessment questionnaire

Dear patients, some drugs and diseases may increase the risk of adverse events caused by the use of iodinated contrast media. Therefore, you are required to conduct this self-assessment before making an appointment. The specific form is as follows:

Are you taking any of the following drugs?		
Hypoglycemic agent: metformin	yes☐	no☐
Antihypertensive drugs: (such as valsartan, metoprolol, perindopril tert-butylamine, etc.)	yes☐	no☐
Non-steroidal anti-inflammatory drugs: (such as aspirin, acetaminophen, ibuprofen, etc.)	yes☐	no☐
Antibiotics: (such as gentamicin, streptomycin, amikacin, etimicin, etc.)	yes☐	no☐
Diuretics: (such as furosemide, tolasemi, etc.)	yes☐	no☐
Chemotherapy drugs: (such as cisplatin, methotrexate, bleomycin, cyclophosphoamine, etc.)	yes☐	no☐
Hypothyroidism: levothyroxine sodium tablets	yes☐	no☐
Hyperthyroidism: methimazole or propylthiouracil	yes☐	no☐
Whether you have renal insufficiency: yes☐ no ☐ unknown ☐		
Whether there is thyroid dysfunction : yes☐ no ☐ unknown ☐		
History of food or drug allergy : yes☐ no ☐ unknown ☐		
I suffer from the following diseases: Diabetic nephropathy ☐ Heart failure ☐ Multiple myeloma ☐ Pulmonary hypertension ☐ Hypoproteinemia / Hypohemoglobin ☐ asthma ☐Homocysteinuria ☐ Myasthenia gravis ☐ Pheochromocytoma ☐ Allergic rhinitis ☐		

If you choose "yes" for one item or do not know your current medication and renal function or thyroid function, please go to room 75, Area 2, 3rd floor of the outpatient clinic and the pharmacist will evaluate the risk of your angiography. Thank you for your cooperation!

Name: Date:

Figure 9.17. Patient allergy screening checklist for contrast media use.

Source: https://www.researchgate.net/figure/Iodinated-contrast-media-risk-self-assessment-questionnaire_fig1_371041913.

These cautionary measures are commensurate with the medical consensus that highly individualized patient care is the best practice, ensuring the safe administration of contrast media with the minimum possible risk of adverse reaction. Additionally, the significance of interprofessional practice among health professionals is underscored in pre-allergy screening. Interdisciplinary practice among radiologists, nurses, and pharmacists is necessary to develop comprehensive protocols that prioritize patient safety before the administration of contrast media (Coalition I for Safety P, 2017). This provides the foundation for creating standardized screening procedures, which can subsequently reduce intra-institutional variability and enable uniform patient care across different healthcare settings. By exchanging knowledge and experience on how to manage allergies, medical professionals can foster a safe environment that prioritizes patient care and is rooted in best practices and clinical expertise. Ultimately, good pre-screening for allergies is the foundation on which safe imaging, scanning, and the use of contrast media both rest.

9.6.2. Monitoring During and After Administration

Intravenous administration monitoring and, later, post-contrast medium administration are critical aspects of ensuring patient safety and quality imaging outcomes. During administration, caregivers need to carefully monitor patients for immediate reactions, particularly when administering iodinated agents or gadolinium-based contrast media. Monitoring at this phase is crucial, as it enables prompt detection of hypersensitivity reactions and other adverse effects. There should be proper protocols for monitoring vital signs and patient comfort, which can include symptoms such as headache, nausea, or allergies. Some populations, for example, with a history of renal impairment, may need to be monitored more intensively to prevent contrast-induced nephropathy complications, thereby again emphasizing the paramount significance of intensive monitoring at this phase of imaging studies (Figure 9.18).

Post-procedure monitoring is also warranted because it produces valuable data on the patient's recovery and the effectiveness of administered contrast. After the imaging study is completed, patients should be observed for signs of delayed reactions, which may appear hours or even days after administration. Such monitoring is particularly critical in the case of iodinated contrast, where studies have indicated that even normal doses are not associated with symptomatic intracranial hemorrhage in specific groups of patients, though vigilance remains the key (Teasdale et al., 2011).

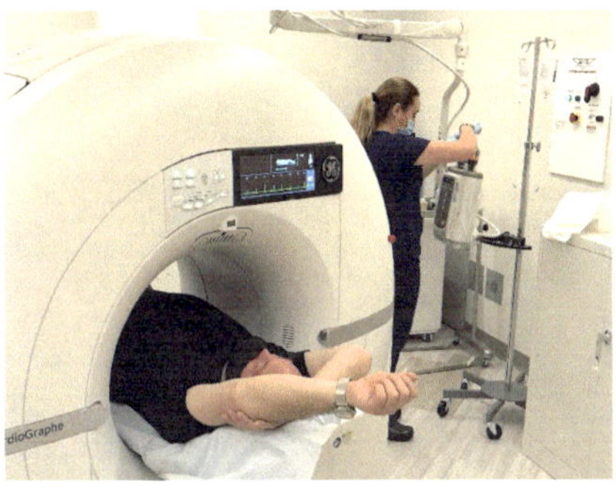

Figure 9.18. Monitoring setup for patients during contrast-enhanced imaging.

Source: https://radiologybusiness.com/sites/default/files/2022-04/ct_patient_pre-contrast_setup_cardiac_duly_df.jpeg.

Additionally, hydration is crucial in patients receiving nephrotoxic agents, as it optimizes renal function and reduces the frequency of side effects. Use of a structured follow-up protocol ensures that any adverse outcomes are identified promptly, promoting a broader continuum of care beyond the immediate administration of contrast media. Lastly, an efficient monitoring protocol during and after contrast media administration depends on interprofessional coordination and excellent communication among treating clinicians. Specifying definite protocols enhances patient outcomes through the potential for timely intervention, should complications arise. This emphasis on collaborative practice is reinforced by advances in imaging technology, which demand a high degree of understanding of both the biological actions of contrast agents and the safety protocols that guide their administration (Bose et al., 2019). Having the patient involved in their own treatment pathways is essential, too, allowing them to report any concerning symptoms post-procedure. As imaging continues to expand, there will be a need for a culture of vigilant oversight to ensure patient safety and confidence in the use of contrast media.

9.6.3. Recommendations For Patients with Renal Impairment

In planning the safety of contrast media injection in patients with renal dysfunction, some recommendations emerge that point to pre-procedure assessment.

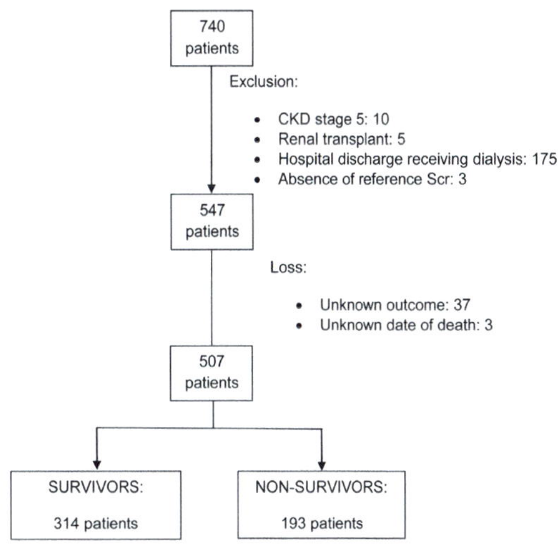

Figure 9.19. Flow-chart showing the selection process. CKD: chronic kidney disease Scr: serum creatinine. doi:10.1371/journal.pone.0047746.g001.

Source: https://www.researchgate.net/publication/232321481/figure/fig1/AS:300564178063360@1448671492260/Flow-chart-showing-the-selection-process-CKD-chronic-kidney-disease-Scr-serum.png.

First, baseline renal function needs to be determined using serum creatinine levels and glomerular filtration rate (GFR) to risk-stratify for contrast-induced nephropathy (CIN). The Kidney Disease: Improving Global Outcomes guidelines emphasize that even subtle rises in serum creatinine can indicate susceptibility, warranting careful management (Kellum et al., 2013). Risk stratification not only informs the choice of contrast agent but also enables personalized procedural tactics, such as the potential for hydration maneuvers to mitigate risk. These assessments become critical as they directly influence clinical decision-making in order to maintain patient safety while ensuring the best imaging results (Figure 9.19).

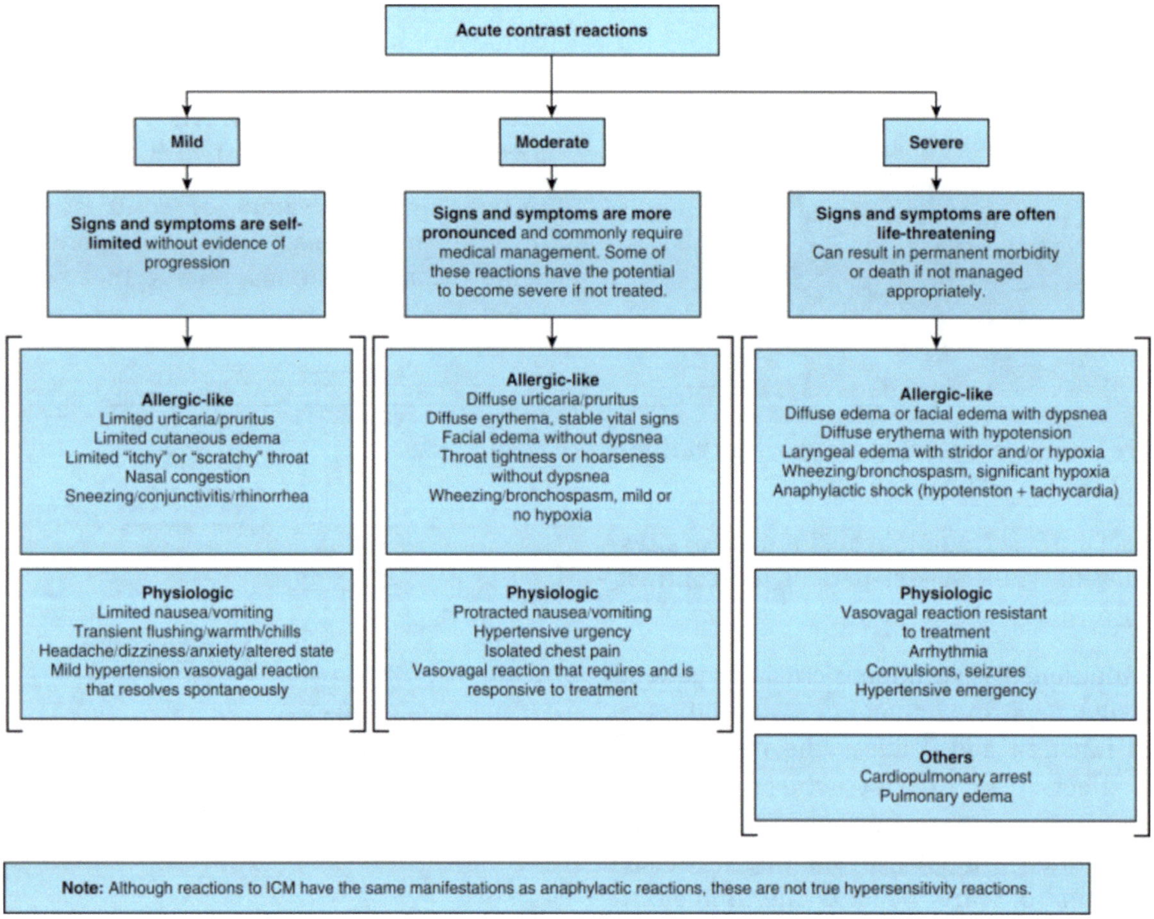

Figure 9.20. Safety recommendations for contrast media administration.

Source: https://radiologykey.com/wp-content/uploads/2018/09/f20-01-9780323462976.jpg

Pre-procedural hydration is crucial for protecting renal function during contrast media administration. Renal impairment patients are generally recommended to receive hydration protocols before and after the administration of nephrotoxic agents. Precautions such as this help dilute nephrotoxins and induce diuresis, presumably lowering the peak contrast media concentration in renal tubules (Bellin et al., 2023). Healthcare providers may also consider administering isotonic intravenous fluid or oral rehydration for patients who tolerate it. Where intravenous fluid administration is contraindicated or ineffective, other interventions, such as the application of low-osmolarity or iso-osmolar contrast media, may also be beneficial, as these products are likely to produce a less distasteful safety profile in at-risk populations. Thus, proper hydration forms the bedrock of preventive strategies for patients at risk with renal impairment. Ongoing surveillance of renal function following a procedure is also important, as it enables early detection of deterioration or signs of acute kidney injury (AKI). Recommendations call for close observation of serum creatinine levels, particularly within the first 48–72 hours following exposure to contrast media. Such vigilance is not only in line with expectations of formalized clinical guidelines but also is critical to implementing timely interventions when necessary (Kellum et al., 2013). Continued communication with patients about their symptoms and any possible changes in their urination habits can further reinforce safety precautions. By applying a holistic strategy encompassing evaluation, hydration, and stringent monitoring, medical personnel can significantly reduce the risks of contrast media administration in renal-impaired individuals and, in turn, improve patient safety and achieve optimal imaging outcomes (Figure 9.20).

SUMMARY

In conclusion, the use of contrast media in imaging is a highlight of diagnostic medicine, enabling improved visibility and tissue differentiation. Iodinated and gadolinium-containing agents are among the various contrast agents developed to achieve optimal diagnostic performance while balancing patient safety. More recent formulations have yielded safer, better-tolerated contrast materials that reduce concerns regarding adverse effects and nephrotoxicity. It is imperative that physicians be informed about the properties and hazards of each contrast agent. As explained, the careful choice of contrast media involves balancing efficiency with potential risks, with patients' welfare given prime consideration during the imaging process. Furthermore, safety protocols and guidelines are an essential element in the application of contrast media. Side effects, while rare, do occur, and knowledge of these hazards allows practitioners to manage them best. Hydration protocols, medication modification, and vigilant monitoring not only enhance safety but also ensure optimal imaging outcomes. Blending evidence-based guidelines with ongoing professional development fosters an ethos of high-level care for patients receiving imaging procedures with contrast media. With advancements in medical practice, it is crucial that radiologists stay up to date on new research and innovations that can be used to improve safety procedures and imaging modalities. Basically, the ongoing evolution of imaging technology necessitates a well-established understanding of contrast media. The evolution of formulations and safety measures is an affirmation of improving diagnostic efficacy while safeguarding patients against injury. Future research and development must continue to enhance the safety profiles of contrast agents, driven by ever-compelling studies and clinical trials. For instance, recent agents such as gadobenate dimeglumine raise questions about the necessity of tailored strategies in imaging situations, particularly sensitive ones like breast MRI, where some characteristics of contrast media can affect diagnostic efficacy (Kirchin et al., 2015). Finally, judicious choice and use of contrast media will lead to better diagnoses, improved patient care, and a long-term impact on the profession of medical imaging as a whole (Cartocci et al., 2017).

CLOSER LOOK

NEXT-GENERATION CONTRAST AGENTS: ENHANCING IMAGING PRECISION WHILE MINIMIZING RISK

Future studies on safety and contrast media are increasingly focused on minimizing adverse effects while maintaining enhanced imaging capabilities. With the increased use of gadolinium-based agents, particularly in NSF-susceptible patients, there is a need for safer alternatives. Altered formulations and dosages are now being proposed as they are likely to reduce risks without compromising diagnostic efficacy. Studies have begun investigating other chelation methods to enhance gadolinium clearance from the body and, in turn, lower the incidence of side effects. Other developments like new-generation formulations of higher biocompatibility and lower osmolality also go some way to highlight the emphasis on safer contrast media further. Current research studies should still address these safety issues, aiming to achieve a balance between the efficacy of imaging and patient well-being, as described in the current literature, with emphasis on cautious evaluations of new contrast agents as they enter the market (Bose et al., 2019). Future research areas will also largely depend on the application of advanced imaging modalities. Emerging directions, such as molecular imaging using targeted contrast agents to specific cellular locations, are at the forefront. This could ultimately allow one to differentiate between benign and malignant tissues more effectively than with traditional contrast agents. Multifunctional agents capable of providing diagnostic information and delivering therapeutic interventions hold much promise. For instance, anti-inflammatory mesenchymal stromal cells or engineered stem cells have shown promising prospects in the treatment of malignancies in preclinical models and thus impact future therapy and imaging interventions (Janes et al., 2015). As capabilities are increasingly exposed through ongoing research, protective safeguards must also evolve to ensure that such sophisticated agents do not adversely impact patient safety while delivering improved diagnostic outcomes. Finally, comprehensive patient management algorithms are essential to ensure appropriate utilization of contrast media, with particular attention to individualized patient care. Future research must prioritize pre-procedure and post-procedure safety, including hydration techniques to protect renal function and individualized medication regimens for patients with known allergies or a history of adverse reactions. Current research has emphasized the importance of surveillance regimens and shown that early response measures can significantly reduce the severity of acute anaphylactoid responses. Additionally, applying machine learning techniques to predict patient risk profiles from rich health data can redefine clinicians' approaches to administering contrast media. By leveraging technology, researchers can facilitate safer practices and improved patient outcomes, ensuring the responsible advancement of diagnostic imaging procedures in a clinical setting.

REFERENCES

1. Aboagye, E., Adams, J., Aerts, H., & Barrington, S. (2016). Imaging biomarker roadmap for cancer studies. https://core.ac.uk/download/79539615.pdf (accessed on 14th July 2025).
2. Valdora, F., Cutrona, G., Matis, S., Morabito, F., Massucco, C., Emionite, L., Boccardo, S., Basso, L., Recchia, A. G., Salvi, S., Rosa, F., Gentile, M., Ravina, M., Pace, D., Castronovo, A., Cilli, M., Truini, M., Calabrese, M., Neri, A., . . . Ferrarini, M. (2016). A non-invasive approach to monitor chronic lymphocytic leukemia engraftment in a xenograft mouse model using ultra-small superparamagnetic iron oxide-magnetic resonance imaging (USPIO-MRI). *Clinical Immunology*, *172*, 52–60. https://doi.org/10.1016/j.clim.2016.07.013Bellin, M. F., Bertolotto, M., Brismar, T. B., & Clement, O. (2023). Waiting times between contrast-enhanced examinations: ESUR guidelines. https://core.ac.uk/download/614214536.pdf (accessed on 14th July 2025).
3. Bose, R. J. C., & Mattrey, R. F. (2019). Accomplishments and challenges in stem cell imaging *in vivo*. https://core.ac.uk/download/287623865.pdf (accessed on 14th July 2025).
4. Burke, L., Jay, M., Ramalho, J., & Ramalho, M. (2016). Gadolinium toxicity and treatment. https://core.ac.uk/download/85005336.pdf (accessed on 14th July 2025).
5. Calabrese, E., Dietrich, C. F., Dirks, K., & Gilja, O. H. (2016). EFSUMB recommendations for GI ultrasound–Techniques and findings. https://core.ac.uk/download/74321241.pdf (accessed on 14th July 2025).
6. Cametti, C., Fratoddi, I., Russo, M. V., & Venditti, I. (2015). How toxic are gold nanoparticles? The state-of-the-art. https://core.ac.uk/download/54248998.pdf (accessed on 14th July 2025).
7. Cartocci, G., Fineschi, V., Frati, P., & Guglielmi, G. (2017). The choice of gadolinium-based contrast agents: A radiologist's responsibility between pharmaceutical equivalence and bioethical issues. https://core.ac.uk/download/153367327.pdf (accessed on 14th July 2025).
8. Catania, F., Cavaliere, A. F., D'Indinosante, M., De Luca, C., Eleftheriou, G., Giorgi, M. G., & Giusti, M. (2022). Contrast agents during pregnancy: Pros and cons when really needed. https://core.ac.uk/download/576927287.pdf (accessed on 14th July 2025).
9. Chui, T. Y. P., Dubow, M., Dubra, A., & Gan, A. (2014). Comparison of adaptive optics scanning light ophthalmoscopic imaging. https://core.ac.uk/download/213079586.pdf (accessed on 14th July 2025).
10. Hoste, E., & Vandenberghe, W. (2019). Contrast-associated acute kidney injury: Reality and management. https://core.ac.uk/download/225020701.pdf (accessed on 14th July 2025).
11. Janes, S. M., & Sage, E. (2015). Anti-tumor effects of TRAIL-expressing mesenchymal stromal cells in a mouse xenograft model of human mesothelioma. https://core.ac.uk/download/29410635.pdf (accessed on 14th July 2025).
12. Kellum, J. A., & Lameire, N. (2013). Contrast-induced acute kidney injury: A KDIGO summary (Part 2). https://core.ac.uk/download/55800526.pdf (accessed on 14th July 2025).
13. Kirchin, M., Luciani, M. L., Pediconi, F., & Telesca, M. (2015). Clinical utility of gadobenate dimeglumine in contrast-enhanced MRI of the breast: A review. https://core.ac.uk/download/141692117.pdf (accessed on 14th July 2025).
14. Larauche, M., Mulak, A., & Taché, Y. (2011). Stress-related alterations of visceral sensation: Animal models for IBS study. https://core.ac.uk/download/323080393.pdf (accessed on 14th July 2025).

15. Maes, B., Rigothier, C., Alison, D., Devos, D., Glowacki, F., Vrtovsnik, F., & Deray, G. (2012). Safety of Gd-DOTA-enhanced MRI vs unenhanced MRI in CKD patients (RESCUE study). https://core.ac.uk/download/pdf/81262116.pdf (accessed on 14th July 2025).

16. Naeem, M. A., Rauf, H., & Razzaq, R. (2021). Frequency of acute and late reaction of non-ionic iodinated contrast media in contrast enhanced computed tomography. https://core.ac.uk/download/427748494.pdf (accessed on 14th July 2025).

17. Nievelstein, R. A. J., van Dam, I. M., & van der Molen, A. J. (2010). Multidetector CT in children: Current concepts and dose reduction strategies. https://core.ac.uk/download/pdf/8425712.pdf (accessed on 14th July 2025).

18. Teasdale, E., McVerry, F., Muir, K. W., MacDougall, N. J. J., Baird, S., Baird, T., & Wilcox, J. (2011). Iodinated contrast media and cerebral hemorrhage after intravenous thrombolysis. https://core.ac.uk/download/110588.pdf (accessed on 14th July 2025).

19. van de Ven, A. J. M., Dekkers, I. A., Laguna, J. J., & van der Molen, A. J. (2024). Hypersensitivity reactions to contrast media and the role of the allergy specialist. https://core.ac.uk/download/653279066.pdf (accessed on 14th July 2025).

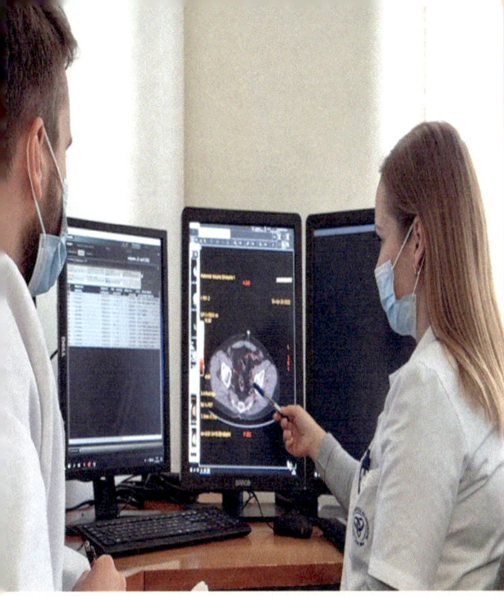

Chapter 10

RADIATION DOSIMETRY AND PATIENT SAFETY

Contents

Introduction

In current medical treatments, the significance of radiation dosimetry cannot be ignored, particularly in attaining patient protection. Radiation dosimetry involves measurement, calculation, and assessment of ionizing radiation doses delivered to patients via diagnostic and therapeutic procedures. The function of this discipline is crucial in optimizing the trade-off between the benefits of medical imaging and the morbidity incurred due to radiation exposure. With an overall understanding of dosimetry concepts, healthcare professionals can minimize damage while maximizing diagnostic efficiency. For instance, knowledge of the difference between absorbed and equivalent doses is useful when examining how various types of radiation affect biological tissue in different ways, pointing to the use of appropriate dosage levels for specific treatments to avoid unnecessary risks (Damilakis et al., 2017). Furthermore, measurements of patient doses obtained using these methods are a fundamental part of effective radiation management and optimization. Contemporary advances in dosimetry, such as in thermoluminescent dosimeters and optically stimulated luminescence devices, offer dramatic enhancements in accuracy and reliability. These instruments make precise determinations of radiation exposure possible, which enhances the capability of healthcare workers to tailor imaging protocols and safeguard patient health. Moreover, adopting new technology fosters a safety culture that emphasizes continuous learning and improvement. By systematically evaluating patient dose measurements and results, healthcare organizations can make necessary adjustments to equipment, procedures, and education, thereby reducing overexposure events and improving overall patient care (Akahane et al., 2017).

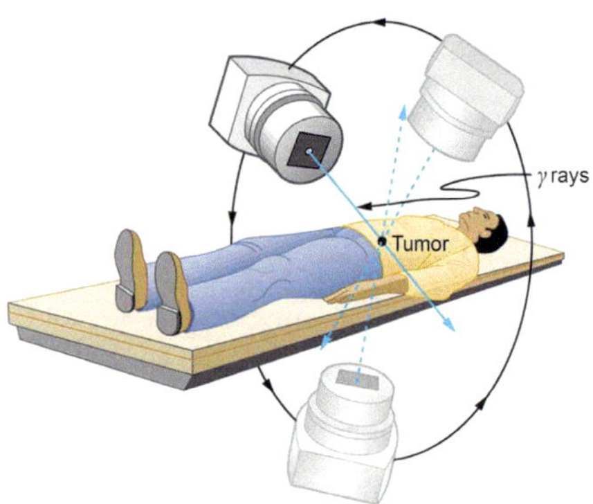

Figure 10.1. Overview of radiation use in modern medicine.

Source: https://philschatz.com/physics-book/resources/Figure_33_03_02a.jpg.

Accordingly, the intersection of radiation dosimetry and patient safety arises as a complex challenge that infuses the technical and human aspects of medicine. It requires a stringent regulatory framework comprising the International Basic Safety Standards and national regulatory agencies, as well as adherence to best practices. Furthermore, developing effective radiation risk communication is essential to empowering patients through mechanisms of informed consent and explicit educational materials. By engaging patients actively in understanding the implications of radiation exposure, healthcare providers can build trust and facilitate collaborative decision-making. Proactive integration of dosimetry principles with safety measures overall puts healthcare systems in a position where they can remove risks and drive the advancement of medical treatment and imaging (Damilakis et al., 2017) (Figure 10.1).

10.1. Fundamentals of Radiation Dosimetry

Understanding the nuances of radiation dosimetry is vital in ensuring patient safety in the clinical setting. The distinction between absorbed dose and equivalent dose is a fundamental aspect of dosimetry. The absorbed dose is a measure of the energy that is deposited in a material per unit mass, in grays (Gy), while the equivalent dose is normalized for the action of radiation upon biology by application of a type-specific quality factor, in units of sieverts (Sv) (Seibert et al., 2018). This is an important distinction as different kinds of radiation, such as alpha and beta particles, have varying abilities to cause biological damage. In addition, understanding the relationship between absorbed and equivalent dose allows clinicians to make appropriate clinical decisions regarding treatments, preventing unnecessary risks from overexposure and, ultimately, improving patient outcomes through tailored radiation treatments. Another fundamental principle of radiation dosimetry is linear energy transfer (LET), a measure of the energy dissipated by radiation passing through a material. LET is important because it is related to the biological effectiveness of various forms of radiation. High-LET radiation, such as alpha particles, causes more cellular damage than low-LET radiation, such as gamma rays, due to its higher energy deposition per unit path length (Vincentis et al., 2019). Therefore, it is of great importance to understand LET in depth when designing treatment schemes that involve radiation therapy. By understanding the reactions of various forms of radiation when they encounter biological tissues, medical physicists can calculate dosages more accurately and assess the potential harm to surrounding healthy tissues. This is important for optimizing the use of radiation therapy, ensuring it achieves its intended therapeutic effects while minimizing unwanted effects on patients. Lastly, dose–response models also enhance understanding of how exposure to radiation is associated with its biological effects. These models make it possible to forecast the impact on health with different doses of radiation and, by extension, a more precise understanding of risks resulting from exposure. Models such as the linear-no-threshold (LNT) model and threshold models provide means of risk estimation and, consequently, inform clinical practice and regulation on the use of radiation (Seibert et al., 2018). Significant improvements in dose-response modeling enable customized patient treatments and simplify the handling of complex variables based on health conditions, age, and other factors. Adding such models to radiation dosimetry enables medical practitioners to make well-informed choices, thereby enhancing patient safety and improving health outcomes.

10.1.1. Types of Radiation Detectors

Radiation detectors are vital instruments for ensuring patient safety by accurately measuring and monitoring radiation exposure in clinical settings. Among the most common detectors used are thermoluminescent dosimeters (TLDs), which use materials that store energy after exposure to ionizing radiation. When these materials are heated, they release the stored energy as light, enabling exposure levels to be quantified. This method not only provides precise readings but also offers stability and recyclability, making TLDs a crucial tool in both clinical and research settings. Additionally, their ability to measure low radiation doses makes them critical for tracking patient exposure during diagnostic treatments, reinforcing the safety protocols needed for effective radiation dosimetry. In addition to TLDs, metal-oxide semiconductor field-effect transistors (MOSFETs) are increasingly used for real-time dosimetry (Figure 10.2).

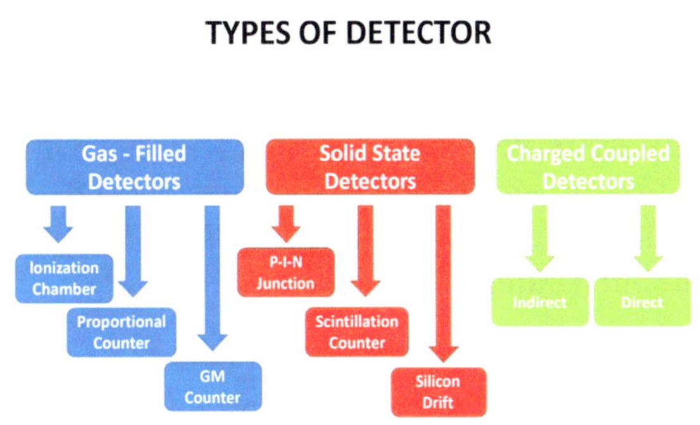

Figure 10.2. Common types of radiation detectors used in clinical settings.

Source: https://image.slidesharecdn.com/radiationdetectors4fx-151125012018-lva1-app6891/95/radiation-detectors-8-638.jpg?cb=1448414632.

These detectors offer several advantages due to their compact size, high spatial resolution, and rapid response to radiation. MOSFETs are particularly valuable when rapid assessment is required, for instance, in radiation therapy. They allow for real-time feedback of radiation levels, which facilitates immediate adjustments to treatment protocols and thus contributes to dose optimization methods. As discussed in recent studies, integrating advanced detection systems, such as MOSFETs, not only helps minimize risks associated with overexposure during procedures but also enhances overall patient safety in health facilities, as clinicians can make informed decisions based on accurate information (Chan et al., 2017). Optically stimulated luminescence (OSL) detectors represent another new technology used for radiation measurement. Similar to TLDs, OSL detectors use phosphors that absorb energy upon irradiation; they are light-stimulated rather than heat-stimulated to release the absorbed energy. This allows more flexibility, as OSL detectors can be read multiple times without significant loss of accuracy, offering reliability in many clinical applications. Their broad sensitivity to a range of radiation types makes them even more valuable for tracking exposure during complex medical procedures. By facilitating improved understanding of exposure levels and aiding incident reporting, OSL detectors primarily support risk mitigation strategies, which ultimately lead to a more secure environment for diagnostic and therapeutic interventions in patients (Damilakis et al., 2017) (Figure 10.3).

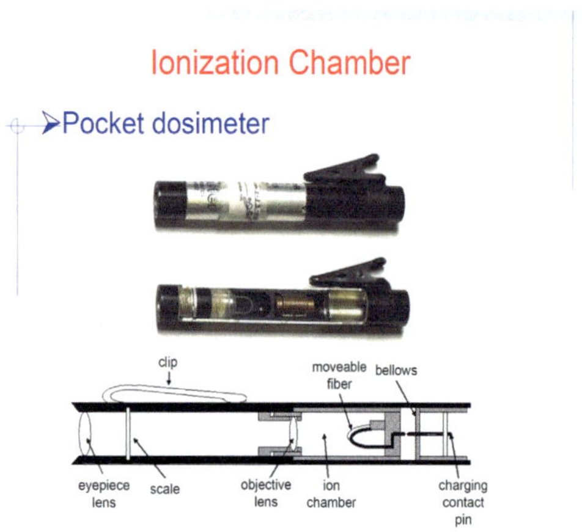

Figure 10.3. Ionization chamber dosimeter used in radiology departments.

Source: https://image.slideserve.com/1441086/ionization-chamber1-l.jpg.

10.1.2. Measurement Units in Dosimetry

In radiation dosimetry, the understanding of the measurement units is crucial to ensure patient safety. The principal unit of the measurement of the absorbed dose is the gray (Gy), which is the energy deposited by radiation per tissue mass unit. On the contrary, the equivalent dose, expressed in sieverts (Sv), accounts for the biological effects of radiation, as it varies depending on the type of radiation and its action on tissues. This differentiation becomes particularly useful when assessing the potential risks of various medical imaging modalities, such as computed tomography (CT) or fluoroscopy, where patient exposure is highly variable. By utilizing these units of measurement, physicians are able to more readily estimate doses in procedures and use practices that minimize unnecessary exposure, thereby enhancing patient safety and quality of care. Also, dosimetry technology has evolved, leading to the development of sophisticated devices that provide greater precision in measuring radiation doses. Thermoluminescent dosimeters (TLDs), metal-oxide semiconductor field-effect transistors (MOSFETs), and optically stimulated luminescence (OSL) dosimeters are examples of devices that measure dose. These devices have varied capabilities; TLDs are typically known to be stable and highly sensitive, while MOSFETs offer real-time tracking. OSL dosimeters, though, both high-resolution dose measurements and the ability to reanalyze. Their integration into clinical practice not only offers better radiation dose measurements but also enables compliance with safety standards as described in guidelines prepared by organizations such as the International Atomic Energy Agency, emphasizing the essentiality of precise measurement of dose towards patient safety (Damilakis et al., 2017). The effects of accurate measurement units in dosimetry go beyond the immediate effect to the patient, with long-term health consequences and healthcare policy also being influenced. Organizational bodies, such as the International Commission on Radiological Protection, stipulate the need for systematic reporting of dose and protocol compliance. It is underscored by the need for healthcare centers to properly address overexposure mishaps and ensure that occurrence frequency is minimized. In this case, ongoing assessment and refinement of radiation safety practices are critical. Health facility feedback systems allow dosage records to be checked ultimately for preventing unnecessary exposure and increasing overall patient protection (Badal et al., 2012). Thus, pressure to understand and apply units of measurement in dosimetry is not a technical necessity but an integral part of ethical patient care (Figure 10.4).

Table 2 Units of Radioactivity and Radiation Dose

Quantity	SI unit and symbol	Non-SI unit	Conversion factor
Radioactivity	becquerel, Bq	Curie, Ci	10 1 Ci = 3.7x10 Bq =37 Gigabecquerels (GBg) 1 Bq = 27 picocurie (pCi)
Absorbed dose	gray, Gy	rad	1 rad = 0.01 Gy
"Dose" (Equivalent dose)	sievert, Sv1	rem	rem= 0.01 Sv1 rem = 10 mSv

Figure 10.4. Standard dosimetry measurement units.

Source: https://cf.ppt-online.org/files/slide/h/h0dAYf5iI7qo6VTky8OFjetZHJLnmDr94Kv2zC/slide-14.jpg.

10.1.3. Dosimetry in Different Medical Applications

Dosimetry is a very important aspect of a variety of medical procedures, specifically in diagnostic imaging and radiation therapy. In radiation therapy, precise dosimetry helps ensure that tumors receive effective doses while minimizing exposure to surrounding healthy tissues. Such techniques, through the use of advanced 3D printing technology, are being used in the goal of designing patient-specific immobilization devices. These technologies can enhance both treatment outcomes and patient comfort by improving alignment during irradiation. Research has indicated that the materials used in 3D printing have different mechanical and radiological properties, and these can be enhanced through proper characterization to improve patient positioning and ensure successful treatments (Ahn et al., 2016). Therefore, an understanding of how dosimetry informs treatment planning profoundly impacts therapeutic effectiveness and patient safety, and makes it essential to maintain good dosimetric practices in the clinic. In diagnostic imaging, dosimetry plays a significant role in ensuring patients receive the lowest possible radiation dose while maintaining good image quality. The use of various dosimetry techniques, such as Thermoluminescent Dosimeters (TLDs) and Optically Stimulated Luminescence (OSL), enables precise dose measurements for radiation treatments, such as X-rays and CT scans. The measurements are crucial for assessing patient safety and ensuring conformity to regulatory standards. Furthermore, the use of dose-optimization techniques, such as protocol adaptation and adaptive exposure controls, can reduce unnecessary radiation exposure. As witnessed in interventional radiology, accidental overexposure is frequent due to training deficits among personnel and a lack of procedural shielding. Recognition and understanding of these elements remain vital for safer diagnostic practice across the healthcare sector (Damilakis et al., 2017), highlighting the interconnected nature of dosimetry, radiation protection, and quality patient care. Furthermore, the relevance of dosimetry extends beyond current treatment perspectives, as it guides the production of effective risk communication regarding radiation risks to patients. On account of the unintended effects associated with radiation exposure, medical professionals must adopt open risk communication processes. These include the informed consent process, whereby patients should be adequately informed about the potential risks and benefits of radiation treatments. Effective risk communication fosters trust among patients and health professionals, thereby enhancing patient compliance and satisfaction. Incident reporting policies concerning radiation are also required to facilitate continuous improvement of safety practices. From learning from regrettable incidents and instituting corrective actions, health facilities can improve protection of patient welfare and create a safety culture in radiation procedures (Damilakis et al., 2017). Therefore, the role of dosimetry is of the highest value not only in direct clinical applications but also in inspiring an overall awareness of patient safety regarding radiation exposure (Figure 10.5).

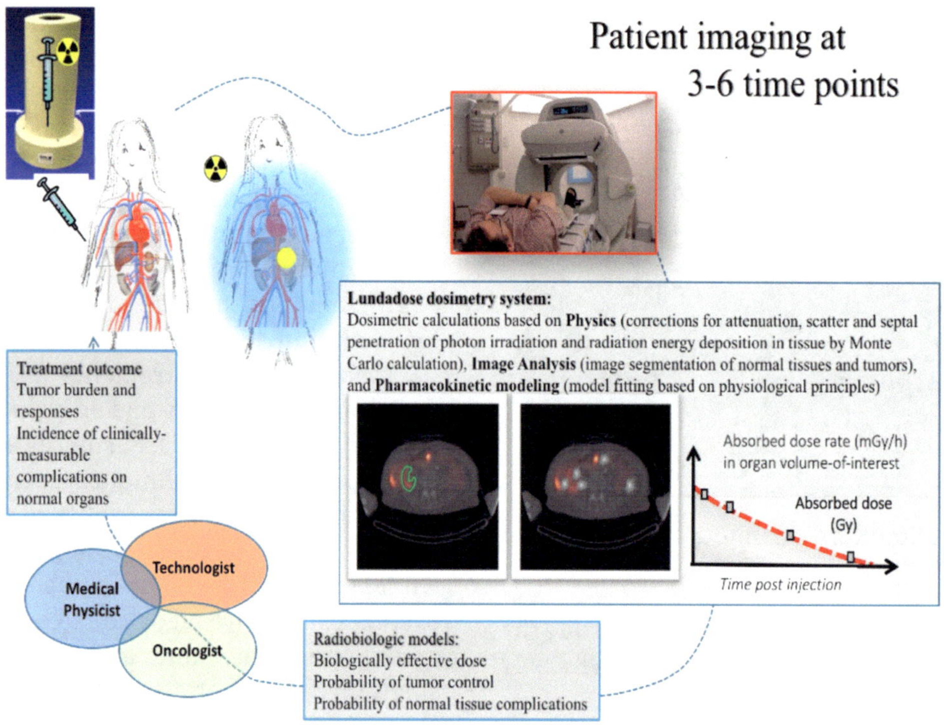

Figure 10.5. Application of dosimetry in diagnostic imaging and radiation therapy.

Source: https://www.mdpi.com/biomedicines/biomedicines-04-00025/article_deploy/html/images/biomedicines-04-00025-g001.png.

10.2. The Role of Dosimetry in Patient Safety

In patient safety, dosimetry takes center stage in the application of radiation for tumor treatment and diagnostic imaging. Measurement and monitoring of radiation dosage ensure that patients receive treatment appropriately without incurring the damage caused by excess exposure. The distinction between absorbed dose and equivalent dose is a fundamental concept in the field, as it helps explain how radiation affects human tissue biologically. The absorbed dose quantifies the energy deposited per unit mass of tissue, whereas the equivalent dose accounts for the nature of the radiation and its capacity to inflict biological injury, underscoring the need for dosimetric measurements tailored to the clinical need. The application of diversified technologies, such as thermoluminescent dosimeters and optically stimulated luminescence devices, significantly enhances the accuracy of dose measurement and therefore enables a safer therapeutic environment for radiation-exposed patients (Cremonesi et al., 2024). Furthermore, techniques of dose optimization are critical in correlating therapeutic aims with the safety of patients. Tailoring protocols refers to modifying radiation exposure parameters based on individual patient attributes, ensuring delivered doses are sufficient for therapeutic effectiveness but not excessive. Real-time adaptation of exposure controls enables radiation delivery to be fine-tuned to the patient's response, thereby enhancing treatment precision while reducing the risk of destructive side effects. The iterative reconstruction advantages in imaging methodologies enhance image quality during diagnosis as the dose of radiation required decreases. This summary approach focuses on implementing advanced dosimetric practices that not only ensure patient safety but also optimize the efficacy of radiation treatments (Antunes et al., 2017). The regulation of radiation dosimetry is essential to securing patient safety standards in medical practices. International Basic Safety Standards provide essential guidelines that healthcare facilities must follow, ensuring consistency in radiation protection measures. Domestic regulatory bodies also implement these standards, with adaptations tailored to the specific contexts and needs of their patient populations. Accreditation requirements often demand implementing full dosimetry protocols, reassuring patients that radiological treatment is up to standards. The convergence of effective dosimetry protocols and regulation, therefore, supports a multifaceted practice of patient safety in radiation therapy, instilling confidence and transparency in health systems (Cremonesi et al., 2024).

10.2.1. Monitoring Radiation Exposure

Monitoring radiation exposure is a crucial aspect of patient safety in environments where radiological tests are performed. Monitoring not only involves quantifying patients' absorbed radiation doses but also developing procedures to minimize potential exposure risks. Effective monitoring systems for radiation have the potential to significantly improve patient safety by identifying potential overexposure and optimizing dosage using advanced methods of measurement. According to International Atomic Energy Agency recommendations, poor staff training in equipment operation and optimization strategies can lead to extreme overexposures, underscoring the importance of strict training programs and adherence to safety protocols during procedures (Damilakis et al., 2017). Furthermore, implementing systematic screening, such as pre-procedure instructions and dose reminders, can be measures of safety that decrease the risk of overdosing with radiation without sacrificing diagnostic and therapeutic effectiveness (Figure 10.6).

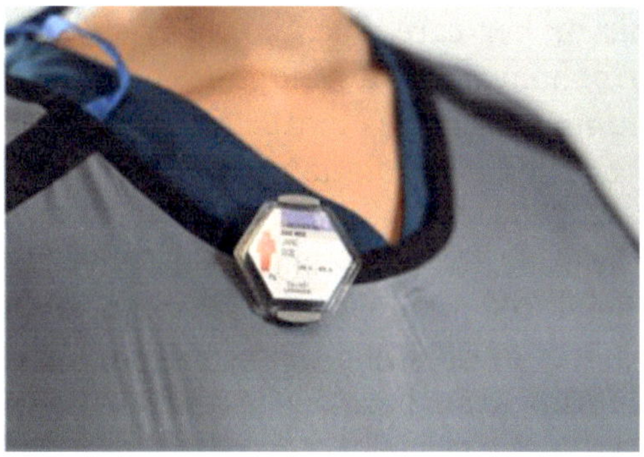

Figure 10.6. Wearable radiation dosimeter badge used for exposure monitoring.

Source: https://www.landauer.com/sites/default/files/inline-images/Landauer%20Luxel%20clipped%20on_0.jpg.

In radiation dosimetry, several methods are used to accurately measure patient exposure levels. Some advanced technologies used in a clinical setting include thermoluminescence dosimeters, metal-oxide semiconductor field-effect transistors, and optically stimulated luminescence detectors. Each of these methods has its own advantages and disadvantages regarding sensitivity, energy response, and calibration requirements. For instance, thermoluminescent dosimeters are highly sensitive to low doses of radiation and can be deployed in environments with varying exposure levels (Seibert et al., 2018). Moreover, new technologies, for instance, the integration of real-time radiation monitoring systems, enable dynamic assessment of exposure and can trigger instant remedial measures as needed. These advancements, in turn, enhance measurement fidelity while improving overall understanding of radiation dosimetry and its impact on patient safety, toward a proactive approach to minimizing the risks associated with radiological procedures. Risk communication due to radiation is essential towards facilitating a safety culture for medical practices. An informed consent process that properly distinguishes the risks and benefits of radiologic procedures is more informative and more engaging for the patient in his or her care. Such active involvement is also enhanced by developing comprehensive patient education materials that address concerns about radiation exposure (Damilakis et al., 2017). Furthermore, organizations such as the American Association of Physicists in Medicine set standards to see best practices in the safety of radiation uniformly implemented, promoting transparency in the dosimetry of radiation across clinical specialties (Seibert et al., 2018). Coupled with effective incident-reporting mechanisms, these interventions promote a culture of learning in healthcare settings, ultimately translating into better patient safety outcomes. By emphasizing clear and efficient risk communication, the medical profession can foster public trust in radiological practice while ensuring the optimal implementation of safety protocols and surveillance practices.

10.2.2. Establishing Safe Dose Limits

Setting safe dose limits is a central concern in radiation dosimetry, particularly in ensuring patient safety in therapeutic procedures. The concept of dose limits is a balance between the therapeutic benefit of exposure to radiation and the potential hazards of ionizing radiation that induce acute and late effects on health. Carefully planned dose calculations are the foundation of this balance, aimed at providing sufficient radiation to destroy cancer cells without causing harmful side effects in normal tissues. A core component of this approach is the establishment of minimum effective and maximum tolerated absorbed doses, taking into account individual patient information, tumor type, and treatment goals, in accordance with (Beşli et al., 2016) (Figure 10.7).

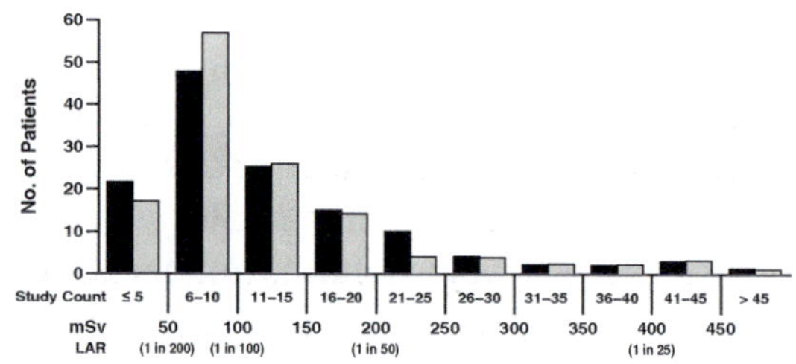

Figure 10.7. Chart showing radiation-associated cancer risk estimates.

Source: https://www.ajronline.org/cms/10.2214/AJR.08.1351/asset/images/04_08_1351_01.jpeg.

By applying these personalized dosimetric strategies, clinicians can optimize patient outcomes without compromising safety. One such successful application of establishing safe dose cutoffs is found in the radioiodine therapy of differentiated thyroid carcinoma. Therapy of this type of cancer involves careful measurement of radiation dose to set appropriate discharge planning for the patient. Research shows that patient outcomes following radioactive iodine treatment are highly variable, indicating that individualized dosimetry regimens are necessary to determine the optimal dose for each case. As an example, patients with higher activities of iodine-131 should have their rates of exposure monitored carefully, as shown by the documented dose rates in a study of 100 patients. Following I-131 therapy, most patients presented with an acceptable dose rate on the day of discharge, indicating that early and accurate assessment can facilitate safe discharge procedures and protect the patient without compromising the treatment effect, as cited in (Asli et al., 2013). More importantly, regulatory mechanisms responsible for radiation dosimetry play a significant role in contributing to the availability of safe levels of doses. Global standards, such as the International Basic Safety Standards, provide a general framework for radiation protective measures in all health care settings. The regional regulatory bodies then modify these standards to account for local health care practices and technological advancements, making them more effective and useful. Compliance with these regulatory guidelines is required to maintain minimal radiation risk without compromising patient care. Health care facilities must give top priority to ongoing review and revision of dosimetry practices to align with contemporary standards, and must also invest in training professionals in radiation protection guidelines. If those principles are observed with commitment, patient safety can be substantially integrated across all areas of radiation therapy, thereby reiterating the need to establish safe dose limits in clinical practice.

10.2.3. Impact on Treatment Planning

In the rapidly changing world of cancer treatment, the incorporation of individualized dosimetry plays a central role in achieving maximum treatment effectiveness and safety. Targeted alpha therapy (TαT) is an innovative manifestation of this potential, promising to deliver maximum tumor control while minimizing damage to normal tissue. This solution underscores the importance of dosimetry-based individualized treatment planning, which modulates radiation dose based on individual pharmacokinetic and tumor-relevant calculations. As evidenced by clinical trials, including the ALSYMPCA trial using radium-223, dose individualization has been shown to enhance overall survival in bone-metastatic prostate cancer patients, underscoring the pivotal link between precise dose assessment and effective treatment outcomes (Vincentis et al., 2019). Integrating sophisticated dosimetry into treatment plans is, therefore, imperative for optimal therapeutic gain along with patient safety (Figure 10.8).

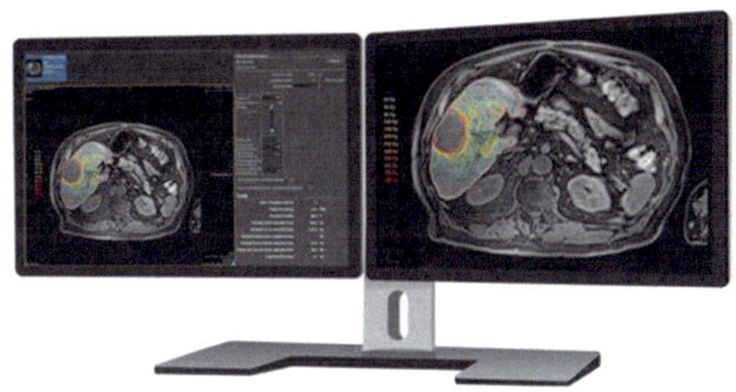

Figure 10.8. Integration of dosimetry in personalized treatment planning software.

Source: https://www.bostonscientific.com/en-US/products/cancer-therapies/simplicit90y-personalized-dosimetry-software/_jcr_content/maincontentpar/image_1908376351.img.simplicit90Y-software-two-screens.png.

The consequences of accurate dosimetry extend far beyond efficacy, shaping patient treatment planning at a fundamental level. Correctly measured doses, enabled by devices like thermoluminescent dosimeters and optically stimulated luminescence, deliver critical information that influences clinical choice. By using these technologies, health practitioners can guarantee that the delivered radiation is tightly matched with intended therapeutic objectives, therefore eliminating underdosage or toxicity potential (Seibert et al., 2018). This optimization not only meets regulatory needs but also enhances overall quality of care for the patient. Further, periodic monitoring and readjustment of the treatment plan based on real-time dosimetry information allow for more responsive, patient-specific, and tailored interventions. Effective communication of radiation risks and treatment options is also crucial in treatment planning, as it allows patients to make informed choices about their treatment. The process of informed consent becomes an interactive discussion where dosimetry data, the risks, and benefits of the treatment are intelligently communicated. Patient education materials that clarify the principles of radiation safety and dosimetry practice can depersonalize the treatment process, instilling confidence and fostering participation in relationships between patients and healthcare workers. This underscores an integrated approach to planning treatments, where technical accuracy in dosimetry is complemented by empathetic patient care. Lastly, synergizing sound dosimetry with sound communication practices guarantees that radiation therapy not only effectively treats cancerous tumors but also prioritizes patient comfort and safety.

10.3. Regulatory Standards and Guidelines

Regulatory rules and standards play a central role in the practice of radiation dosimetry by providing significant frameworks that ensure patients' and healthcare professionals' safety. The [International Basic Safety Standards (IBSS)] sets the foundation upon which national regulations for ionizing radiation have been fashioned, protection and safety principles being put forward as ought to be adopted by member states. This worldwide strategy ensures cross-border cooperation, allowing countries to implement these regulations within their respective healthcare systems while preserving essential safety protocols. Most of these regulations mandate that medical facilities adhere to specific radiation dose levels for patients and tolerable exposure rates for staff, thereby minimizing the probable health risks associated with radiation exposure. It is the duty of local regulatory bodies to implement and enforce these international standards. Local regulatory bodies tend to develop policies based on IBSS' broader principles, which are then tailored to regional healthcare and technological needs. The customization and breakdown of these standards into local legislation are also important, as they address regional variations in radiation procedures and patient care. Furthermore, local governments have the responsibility to ensure compliance, conduct inspections, and implement training programs that educate medical staff on best practices in radiation safety. This regulatory oversight enhances not only the quality of care but also public trust in medical facilities by demonstrating a commitment to patient safety and adherence to internationally recognized best practices. Accreditation standards further identify the function of regulatory standards in radiation dosimetry. Accreditation is one way to ensure that health facilities adhere to established safety standards and clinical practices, which is important for delivering high-quality patient care. Organizations such as the American Association of Physicists in Medicine support maintaining best practices through their medical physics practice guidelines (MPPG) (Seibert et al., 2018). These regulations are regularly reviewed and updated to reflect technological changes and new information in the field, keeping the standards current and effective. Additionally, implementing continuous quality improvement programs in radiation practices enhances dosimetry, thereby improving patient outcomes. Implementing these regulatory systems together helps healthcare facilities systematically control and avert radiation exposure hazards, thus ensuring patient safety.

10.3.1. National and International Dosimetry Standards

National and international dosimetry standards

play a key role in ensuring patient safety in radiological procedures. The standards provide guidelines for determining protocols that dictate the measurement and control of radiation doses given to patients.

Target organ	Radiation dose (μGy/MBq)
Adrenals	3.4
Brain	5.5
Breasts	1.9
Gallbladder wall	35.6
Lower large intestine wall	2.4
Small intestine	4.1
Stomach wall	2.6
Upper large intestine wall	2.8
Heart wall	12.8
Kidneys	13.5
Liver	13.8
Lungs	11.2
Muscle	2.1
Ovaries	2.5
Pancreas	3.5
Red marrow	5.0
Osteogenic cells	4.5
Skin	1.5
Spleen	11.9
Testes	1.8
Thymus	2.3
Thyroid	1.9
Urinary bladder wall	15.7
Uterus	2.8
Total body	2.8
Effective dose (μSv/MBq)	5.0

Figure 10.9. Radiation dosimetry estimates for 11 C-NOP-1A in standard reference man.

Source: https://www.researchgate.net/profile/Sami-Zoghbi/publication/51608278/figure/tbl1/AS:669356577021976@1536598452822/Radiation-Dosimetry-Estimates-for-11-C-NOP-1A-in-Standard-Reference-Man.png.

International organizations such as the International Atomic Energy Agency (IAEA) and the World Health Organization (WHO) have developed regulations to control dosimetry practices and ensure consistency and accuracy worldwide. Specifically, the IAEAs safety standards allude to the need for extensive training and optimization procedures for radiology staff in a bid to limit risks of possible exposures, as elucidated in various technical meetings where authorities shared experience and best practices (Damilakis et al., 2017). By adhering to these standards, healthcare institutions can limit overexposure incidents to an absolute minimum, thereby improving patient outcomes and safety. In addition to establishing a regulatory environment, dosimetry standards provide a foundation for medical physicists' and practitioners' accreditation requirements (Figure 10.9).

The American Association of Physicists in Medicine (AAPM) has a significant role in making and distributing updated practice guidelines that adapt to the evolving environment of dosimetry (Seibert et al., 2018). These practices aim to ensure that healthcare practitioners use appropriate means and devices to measure radiation doses, such as thermoluminescent dosimeters and optically stimulated luminescence. To this end, the guidelines are regularly updated and revised, and with due consideration to advancing technology and methodology, thereby maintaining the highest level of safety in the practice of medicine. The rigorous consensus process used to develop the guidelines ensures they are not only comprehensive but also transferable across various clinical settings, fostering an organizational culture of quality and safety in care delivery. Regular communication regarding the risks of radiation, based on standardized dosimetry standards, enhances patient safety and aids in informed consent procedures. Proper educational materials must be developed that address radiation doses in diagnostic and therapeutic scenarios. Medical professionals must also address patients regarding potential hazards and the protective procedures taken to reduce them. As outlined in IAEA recommendations, proactive measureshandling overexposures are essential for building accountability within healthcare organizations

(Damilakis et al., 2017). By fostering a culture of transparency, practitioners can not only increase patient understanding and confidence but also work together to reduce the stigma that may be associated with radiation exposure in the medical environment.

10.3.2. The Role of Organizations like the ICRP and NCRP

Under dosimetry and radiation safety, organizations such as the International Commission on Radiological Protection (ICRP) and the National Council on Radiation Protection and Measurements (NCRP) establish guidelines that establish clinical practices globally. These organizations conduct extensive research and provide evidence-based recommendations to establish radiation protection standards that ensure patient safety (Figure 10.10).

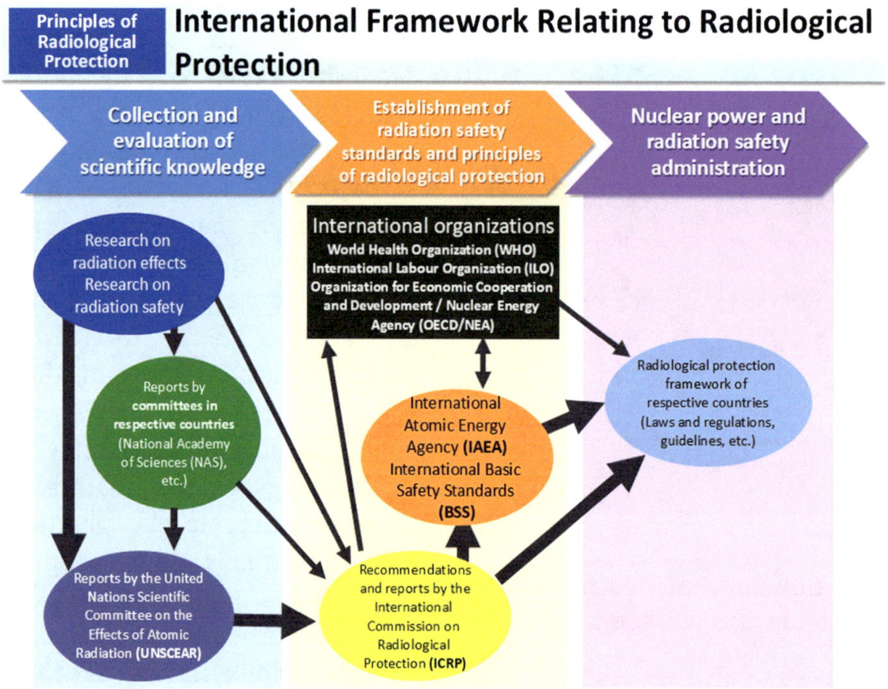

Figure 10.10. Radiological protection system [MOE].

Source: https://www.env.go.jp/en/chemi/rhm/basic-info/1st/img/img-04-01-01.png.

ICRPs guidelines, for instance, are crucial in establishing the criteria for dose limits and risk assessments that are fundamental to ensuring safe uses of radiological technologies. Furthermore, their ongoing efforts to raise public awareness of radiation hazards underscore the importance of informed consent and patient education in alleviating anxiety about imaging studies and the associated radiation exposure. Secondly, the activities of these bodies cover quantifying acceptable doses in a majority of medical situations, encouraging optimized protocol usage in radiation practice. For example, the NCRP has provided detailed guidance on optimal procedures for minimizing patient radiation exposure during diagnostic imaging. Their reports indicate that, with emerging imaging technology, there is potential for both greater efficacy and the risk of higher doses if not properly controlled. It speaks to the need for constant monitoring and standardization, as well as what the NCRPs promotion of national standards specifically recommends, particularly in nations such as Nigeria, where differences in radiological practice create variable patient doses. This desire for regulatory consistency reflects an overall intent of keeping radiation doses as low as reasonably achievable yet still achieving clinical objectives (Olarinoye et al., 2010). In addition, the dynamic nature of radiation protection standards reflects the evolving nature of medical imaging. Both the ICRP and NCRP provide immediate guidelines and highlight the need for an adaptive regulatory framework capable of addressing technological advances and emerging research evidence. Their collective action aims to engage the stakeholders along the healthcare continuum, creating a culture of safety in the patient care settings. This is particularly the case as guidelines for practices like patient contact shielding are updated; for instance, the NCRPs stance against shielding gonads and thyroid glands from specific imaging procedures indicates an increasing trend towards evidence-based practice (Benavides et al., 2023). Ultimately, the efforts of bodies such as the ICRP and the NCRP play a crucial role in keeping the complexity of radiation dosimetry in check, ensuring patient safety even amid rapid technological developments.

10.3.3. Compliance and Enforcement Mechanisms

Compliance mechanisms and enforcement frameworks are critical in radiation dosimetry and patient protection, as they ensure that guidelines and regulations are adhered to. These are not only engaged in developing regulatory frameworks but also with active surveillance and monitoring of practices within healthcare facilities. Regulatory bodies at the international and national levels play important roles by setting standards that limit radiation exposure and establish safety criteria. International Basic Safety Standards (IBSS) act as a model for these jurisdictions and ensure protection for patients and health workers against undue exposure to radiation. In addition, compliance is typically measured through ongoing audits and inspections to ensure that medical facilities adhere to rigorous safety protocols. Proper governance in this manner helps sustain public confidence in medical imaging and therapeutic services. Regulations aside, compliance and implementation largely depend on medical staff training and education. Routine professional development courses are employed to reaffirm the information and skill of healthcare workers in the field of radiation safety procedures (Figure 10.11).

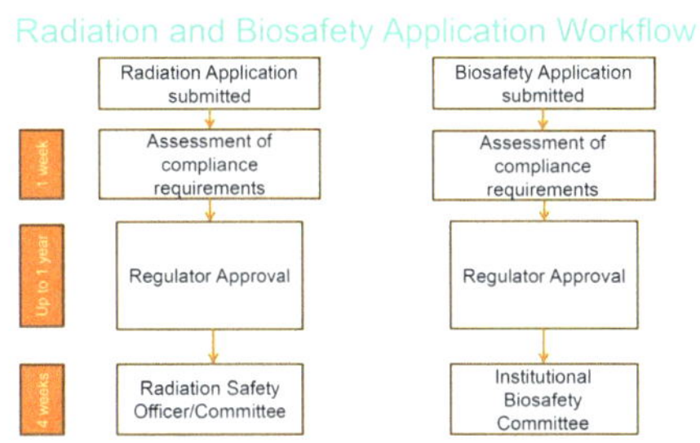

Figure 10.11. Inspection and compliance workflow for radiation safety protocols.

Source: https://slideplayer.com/slide/17517779/103/images/14/Radiation+and+Biosafety+Application+Workflow.jpg.

The use of accreditation standards ensures that facilities not only possess the needed technology but also follow the operational standards needed to ensure patient safety. For instance, regular training can keep employees up to date on current developments in the application of dosimetry methods and safety measures, thereby promoting a culture of safety in the health environment. This proactive approach to learning is also used in analyzing accidents or near-misses, so institutions can learn from them and change their practices to avoid future hazards. Furthermore, continuous monitoring and reporting on incidents are also key facilitators in being compliant. Facilities use dosimetry equipment and ongoing sampling to track radiation doses and test compliance with safety standards. Investigations have shown varying radiation doses across various areas of radiological practice, including CT-Scan and standard X-ray rooms, indicating the need for ongoing monitoring (Andriati et al., 2024). Measurement is utilized by departments to discover how much radiation they are exposed to and where compliance is poor. By addressing such inefficiencies, health institutions are able to take corrective action and rationalize their pattern of utilization of radiation. Lastly, an effective compliance and enforcement system not only safeguards patient health but also enhances the integrity of radiation practice within the health profession, in line with the guiding principle of safety in health procedures.

10.4. Advances in Dosimetry Technology

Technological advancements in dosimetry have significantly transformed radiation safety and patient management. New methods, such as Thermoluminescent Dosimeters (TLD) and Optically Stimulated Luminescence (OSL), enable the precise measurement of radiation doses received by patients during treatment. TLDs operate on the principle of capturing energy from ionizing radiation, which is emitted as light when heated, to give a true reading of absorbed dose. But OSL technology harnesses the excitation of electrons trapped within a crystal matrix, which subsequently emits measurable light after photo- or laser stimulation. The new dosimetry equipment has improved sensitivity compared to traditional methods, thereby allowing medical professionals to provide more accurate measures of exposure and adapt therapeutic interventions to specific patients' needs without excess risks of unwarranted radiation (Zainuddin et al., 2018). Furthermore, Metal-Oxide Semiconductor Field-Effect Transistors (MOSFET) technology in dosimetry enables real-time monitoring of radiation therapy. MOSFETs are significantly radiation-sensitive and can directly convert ionizing radiation into an electrical signal. Instant feedback on dose delivery is possible with this technology, enabling timely adjustment during treatment sessions and enhanced patient safety. Dynamic radiation exposure monitoring enables more responsive treatment delivery management, especially in achieving precise dosimetry, which can lead to improved therapeutic results. As healthcare advances, such advanced dosimetric tools are central to ensuring patient safety at the core of radiation treatment modalities (Blancafort et al., 2023). Finally, the integration of more sophisticated dosimetric equipment into clinical operations raises significant regulatory and accreditation considerations. For instance, requirements such as those established by the International Basic Safety Standards emphasize ongoing training and education throughout the application of higher-level technologies. To properly utilize high-level dosimetry equipment, healthcare facilities must align with local regulatory bodies to ensure compliance with required safety standards. Such a correspondence not only contributes to operating capacity but also reiterates the commitment to patient safety and the reduction of radiation exposure. As the medical world gets to feel these advancements transform, there needs to be navigation through the regulatory landscape well in advance, with facilities and practitioners adequately informed and compliant with evolving safety guidelines (Zainuddin et al., 2018).

10.4.1. Digital Dosimetry Systems

Digital dosimetry systems are a significant advancement in radiation dosimetry technology to measure and monitor radiation exposure accurately. Digital dosimetry systems utilize advanced technologies, such as semiconductor detectors, that facilitate real-time data analysis and improved dose measurement compared to other dosimetry methods. Use of digital platforms enables improved data management, immediate visualization of dose distributions, and enhanced patient monitoring. As a result, health care providers can better tailor radiological tests to patients' individual needs, achieving maximum diagnostic efficacy and safety. Digital dosimetry systems also ensure compliance with legislative standards by comparing doses with prescribed safety levels, enabling the implementation of patient safety programs (Seibert et al., 2018). Another landmark benefit of digital dosimetry systems is their capacity to automatically collect data and report it. These systems can rationalize clinical workflow processes, significantly reducing the prospect of human error associated with manual data capture. Increased traceability of doses delivered to patients is critical for quality assurance and regulatory compliance, as it establishes a culture of transparency in radiation practice. Besides, digital dosimetry systems can facilitate easy communication between medical teams, enabling real-time data transmission and timely decision-making and quick action in response to any dose concerns. Such heightened observation is vital while dealing with potential overexposures, justifying the need for monitoring strategies that emphasize patient safety and well-being (Damilakis et al., 2017). The implementation of digital dosimetry systems also poses new challenges that must be overcome to fully optimize patient safety. As these systems are designed on sophisticated hardware and software components, regular training and technical support are mandatory for clinical staff so that correct usage is ensured and mistakes in dose calculation and interpretation are minimized. Additionally, the systems must undergo frequent maintenance and updates to ensure accuracy and effectiveness across various clinical settings. It is through constant monitoring of the functionality and robustness of digital dosimetry systems that they can be effectively incorporated into clinical routines. It is critical that health centers not only invest in the systems but also develop guidelines for their use, with strict adherence to safety standards and patient care objectives (Seibert et al., 2018) (Figure 10.12).

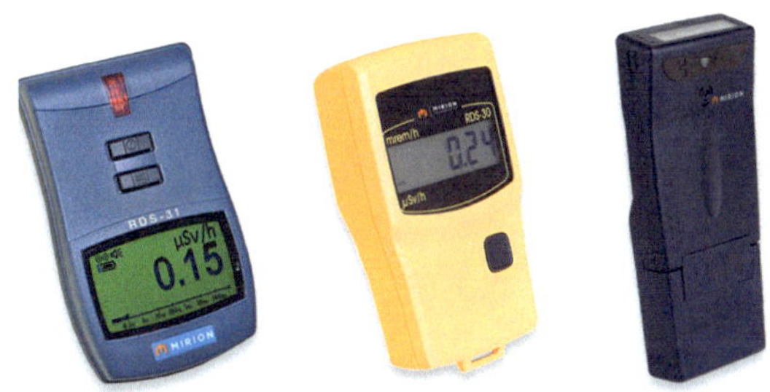

Figure 10.12. Handheld digital dosimeter used for on-site radiation measurement.

Source: https://www.southernscientific.co.uk/data/image/7/c/7c716722851a9fbe04ee892d99bcf956.1625145821.png.

10.4.2. Real-Time Monitoring Methods

The application of real-time monitoring techniques in radiation dosimetry significantly enhances patient safety in the clinical setting by providing immediate feedback on radiation dose levels. These techniques utilize advanced technologies, such as integrated dosimeters in imaging equipment and continuous monitors, to ensure doses fall within previously set safety thresholds. By providing real-time information, physicians can respond quickly to any deviation from optimal dose levels, thereby minimizing the risk of overexposure. The ongoing surveillance of exposure not only protects patients but also fosters a culture of safety and vigilance among healthcare teams, in line with the AAPM guidelines that emphasize ongoing learning and adherence to updated guidelines in practice (Seibert et al., 2018). Real-time monitoring techniques also play a crucial role in the training and education of health care personnel, who must be skilled at operating imaging equipment and be familiar with radiation protection guidelines. By utilizing these monitoring systems by personnel, health care organizations are able to maximize their dose and risk management capabilities (Figure 10.13).

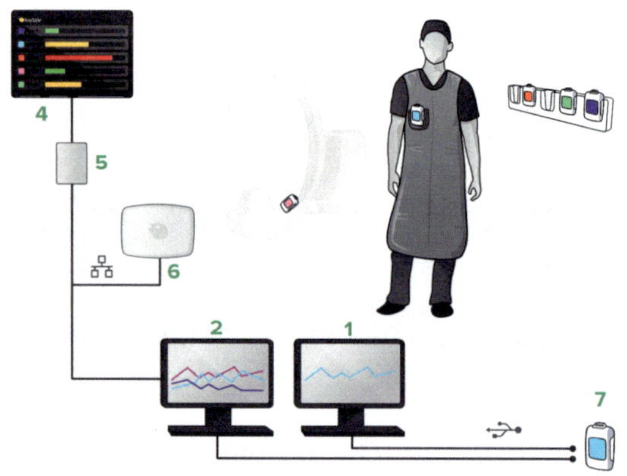

Figure 10.13. Real-time dosimetry dashboard display in a radiation therapy center.

Source: https://www.raysafe.com/sites/default/files/2020-08/raysafe_i3_configuration2.png.

The instant feedback enhances understanding of the physics of radiation and potential effects of exposure, as integrated into suggestions advocating the integration of practicum training sessions with technological support (Damilakis et al., 2017). Training of this nature ensures staff can better detect and handle potential overexposure accidents, leading to improved patient safety and quality care. Moreover, integration of bio-surveillance into clinical procedures synchronizes with contemporary bio-surveillance legislation whose intention is to safeguard patients. As healthcare infrastructure increasingly focuses on patient-centered care, these devices are not only safety measures but also compliance tools that meet national and global standards. With the potential to present thorough records of exposure degrees with on-time tracking, there is assistance for regulatory bodies' requirements of transparency and accountability in radiation therapy. Systematic record-keeping not only aids compliance with safety standards but also facilitates informed consent protocols, upholding the belief that patients should be made aware of their risk of exposure and the safety protocols related to their treatment. The integrated approach of radiation protection upholds the ethos of enhanced patient care and rigorous regulatory adherence (Seibert et al., 2018).

10.4.3. Innovations in Imaging Modalities

Advancements in imaging modalities have significantly impacted radiation dosimetry, enhancing diagnostic quality and protecting patients. Advancements in medical imaging, such as computed tomography (CT) and magnetic resonance imaging (MRI), have revolutionized medical imaging by providing complete anatomical and functional information. The elevated rate of imaging, however, has brought concerns about the associated radiation exposure in patients. This problem necessitates the inclusion of new dose-optimization techniques capable of balancing diagnostic benefits with risks. With the development of advanced dosimetry techniques, such as iterative reconstruction algorithms and adaptive exposure control, medical professionals can reduce radiation doses without compromising image quality, thereby moving towards the basic principles of radiation protection established by Seibert et al. (2018). One of the integral components of the innovations is the construction and use of advanced dosimetry devices. Thermoluminescent dosimeters (TLDs) and optically stimulated luminescence (OSL) dosimeters are increasingly used to assess patient radiation exposure. These devices offer higher sensitivity and precision with real-time feedback in clinical settings. Consequently, healthcare providers can tailor image protocols to optimize, justify, and ensure compliance with organizations' guidelines, including those of the American Association of Physicists in Medicine (Figure 10.14).

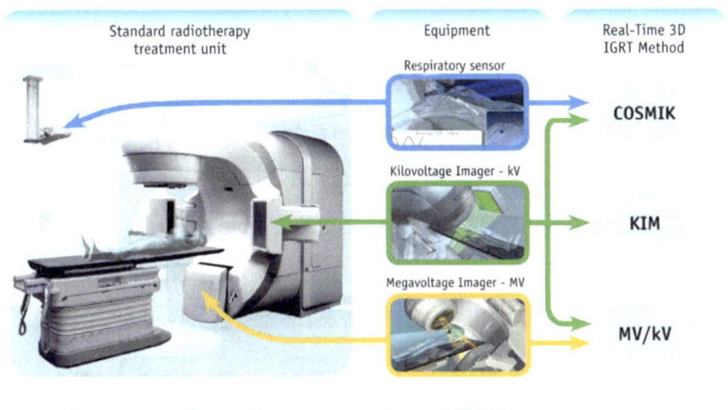

Figure 10.14. Image-guided radiotherapy system enhancing dosimetry accuracy.

Source: https://www.redjournal.org/cms/attachment/4b0ab067-c31f-4f57-97e7-ebd2be382705/gr2_lrg.jpg.

The incorporation of these new practices into routine practice is a giant leap towards ensuring patient safety in radiation-based imaging, thus necessitating continuous training and education within the practice, as highlighted by Seibert et al. (2018). Furthermore, regulatory systems have an essential role to ensure monitoring of incorporation of innovations within imaging modalities without jeopardizing patient safety. Local regulations and the International Basic Safety Standards are complemented and synergized by regulatory bodies to ensure safe practices in medical imaging. Accreditation requirements supplement this process by creating a formalized plan under which facilities operate in accordance with best radiation dosimetry practices. Continuous monitoring and revision of these standards are critical to enable technological advancements and to reflect the realities of actual healthcare practice. Documenting activities and the appropriate distribution of patient educational materials are also vital components of awareness and understanding radiation exposure consequences. Embracing a holistic approach to radiation safety, the medical profession aims to foster an environment of informed consent and proactive risk communication, as outlined by Zainuddin et al. (2018).

10.5. Challenges in Radiation Dosimetry

In radiation dosimetry, there are a number of issues that make accurately measuring and controlling the radiation absorbed by patients hard. They include inconsistencies in measurement processes, leading to differences in reported doses. Some dosimetry methods, for instance, TLD and OSL, can yield different results when tested under the same conditions. These variations can be due to variations in calibration, environmental conditions, and natural detector sensitivity when detectors are used. Furthermore, variation in patient anatomy and patient position during imaging or treatment increases the difficulty of estimating the dose. These uncertainties necessitate improved calibration standards and advanced techniques to ensure uniformity and reliability in dosimetry, which is crucial in protecting the patients and ensuring effective treatment. Dose optimization is another critical aspect of radiation dosimetry, particularly in terms of patient protection. Coupled with advanced imaging and treatment technologies, though beneficial, they introduce complexity in the management of radiation exposure. As methodologies improve, clinicians must tailor radiation protocols to individual patient requirements without compromising safety.

Adaptive exposure control and iterative reconstruction methods can help to optimize dose delivery but come with challenges. The personnel must be adequately trained to use these technologies proficiently to ensure minimal patient doses while achieving optimal therapeutic results. Frequent monitoring and evaluation of the dose distribution must also be conducted to prevent hazards caused by incidental overexposure. In the absence of such optimization challenges, the threat of adverse effects still remains a concern for radiation treatment and diagnostic imaging. Governmental systems are also vital in solving problems in radiation dosimetry. International and national regulations control practices according to radiation exposure and ensure that safety protocols are upheld. Enforcement and compliance with such standards, however, vary considerably from institution to institution and by locations, primarily based on the available resources and technology. Such variability could lead to inconsistent dosimetry methods, potentially putting patients at risk. Moreover, the technical nature of radiation protection regulations could pose barriers to healthcare practitioners in understanding and implementing required protocols. Strengthening these control systems and encouraging better education about the risks of radiation are needed to improve safety protocols associated with radiation dosimetry and to develop a culture of safety in healthcare environments. More research on practical techniques of risk communication will further improve informed decision-making for patients and practitioners.

10.5.1. Variability in Patient Anatomy

Variability in patient anatomy is a severe threat to the dosimetry of radiation and the delivery of treatment. Differences in organ size, shape, and position among patients can affect the dosimetric accuracy of radiation therapy. Differences in lung volume due to disease states, such as atelectasis, can significantly alter the positions of tumors throughout the treatment period. Studies have indicated that atelectasis patients had greater tumor displacements outside normal setup margins, necessitating repeated imaging to enable adequate patient management (Tennyson et al., 2017). Anatomical variability such as this underscores the importance of personalized treatment plans that account for each patient's unique characteristics to enhance treatment accuracy and safety. In addition to affecting treatment delivery, anatomical variability also complicates accurate dose measurement. Techniques such as thermoluminescent dosimeters and optically stimulated luminescence are essential for dose calculation, but their accuracy can be influenced by variable anatomical features. The fluid-filled nature of certain organs, including the urinary bladder, further complicates dosimetric accuracy because organ position and volume vary throughout the course of treatment. These issues require combining invasive and non-invasive measurement methods to obtain comprehensive information on delivered thermal doses and to improve treatment outcomes in diseases such as bladder cancer (Bakker et al., 2016). To address these issues, adaptive methods in radiation therapy are needed to achieve optimal dosimetry and patient protection. Real-time imaging and adaptive exposure control protocols can adjust treatment plans to accommodate anatomical changes encountered during radiation delivery. Better iterative reconstruction algorithms also enhance treatment precision by reducing unnecessary radiation exposure to normal tissues. By implementing such adaptive methods in the clinical environment, medical practitioners can better address the variability in patient anatomy, ultimately achieving greater therapeutic efficiency with lower radiation-related complications. Emphasis on the need for ongoing evaluation and readjustments is essential to ensure high-quality radiation protection and patient management (Figure 10.15).

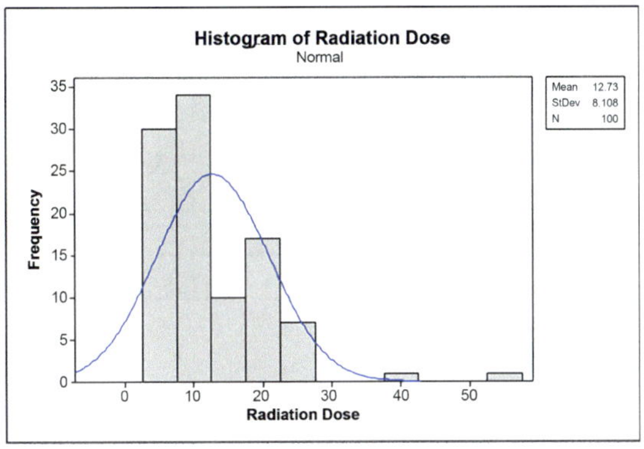

Figure 10.15. Comparison of radiation dose distribution in patients of varying body sizes.

Source: https://www.researchgate.net/figure/Radiation-dose-distribution-among-patients_fig1_320557011.

10.5.2. Limitations of Current Dosimetry Methods

The malfunction of current dosimetry technologies offers an enormous challenge in the successful control of radiation in healthcare facilities. Conventional dosimetry devices, such as the thermoluminescent dosimeters (TLD) and optically stimulated luminescence (OSL) dosimeters, are frequently not able to provide immediate dose feedback following exposure to radiation.

Technique	Pros	Cons
Planar scintigraphy	Easily accessible and cost effective	Lack of anatomical information results in relatively low accuracy
	Suitable for routine clinical use	Organs with a high ^{177}Lu uptake, such as the kidneys, may receive an underestimated dose
	Easy to perform and simple to understand	Inaccurate when organs overlap
SPECT	Better spatial resolution than planar scintigraphy	Specialized equipment is required
	Determine the activity distribution in three dimensions accurately	Complex and time-consuming process compared to planar scintigraphy
	An improved dose estimation method	Patient motion can affect measurements
		Inaccurate when organs overlap due to Partial Volume Effect (PVE)
Time activity curve analysis	Improves the accuracy of time activity curves for each organ	More frequent blood sampling and imaging is required
	Estimation of radiation absorbed dose is better than planar scintigraphy and SPECT	Results may vary between different institutions according to calculation methods
Monte Carlo simulation	Simulating radiation behavior in tissues with high accuracy	Computationally demanding and time-consuming
	Calculates the dosimetry accurately	Expertise and specialized software are required
		Simulation sensitivity to input parameters
Hybrid imaging	Enhances accuracy by combining anatomical and functional information	Equipment and expertise are required
	Better radiation absorbed dose estimation than planar scintigraphy or SPECT alone	Time-consuming and costly imaging
		Inaccurate when organs overlap

Figure 10.16. Advantages and disadvantages of different dosimetry techniques.

Source: https://www.researchgate.net/publication/372800941/figure/tbl2/AS:11431281178366307@1690900908123/Advantages-and-disadvantages-of-different-dosimetry-techniques.png.

A lack of immediate dose monitoring may lead to accidental overexposure, as sudden fluctuations in radiation levels are the norm, particularly during complex interventional procedures. For instance, incompetence in training staff in the operation of equipment and optimization protocols has been reported as one of the main causes of exacerbating overexposure accidents, which demand a serious reevaluation of dosimetry protocols aimed at enhancing patient safety and preventing associated risks of stochastic consequences (Damilakis et al., 2017). Moreover, interference from passive dosimetry methods can affect accurate measurement of occupational exposure for anesthesia professionals and ancillary staff working close to the radiographic equipment. Unlike surgeons and interventionalists, anesthesia professionals generally do not have access to protective barriers and monitoring equipment that can limit exposure during fluoroscopically guided procedures (Figure 10.16).

In the absence of adequate precautions and data about radiation hazards, such workers may be exposed to more health hazards, including radiation-induced cataracts and other adverse health consequences. Past research indicates a gross deficiency in awareness and training among such workers, underscoring the need for enhanced education interventions and appropriate equipment to ensure workplace safety (Filbert et al., 2022). Finally, the limitations of existing dosimetry techniques highlight the need for more sophisticated methods to measure radiation exposure, such as integrating dosimetry with emerging imaging modalities. Existing practices are often based on broad risk models that do not account for patient-specific susceptibility to radiation injury. Consequently, this jack-of-all-trades technique can inaccurately define the risks posed to specific patient populations, for example, pregnant women or children. To address these limitations, additional research is needed to further enhance dosimetry techniques and improve dose measurement precision. These improvements are essential for developing optimized radiation protection guidelines and enhancing regulatory policies aimed at patient and occupational protection in radiation dosimetry (Damilakis et al., 2017).

10.5.3. Addressing Human Error in Dosimetry

Human dosimetry mistakes are critical for patient safety, particularly in cases of radiation exposure due to therapeutic and diagnostic interventions. Inaccurate dose delivery can lead to adverse overexposure or underexposure, jeopardizing treatment efficacy and safety. Such issues require a multi-pronged approach that includes rigorous training programs for health professionals, ongoing audits of dosimetry practices, and the creation of a safety culture within hospitals. These measures aim to reduce the risk of human miscalculation by ensuring that all stakeholders are well informed about the intricacies of dosimetry and the consequential implications in the event of mistakes. The incorporation of technology, including automated dose calculation and real-time monitoring systems, is aimed at reducing the margin of error further to improve patient safety in radiation-associated procedures (Figure 10.17).

To properly address human error in dosimetry, continuous education and awareness programs for medical practitioners need to be implemented. Such programs would emphasize concepts of radiation physics, proper dose measurement, and adherence to specified protocols. Regular training programs can equip people to guard against potential errors and provide exposure to state-of-the-art dosimetry devices, such as thermoluminescent dosimeters and optically stimulated luminescence sensors. Such a human capital investment not only enhances the competence of healthcare teams but also reinforces a culture of responsibility and a commitment to patient safety. In a compliance environment, the inclusion of guidelines from authoritative bodies can enhance procedural stringency, thereby reducing the likelihood of human error in the dosing of ionizing radiation. Also, the standards that are instituted by local and international bodies are essential in minimizing human error in dosimetry. Bodies such as the International Atomic Energy Agency establish safety standards that are implemented at the local level through adaptation and operationalization. Compliance with these standards by health units ensures that their dosimetry standards align with existing safety guidelines, thereby minimizing the risk of errors. Routine compliance audits and accreditation standards strive to further assist the implementation of these models by encouraging excellence in the workforce. Continuous improvement is not only encouraged for technical performance in dosimetry but also includes avenues for feedback on continuous improvement of patient safety practice. Hence, the intersection of human factors and regulation compliance is crucial to addressing the complexity of dosimetry errors, supporting the importance of a system-oriented approach to ensuring patient health and well-being (Impens et al., 2019).

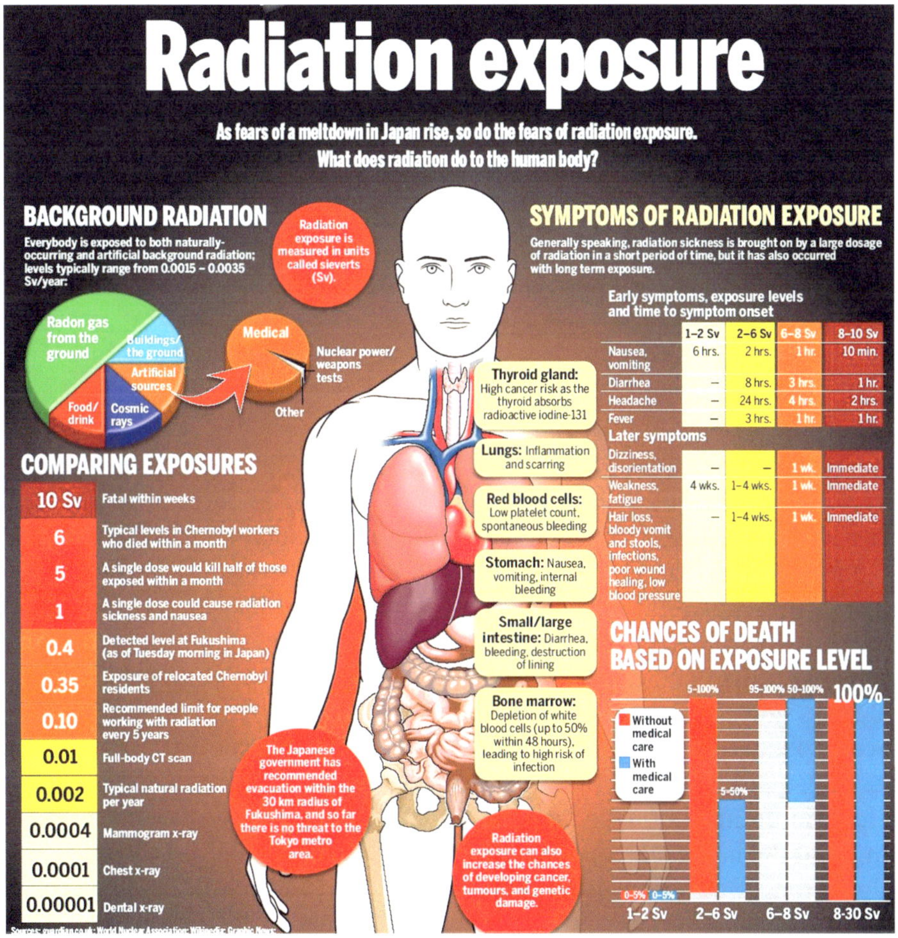

Figure 10.17. What effect does radiation have on the body?

Source: https://iccareprodstorage.blob.core.windows.net/prod-20220426/cms4_instadose/files/blog-images/what_effect_does_radiation_have_on_the_body.jpg?1565297052.

10.6. Case Studies in Patient Safety

While searching case studies on patient safety with regard to radiation dosimetry, significant attention must be devoted to the developments in imaging technologies that have taken place to enhance both safety and performance in clinical practice. For instance, a recent study reported that a new X-ray system for coronary angiography procedures led to a remarkable 75% decrease in patient radiation exposure without compromising diagnostic image quality. This technique illustrates the potential of technology to minimize the risk posed by high radiation doses. Through careful calibration and optimization of acquisition parameters, clinicians can substantially reduce the kerma-area product without compromising the high level of detail required to enhance clinical decision-making. These observations highlight the need for ongoing technological advancements in improving patient safety and outcomes, consistent with the broader objective of reducing risk in medical radiation use (Bacher et al., 2015). Additionally, proper handling of radiation exposure accidents is critical to protecting patient safety. Injuries arising from overexposure can be severe. Thus strict protocols and staff training are needed for diagnostic and interventional radiology. A combination of international guidelines highlights the need to implement preventive measures, such as checklists and time-outs, to improve procedural safety. This minimizes the potential for overexposures and ensures that staff members are adequately trained in the use of equipment and dose-optimization techniques. Accident learning is of the highest priority since it aids in the detection of potential loopholes in procedures and enhances practices better to reduce the risks of stochastic effects from radiation exposure. Here, an interdisciplinary strategy among healthcare professionals can go a long way towards enhancing patient safety, instilling an atmosphere of vigilance and continuous improvement (Damilakis et al., 2017). Finally, patient safety research through the lens of radiation dosimetry requires a multidisciplinary effort that integrates regulatory principles and effective communication strategies. Following international safety standards and country-specific regulations is critical to ensuring high-quality patient care. Secondly, the informed consent process is crucial for educating patients about the risks and benefits of radiological procedures. A clear explanation of radiation exposure and safety precautions enhances patients' knowledge and reaffirms their confidence in the health professional. Extensive patient education tools can enable patients to be active participants in their care, with an understanding of possible hazards. Coordination of these factors with an apparatus system actually leads to improved outcomes and a remarkable reduction in adverse events related to radiation exposure (Bacher et al., 2015).

10.6.1. Analysis of Radiation Overexposure Incidents

In research on cases of radiation overexposure, it is essential to understand the multifaceted nature of these events, particularly in diagnostic and interventional radiology environments. Overexposures may result in uncomfortable effects, such as tissue reactions, particularly during high-dose procedures like computed tomography (CT) scans and interventional radiology procedures. These events are often the result of various deficiencies, including poor personnel training and improper equipment use, underscoring the importance of sound quality assurance procedures. The creation of detailed guidelines and the implementation of systematic checks, such as pre-procedure time-outs and dose warnings, are crucial for limiting the adverse effects of radiation exposure. Awareness of such risks and learning from previous errors will aid healthcare organizations in strengthening their procedures and furthering patient safety outcomes significantly, as well as indirectly reducing corresponding psychological issues regarding the risk of radiation that patients may have (Damilakis et al., 2017). Furthermore, the continuous evolution of radiological apparatus necessitates continual reassessment of quality assurance protocols to prevent overexposure. In radiotherapy, where accurate dose delivery is at stake, conventional QA procedures risk unnecessarily putting patients in harm's way. The exploration of new tools for patient-specific quality assurance has become the most vital role in keeping up with the rapid evolution of technology in this field. New methods, such as independent monitor unit verification and time-resolved dosimetry, can enhance accuracy during treatment planning and delivery. Also, the incorporation of statistical process control frameworks allows for a serious investigation of these systems in several centers, which demonstrates a concern with patient safety. Lastly, the inclusion of sophisticated technologies and regular checks in the radiation framework reduces the potential for overexposure but increases the efficiency of treatment (Nordström et al., 2012). An investigation of overexposure incidents extends beyond technical analyses; it should incorporate detailed risk communication procedures and regulatory criteria. Correct communication during the informed consent process is essential to ascertain that patients understand the risks associated with radiation. Patient education literature can put those risks into perspective and highlight the importance of adhering to safety protocols. Regulatory bodies must also develop guidelines and oversight procedures to ensure that facilities obtain accreditation and maintain operational best practices. By adopting an accountability and transparency culture, medical practitioners are better positioned to address incidents of overexposure while building public confidence. Finally, the marriage of good communication and rigorous regulatory frameworks is most critical in ensuring optimal patient safety and reducing the incidence of radiation overexposure events in clinics (Damilakis et al., 2017) (Figure 10.18).

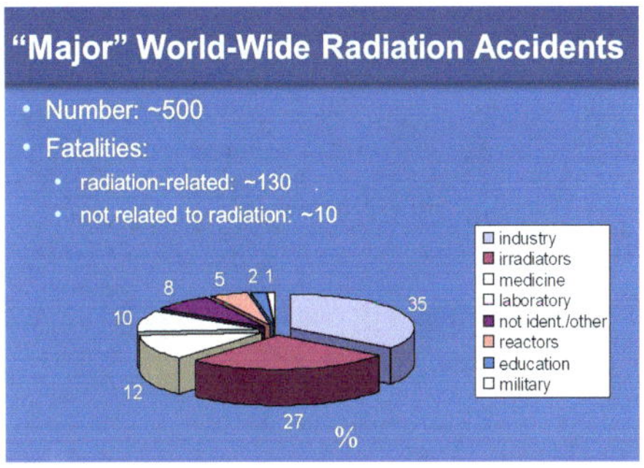

Figure 10.18. Major radiation overexposure incidents worldwide.

Source: https://slideplayer.com/slide/17926078/105/images/3/Major+World-Wide+Radiation+Accidents.jpg.

10.6.2. Successful Implementation of Dosimetry Protocols

Proper implementation of dosimetry protocols is key to enhancing patient safety throughout radiation therapy and imaging diagnostics. Development of integrative dosimetry protocols not only enables precise dosimetry of radiation doses but also ensures that the doses are linked with clinical results. Protocols must be tailored to the distinct needs of each procedure, employing sophisticated technology to increase exposure while reducing risks. For instance, utilization of devices like thermoluminescent dosimeters and metal-oxide semiconductor field-effect transistors enhances the dose accuracy, thus avoiding harm to both patients and medical professionals. Furthermore, the development of a culture of safety through collaboration among radiologists, medical physicists, and radiographers facilitates the implementation of shared, agreed-upon dosimetry standards, thereby leading to improved patient treatment outcomes and care. Apart from technicalities, the application of dosimetry protocols in practice largely relies on ongoing training and education.

As Current guidelines highlight, training deficits among staff may result from excessive exposure, particularly to complex procedures such as interventional radiology (Damilakis et al., 2017) (Figure 10.19).

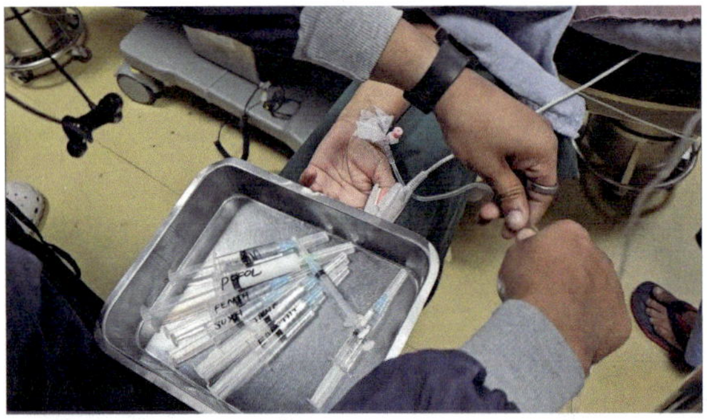

Figure 10.19. Hospital implementing electronic dosimetry protocol with staff training.

Source: https://i.ytimg.com/vi/jPlfqGkUVus/maxresdefault.jpg?sqp=-oaymwEmCIAKENAF8quKqQMa8AEB-AH-CYAC0AWKAgwIABABGGUgWSg-MA8=&rs=AOn4CLAY9YLr86REBnCVlPyVai63YaSWVw.

Thus, inpatient departments of organizations should prioritize professional development programs that allow employees to possess skills needed for the use of equipment, along with optimization procedures. The programs must also include training for real-world situations, emphasizing the importance of adhering to the provided protocols and understanding the impact of radiation exposure. Along with checklists and time-out procedures before clinical procedures, health teams are being prepared to actively avoid risks through emphasizing the importance of precise procedural adherence to patient safety. The creation of a strict regulatory framework is also key to ensuring effective deployment of dosimetry protocols. Organizations need to align their protocols with international standards, including those set by the International Atomic Energy Agency (IAEA). Alignment also enhances safety policies as well as creates a clear framework for managing exposure to radiation accidents. As observed in practices across various healthcare institutions, communicating the hazards of radiation and implementing clear policies for managing overexposures facilitate compliance with dosimetry protocols (Bar-Ad et al., 2019). Accreditation agencies also play critical roles in ensuring that they apply these standards and offer advice on best practice in dose optimization. By combining trained staff, technological innovation, and close compliance with regulatory guidelines, institutions have the potential to significantly enhance the efficacy and safety of medical procedures conducted using radiation.

10.6.3. Lessons from Previous Failure

Past radiation dosimetry errors are learning milestones that underscore the importance of high-quality safety precautions in patient care. Past events, particularly those involving excessive radiation exposure, remind us of the importance of high-quality assurance. Such mistakes show that old ways can lead to highly catastrophic outcomes and prompt the re-examination of existing systems and standards. For instance, the history of experience has driven technological innovation and quality assessment, emphasizing the need to adopt new solutions. Based on recent literature, support for the production of standardized practice, particularly in the low- to middle-income countries, must be cautious about quality and safety concerns in order not to repeat past errors (Meghzifene et al., 2016). Hence, conscientiously studying and reviewing past mistakes is a prerequisite for establishing a culture of safety in radiation therapy, prompting professionals to demand higher levels of practice. In radiation dosimetry, learning from past mistakes underscores the need for continuous education and training for health workers. A typical trend among documented cases is the collapse of communication and inadequate training, leading to errors in treatment delivery. The development of holistic training courses that cover both the technical aspects of dosimetry and the ethical facets of patient handling becomes crucial. Evidence indicates that health professionals must remain abreast with emerging technologies and best practices to ensure adequate patient safety (Nordström et al., 2012). Developing an informed workforce with the knowledge to identify potential errors before they result in adverse outcomes can significantly lower risks (Figure 10.20).

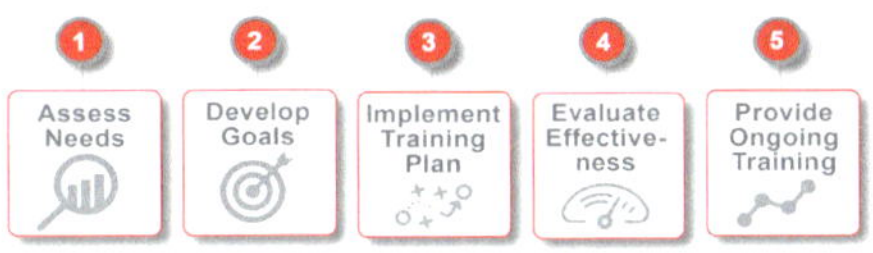

Figure 10.20. Creating a comprehensive system training plan.

Source: https://www.bwf.com/wp-content/uploads/2021/03/five-ways-training-strategies.jpg.

By establishing a culture that promotes continuous learning, healthcare organizations are better positioned to prepare staff to address emergent challenges related to radiation exposure and patient safety. In addition, the building of sound regulatory frameworks based on past blunders enhances the overall safety and performance of radiation therapy. Regulatory bodies have a crucial role in setting and refining standards that healthcare practitioners must meet, particularly in the wake of past failures that have compromised patient safety. International Basic Safety Standards and national laws should not focus solely on compliance but also on promoting a proactive approach to risk management. The effectiveness of accreditation processes in assessing practice and institutions has been emphasized by previous experience, with increased accountability for radiation practices being introduced (Meghzifene et al., 2016). Such frameworks should ensure transparency in incident reporting and enhance collaboration among stakeholders to promote patient safety. Experience gained from the past is used to create more robust systems focused on the well-being of individuals receiving radiation therapy.

SUMMARY

In summary, the interface between radiation dosimetry and patient safety is crucial for reducing the risks associated with medical imaging and treatment. As the above discussion highlights, precise dose measurement and optimization techniques are required to ensure patients receive the minimum amount of radiation exposure. The development of dosimetry technologies and methods, including thermoluminescent dosimeters and Monte Carlo simulations, enables clinicians and medical physicists to have the tools required to assess and control patient doses appropriately. For instance, studies have confirmed the potential to achieve linear relationships between effective doses and dose-area products, enabling the application of responsible dose management practices that ensure patient safety is a core issue while still allowing effective diagnosis and treatment (Cannavale et al., 2015). Even more importantly, the importance of open communication regarding radiation risks can never be overstated; it plays a crucial role in guaranteeing patient satisfaction and compliance with safety standards. Engaging patients in informed consent and providing educational materials make the procedures they undergo less mysterious and foster trust among patients in healthcare professionals. As with the situation with iodine-131 treatment for differentiated thyroid cancer, if patients also understand the reasonableness of their treatment and efforts made to ensure their safety, they will be more adherent to treatment protocols and discharge instructions, such as waiting for their exposure rates to be evaluated enough before their release from the hospital (Asli et al., 2013). This interactive capability underscores the critical need for complete radiation risk communication in the clinical setting. Ultimately, the regulatory frameworks that govern radiation dosimetry—and their enforcement at local and international levels—are the cornerstone of patient protection. Effective regulatory agencies and stringent accreditation requirements create environments where education, training, and technological innovation converge to minimize radiation exposure and enhance safety standards. Periodic review of these guidelines, based on new evidence and optimal practice, is necessary to keep pace with innovation in medical imaging technology and patient treatment. By affirming dosimetry principles and diligent care to ensure patient safety and health, health organizations can guarantee that the benefits of radiation application in medicine far outweigh its risks, resulting in improved patient outcomes.

CLOSER LOOK

EMERGING TRENDS IN DOSIMETRY: AI INTEGRATION, PATIENT AWARENESS, AND REGULATORY COMPLIANCE

As the field of radiation dosimetry evolves, technical advances and analytical methods will likely play a major role in shaping future trends. New dosimetry systems, such as real-time dosimeters, have the potential to be more precise in measuring absorbed doses. Such systems have the potential to replace traditional dosimetry techniques, enabling more precise radiation delivery in therapeutic treatments. In addition, integration of artificial intelligence and machine learning in dosimetric calculations can enable adaptive treatment planning and improve patient safety. AI, through large databases of patient outcomes and radiation exposure, will allow doctors to tailor dosing regimens to the patient, thus mitigating risks of radiation exposure while not compromising on effective treatment regimens. In light of technological developments, greater emphasis is being placed on raising patients' awareness of the use of radiation in imaging and therapy. Developing comprehensive patient education materials can lead to a better understanding of the risks and benefits of radiation procedures. There must be a top priority on well-informing patients about new developments in practices, such as the reduced requirement for lead x-ray vests due to improved radiographic technology (Deker et al., 2020). Educating health practitioners and informing patients about developments in radiation security measures will foster an open, safety culture in health facilities, thereby promoting improved patient outcomes. Furthermore, the formation of a robust system for communication of radiation risk, like informed consent procedures, will allow patients to make informed choices in radiation exposure treatments. Further, another crucial area of future radiation dosimetry will definitely be regulation and compliance with accreditation standards. More stringent compliance with international safety standards, such as those issued by the International Atomic Energy Agency, will be a primary contributor to providing safety in the practice of radiation. Regulatory bodies at the local level must update and enact guidelines that are sensitive to present dosimetric techniques and technology, so that practitioners can provide safe and effective care. Concurrently, ongoing evaluation of the efficacy of new radiation treatment modalities, including intensity-modulated radiation therapy (IMRT) (Duthoy et al., 2006), underscores the need for regulatory updates to enable the productive integration of novel methodologies into standard clinical practice. This integrated approach will ensure patient safety always takes precedence in the ever-evolving field of radiation dosimetry and treatment.

REFERENCES

1. Lamb, J., Cao, M., Kishan, A., Agazaryan, N., Thomas, D. H., Shaverdian, N., Yang, Y., Ray, S., Low, D. A., Raldow, A., Steinberg, M. L., & Lee, P. (2017). Online Adaptive Radiation therapy: Implementation of a new process of care. *Cureus, 9*(8), e1618. https://doi.org/10.7759/cureus.1618Ahn, S., D'Hollander, A., Attix, F. H., Barker, J., Barten, D., & Bazalova, M. (2016). Towards 3D printed multifunctional immobilization for proton therapy: Initial materials characterization. *Medical Physics, 43*(6), 3270–3278. https://doi.org/10.1118/1.4951732 (accessed on 14th July 2025).
2. Akahane, K., Balter, S., Cantone, M. C., Dauer, L. T., & Vano, E. (2017). Report of IRPA task group on the impact of the eye lens dose limits. *Journal of Radiological Protection, 37*(3), 527–542. https://doi.org/10.1088/1361-6498/aa6e2eIOPscience+1PubMed+1 (accessed on 14th July 2025).
3. Al-Ibraheem, A., Baum, R. P., Ben-Haim, S., Blay, J. Y., & Herrmann, K. (2024). Guiding principles on the education and practice of theragnostic. *European Journal of Nuclear Medicine and Molecular Imaging, 51*(1), 1–5. https://doi.org/10.1007/s00259-023-06345-6 (accessed on 14th July 2025).
4. Andriati, S., Fardela, R., Firmawati, N., & Irka, M. (2024). Determination of radiation dose rate in radiology installations using Raysafe X2 surveymeter. *Journal of Radiation Research and Applied Sciences, 17*(1), 1–8. https://doi.org/10.1016/j.jrras.2024.01.001 (accessed on 14th July 2025).
5. Azizmohammadi, Z., Tabei, F., Shafiei, B., Babaei, A. A., Jukandan, S. M., Naghshine, R., & Assadi, M. (2013). A study of the time of hospital discharge of differentiated thyroid cancer patients after receiving iodine-131 for thyroid remnant ablation treatment. *Iranian Journal of Nuclear Medicine, 21*(1), 1–7. https://irjnm.tums.ac.ir/article_37650.html (accessed on 14th July 2025).
6. Badal, A., Kyprianou, I., Rupcich, F., Schmidt, T., & Seibert, J. A. (2012). A database for estimating organ dose for chest and head CT scans for arbitrary spectra and angular tube current modulation. *Medical Physics, 39*(11), 6580–6591. https://doi.org/10.1118/1.4754797 (accessed on 14th July 2025).
7. Bakker, A., Balidemaj, E., Chopra, R., & Crezee, J. (2016). Thermal dosimetry for bladder hyperthermia treatment: An overview. *International Journal of Hyperthermia, 32*(4), 398–408. https://doi.org/10.3109/02656736.2016.1144055 (accessed on 14th July 2025).
8. Benavides, E., Bhula, A., Gohel, A., Lurie, A. G., & Tadinada, A. (2023). Patient shielding during dentomaxillofacial radiography: Recommendations from the American Academy of Oral and Maxillofacial Radiology. *Oral Surgery, Oral Medicine, Oral Pathology and Oral Radiology, 135*(2), 129–136. https://doi.org/10.1016/j.oooo.2022.11.004 (accessed on 14th July 2025).
9. Beşli, L. U., & Demir, M. (2016). Radiation dosimetry in thyroid cancer patients. *Molecular Imaging and Radionuclide Therapy, 25*(3), 93–98. https://doi.org/10.4274/mirt.2016.45678 (accessed on 14th July 2025).
10. Chan, M. F., Deasy, J. O., Lim, S. B., & Scheuermann, R. (2017). IMRT QA using machine learning: A multi-institutional validation. *Medical Physics, 44*(4), 1614–1623. https://doi.org/10.1002/mp.12151 (accessed on 14th July 2025).

11. De Vincentis, G., Gerritsen, W., Gschwend, J. E., Hacker, M., & Sartor, O. (2019). Advances in targeted alpha therapy for prostate cancer. *Annals of Oncology, 30*(11), 1728–1739. https://doi.org/10.1093/annonc/mdz194 (accessed on 14th July 2025).

12. Filbert, E. A., & Valdes, J. (2022). An educational intervention on occupational radiation exposure and risk of cataract development. *Radiologic Technology, 93*(4), 345–354. https://www.radiologictechnology.org/content/93/4/345 (accessed on 14th July 2025).

13. Gloi, A. M., & Kibisu, P. L. (2024). A note on electrometer intercomparison: A routine quality assurance check. *Journal of Applied Clinical Medical Physics, 25*(1), 45–50. https://doi.org/10.1002/acm2.13567 (accessed on 14th July 2025).

14. Longo, M., Marchioni, C., Insero, T., Donnarumma, R., D'Adamo, A., Lucatelli, P., Fanelli, F., Salvatori, F. M., Cannavale, A., & Di Castro, E. (2016). Non-vascular interventional procedures: Effective dose to patient and equivalent dose to abdominal organs by means of DICOM images and Monte Carlo simulation. *Radiation Protection Dosimetry, 168*(4), 509–515. https://doi.org/10.1093/rpd/ncv362Iris (accessed on 14th July 2025).

15. Martin, C. J., Vassileva, J., Vano, E., Mahesh, M., Ebdon-Jackson, S., Ng, K. H., Frush, D. P., Loose, R., & Damilakis, J. (2017). Unintended and accidental medical radiation exposures in radiology: Guidelines on investigation and prevention. *Journal of Radiological Protection, 37*(4), 883–906. https://doi.org/10.1088/1361-6498/aa881ePubMed+3IOPscience+3IAEA+3 (accessed on 14th July 2025).

16. Meghzifene, A., & Van Dyk, J. (2016). Radiation oncology quality and safety considerations in low resource settings: A medical physics perspective. *Medical Physics International, 4*(1), 1–9. https://www.mpijournal.org/pdf/2016-01/MPI-2016-01-p001.pdf (accessed on 14th July 2025).

17. N/A. (2000). *Focal Spot, Fall/Winter 2000. Focal Spot Magazine, 2000*(Fall/Winter), 1–20. https://core.ac.uk/download/129069319.pdf (accessed on 14th July 2025).

18. Nordström, F. (2012). *Quality Assurance in Radiotherapy: Development and Evaluation of New Tools for Improved Patient Safety* (Doctoral thesis). Umeå University. https://www.diva-portal.org/smash/get/diva2:511589/FULLTEXT01.pdf (accessed on 14th July 2025).

19. Olarinoye, I., & Sharifat, I. (2010). A protocol for setting dose reference level for medical radiography in Nigeria: A review. *Radiation Protection Dosimetry, 140*(1), 91–94. https://doi.org/10.1093/rpd/ncp234Iris (accessed on 14th July 2025).

20. Pladevall Blancafort, A. (2023). *Analysis of the Existing Technologies in Intraoperative Radiotherapy* (Bachelor's thesis). University of Barcelona. https://diposit.ub.edu/dspace/bitstream/2445/199592/1/TFG%20Pladevall_Blancafort_Adria.pdf (accessed on 14th July 2025).

21. Seibert, J. A., Baird, C. T., Clements, J. B., & de Boer, S. F. (2018). AAPM medical physics practice guideline 10.a.: Scope of practice for clinical medical physics. *Journal of Applied Clinical Medical Physics, 19*(6), 11–17. https://doi.org/10.1002/acm2.12470 (accessed on 14th July 2025).

22. Tennyson, N., Weiss, E., Sleeman, W., & Rosu, M. (2017). Effect of variations in atelectasis on tumor displacement during radiation therapy for locally advanced lung cancer. *Journal of Applied Clinical Medical Physics, 18*(5), 89–96. https://doi.org/10.1002/acm2.12145 (accessed on 14th July 2025).

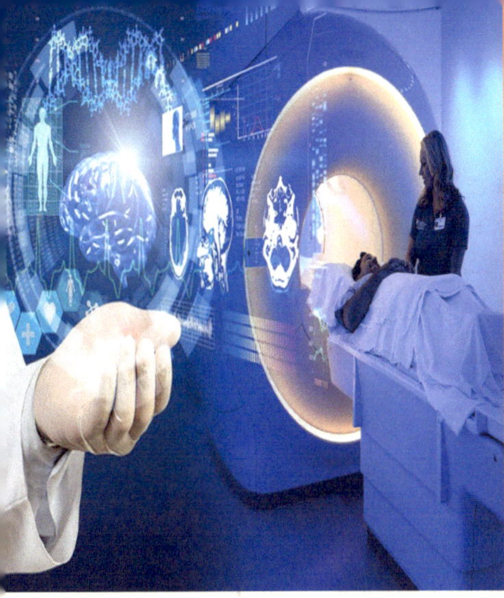

Chapter 11

DIGITAL IMAGE ACQUISITION AND QUALITY CONTROL

Contents

Introduction

In the era of high-tech, computer-based digital image acquisition is now a mainstay of modern medical imaging, revolutionizing the way doctors diagnose and monitor disease. The move away from traditional film-based systems towards digital technology provides unparalleled access, enhances image quality, and simplifies the storage and retrieval of imaging data. of modalities, such as computed tomography (CT), magnetic resonance imaging (MRI), and ultrasound, are complemented by advances in image acquisition, enabling resulting images to indeed assist clinical decision-making. Advances come at a price, however, in terms of the requirement for strict quality control to guarantee that resulting images are not impaired in integrity or diagnostic validity. Implementing such protocols is important to avoid errors that may be induced by variations of the imaging process and technological limitations, demonstrating the necessity for continuous improvement of acquisition processes and quality assurance practice. Ensuring that the images obtained are not only of good quality but also a true representation of the patient's condition is an important aspect of medical image acquisition using digital imaging. It is imperative where therapy is dependent on precise imaging, like the diagnosis of neurodegenerative disease. The availability of atrophy evaluation techniques, for instance, helps to highlight the complexity of brain health evaluation when more traditional methods cannot be trusted across different patient populations. According to Camara et al. (2006), the generation of ground-truth data plays a pivotal role in the development of these techniques, and the development of sophisticated simulation methods is crucial for the verification of the performance of various imaging practices.

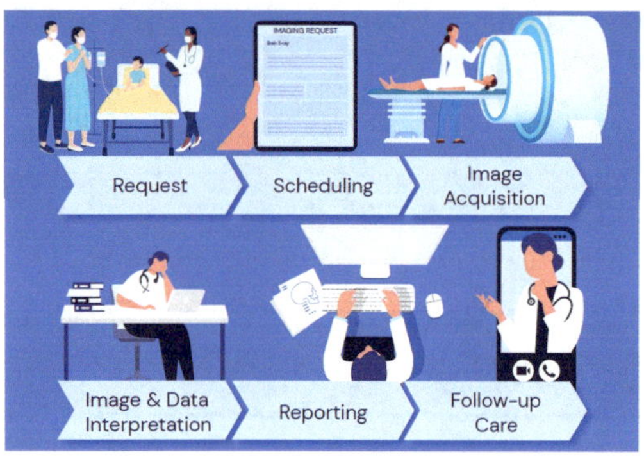

Figure 11.1. Overview diagram of digital image acquisition workflow.

Source: https://enlitic.com/wp-content/uploads/MicrosoftTeams-image-97-640x427.jpg.

With the development of a framework to simulate changes in brain images, researchers can evaluate tools applied to atrophy measurement and the effects they have on clinical outcomes more effectively. Quality control of digital image acquisition is not simply a question of maintaining aesthetic criteria; it also encompasses the achievement of accuracy and reliability in medical imaging. It is critical that imaging protocols comply with established standards and that defects, if any, are diagnosed and corrected systematically. Including robust quality assurance protocols enables the assessment of registration accuracy and quality, which is important for combining images of the same anatomical structure from different views or at different time points. Image registration processes play a crucial role in the diagnostic power of medical imaging modalities, as elaborated in (Nag et al., 2017). become integral to routine imaging practice so that holistic and accurate patient assessments can be achieved and ultimately improve health results, along with encouraging the proper use of medical imaging technologies (Figure 11.1).

11.1. Fundamentals of Digital Image Acquisition

The concepts of digital image capture are an integral part of learning the dynamics of medical imaging, where the precision of captured images is paramount for proper diagnosis. Digital image capture is capturing, processing, and storing images via an array of sensors and imaging modalities. In the medical setting, these systems are more likely to use complementary metal-oxide-semiconductor (CMOS) technology for their image sensor. CMOS sensors have increasingly replaced traditional film and charge-coupled device systems due to their promising characteristics, including lower cost, lower power consumption, and better integration capabilities. Pixel miniaturization is leading to higher image resolution, thereby enhancing the detail and accuracy of medical images. This innovation has also made CMOS a popular technology across various applications and has significantly advanced medical diagnostics through improved, more precise imaging. The advent of the CMOS image sensor has also fueled numerous technological advances that are at the heart of the future of medical imaging. Over the last decades, improvements in image quality—higher resolution, higher capture speed, and improved light sensitivity—have been critical to responding to the needs of the medical community. These improvements enhance visualization of anatomical information and pathology, enabling earlier diagnosis and intervention. Furthermore, improvements in computational imaging enhance the ability to compute images on-chip, with real-time analytics and image processing integrated directly into sensor hardware. These developments not only improve the quality of images acquired but also aim to address the growing demand for accelerated imaging techniques at affordable prices, thereby making medical imaging more efficient and affordable. Despite the revolutionary CMOS developments, differentiation between competing sensor manufacturers is still a problem. With the marketplace awash with high-res and low-cost imaging products, drawing attention to the differentiating factors of new products is becoming a significant challenge. Manufacturers need to be in settings where the end objective is to enhance metrics such as resolution, speed, and power efficiency, while containing manufacturing costs (Choubey et al., 2014). In addition, embedding sophisticated processing techniques has also remained a primary area of competition (Gouveia et al., 2016). Pursuing disruptive growth trajectories in CMOS sensor technology is essential in enabling innovation within the sector (Gouveia et al., 2016). With progress in digital image acquisition continuing, the general goal remains clear: to enhance the quality of medical images and ensure that these improvements benefit patient care and healthcare efficiency.

11.1.1. Types of Digital Imaging Modalities

Digital imaging modalities encompass a variety of approaches employed to image the internal human body structures in support of proper diagnosis and monitoring of medical conditions by health practitioners. The chief primary modalities are X-ray imaging, computed tomography (CT), magnetic resonance imaging (MRI), ultrasound, and nuclear medicine. X-ray imaging remains one of the most widely applied technologies due to speed and image quality, particularly for bone fracture and dental diagnostic imaging. CT scanning, with high-quality cross-sectional images generated by integrating numerous X-ray images, has proven invaluable in the evaluation of trauma and severe disease. All of these modalities possess unique advantages and limitations, which are crucial for prudent selection of the appropriate imaging technique based on clinical indications and patient safety (Figure 11.2).

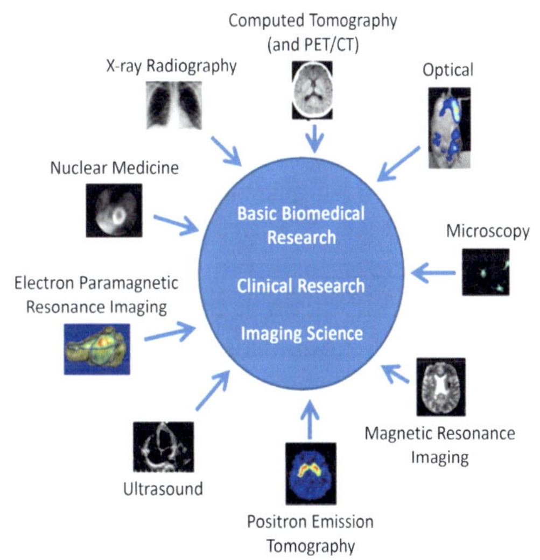

Figure 11.2. Digital imaging modalities.

Source: https://d1hj7uubji8r0c.cloudfront.net/sites/radiology/files/styles/large/public/2019-10/ImagingModalityChart.png?h=2f4de4dc&itok=fQMZzJpW.

Ultrasound scanning, utilizing sound waves to create live images of soft tissues and organs, is essential in obstetrics, cardiology, and most other specialties because it is non-invasive. Unlike CT scans and X-rays, ultrasound does not employ ionizing radiation and is thus safer for certain groups, for example, pregnant women. Furthermore, advances in ultrasound technology, including three-dimensional imaging, have significantly enhanced its diagnostic potential. At this point, nuclear medicine employs radioactive tracers to image the body's metabolic function, enabling functional imaging that contrasts with anatomical imaging techniques such as CT and MRI. As these modalities advance, often incorporating digital technology, they are not only used for diagnosis but also to guide targeted therapies, thereby improving patient care. In recent years, the field of digital imaging has also witnessed a significant shift towards integrating modalities to enhance diagnostic potential. Computer-Aided Medical Interventions (CAMI) provide an example in this direction, specifically in the manipulation of soft tissues that cause difficulties due to their mobility and deformation in procedures. The application of image fusion technology and minimally invasive robotics, most notably in urology, is a clear example of the enhanced outcomes possible through the synergy among different imaging modalities. Such convergence enables a more comprehensive understanding of the anatomical and functional changes in a patient. As described in recent literature, the priority given to establishing support systems using newer imaging modalities, such as surgical navigation and robot-assisted surgery, reflects a new situation in medical imaging in which precision and performance are continually advanced by technology (Alimin et al., 2001; Bart et al., 2006).

11.1.2. Principles of Image Formation

The fundamental physics of light and imaging modalities underlies medical image formation. These principles govern image formation, processing, and interpretation, and they all contribute to the diagnostic quality and value of medical images. For instance, X-ray imaging is based on differential X-ray absorption by different tissues, while magnetic resonance imaging (MRI) exploits magnetic differences to generate contrast between different classes of biological tissues. These concepts not only serve to enhance image acquisition procedures but also are critical in quality control processes in clinical uses. The intricate interaction between imaging technology and biological structure is crucial for creating accurate, reliable images that aid diagnosis and treatment planning. In digital image capture, the interaction between data faithfulness and resolution is paramount. Imaging methods such as computed tomography (CT) and ultrasound employ advanced computational methods for reconstructing images from unprocessed data, revealing intricate details that inform clinical decisions (Figure 11.3).

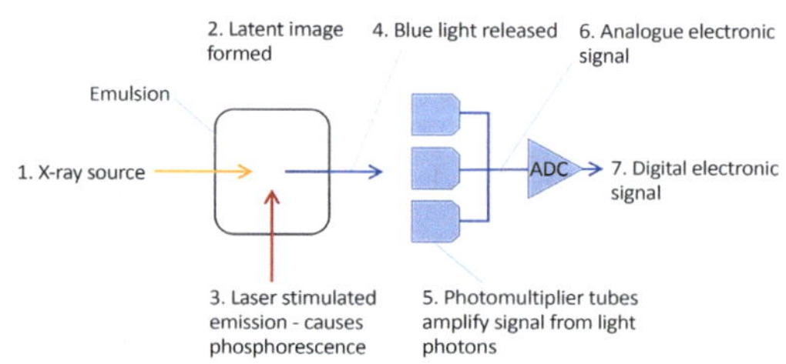

Figure 11.3. Schematic of image formation process in digital radiography.

Source: https://www.radiologycafe.com/wp-content/uploads/2021/04/xray-imageprocess.png.

These techniques are highly efficient but depend on parameters such as sampling frequency and signal-to-noise ratio, which may influence image quality and diagnostic performance. Moreover, novel developments like iterative reconstruction approaches have emerged to mitigate motion artifacts and render the medical images more diagnostically pertinent and clear. By addressing inherent limitations in conventional imaging practices, these developments lay the foundation for improved medical imaging standards necessary for patient management and care. Yet, the ongoing progression of the medical imaging process ensures that there remains a need for extensive training and standardization of practitioners. Technology has advanced considerably, yet issues remain concerning access to and the quality of medical imaging information. As reported at the First Conference on Machine Intelligence in Medical Imaging, there is global recognition of the data-limited issue across medical imaging evaluation. International cooperation among medical imaging informaticists, clinical researchers, and government institutions is critical to establishing best practices for collecting and annotating medical images. Better communication and cooperation on the sharing of resources may lead to the development of reusable medical image datasets, and hence improve the quality of machine learning in healthcare settings, as indicated by studies into Digital Volume Correlation (DVC) and iterative CT reconstruction (Geis et al., 2017; Boone et al., 2018).

11.1.3. Role of Sensors in Image Acquisition

The role of sensors in image acquisition is pivotal in medical imaging, as the precision of the acquired images determines diagnosis. Sensors such as charge-coupled devices (CCDs) and complementary metal-oxide semiconductors (CMOS) convert analog light signals into digital data that clinicians use for analysis. These elements are widely utilized in capturing the minute anatomical details, thus enabling medical practitioners to make well-informed clinical decisions. Progress in technology in sensors has significantly enhanced image quality, enabling high-resolution imaging that was not possible before. This enhancement is not only vital to diagnosis but also to monitoring disease development and treatment success, thereby entrenching the role of sophisticated sensor technology in the ongoing development of medical imaging technologies, underpinning improved techniques documented in the development of dental surgery and other branches of medicine (Camilleri et al., 2004). Moreover, the inclusion of sophisticated sensors improves image acquisition rates and reduces exposure time, thereby enhancing patient comfort and safety (Figure 11.4).

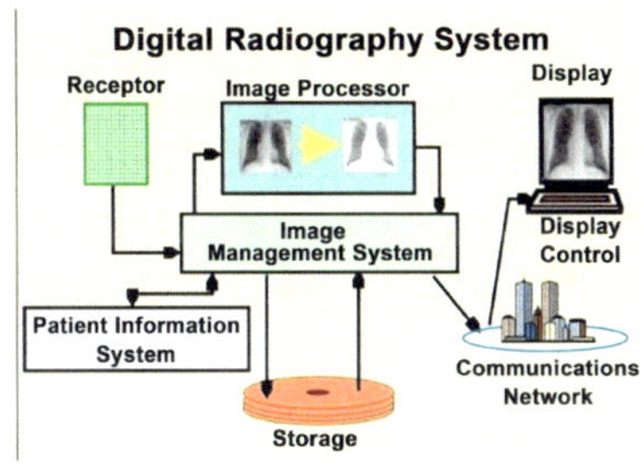

Figure 11.4. Diagram showing sensor components used in digital imaging.

Source: https://ffden-2.phys.uaf.edu/104_2012_web_projects/Elizabeth_Goldsmith/Digital_Radiography.html.

Modern medical imaging devices employ sophisticated sensors and advanced algorithms to provide high-quality images. For instance, sensors that incorporate electrical impedance tomography (EIT) have shown promise in producing real-time images with minimal invasiveness, as reflected in their application beyond traditional imaging settings (Hill et al., 2025). This flexibility in sensor design not only enables new imaging modalities but also enables real-time monitoring of physiological changes. With the growing need for rapid diagnosis, the pivotal importance of sensors in meeting this need cannot be overstressed, and continuous improvement in sensor design and operation is imperative to improve healthcare outcomes. Lastly, the quality of medical imaging depends entirely on the performance and integrity of the sensors employed during image formation. Without consistent sensors that produce high-quality images, the performance of the imaging modalities can be lost. Constant advancements in sensor technology are necessary not only to maintain image quality but also to establish quality-control standards crucial to clinical practice. For example, sensors must be maintained in calibration and precision to the point of taking accurate anatomical images. The integration of high-quality sensor technologies and control methods ensures the best diagnostic performance and eliminates the pitfalls of misdiagnosis in medical images. The integration of the symbiotic relationship among sensors, image acquisition methods, and quality control procedures underscores their combined importance in advancing medical imaging methods.

11.2. Image Processing Techniques

The advancement of digital image acquisition in medical imaging largely relies on reasonable image processing techniques. The techniques enhance image quality, contribute to better diagnosis, and enable efficient treatment planning. Some of the key processes used include image enhancement and restoration, which aim to improve the visual appearance and structural integrity of images. Image enhancement aims to improve notable features in medical images, such as edges and textures, typically through the application of filters and contrast manipulation methods. Restoration attempts to reverse the effects of noise or distortion by applying algorithms to minimize issues encountered during image capture. Collectively, these techniques enhance the visual experience and play an essential role in ensuring diagnostic accuracy, solidifying their vital role in the medical imaging field. Another intrinsic aspect of image processing techniques is image registration, which involves aligning multiple images of the same object to provide complete information. This process is particularly crucial for medical imaging when images from various modalities, such as MRI and CT scans, are to be superimposed for the right analysis. Image registration enables one to monitor anatomical changes over a duration of time, thereby informing treatment and improving patient outcomes. Numerous algorithms exist for registration, each with its own strengths and weaknesses, enriching the field of study and application in medicine. Performance measures must be used to quantify the efficacy of such registration techniques; they provide precise alignment and enable clinical interpretation. As medicine advances, continued innovation in image registration technology can further enhance the usefulness and quality of medical images and result in improved patient care. Furthermore, medical imaging quality control cannot be overlooked as it directly correlates with the effectiveness of image processing techniques. Quality control involves systematic examination of imaging equipment to determine if they consistently produce high-fidelity outputs. This involves regular calibrations, examination of imaging parameters, and adherence to prescribed standards to minimize diagnostic errors. The integration of image processing techniques, such as denoising and artifact removal, is crucial to ensuring high-quality images. Therefore, institutions are increasingly adopting these steps to guarantee the reliability of their imaging systems. The outcomes of most studies have shown that , reasonable quality control not only enhances image acquisition but also enhances the overall integrity of the medical imaging process, with a final impact on patient diagnosis and treatment efficiency significantly.

11.2.1. Pre-Processing Methods

In medical imaging, pre-processing strategies play a central role in enhancing image quality, which directly affects diagnostic accuracy. Pre-processing strategies are formulated to improve image definition, remove noise, and facilitate feature extraction, and thereby lay a solid groundwork for analyses conducted thereafter. Noise reduction algorithms, contrast enhancement, and image normalization are among the most widely used preprocessing strategies. Using preprocessing filters, such as Gaussian or median filters, practitioners can effectively counteract irrelevant variations caused by factors such as equipment failures or external environmental conditions. Furthermore, techniques of contrast enhancement, such as histogram equalization, allow for the improved visibility of concealed structures, which is significant when detecting abnormalities. In general, using robust preprocessing techniques ensures that the resulting images are of high quality, ultimately resulting in good clinical outcomes. One of the essential elements in pre-processing is image registration, a method that aligns multiple images of a single object captured at different times or angles (Figure 11.5).

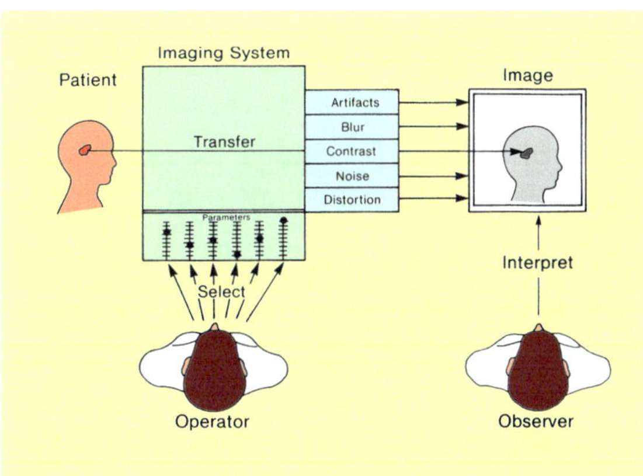

Figure 11.5. Flowchart illustrating typical image pre-processing stages.

Source: https://th.bing.com/th/id/R.c0463ae12f0b87e79d63b8fae0385f5d?rik=xNl1NDvmCAZJjw&riu=http%3a%2f%2fwww.sprawls.org%2fppmi2%2fIMGCHAR%2f1IMCHAR01.gif&ehk=DTl0n1SYErJIlyEsSnqifSbRaxyKguSizDGozxlgkVo%3d&risl=&pid=ImgRaw&r=0.

Such registration is particularly vital in longitudinal and multi-modal imaging, where homogeneity is essential when tracking changes over time. As explained in the literature, image registration enhances the ability to diagnose and analyze temporal changes and spatial correlations within the same anatomical structures, thus enabling proper diagnosis and treatment planning in medical fields (Nag et al., 2017). Different registration methods, ranging from fixed to elastic, are beneficial depending on the type of imaging data. Having knowledge and selecting the appropriate registration method, therefore, might have a significant impact on the overall accuracy of the imaging solution, underscoring the importance of pre-processing in medical imaging. In addition to image registration, dimension reduction techniques also form an essential aspect of image pre-processing. These methods condense the data without sacrificing meaningful features and can significantly reduce computational load in later processing stages. Principal component analysis (PCA) and singular value decomposition (SVD) are popular tools with widespread application for extracting significant patterns from high-dimensional data. Medical practitioners can thus deal with high-dimensional problems more effectively, such as overfitting and computational inefficiency. The integration of dimensionality reduction not only enhances data interpretability but also streamlines the image acquisition-to-analysis pipeline, thereby underscoring the importance of good pre-processing methods for generating high-quality imaging results in clinical practice (Alimin et al., 2001).

11.2.2. Image Enhancement Techniques

Image enhancement techniques play a significant role in medical imaging, improving the visual quality of images acquired across many modalities. The enhancements ensure diagnostic information is accurately conveyed, enabling enhanced patient management. Techniques such as histogram equalization, contrast stretching, and spatial filtering help eliminate noise while enhancing critical anatomical information. Better images assist radiologists in identifying abnormalities and also aid the development of Computer-Assisted Diagnosis (CAD) systems (Figure 11.6).

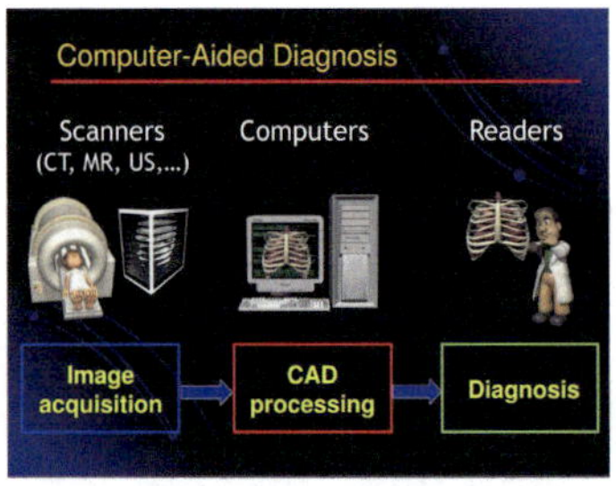

Figure 11.6. Computer-assisted diagnosis (CAD) systems.

Source: https://image3.slideserve.com/5986346/computer-aided-diagnosis-l.jpg.

Using sophisticated algorithms, such systems can scrutinize images for subtle abnormalities and provide additional information that would be lost with traditional imaging methods, underscoring the importance of image enhancement in healthcare settings. In addition, the availability of new digital sensors and methodologies necessitates aggressive image improvement approaches. Digital mammography, for instance, has revolutionized breast cancer diagnosis with the implementation of leading-edge direct digital detection techniques. But this also imposes complexity issues around image processing, for example, demanding proper noise reduction and enhancement protocols. Advanced methods must be established to handle the vast volume of data generated by digital mammography systems, thereby maximizing diagnostic resolution and image quality. As noted, the role of compression algorithms thus becomes critical in handling these large data sets, balancing image fidelity against system performance. The intersection of these technologies presents new challenges and opportunities, opening the door to advances in image improvement (Blaine et al., 2025). In orthopedic surgery, image improvement methods play a key role in raising the accuracy and safety of surgical procedures. CAOS systems utilize volumetric imaging—for example, MRI and CT scans—to create precise surgical plans. Such improvements ensure surgeons have a clear understanding of patient anatomy before performing procedures. Image enhancement technologies not only improve image quality but also enhance tracking and navigation during surgery, thereby significantly influencing patient outcomes. With the developments in CAOS systems that incorporate a variety of imaging modalities, enhanced enhancement methods are required, highlighting their crucial aspect as facilitators of successful surgical outcomes (Kalová et al., 2019).

11.2.3. Image Reconstruction Algorithms

The application of image reconstruction algorithms in medical imaging is pivotal because they directly influence the quality of images acquired digitally. The applications are deployed to enhance and purify the raw imaging data to yield clear and precise diagnostics to healthcare providers. By employing sophisticated techniques, such as iterative reconstruction, these applications can effectively minimize artifacts and improve visualization of anatomical structures. This becomes particularly important in dynamic imaging scenarios where motion artifacts can have the capacity to obscure valuable information, perhaps leading to misdiagnosis or ineffective treatment protocols. Thus, integrating sophisticated image reconstruction algorithms is important for enhancing image fidelity and credibility in medical testing, thereby contributing to better patient outcomes across various healthcare settings. In novel image quality improvement solutions, iterative image reconstruction algorithms are highly effective, particularly in applications such as in optoacoustic tomography (OAT). Unlike traditional methods based on analytic forms, iterative approaches include explicit models of imaging physics, instrument responses, and intrinsic measurement noise, which tends to yield improved output. For instance, recent research has employed penalized least-squares methods that incorporate smoothness penalties and total variation norms, demonstrating reduced image artifacts while preserving spatial resolution. These advances indicate that such algorithms can potentially revolutionize imaging protocols and increase diagnostic accuracy (Figure 11.7).

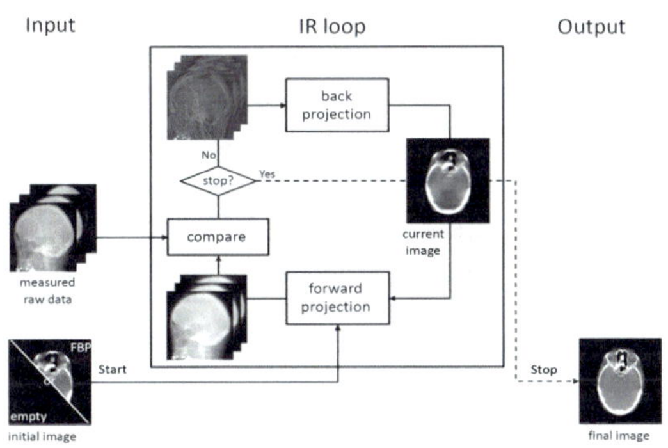

Figure 11.7. Algorithm pipeline for tomographic image reconstruction.

Source: Reconstructed from scientific publication.

With ongoing advancements in medical imaging, constant innovation and enhancement of these algorithms are also imperative for achieving improved visualizations and decision-making information from challenging datasets (Alexander et al., 2012). This combination of digital volume correlation and iterative CT reconstruction also evidences the synergy between these technologies in enhancing image quality. This hybrid method suppresses motion artifacts even during a single 360° rotation, enabling high-resolution dynamic X-ray CT imaging and quantitative 3D strain map creation. These maps not only correspond to tissue material properties but also enable us to better understand how they behave under various conditions. These advanced analysis techniques are particularly important for medical applications in biomechanics and materials science, demonstrating the power of interdisciplinary applications of image reconstruction algorithms to make significant contributions. This methodology also emphasizes the need for continued investment in image processing technology to improve diagnostic accuracy and facilitate more efficient patient care through appropriate image enhancement (Boone et al., 2018).

11.3. Quality Control Standards in Medical Imaging

Standards of quality control in medical imaging are crucial to maintaining diagnostic accuracy and patient safety. These are not regulatory initiatives per se; they are a framework of standards for the maintenance of the integrity of imaging processes. By adhering to established quality assurance protocols, medical centers can implement systematic assessment and improvement of imaging practices. As technology advances, the complexity of digital image capture increases, and institutions have to implement stringent quality control measures. Regular calibration of the imaging devices and adherence to dosimetry standards enable the detection of potential faults or abnormalities and thereby ensure better overall imaging quality. In addition, the need for best practices aligns with ongoing discussion among medical imaging experts about the merit of developing collaborative best practices shared between institutions, as exemplified in recent conferences on machine learning and medical imaging data (Geis et al., 2017). Professional organizations, like the American Association of Physicists in Medicine (AAPM), play an integral role in establishing quality control standards in medical imaging. The AAPM provides broadly peer-reviewed medical physics practice guidelines, which are professional guidebooks for practitioners. These guidelines emphasize the value of specialty training and expertise needed for safe imaging practice. Each guideline is reviewed periodically to ensure that it remains up to date, considering new technologies and techniques. The AAPM's commitment to a culture of safety and efficacy is echoed through its efforts to harmonize its guidelines with the regulatory paradigms that oversee healthcare practice. In endorsing a consensus-based mechanism for quality control, the AAPM enables building blocks for continuous improvement, thereby improving patient care across the medical imaging sector (Seibert et al., 2018). As the medical imaging landscape continues to evolve, the convergence of quality-control requirements with technological advancements is increasingly paramount. As machine learning-driven solutions increasingly apply to imaging diagnosis, organizations have an essential responsibility to prioritize the creation of high-quality, reusable imaging datasets. Data availability, data quality, and data annotation issues underscore the gravity of the need for industry players, data scientists, and regulatory bodies to come together for collective action. Creating detailed guidelines for the use and collection of medical imaging data is important for properly training machine learning models. Quality control practices must adapt to accommodate these new realities, serving as the blueprint for the proper use of digital technologies in the clinic. Ultimately, the successful synergy of quality standards and new imaging tools will significantly enhance diagnostic performance and patient health and access to a more reliable healthcare delivery system (Geis et al., 2017).

11.3.1. Regulatory Bodies and Guidelines

The role of medical imaging regulatory agencies is fundamental in ensuring high-quality standards in digital image acquisition and quality control. Regulatory agencies play a role in establishing specific guidelines that oversee the practice of medical physics, which are crucial to making patient diagnosis and treatment effective and safe. A key organization in this category is the American Association of Physicists in Medicine (AAPM), which regularly issues medical physics practice guidelines (MPPGs). Not only are they grounded in modern scientific consensus, but they also transcend peer review and public commentary, undergoing rigorous testing before application. By encouraging adherence to these guidelines, regulation aims to provide assurance of the safe use of diagnostic and therapeutic modalities in medical imaging and to harmonize the unique challenges associated with new technologies in the practice of medical physics, according to their policy statements (Seibert et al., 2018) (Figure 11.8).

AMERICAN ASSOCIATION *of* PHYSICISTS IN MEDICINE

Figure 11.8. American association of physicists in medicine (AAPM).

Source: https://www.newswise.com/images/institutions/logos/AAPM_Logo_Name_stacked_FINAL_AAPMBlue_CMYK20210811100952.jpg.

In digital imaging, particularly in pathology, the lack of a standardized approach to image quality evaluation makes it difficult to develop uniform guidelines. As a result, regulatory bodies face the added challenge of establishing viable frameworks for evaluating clinical image quality (cIQ) and perceived image quality (pIQ). The distinction between these two measures of quality is critical: cIQ is the ability of images to aid clinical decision-making, whereas pIQ focuses on image quality as subjectively assessed. The American Association of Physicists in Medicine recognizes the need for strict protocols to establish relationships between the two types of quality assessment measures. For instance, recent studies have identified conflicting results across different quality evaluation approaches, necessitating clear concepts and concordance in quality guidelines for digital pathology (Ducatelle et al., 2017). Ultimately, regulatory control of digital image capture and quality control extends beyond mere compliance; their guidelines establish the practice of medical imaging itself. Consistent coordination between rule-making authorities and clinicians strengthens the regime governing imaging, fostering a culture that prioritizes patient safety and care quality. As technologies evolve, these organizations must be agile, revising guidelines continuously to adapt to emerging practices and thelatest research. Ongoing training and education, underscored through MPPGs, are imperative for professionals to adjust to such changes effectively. With the integration of systematic regulatory norms into medical imaging applications, the field can be developed, with patients being afforded the best possible care in diagnostic testing (Seibert et al., 2018).

11.3.2. Importance of Standardization

Standardization is important in the field of digital image acquisition and medical imaging quality control, as it provides a consistent framework that ensures uniformity across all imaging modalities. With all the development of technologies, which translates to varied imaging methods, the lack of a consistent standard can lead to differences in the quality of images as well as in interpretation. Standardization facilitates interoperability among several systems and devices and the seamless integration of imaging data in healthcare systems. Additionally, the creation of comprehensive guidelines and protocols not only reduces heterogeneity in clinical processes but also enhances the reliability of diagnoses derived from medical images. Such consistency is critical for building confidence between healthcare service providers and patients, thereby enhancing overall patient outcomes. Furthermore, uniform practices are essential to enhance the education and training of healthcare providers. Since uniform imaging practices are followed, it is easier to train practitioners regarding digital image interpretation and use (Figure 11.9).

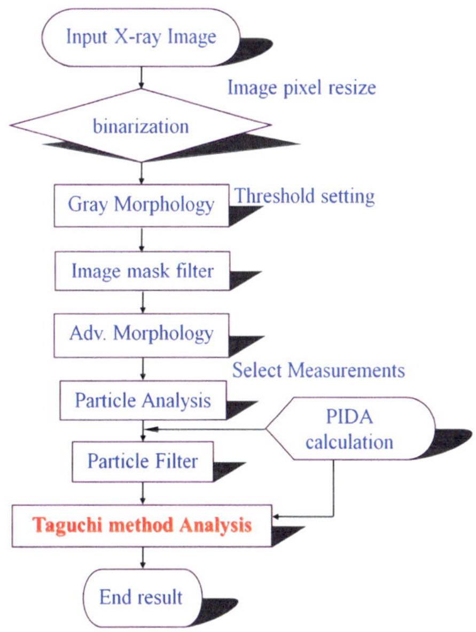

Figure 11.9. Flowchart for processing X-ray images.

Source: https://www.researchgate.net/publication/323122651/figure/fig5/AS:11431281155453103@1683190772599/Flowchart-for-processing-X-ray-images.tif.

Standardized imaging acquisition and analysis procedures ensure that all members of healthcare are on the same page regarding the expected image quality. This uniformity is particularly important when adopting new imaging modalities or methods. By applying well-defined standards, organizations can accelerate professionals' learning and adoption of newer technologies, reducing the risk of errors caused by irregular training processes. As noted in discussions about the INCF Digital Atlasing Program, well-designed standards can truly make a tangible impact in the academic and medical communities, enabling better research and more methodologies (Burger A et al., 2009). Also crucial is standardization's influence on the evaluation processes of imaging quality in medical imaging. With the rapid expansion of digital pathology, for instance, there has been agreement but no consensus on how to assess image quality (Ducatelle et al., 2017). The development of standardized assessment measures—such as clinician success rates on tasks or other quality ratings—enables healthcare providers to better gauge the effectiveness of imaging systems and approaches. These assessments not only help establish benchmarks but also facilitate continuous quality improvement in medical imaging procedures. By ensuring image quality assessments are grounded in standard methods, healthcare organizations can support continuous improvement in diagnostic imaging, thereby contributing to patient care through greater accuracy and reliability in clinical practice.

11.3.3. Common Quality Control Metrics

The use of universal quality control procedures is of utmost importance in the pursuit of the stability of medical image acquisition with digital imaging. One such measure is the diagnostic accuracy of an image, which quantifies an imaging system's ability to acquire images that satisfactorily depict the underlying pathology. For instance, recent research has demonstrated the efficacy of utilizing advanced algorithms, such as the deep learning architecture AlexNet, in discriminating between diagnostic and non-diagnostic images. In one confocal laser endomicroscopy study with an overall model accuracy of 91%, this technique was shown to be very promising in enhancing the diagnostic yield of images taken during surgery (Figure 11.10).

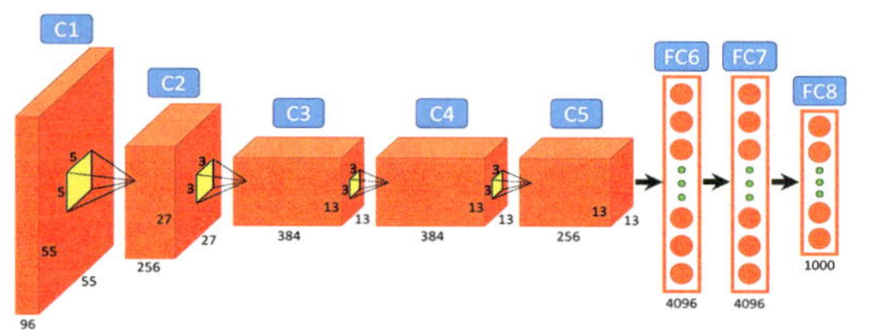

Figure 11.10. AlexNet: A revolutionary deep learning architecture.

Source: https://viso.ai/wp-content/uploads/2024/04/alexNet-architecture.png.

These findings underscore the importance of integrating auto-analysis into the quality control process to boost efficiency and reduce the manual workload of image evaluation for medical professionals (Belykh et al., 2018). The second quality control characteristic of significant relevance is image registration accuracy, particularly in cases where a series of images of the same anatomical region is captured over time or under varying conditions. Accurate image registration enables medical professionals to identify temporal changes, which are indispensable in following the progression of disease or response to treatment. It is an alignment process for images acquired with various modalities or views, and hence requires a robust quality check to assess alignment accuracy. Some performance measures have been developed to quantify image registration quality, focusing on precision, recall, and the overall fidelity of the registered images. Clinicians can use such measures to ensure that the software used to interpret medical images is of the highest quality, thereby saving patient lives (Nag et al., 2017). Lastly, noise level analysis and artifacts are another significant quality control parameter in digital imaging. Noise from system electronics or from external sources can obscure diagnostic detail and lead to misdiagnosis of medical images. Measurement of the signal-to-noise ratio (SNR) is thus critical for assessing image quality. In addition, the identification and eradication of artifacts, such as motion blur or beam hardening, must be addressed to ensure that diagnostic images remain intact. Regular quality control tests that incorporate these factors allow medical facilities to maintain equipment levels and ensure imaging protocols yield consistently high-quality results. By placing greater focus on these interdependent measures, medical professionals can enhance the consistency of imaging findings, which is at the heart of clinical decision-making algorithms.

11.4. Factors Affecting Image Quality

Also impacting medical image quality are a wide array of technical and environmental factors that must be considered when acquiring images. Resolution of the imaging device is a key factor in that it is linked to detail and clarity achieved in an image. Higher-resolution systems yield more precise images with improved visualization of anatomical structures. For instance, advances in dental imaging technology have greatly improved resolution compared to earlier methods, highlighting the revolutionary impact of technology in the field. Further, parameters such as imaging modality, patient positioning, and the use of appropriate filters play a crucial role in determining final image quality. As reported in the literature, advances in medical imaging technology have brought about a quantum leap in the sophistication of procedures, highlighting the importance of these parameters in obtaining high-quality images (Camilleri et al., 2004). A second important parameter that affects image quality in medical imaging is noise handling during imaging. Noise, in the form of unwanted variation in the image signal, obscures critical diagnostic detail and thus demands successful de-noising of the images. Some recent research has established that the application of advanced algorithms, such as deep learning, can significantly enhance the image quality by reducing the noise in optical coherence tomography (OCT) scans. Using a custom deep learning network, single-frame B-scan scans of the optic nerve head were effectively denoised, increasing the signal-to-noise ratio (SNR) from 4.02 dB to 8.14 dB and improving contrast-to-noise ratio (CNR). Findings emphasize the pivotal contribution of noise control to image quality and affirm the need for reliable image processing methods in the clinic (Aung et al., 2018).

Post-acquisition processes, including image processing and enhancement techniques, also contribute significantly towards maximizing image quality. Such process methods include algorithms for the correction of brightness, contrast, and sharpness to ensure better visibility of anatomical structures and pathological results. The efficacy of such processes heavily relies on the initial quality of the acquired images. Thus, an image that is already of maximum resolution and low noise can be significantly enhanced through processing. Moreover, clinicians and radiologists must participate in rigorous quality control procedures to ensure that images produced are of diagnostic quality. An interdisciplinary approach that incorporates technological advancements and stringent quality assurance procedures is essential to maximizing the operation of medical imaging systems. Ultimately, consideration of these parameters will lead to improved patient outcomes by increasing diagnostic accuracy and reliability.

11.4.1. Equipment Calibration and Maintenance

In the context of digital image capture and image quality assurance in medical imaging, equipment calibration and maintenance are pivotal for achieving optimal performance and precision. Calibration refers to the process of setting a medical imaging machine to meet predetermined standards, which is important for the accurate measurement of images and their reproducibility for diagnosis. Over time, equipment can stray from these standards due to a variety of conditions, such as environmental changes, aging of components, or software modifications. Multiple calibration sessions enable the detection and correction of these deviations, thereby allowing imaging equipment to yield consistent results on which clinicians may depend. The American Association of Physicists in Medicine (AAPM) emphasizes that strict adherence to calibration protocols on a routine basis is essential, not only for regulatory requirements but also to support continuous improvement in the quality of patient care by enhancing diagnostic accuracy (Seibert et al., 2018). Regular hardware maintenance on imaging equipment is also a key factor in ensuring the devices' lifespan and performance (Figure 11.11).

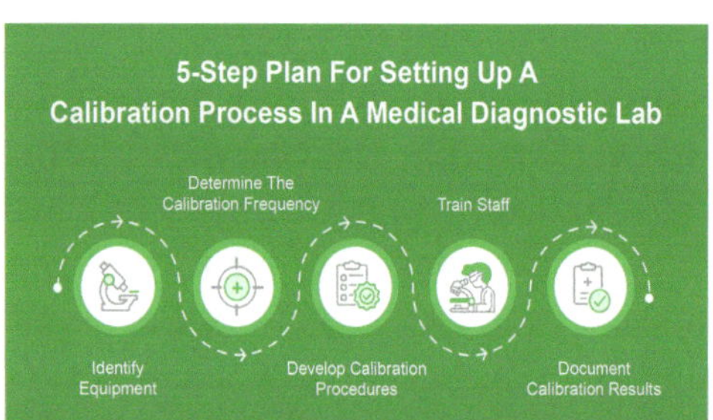

Figure 11.11. Medical equipment calibration for labs.

Source: https://i0.wp.com/blog.creliohealth.com/wp-content/uploads/2023/03/Section-Image.png?resize=640%2C348&ssl=1.

Preventive maintenance plans, including processes such as cleaning, hardware checks, and software updates, are important for reducing the likelihood of failure. Properly maintained imaging equipment is less likely to malfunction and affect the image quality obtained. Additionally, timely performed maintenance can also prevent unplanned downtime, which can lead to clinical process disruption and adversely affect patient treatment. The AAPM outlines maintenance practices that enable practitioners to conduct regular inspections and address potential issues before they escalate, thereby fostering a culture of reliability and safety in healthcare facilities (Seibert et al., 2018). Ultimately, the relationship among calibration, maintenance, and quality control plays a critical role in fostering an environment where high-quality imaging standards are consistently achieved. Every imaging modality, whether magnetic resonance imaging, computed tomography, or ultrasound, requires specific calibration and maintenance procedures to ensure the integrity of the resulting digital images. Additionally, as technology evolves, new research methodologies and practices for equipment maintenance and calibration emerge constantly, driven by innovations in research and technology —for example, those resulting from NASA's research and development. By embracing these evolving practices, healthcare facilities' medical imaging systems can remain at the forefront of precision, thereby improving patient outcomes and meeting the stringent standards imposed in medical imaging.

11.4.2. Operator Training and Expertise

The correct operation of medical imaging devices is highly dependent on employee training and capability. Inadequate training can pose severe hazards to the operator and the patients being examined. Operator knowledge deficits generally result in suboptimal image acquisition and quality control, at the expense of diagnostic accuracy. This risk is compounded by sophisticated imaging modalities, such as interventional procedures, where the operator must skillfully navigate technical and ethical issues. The inclusion of robust training programs focused on operational skills and optimization techniques can help minimize these risks. Moreover, the use of techniques such as checklists and time-outs during operations can further enhance safety by keeping operators acutely aware of potential risks (Damilakis et al., 2017). Operator training expenditure is not only an industry best practice; it is also crucial for compliance with health and safety legislation. Long courses of instruction cannot only teach the technical skills of operating imaging equipment but must also cover the impact of radiation exposure and patient protection (Figure 11.12).

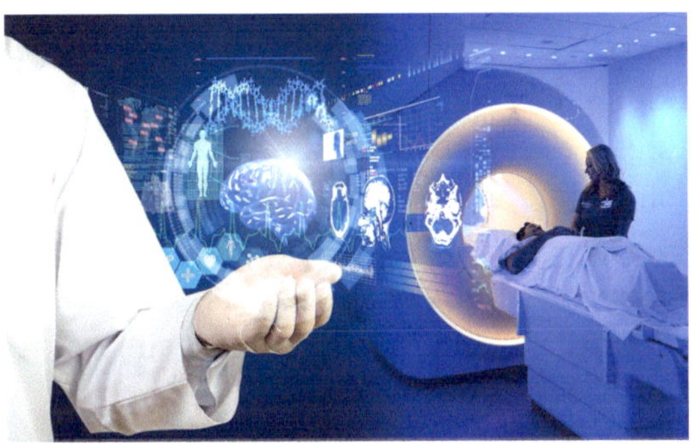

Figure 11.12. Insufficient training of operator can lead to significant risks not only for the operator but also for the patients being examined.

Source: https://admissionxpert.in/wp-content/uploads/2020/09/Medical-Imaging-min.jpg.

For example, the standards place strong emphasis on learning about dose management, as overexposure can harm one's health. Focusing on theoretical knowledge alongside practical experience can equip operators with the skills to make data-driven decisions that ensure patient welfare throughout imaging procedures. A well-trained operator is essential in optimizing the imaging process and obtaining correct diagnostics, especially in situations where accuracy is of high importance (Damilakis et al., 2017). As the medical imaging environment continues to change, with developments such as MRI guidance becoming more widespread, professional competence and competence maintenance through ongoing professional development are essential to ensuring top standards of practice. Ergonomics is also crucial in operator competence and productivity within the medical imaging discipline. As procedures get more complex, the physical and mental stress on operators increases proportionately. Greater exposure to unergonomic settings is also possible to provide for musculoskeletal traumas that impact an operator's performance in the long term. There is a correlation that is found between ergonomic improvements and operators' reduced fatigue, and this means enhanced accuracy in image capture. Training programs that address these ergonomic issues can provide professionals with improved skills for negotiating their workplace. As imaging technologies continue to develop, such as MRI-guided interventions, incorporating ergonomic training into day-to-day procedures will increase sustainability and long-term viability in the careers of healthcare imaging practitioners. Educating on the multifaceted nature of operator training ensures that technology is not the sole definition of expertise, and that it encompasses health and safety, ultimately translating into better outcomes for both practitioners and patients.

11.4.3. Environmental Influences on Imaging

Environmental impacts on imaging in health settings extend beyond the mere physical factors that are usually discussed, encompassing a complex interplay of technical, organizational, and social processes. For instance, the acute care environment is a critical context that initiates the use of imaging modalities. Contextual factors must be thoroughly understood to reduce digital image acquisition. Imaging system performance largely depends on the infrastructure provided by an institution, including the reliability of power and network connectivity. These ecological variables not only dictate the quality of images produced but also drive the urgent dissemination of imaging results, thereby impacting patient outcomes. In addition, inequality in resource access among hospitals may lead to variation in the efficacy of imaging, hence validating the need for a practical quality assurance framework for medical imaging modalities, as noted in earlier research that has taken into account the healthcare systems and deployment tactics at clinics (Abbas-Zadeh et al., 2014). External factors also manifest in the use of imaging technology and techniques for image assessment (Figure 11.13).

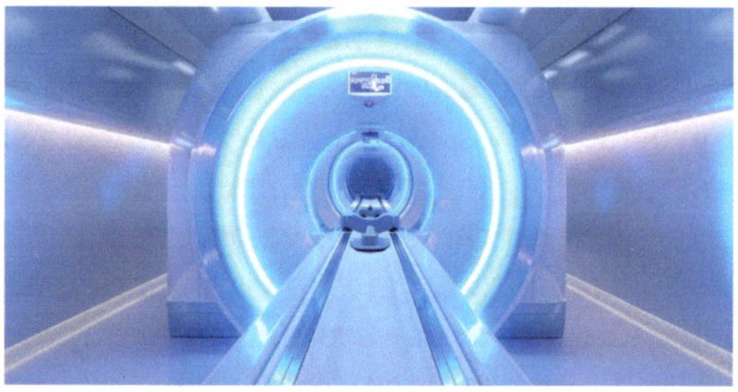

Figure 11.13. Hightech MRI room with blue neon lights and advanced medical imaging.

Source: https://www.freepik.com/.

Root system quantification, for example, demonstrates how environmental conditions influence imaging technologies and the resulting data. Present development indicates that imaging technologies are able to capture root morphology and interactions with soil effectively, yet results are influenced by many environmental factors like soil type and moisture content. This relationship concerns the requirement to appreciate both extrinsic and intrinsic factors in the integration of imaging in clinical use. With scientists coming up with better image acquisition techniques, they are faced with the challenge of resolving sample throughput, resolution, and integrity of data. Such a compromise not only demonstrates the complexities involved in image analysis but also the immense contribution that a controlled environment can make in unshackling the potential of imaging tools for successful measurements (Abbas-Zadeh et al., 2014). The integration of environmental factors into imaging extends to the social dynamics within healthcare facilities, particularly the relationships between clinical staff. Introduction of new imaging technologies typically requires additional reorganizations of assigned roles and processes between radiologists, radiographers, and other clinical stakeholders. As evident from many studies, including those in Malaysian hospitals, the organizational context—such as the influence of external entities like the Ministry of Health—determines how imaging technologies are adopted and used in medical settings. These dynamics affect staff cooperation, which ultimately affects the quality of patient care. The evolution of these dynamics, driven by reliance on advanced imaging, necessitates a holistic approach to quality control that accounts for technological integration as well as the human dimensions of healthcare delivery (Nor et al., 2010).

11.5. Advances in Digital Imaging Technology

Recent technological innovations in digital imaging have significantly enhanced the accuracy and efficiency of medical image acquisition. Technological advances in image sensors, particularly those based on complementary metal-oxide-semiconductor (CMOS) technology, have fundamentally changed how medical images are captured and processed. The sensors have made incredible progress regarding resolution, speed, and sensitivity, which are all critical elements in ensuring high-quality imaging in healthcare settings. Through this, physicians can now capture detailed images to aid in proper diagnosis. The ongoing development of such technologies highlights a growing trend: more power-efficient use and cost-effective solutions. Not only do these advancements improve patient outcomes, but they also make the workflow in healthcare facilities more efficient, a testament to the profound impact of digital imaging on effective medical practice. Moreover, the inclusion of computerized imaging techniques has further improved medical imaging quality. By incorporating advanced algorithms and processing methods, medical professionals can modify digital images in real time, adjusting features such as contrast and clarity. Not only is this useful for diagnostic determination, but it is also paramount in surgical procedure planning and treatment. The ability to rapidly process and tweak images enables a more thorough understanding of patient conditions, which is paramount in fields such as radiology and cardiology. With continuous research and development in computational imaging, the possibility of unparalleled image quality is at our doorstep. As these technologies advance further, they hold the potential to not only improve diagnostic efficacy but also revolutionize the patient care landscape in profound terms. Beyond healthcare innovation, quality control in medical imaging has become even more critical with advancements in imaging acquisition technologies. Maintaining the uniformity of medical images requires rigorous calibration and maintenance of imaging devices to minimize fluctuations in results. Given the notable developments in imaging techniques, maintaining consistent quality is a priority to avoid misinterpretation, which can lead to unjustified clinical decisions. Rigorous quality control procedures can prevent hazards in digital imaging processes. Moreover, the education of healthcare professionals in the effective use of these technologies is essential to maintaining standards. By developing an environment in which quality assurance is integrated into the imaging process, the healthcare sector can best capitalize on the advantages of digital imaging technologies, thereby enhancing patient safety and the quality of care.

11.5.1. Innovations in Imaging Hardware

The future of digital image acquisition and quality control in the medical imaging industry is anchored on advances in imaging equipment. With the introduction of high-tech technology, revolutionary imaging machines have been developed that produce high-quality images with stupendous clarity. For example, breakthroughs in sensor technology, particularly the development of CMOS Image Sensors (CIS), enable significant improvements in image quality through reduced noise and enhanced dynamic range.

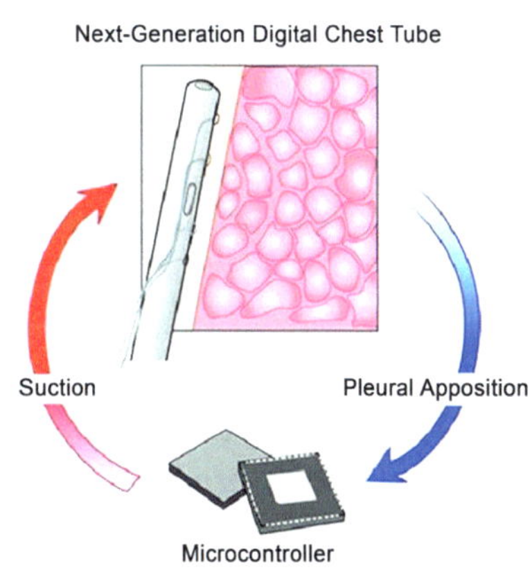

Figure 11.14. Illustration of next-generation digital detectors.

Source: https://th.bing.com/th/id/OIP.lPvLYeUOdpkAvMdFpDj0kAHaHa?rs=1&pid=ImgDetMain.

These sensors, which form the backbone of several imaging modalities, are built with components that emphasize calibration processes and error correction to ensure that the images generated are accurate and trustworthy. This development in imaging hardware is perfectly aligned with the industry's need for more precise diagnostics, resulting in better patient care and outcomes. Additionally, developments in medical imaging hardware are moving towards harnessing artificial intelligence and machine learning to a greater extent to achieve maximum efficiency. One of the key developments is the creation of Computational Vision Sensors (CVIS), which not only capture images but also process them by deriving useful features (Figure 11.14).

Unlike traditional CIS, CVIS is designed to derive conclusions from the data it acquires, enabling doctors to make timely and well-informed decisions. Such innovative imaging equipment prioritizes the path to a more integrated medical diagnostic approach, with increased emphasis on interpreting data rather than image acquisition. Employing such sophisticated systems, experts can improve diagnostic accuracy and workflow optimization, ultimately leading to better quality control of medical imaging procedures. Furthermore, the implementation of Medical Reverse Engineering (MRE) techniques offers new opportunities to significantly enhance medical imaging applications. MRE applies reverse-engineering technology to create three-dimensional models of anatomical structures to enable the design of personalized medical products and support biomedical research. The novel hardware and software methodology employed in MRE allows clinicians to to view detailed anatomical details more accurately than ever before. These innovations are particularly critical for disciplines such as tissue engineering and orthopedics, whose high accuracy is paramount. The ongoing development of such imaging technologies accentuates the essential interdependence of hardware innovation, quality control, and clinical intervention efficacy, as highlighted by Jos et al. (2010). Together, such innovations push the medical community toward a future characterized by advanced imaging and patient-specific therapeutic applications.

11.5.2. Software Designed for Image Analysis

The area of software advancements in image analysis has developed dramatically, particularly within the field of medical imaging. Advanced algorithms have been developed in order to further enhance the capabilities of systems in managing complex image data, which is especially applicable in modalities such as mammography.

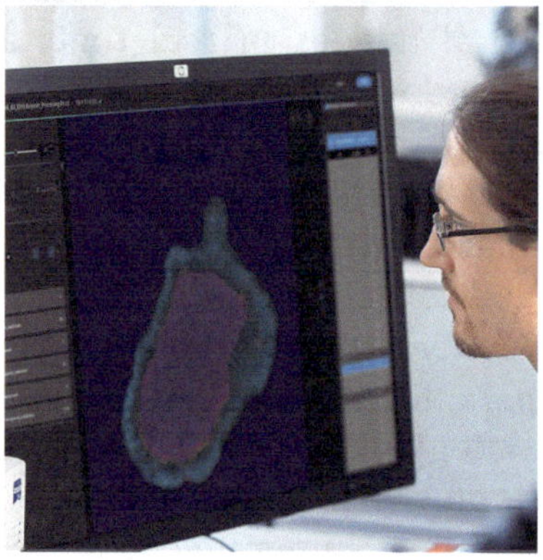

Figure 11.15. Screenshot of advanced image analysis software interface.

Source: https://www.zeiss.com/content/dam/rms/reference-master/products/software/arivis-cloud/czmi_23-arivis-cloud-cover-with-person.jpg/_jcr_content/renditions/original.image_file.851.851.867,0,1718,851.file/czmi_23-arivis-cloud-cover-with-person.jpg.

Traditional approaches are now complemented or replaced by computer-aided diagnosis (CAD) systems that use sophisticated pattern recognition techniques to improve diagnostic accuracy and reduce the impact of image noise. As a result, these developments paved the way for more accurate and reliable assessment of medical images, and thus ultimately contributed to improved quality patient care and diagnosis. The integration of novel digital sensors and these software technologies offers stable processing capabilities that can support greater data from higher-resolution imaging modalities, underscoring the need to handle and analyze this data effectively (Blaine et al., 2025) (Figure 11.15).

In addition to enhancing diagnosis, new software tools are also advancing image compression algorithms needed for the economic storage and transmission of data. As digital imaging becomes more popular in healthcare delivery, image creation volumes are rising, calling for effective compression methods to manage bandwidth without degrading image quality. Here, whether the compression is lossy or virtually lossless depends on need, as it determines how much information from a diagnosis is preserved. Advanced algorithms have been developed that can adaptively compress images without losing significant characteristics, enabling images to be exchanged and examined regularly across platforms. Such uses also play a vital part in telemedicine, in which high-quality images viewed from a distance remain of utmost importance for specialist consultations (Blaine et al., 2025). Such innovations ensure that healthcare professionals can deliver high standards of care even when physical distance separates them from patients. Moreover, modern software packages have expanded to address problems concerning root-soil interaction, which, as seemingly peripheral at best, indicate the range of use for image analysis technology. The techniques emerging in this field apply state-of-the-art imaging methods to quantify root systems and relate several morphometric characteristics to environmental factors. Notably, technology advancements in analysis software for imaging allow researchers to extrapolate high-resolution data linking phenotyping to environmental impact—an endeavor that can benefit agriculture and forecast yield. The trade-offs in this imaging space, namely resolution and sample throughput, also mirror those encountered in medical imaging, further underscoring the interdisciplinarity of technology. Therefore, as image analysis software advances, so does its impact in both the medical and agricultural fields.

11.5.3. Artificial Intelligence Impact on Imaging

The addition of artificial intelligence (AI) to medical imaging has transformed digital image capture, enabling significant improvements in both speed and accuracy. Using machine learning algorithms, radiologists can now interpret and process vast volumes of imaging data at unprecedented speeds.

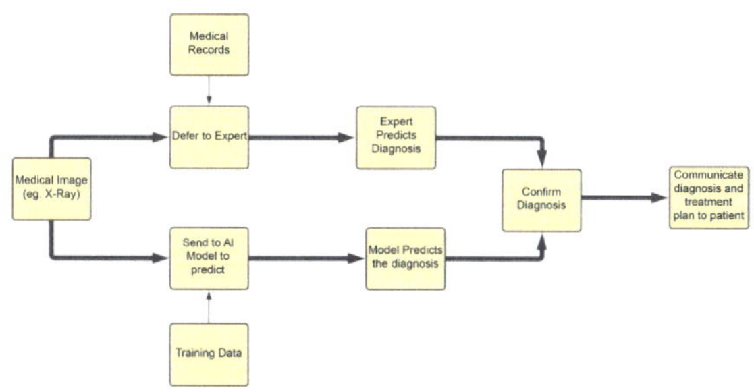

Figure 11.16. Flowchart of AI-driven diagnostic imaging analysis.

Source: https://www.researchgate.net/figure/The-Process-Flow-Representation-of-Medical-Image-Diagnosis-using-AI_fig5_355954943.

AI programs can detect patterns and anomalies in images that even experienced practitioners might miss. This capability not only enhances diagnostic accuracy but also reduces the possibility of human mistakes. Moreover, the assistance provided by AI allows clinicians to focus their talent on higher levels of decision-making rather than getting bogged down by tedious image analysis, effectively raising their productivity and improving patient outcomes.

Thus, the application of AI in medical imaging represents a paradigm shift that heralds a more integrated and robust healthcare system, with an optimized future for patient treatment and diagnosis. Apart from increasing the accuracy of diagnosis, AI also plays a key role to play in the quality control in the case of medical imaging (Figure 11.16).

Quality control processes traditionally reliant on human oversight can be augmented by AI-driven software that continuously monitors image quality in real time. Such systems can detect inconsistencies or deviations from established quality standards, ensuring that healthcare professionals produce optimal imaging results. For instance, AI can automatically verify attributes such as contrast, resolution, and signal-to-noise ratio, making it easier for technicians to correct defects before they impair patient care. Not only does this maximize workflow, but it also acts as a safeguard against low-quality image acquisition. AI-facilitated quality control processes, through high-quality imaging, enhance diagnostic accuracy, inspiring confidence in imaging technology and enabling its preeminent role in modern medicine. Lastly, the extent to which AI can be applied to imaging is limited by what can currently be learned with it, as studies continue to explore its potential intersection with other treatment disciplines, including centuries-old therapies like Qigong. The possibility of AI uniting Eastern and Western schools of medicine has interesting opportunities for personalized treatment. For example, the development of tools to read patient-specific respiratory patterns, as proposed using machine learning in AI-Medicine, can further improve the practice of medical imaging. By understanding how physiologic patterns map to imaging findings, AI can guide interventions more specifically. This convergence of technology and holistic principles is a revolutionary field that can provide a broader view of health and disease and emphasize the disruptive but beneficial impact of artificial intelligence on imaging and overall medical practice (Deng et al., 2013; Dethlefs et al., 2019).

11.6. Challenges to Quality Control

Medical image quality control is marked by challenges stemming from the technical complexity of image acquisition protocols, particularly in the context of digital technologies. For diagnostic purposes, radiologists and technologists must address issues such as equipment calibration, operator variability, and environmental factors. The temperamental nature of imaging techniques, along with human heterogeneity of perception and processing, can lead to variability in image quality. Further, the rapid evolution of imaging technology requires continued adaptation in quality control procedures. Lack of consistency in image quality assessment across institutions, owing to the lack of standard procedures, is a significant challenge in the profession. This requires not only robust personnel training but also the establishment of standardized measures to cover the diverse factors affecting image quality. Furthermore, medical imaging has significantly relied on large datasets, particularly when using machine learning algorithms for analysis and diagnosis. However, as has been highlighted at the first annual Conference on Machine Intelligence in Medical Imaging (C-MIMI), the medical imaging field is faced with an astounding lack of available and appropriately annotated datasets that have been referred to as data-starved (Geis et al., 2017). The challenge is not merely to collect data but also to ensure that it is of a certain quality level for reuse in training machine learning algorithms. Bad data quality may result in bad algorithm performance, which can adversely affect patient outcomes. This underscores the need for a collaborative effort from experts across fields to develop best practices for image dataset development, annotation, and dissemination, thereby making diagnostic equipment based on large-scale imaging information more trustworthy. Another emerging quality control challenge is implementing novel methods, such as compressed sensing, which can potentially make imaging less cumbersome but must be carefully analyzed for their impact on quality assurance. Because new technologies are unlikely to resemble traditional imaging paradigms, they challenge validation and implementation; when they do, they challenge validation and integration into settled mores (Vogt et al., 2017). Implicating non-nomological ideas requires re-evaluation of quality control methods designed initially for legacy imaging techniques. Consequently, the medical imaging sector must be dynamic in research and development in an effort to establish new standards and guidelines in support of new, innovative modalities of imaging and maintain high-quality output. This meeting of technology and strict quality control must be addressed by multidisciplinary forces in an effort to make medical imaging advances without compromising diagnostic integrity.

11.6.1. Variability in Imaging Systems

Imaging equipment variability is a critical variable influencing the quality of medical images. Variability originates from numerous sources, including differences in equipment, differences in operator technique, and environmental variations. For instance, two imaging units, even from the same company, may differ in their outcomes owing to the differences in calibration and variations in aging components. Additionally, technical parameters — including resolution, contrast, and noise levels — are affected by the imaging modality used—whether CT, MRI, or ultrasound. These differences can have a tremendous bearing on diagnostic accuracy, leading to different treatment plans (Figure 11.17).

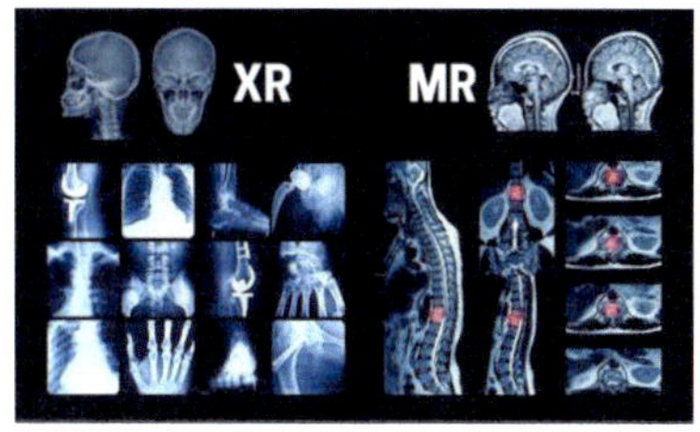

Figure 11.17. Chart showing variability in image output across systems.

Source: https://th.bing.com/th/id/OIP.-zD_w-xTIa_M4DThaSutWQHaEW?rs=1&pid=ImgDetMain.

Thus, controlling such variability through strict quality control measures is required to deliver uniformity and trust in medical imaging, ultimately enhancing patient outcomes and safety in a clinic setting. The need for standards in digital image acquisition has been particularly pronounced in the context of machine learning applications in medical imaging. As the Conference on Machine Intelligence in Medical Imaging recommendations state, among the pressing requirements is the availability of and standardization of medical image data sets. Heterogeneity in imaging responses further exacerbates the challenge of training learning machines to their full potential. The documentation of the data sets must account for the inherent variability of heterogeneous imaging systems, thereby requiring collaboration between data scientists and medical imaging experts. Cooperative collaboration is essential to mitigate the data scarcity problem and promote best practices in imaging data annotation and collection, so that machine learning models can be trained on high-quality, representative datasets that reflect the imaging system diversity used clinically (Geis et al., 2017). The intricate nature of imaging modality characteristics and surgical applications showcases the diversity within medical imaging systems. For example, computer-assisted orthopedic surgery (CAOS) systems utilize different imaging modalities—volumetric ones such as CT or MRI, and 2D or 3D fluoroscopic images. Each of these modes has unique benefits and drawbacks that can introduce variability into the accuracy and result of surgery. Furthermore, integrating kinetic and morphological data into such systems can increase navigation precision but varies significantly across configurations (Kalová et al., 2019). Therefore, understanding variability across imaging systems not only provides insight into technological innovation but also underscores the need for proper training and quality control measures to ensure standardization in the use of various imaging modalities in clinical environments.

11.6.2. Cost Implications of Quality Control Measures

It is costly, both directly and indirectly, to apply quality control (QC) techniques in digital image acquisition. The expenses of QC protocols range from software tools purchase at the highest end to training employees in QC processes.

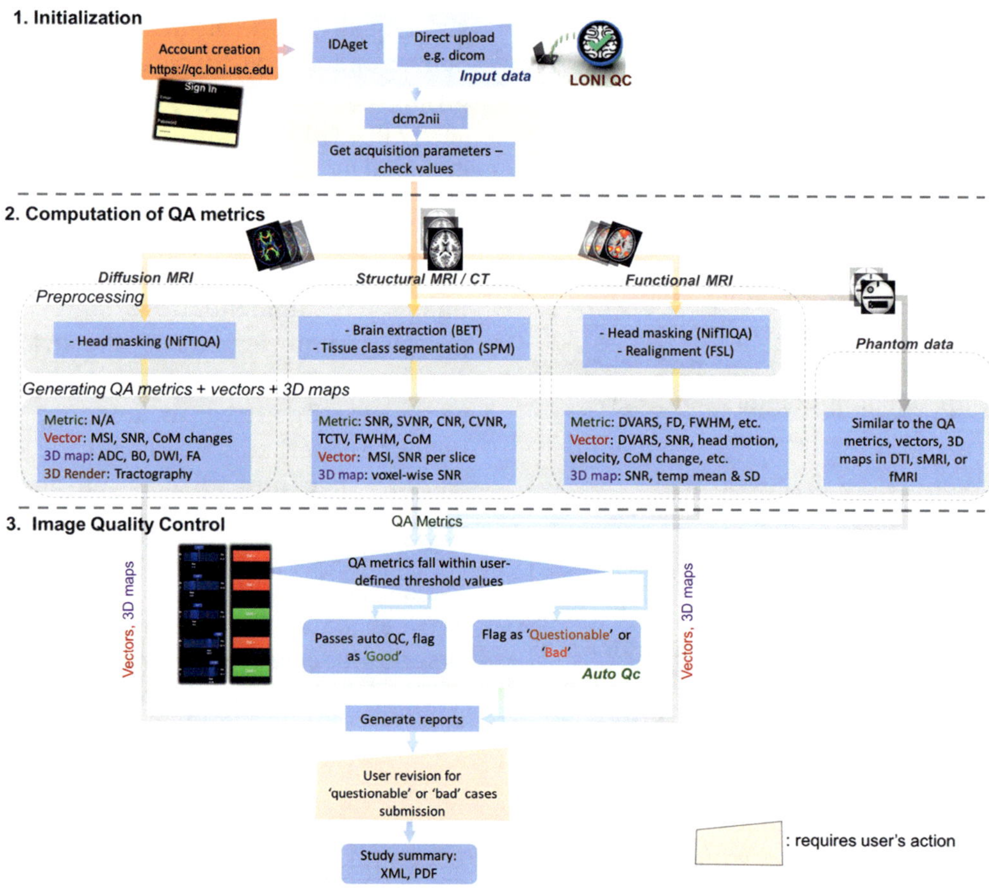

Figure 11.18. Overall workflow for the LONI QC system.

Source: https://www.researchgate.net/publication/335455151/figure/fig1/AS:11431281153850107@1682590913499/Overall-workflow-for-the-LONI-QC-system-The-LONI-QC-system-consists-of-the-three-main.tif.

High-end imaging systems that deliver better, more detailed images can be costly initially but, over the long term, reward the organization by reducing repeat scanning caused by poor-quality images. Furthermore, it would be worthwhile to invest in standardized QC processes, such as the LONI-QC system, which can streamline workflows, yield more valid neuroimaging data, and potentially save resources and time in the long run (Blanco et al., 2019). As a result, while initial costs may be prohibitive, the long-term benefits of reduced errors and improved outcomes are critical factors in planning for quality control in healthcare organizations' budgets. Yet another key cost consideration is the impact of QC actions on treatment effectiveness and patient safety (Figure 11.18).

Poor-quality imaging can lead to misdiagnosis, treatment by proxy, and, finally, extra healthcare costs arising from complications or other procedures. As noted in many studies, rigid QC procedures help ensure the accuracy of diagnostic imaging, thereby reducing costly adverse events from misdiagnosis (Blanco et al., 2019). The investment in the practice of QC, therefore, is not only a cost but also an integral part of patient care. The economic rationale for the imposition of such QC practices thus extends beyond explicit fiscal expenditure to encompass the overall impact on healthcare quality and the confidence of patients in diagnostic tests. Organizations should ultimately incorporate the routine operational costs run by quality control practices into their budgets. Such may entail regular audits, maintenance of QC systems, and adherence to evolving industry standards, all of which involve a continuous allocation of resources. OPTIMAX 2016 demonstrated that collaborative work in academia to optimize imaging practice is possible, illustrating how cooperation can also improve cost-effectiveness in training and research. By providing knowledge and resources, institutions can reduce QC-related costs while maintaining high imaging quality. Cost impacts of QC interventions are consequently multifaceted and need careful planning to balance short-term costs with long-term gains in imaging effectiveness as well as patient safety.

11.6.3. Addressing Human Factors in Imaging

Human factors play a crucial role in the effectiveness of digital image acquisition and quality control in medical imaging. Since medical imaging technologies are rapidly evolving, it is important to understand how humans interact with these systems. The operators often have multiple imaging protocols to perform, which require skilled interpretation and technical expertise. Human factors incorporation into the imaging process can be extremely useful for diagnostic accuracy.

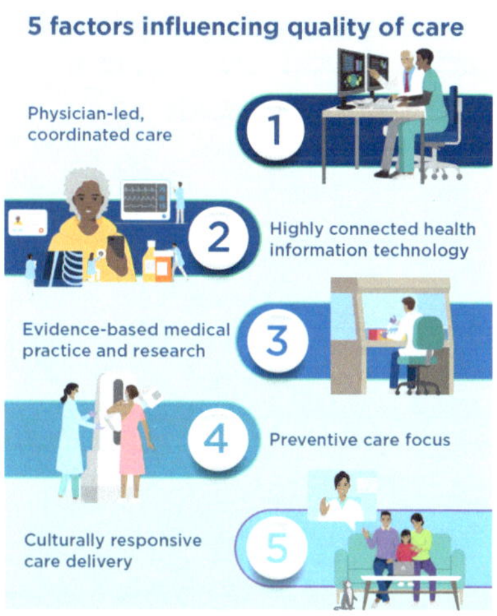
5 factors influencing quality of care
Physician-led, coordinated care
1
2
Highly connected health information technology
Evidence-based medical practice and research
3
4
Preventive care focus
Culturally responsive care delivery
5

Figure 11.19. Discrepancies can arise between perceived image quality (pIQ) and clinical image quality (cIQ) due to individual bias and subjective interpretations by radiologists and pathologists.

Source: https://permanente.org/wp-content/uploads/2023/04/Quality-care-infographic.png.

For instance, the method of image quality assessment has shifted towards the evaluation of clinical performance outcomes, reiterating the importance of clinician interaction and their ability to utilize imaging information effectively. Enhancing these human factors can lead to optimized imaging protocols and, in turn, improved standards and outcomes in patient care (Figure 11.19).

In quality control, accounting for human factors also requires an understanding of perceptual and psychological factors that influence image interpretation. Research reveals that perceived image quality (pIQ) and clinical image quality (cIQ) can differ due to individual bias and subjective judgment by radiologists and pathologists. Differences in methodology for evaluating image quality further exacerbate these problems, underscoring the need to standardize evaluation procedures. In their exploration of these variations, it is observed that pIQ scores on task-specific tasks earned as part of specific clinical tasks can more accurately parallel cIQ, thereby maximizing diagnostic precision. This hints at the potential for critical thinking and image interpretation skills in instructional design for healthcare workers as a mechanism for bridging subjective impressions and clinical efficacy. Secondly, technological applications in medical imaging need to be considered from a human factors perspective to optimize functionality and usability. The user interfaces of imaging systems, including the interpretation software, need to be carefully designed to match the cognitive burden imposed on radiologists and technicians. For example, in explosive detection in luggage through X-ray imaging, image data quality adjustment by adaptive scan parameters is literally dependent upon how users engage imaging technology. Textural signature studies have established that modifying image properties can improve material characterization and identification, outcomes depending upon operators expertise in handling available tools. Therefore, integrating human factors into imaging system design and training is essential to provide a better imaging environment, leading to better diagnostic results and more effective workflows.

SUMMARY

In emphasizing the key importance of digital image acquisition and quality control in medical imaging, it is important to recognize that technological advancements have significantly enhanced the diagnostic capabilities of medical practitioners. Higher-resolution images obtained through sophisticated digital methods allow for earlier diagnosis and proper assessment of medical conditions, with great advantage to the patient. Integration of various imaging modalities with rigorous quality control procedures ensures that medical images not only provide accurate information about the underlying anatomy but are also critical to decision-making in subsequent patient care. This union of technology and quality assurance has revolutionized medical imaging, creating a more efficient healthcare delivery system. Moreover, the role of image registration in medical imaging has a pivotal part to play in the enhancement of the diagnostic process. By registering images from multiple viewpoints or at different times, image registration enables better analysis of temporal changes in morphology, a key consideration in monitoring disease progression or therapy response. As observed, the application of different image registration methods has its merits and demerits, underscoring the need for ongoing innovation in this field. Performance measure assessment is necessary to assess the accuracy and quality of registration processes, as discrepancies may lead to misinterpretation, underscoring the importance of quality control in the delivery of effective diagnostic results (Nag et al., 2017). Lastly, the ongoing evolution of technology requires a responsive approach to the quality control of digital imaging. As medical imaging increasingly relies on artificial intelligence and machine learning algorithms, maintaining stringent standards will be crucial to prevent such advances from compromising diagnostic integrity. Results indicate that factors from outside the imaging process, such as system infrastructure and stakeholders' roles, impact the effectiveness of image acquisition and quality control processes (Alimin et al., 2001). Therefore, the development of a culture of excellence in digital image practice will be essential to sustaining improvements in patient care. In conclusion, with evolving medical imaging, practices in both adopting innovation and applying stringent quality control measures will contribute substantially to health systems and patients.

CLOSER LOOK

With advances in digital imaging science, the future appears promising since it can potentially enhance both acquisition procedures and quality control procedures in medical imaging. One of the primary ways is the integration of advanced machine learning algorithms, which can enhance image interpretation by recognizing patterns and automating tasks. These newer systems have the potential to assist radiologists in identifying abnormalities with unprecedented accuracy, thus facilitating quicker diagnoses and patient-tailored treatment plans. By enhancing algorithms that assess image quality in real time, health providers can respond promptly, ensuring that medical imaging data is wholesome and accurate throughout the diagnostic process. In this directionwill be required multidisciplinary work , multidisciplinary work will be required to develop and evaluate models for implementing machine learning in clinical practice. Another crucial variable shaping the destiny of digital imaging is the evolution of hardware technologies designed for optimized image acquisition. Technological improvements, such as the development of more highly resolved cameras with more sensitivity to various wavelengths of light, should widen the capability of imaging modalities for medical use. Improvements in X-ray and MRI technologies, for instance, will provide more accurate visualization of function and structure at a cellular level, significantly increasing diagnostic capability. In addition, investigation of new imaging modalities, such as photoacoustic imaging, could revolutionize the way physicians image tissue function. While these technological advancements are happening, they then need to be combined with robust quality control systems so that imagery does not vary. The task in the future is to demonstrate these new technologies through rigorous testing, ultimately bringing them to the level of scrutiny necessary for clinical diagnosis and treatment. Along with these advances in technology and acquisition, the future of digital imaging will also feature greater emphasis on its ethical and regulatory aspects. As imaging technologies become increasingly integrated into AI and machine-learning systems, patient privacy, data protection, and the ethics of automated diagnosis will have to be taken seriously. Regulatory agencies are mandated to keep up with the explosive proliferation of imaging technologies so they can be appropriately evaluated before they are used in medical practice. Moreover, healthcare providers' continuing education on these new technologies and their potential implications will be essential to maintaining high standards in medical imaging practice. Formulating comprehensive guidelines and frameworks will facilitate the ethical development of digital imaging, ultimately enhancing patient outcomes in the ever-evolving healthcare system.

REFERENCES

1. Downie, H. F., Adu, M. O., Schmidt, S., Otten, W., Dupuy, L. X., White, P. J., & Valentine, T. A. (2014). Challenges and opportunities for quantifying roots and rhizosphere interactions through imaging and image analysis. *Plant Cell & Environment*, *38*(7), 1213–1232. https://doi.org/10.1111/pce.12448Albaugh, M. D., Botteron, K. N., Ducharme, S., Evans, A. C., et al. (2016). Anxious/depressed symptoms are related to microstructural maturation of white matter in typically developing youths. https://core.ac.uk/download/70385585.pdf (accessed on 14th July 2025).
2. Alimin, A. J., Hushim, M. F., Mohd Rohi, N., Muslim, M., et al. (2001). Kajian motivasi ekstrinsik di antara pelajar lepasan sijil dan diploma Politeknik Jabatan Kejuruteraan Awam KUiTTHO. https://core.ac.uk/download/12007369.pdf (accessed on 14th July 2025).
3. Aung, T., Devalla, S. K., Girard, M. J. A., Perera, S. A., et al. (2018). A deep learning approach to denoise optical coherence tomography images of the optic nerve head. http://arxiv.org/abs/1809.10589 (accessed on 14th July 2025).
4. Bart, S., Baumann, M., Berkelman, P., Bolla, M., et al. (2006). Medical image computing and computer-aided medical interventions applied to soft tissues. Work in progress in urology. http://arxiv.org/abs/0712.2100 (accessed on 14th July 2025).
5. Belykh, E., Eschbacher, J., Izadyyazdanabadi, M., Martirosyan, V., et al. (2018). Improving utility of brain tumor confocal laser endomicroscopy: Objective value assessment and diagnostic frame detection with convolutional neural networks. http://arxiv.org/abs/1801.02101 (accessed on 14th July 2025).
6. Blaine, G. J., Brown, G. S., Clarke, L. P., Doi, K., et al. (2025). Digital mammography, cancer screening: Factors important for image compression. https://core.ac.uk/download/pdf/42807614.pdf (accessed on 14th July 2025).
7. Blanco, R. E. C., Clark, K., Crawford, K. L., Duffy, B. A., et al. (2019). The LONI QC system: A semi-automated, web-based and freely-available environment for the comprehensive quality control of neuroimaging data. https://core.ac.uk/download/323063233.pdf (accessed on 14th July 2025).
8. Boone, M., Boone, M., De Schryver, T., Dierick, M., et al. (2018). Motion compensated micro-CT reconstruction for *in-situ* analysis of dynamic processes. https://core.ac.uk/download/158346784.pdf (accessed on 14th July 2025).
9. Buissink, C., Hogg, P., & Thompson-Hogg, R. (2016). Optimizing image quality for medical imaging. https://core.ac.uk/download/77067051.pdf (accessed on 14th July 2025).
10. Burger, A., Verbeek, F., Johnson, G. A., Zaslavsky, I., Nissanov, J., Boline, J., Puelles, L., et al. (2009). The INCF Digital Atlasing Program: Report on digital atlasing standards in the rodent brain. https://core.ac.uk/download/pdf/288929.pdf (accessed on 14th July 2025).
11. Camara, O., Cash, D. M., Crum, W. R., Fox, N. C., et al. (2006). Phenomenological model of diffuse global and regional atrophy using finite-element methods. https://core.ac.uk/download/1682070.pdf (accessed on 14th July 2025).
12. Camilleri, A., Camilleri, G. E., Camilleri, J., Camilleri, M., et al. (2004). Dentistry. https://core.ac.uk/download/46601883.pdf (accessed on 14th July 2025).

13. Carmona Galán, R., Fernández Berni, J., Leñero Bardallo, J. A., Rodríguez Vázquez, Á., et al. (2018). CMOS vision sensors: Embedding computer vision at imaging front-ends. https://core.ac.uk/download/227044215.pdf (accessed on 14th July 2025).

14. Choubey, B., & Gouveia, L. (2014). On evolution of CMOS image sensors. https://core.ac.uk/download/42354684.pdf (accessed on 14th July 2025).

15. Ciortan, I., Daffara, C., Giachetti, A., Gobbetti, E., et al. (2017). A novel framework for highlight reflectance transformation imaging. https://core.ac.uk/download/86520765.pdf (accessed on 14th July 2025).

16. Cox, B. F., Fatahi, M., Fernandez-Gutierrez, F., French, J., et al. (2015). Comparative ergonomic workflow and user experience analysis of MRI versus fluoroscopy-guided vascular interventions: An iliac angioplasty exemplar case study. https://core.ac.uk/download/228177186.pdf (accessed on 14th July 2025).

17. Damilakis, J., Ebdon-Jackson, S., Frush, D. P., Loose, R., et al. (2017). Unintended and accidental medical radiation exposures in radiology: Guidelines on investigation and prevention. https://core.ac.uk/download/96883276.pdf (accessed on 14th July 2025).

18. Deng, Y., Li, Y., & Liu, J. (2013). A brief network analysis of artificial intelligence publication. http://arxiv.org/abs/1311.5998 (accessed on 14th July 2025).

19. Department of Innovation, Industry, Science and Research. (2025). *2011 Strategic Roadmap for Australian Research Infrastructure*. https://core.ac.uk/download/pdf/30672610.pdf (accessed on 14th July 2025).

20. Dethlefs, B. A., Lee, K. L., Li, S. C., Loudon, D., et al. (2019). Breathing signature as vitality score index created by exercises of Qigong: Implications of artificial intelligence tools used in traditional Chinese medicine. https://core.ac.uk/download/323075335.pdf (accessed on 14th July 2025).

21. Ducatelle, R., Kumcu, A., Philips, W., Platisa, L., et al. (2017). Influence of study design on digital pathology image quality evaluation: The need to define a clinical task. https://core.ac.uk/download/84044422.pdf (accessed on 14th July 2025).

22. Geis, J. R., Kohli, M. D., & Summers, R. M. (2017). Medical image data and datasets in the era of machine learning—Whitepaper from the 2016 C-MIMI Meeting Dataset Session. https://core.ac.uk/download/323063057.pdf (accessed on 14th July 2025).

23. Gouveia, L. (2016). Advances on CMOS image sensors. https://core.ac.uk/download/42370565.pdf (accessed on 14th July 2025).

24. Hill, G., Holliday, R., Maddock, I., Visser, M., et al. (2025). Assessing the viability of complex electrical impedance tomography (EIT) with a spatially distributed sensor array for imaging of river bed morphology: A proof of concept (study). https://core.ac.uk/download/50363.pdf (accessed on 14th July 2025).

25. Kalová, M., Kubíček, J., Oczka, D., Tomanec, M., et al. (2019). Recent trends, technical concepts and components of computer-assisted orthopedic surgery systems: A comprehensive review. https://core.ac.uk/download/287649034.pdf (accessed on 14th July 2025).

26. Mohd Nor, R. (2010). The organizational implications of medical imaging in the context of Malaysian hospitals. https://core.ac.uk/download/1588563.pdf (accessed on 14th July 2025).

27. N/A. (2025). *NASA Tech Briefs Index, 1977, Volume 2, numbers 1–4.* https://core.ac.uk/download/pdf/10345595.pdf (accessed on 14th July 2025).

28. Nag, S. (2017). Image registration techniques: A survey. http://arxiv.org/abs/1712.07540 (accessed on 14th July 2025).

29. Oraevsky, A. A., Barrett, H. H., Elbau, P., Wang, K., Kunyansky, L. A., Anastasio, M. A., Pan, X., et al. (2012). Investigation of iterative image reconstruction in three-dimensional optoacoustic tomography. http://arxiv.org/abs/1207.1028 (accessed on 14th July 2025).

30. Seibert, A. J., Baird, C. T., Clements, J. B., de Boer, S., et al. (2018). AAPM medical physics practice guideline 10.a.: Scope of practice for clinical medical physics. https://core.ac.uk/download/286729023.pdf (accessed on 14th July 2025).

31. Speller, R., & Uroukov, I. (2015). A preliminary approach to intelligent X-ray imaging for baggage inspection at airports. https://core.ac.uk/download/42358441.pdf (accessed on 14th July 2025).

32. Vander Sloten, J., Lam, K., Le, C., Le, T., et al. (2010). Medical reverse engineering applications and methods. https://core.ac.uk/download/42389848.pdf (accessed on 14th July 2025).

33. Vogt, T. (2017). Compressed sensing–A new mode of measurement. https://core.ac.uk/download/186329942.pdf (accessed on 14th July 2025).

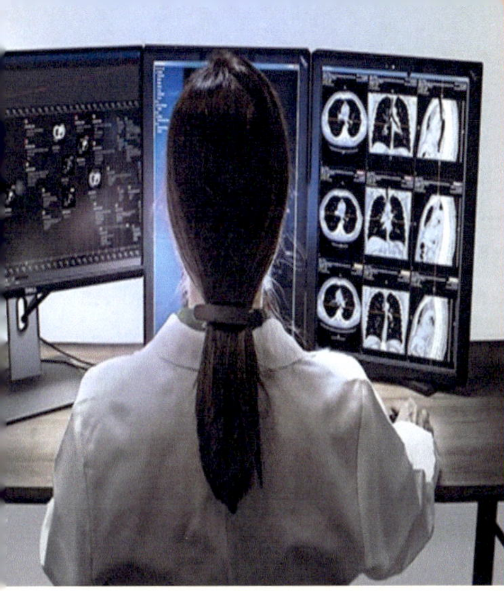

Chapter 12

PICTURE ARCHIVING AND COMMUNICATION SYSTEMS (PACS) IN MEDICAL IMAGING

Contents

Introduction

In the new era of medical imaging, Picture Archiving and Communication Systems (PACS) are fundamental systems that accelerate the pace and improve the availability of diagnostic imaging. PACS enable the storage, reception, and communication of medical images, a tremendous leap from traditional analog methods to sophisticated digital systems. Transitioning to PACS not only optimizes radiology department workflow but also contributes to significant advances in patient care. As put into perspective in the current literature, the introduction of digital PACS transformed the way images were handled, with improved diagnostic accuracy and streamlined processes achieved within healthcare settings (Duerinckx et al., 1983). This essay tries to analyze the complexity and innovation of PACS, focusing on their architectural designs, mechanism of integration, and their game-changing role in medical imaging. Understanding PACS' architecture is important to appreciate its effectiveness in the medical image domain fully. From traditional client-server to modern cloud-native architectures, PACS architecture comprises multiple configurations that serve specific functions. Client-server architectures cache data locally on a central server and are effective in data handling but require large quantities of local infrastructure. In contrast, web-based and cloud-native PACS offer greater accessibility and scalability, enabling medical professionals to utilize real-time diagnosis and collaboration capabilities (Duerinckx et al., 1983). These advances represent a shift towards more flexible, user-oriented systems designed to meet the growing demands of medical imaging. A critical examination of these architectures offers valid data regarding their operational efficiencies and possible effects on future advances in the field. Integration of PACS with HIS and RIS is a prime example of the need for end-to-end data interoperability in today's healthcare. PACS-HIS/RIS interoperability simplifies narrative reporting, order entry, and patient tracking, enhancing communication between departments. Moreover, utilization of Health Level Seven (HL7) interfaces facilitates easy data exchange, and clinicians become proficient in accessing real-time information. Present-day studies have established that such integrations facilitate an enhanced approach to patient management, reducing diagnostic turnaround times by half (Pérez-Sanpablo et al., 2025). Despite this, there are still challenges, particularly in data interoperability and compliance with privacy standards. These challenges will be overcome, which will make maximizing the benefits of PACS in the healthcare setting eventual, eventually leading to improved quality healthcare delivery through more efficient imaging procedures.

12.1. Historical Development of PACS

The history of Picture Archiving and Communication Systems (PACS) is marked by significant technological advances and the gradual development of medical imaging protocols. Conceived in its initial form in the 1980s, PACS aimed to computerize the storage and retrieval of medical images, eliminating the time-consuming film-based archives. As digital imaging devices such as computed tomography (CT) and magnetic resonance imaging (MRI) emerged, high-capacity systems were required to manage the volumes of data they generated. Hospital early adopters began to install the systems, triggering further studies and innovation. The earliest PACS architecture involved combining imaging systems, storage systems, and user interfaces under a single umbrella, which set the stage for the sophisticated systems we use today in a clinical environment (Nor et al., 2010) (Figure 12.1).

As hospitals adopted these technologies in greater numbers, they also recognized the need for standardization, which led to the creation of regulatory frameworks. As PACS evolved, interoperability became the primary issue, which led to the development of the Digital Imaging and Communications in Medicine (DICOM) standards during the 1990s. These norms provided a common platform for managing, storing, and transferring medical images across various systems and devices, which was crucial for improving workflow efficiency in healthcare settings. Most importantly, DICOM was instrumental in offering guarantees that images from multiple modalities would be interconnected seamlessly, facilitating the cooperative work among healthcare professionals (Batenburg et al., 2008). With the ongoing development of DICOM, PACS can now be designed with additional features, such as security protocols, which are essential for protecting patient information in these systems. Thus, the emphasis on standardization over time not only helped develop PACS but also enhanced the overall quality of patient care. Global PACS system implementation has not been uniform, with differences in organizational readiness and external pressures, particularly in the developing nations. Research indicates that government policies, resource availability, and hospital culture influence the adoption and success of PACS technologies to a substantial degree (Nor et al., 2010). Hospitals must navigate such challenges by aligning their business processes with strategic objectives, as demonstrated in frameworks such as the PACS integrated situational alignment (PISA) (Batenburg et al., 2008). The need for continuous assessment and improvement aligns with the dynamic pace of PACS implementation. As systems become increasingly more complex and interconnected to other health information technologies, it is important that healthcare facilities commit to user education, system administration, and monitoring performance in order to bring in the best returns with PACS-enhanced medical imaging capabilities.

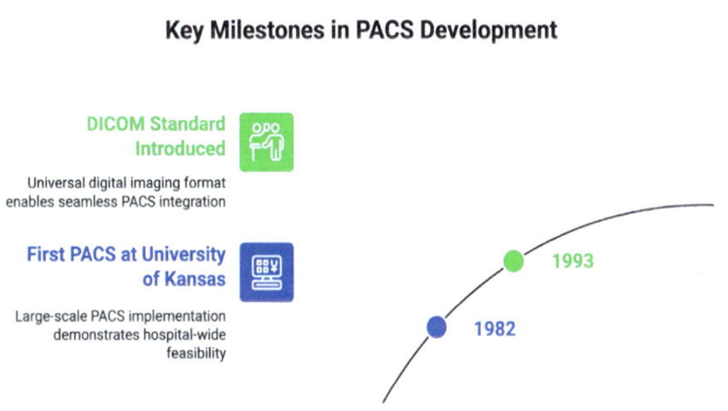

Figure 12.1. Timeline illustrating the evolution of PACS from analog to digital imaging systems.

Source: https://radsource.us/wp-content/uploads/2025/05/The-Origins-of-PACS-in-Radiology-scaled.jpg.

12.1.1. Early Imaging Technologies

The development of early imaging technologies provided the groundwork for today's Picture Archiving and Communication Systems (PACS) by revolutionizing medical professionals' method of visualizing and diagnosing conditions. Diagnostic approaches such as X-rays, developed in the late 19th century, transformed diagnostic medicine by providing non-invasive exploration of the human body. Following X-rays, advances in imaging technologies such as computed tomography (CT) and magnetic resonance imaging (MRI) further enhanced diagnostic capabilities by providing cross-sectional and soft-tissue images. These advances, besides improving diagnostic accuracy, also increased the efficiency of patient care by enabling quicker analysis and decision-making. Consequently, as early imaging technologies evolved, they needed improved means of storing and communicating, giving rise to technologies that would support and store the vast quantities of imaging data produced, providing a valuable bridge to the eventual implementation of PACS technology. As demand for effective management of imaging data rose, early imaging modalities were a driving force behind the development of systems intended to simplify workflows and enhance interdepartmental collaboration. Radiology departments initially relied on physical film, which required time-consuming procedures for storing and retrieving images (Figure 12.2).

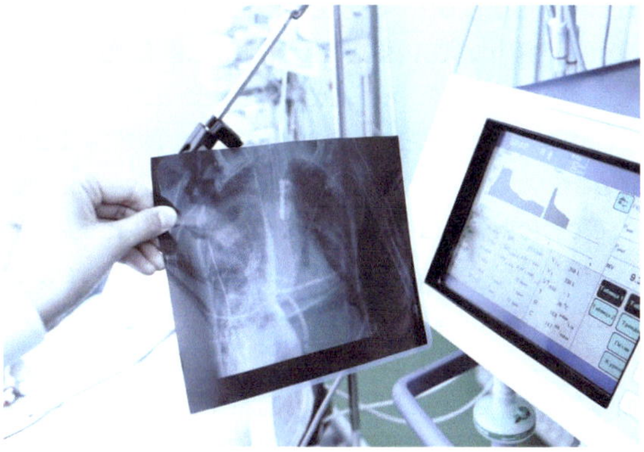

Figure 12.2. Example of an early X-ray film viewer used before PACS.

Source: https://nmchealthcare.com.my/wp-content/uploads/2021/03/Depositphotos_95338682_s-2019.jpg.

The emergence of digital imaging modalities alleviated many of these issues by producing electronic images, opening new possibilities for data storage and communication. For instance, the application of Picture Archiving and Communication Systems sought to digitize these operations so that images could be easily accessed, distributed, and stored securely across different healthcare institutions. This shift to computer-based systems was vital in facilitating interdisciplinary communication, ultimately paving the way for integrated healthcare communication models that maximize patient care and operational efficiency (Nor et al., 2010). Conceptualizing the initial imaging technologies was also made necessary by the need for standardized protocols to ensure interoperability across different systems and devices. The development of the Digital Imaging and Communications in Medicine (DICOM) standard provided a template for formalizing image formatting, network services, and security protocols, which were then incorporated into PACS development. The standardization not only helped various imaging modalities become interoperable but also enabled the integration of imaging systems with Hospital Information Systems (HIS) and Radiology Information Systems (RIS). As healthcare centers began adopting these protocols widely, they created a more cohesive data environment that facilitated the smooth exchange of information essential to diagnosis and treatment planning. The advancements enabled by pioneering imaging technology and DICOM standards reflect the need for continued development in medical imaging to address the complexity of today's patient care (Bastião et al., 2020).

12.1.2. Evolution of Digital Imaging

The digital imaging revolution has significantly transformed medical diagnostics, with developments in Picture Archiving and Communication Systems (PACS) at the forefront. Film-based early imaging set ceilings on access and efficiency as radiologists had to contend with and interpret films firsthand. Digital imaging ushered in a new era, enabling high-quality image storage and transfer over digital networks. This transformation not only improved workflow productivity in healthcare settings but also enabled remote consultations and physician collaboration. With the widespread adoption of PACS, it was clear that integrating computer imaging with healthcare information systems was the future.

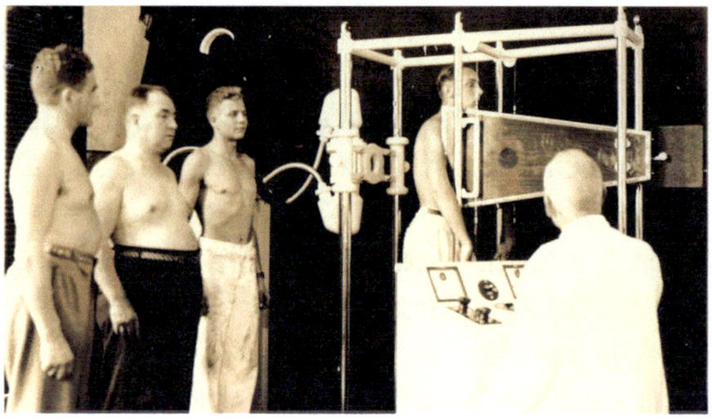

Figure 12.3. Manoel de Abreu's photofluorography unit was the first device to successfully implement the idea of capturing X-ray images with a photographic camera for use in lung screening.

Source: https://www.medmuseum.siemens-healthineers.com/en/stories-from-the-museum/lung-screening.

The use of digital databases and effective telecommunications infrastructure enhanced networking capabilities, ultimately transforming patient care in medical facilities (Nor et al., 2010). Web-based solutions, and more so, have become core to the evolution of digital imaging in PACS. The growth of the internet has driven an evolution toward increasingly scalable, cloud-native solutions, enabling healthcare organizations to leverage remote storage and access capabilities. Over the years, advancements have enabled additional functionalities, such as real-time sharing of imaging data among healthcare providers, allowing streamlined workflows and increased interdepartmental collaboration. Successful image processing technology, such as that used in software like MammoApplet, has also streamlined the diagnostic process by enabling interactive interfaces that facilitate better visualization and annotation of mammogram cases (Figure 12.3).

The integration of these programs into PACS facilitates radiologist training. It makes medical database management easier, a factor that confirms the far-reaching impact of digital technology on medical imaging practice (Martí Bonmatí et al., 2012). Furthermore, as digital imaging advances, the importance of existing standards, such as DICOM (Digital Imaging and Communications in Medicine), continues to grow. DICOM is a key standard for interoperability between imaging devices and systems, enabling the exchange of data across heterogeneous environments. The arrangement, in accordance with the standards for the definition of data objects, network services, and security extensions, enables medical images to be accessible and secure at the same time. These standards also promoted PACS integration with Hospital Information Systems (HIS) and Radiology Information Systems (RIS), therefore streamlining order management and reporting processes. As healthcare continues to adopt and respond to digital imaging technologies, the interplay between robust standards and emerging technologies is also set to shape the future of medical imaging and PACS (Nor et al., 2010).

12.1.3. Milestones in PACS Implementation

The successful implementation of Picture Archiving and Communication Systems (PACS) has been paralleled by significant milestones reflecting progress in medical imaging technology. One of the important early objectives was to achieve interoperability among diverse imaging modalities. Achieving this milestone involved DICOM (Digital Imaging and Communications in Medicine) standards, which govern medical image format and transmission (Figure 12.4).

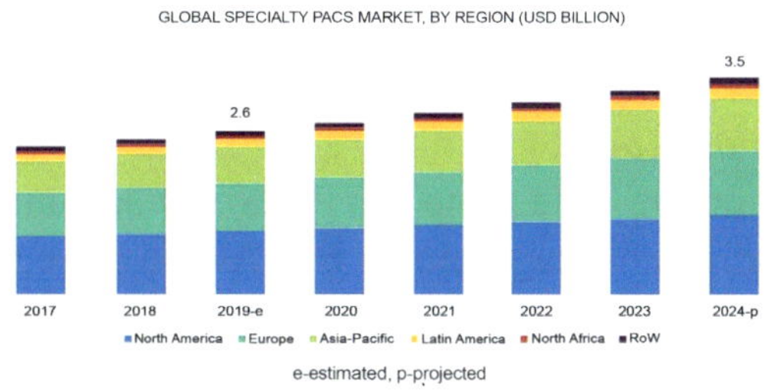

Figure 12.4. Global milestones in PACS implementation across different decades.

Source: https://www.marketsandmarkets.com/Images/specialty-pacs-market1.jpg.

The establishment of robust network infrastructure, along with the seamless integration of imaging devices into the hospital workflow, created effective data access and sharing. These were not only technological feats that enhanced the speed of information retrieval but also boosted the quality of patient care through prompt diagnoses, thereby setting an example for the future regarding PACS implementation. A milestone in PACS development was the transition away from traditional film-based procedures towards digital systems. This transition enabled greater flexibility in data handling and retrieval, underscoring the importance of data storage and archiving strategies. Hospitals began adopting tiered storage systems that addressed the need for fast access while still providing cost-effective long-term archiving. The application of compression mechanisms also optimized storage capacity, enabling huge imaging files to be stored without loss of image quality. With medical systems evolving, so has the necessity for comprehensive disaster recovery planning become, now a necessity for protecting patient data in the case of unforeseen disasters or technical failure. Establishing such milestones not only addressed urgent operational issues but also reaffirmed the ongoing commitment to quality assurance and systematic enhancements in medical imaging. Integration with existing Health Information Systems (HIS) and Radiology Information Systems (RIS) was another significant milestone in PACS development. Seamless integration between different healthcare systems required the use of HL7 interfaces to expedite communication and data transfer across platforms. By streamlining order management and reporting processes, PACS became an integral component of the general operations of healthcare IT systems. This integration streamlined workflows, allowing medical staff to focus on patient care rather than paperwork. Continuous performance monitoring and user training were paramount in ensuring that the benefits of such integrations were maximized. With the development of PACS, the focus on user interfaces —including advanced visualization tools and smartphone applications —further demonstrated the importance of user experience in enabling effective PACS adoption, leading to improved clinical outcomes and business efficiencies (Figure 12.5).

12.2. Components of PACS

In medical imaging, PACS design serves as the foundation for seamless image management and retrieval. The most important components are the imaging device, the secure network, the display stations, and the storage devices. All segments coexist to enhance workflow effectiveness and accuracy in diagnosis. The imaging devices, which include modalities such as MRI and CT scanners, capture digital images that must be transmitted in a timely manner over secure networks to viewing sites where medical professionals can interpret them. Such an arrangement reduces both communication delays for patients and radiologists and streamlines care delivery. Notably, as seen, PACS are built upon communicating components that, in combination, make things easier, reaffirming the necessity of embedding technology within healthcare systems in order to improve patient management results (Hristova et al., 2020). The application of the DICOM standard within PACS cannot be overstated in that it defines the data formats and network protocols needed for the seamless transport of medical images and associated data. DICOM is a vast collection of functionalities, including data object definitions that specify the content of images and network services, which facilitate communication among PACS components. DICOM's security extension also plays an important role in ensuring the confidentiality and integrity of sensitive medical data during storage and transmission. As imaging procedures become increasingly digitized, compliance with DICOM is the call of the day for institutions keen on enhancing interoperability among different health information systems. The ongoing evolution of DICOM standards helps address new challenges in medical imaging, further strengthening PACS as a vital piece of equipment in modern radiology (Hristova et al., 2020). Lastly, PACS integration with HIS and RIS improves the operational capabilities of healthcare facilities. HL7 interfaces, when applied, facilitate smooth communication between systems to ensure easy order management and reporting. The integration not only accelerates patient care procedures but also reduces error rates associated with manual data capture, thereby ensuring the integrity of patient data. In addition, efficient reporting processes allow radiologists to report faster, hence improving clinical judgment and patient care. PACS' integration with HIS and RIS represents a paradigm of technologically driven changes in healthcare delivery, indicating the need for institutions to prioritize and operate these systems optimally to counter the growing demand for medical imaging services (Hristova et al., 2020) (Figure 12.5).

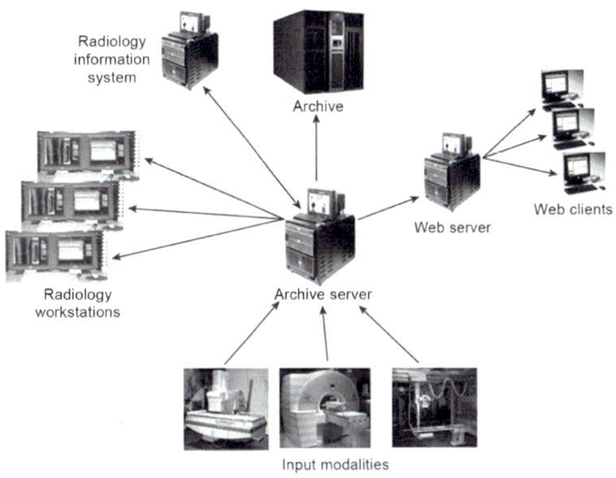

Figure 12.5. Key hardware and software components of a standard PACS system.

Source: https://radiologykey.com/wp-content/uploads/2016/02/F000090f009-001-9780323086448.jpg.

12.2.1. Imaging Modalities

In Picture Archiving and Communication Systems (PACS), imaging modalities play a critical role in enhancing diagnostic capability and workflow effectiveness in medical imaging. Traditional modalities such as X-ray, computed tomography (CT), and magnetic resonance imaging (MRI) have been a standard in clinical practice for years, providing rich information on patient conditions. However, with PACS digitizing these images, it not only enhances access and storage speed but also enables interoperability between modalities and health systems. PACS facilitates the seamless integration of various imaging modalities, enabling health professionals to easily share, access, and analyze information. This shift has far-reaching implications for patient care since timely and correct imaging goes hand-in-hand with higher diagnostic accuracy and treatment outcomes, thereby aligning with the common goal of efficient provision of healthcare (Canguit et al., 2025). Additionally, recent innovations in imaging modalities have also highlighted the importance of PACS implementation in medical imaging. New technologies, including ultrasound and advanced nuclear imaging techniques, are improving the quality and extent of information presented to health professionals (Figure 12.6).

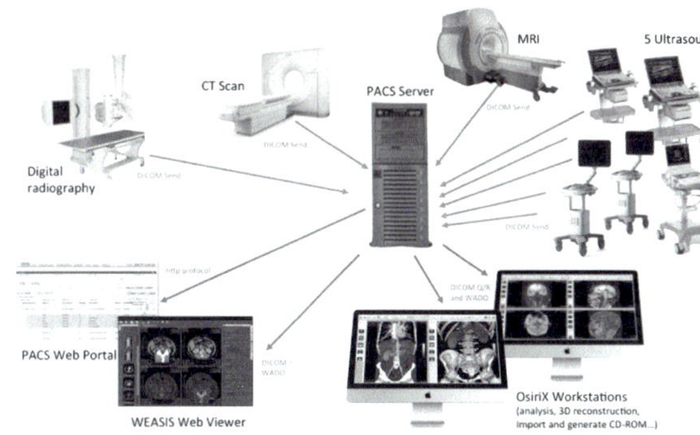

Figure 12.6. Different imaging modalities interfaced with PACS, including CT, MRI, and ultrasound.

The evolution of hybrid imaging devices, such as PET/CT and SPECT/CT, is a prime illustration of this shift, for they provide comprehensive information that can lead to better clinical decisions. As these new imaging modalities become increasingly prevalent, so too does the demand for sophisticated PACS solutions that support diverse data types and formats. Integration of these features into a holistic PACS framework enhances workflow efficiency and enables cooperative decision-making among multidisciplinary teams (Albert et al., 2024). It not only maximizes resource use but also underscores the value of ongoing education and training in new imaging technologies, empowering medical practitioners to optimize their use. In addition to improving accessibility and integration of imaging modalities, PACS significantly influences medical education. By providing access to an extensive library of images produced from various modalities,

PACS advances the training of medical students and radiologic technologists. Through exposure to real-life imaging situations, the students can sharpen diagnostic skills within a mock-up environment, supplementing theoretical knowledge with practical experience. Besides, the ability to implement PACS in research settings promotes interdisciplinary collaboration, and it is thus possible to examine large datasets to research disease development and treatment efficacy. This collaboration is increasingly vital as medical education responds to the rapidly evolving healthcare technology environment. In general, the synergy of imaging modalities and PACS not only improves patient outcomes but also advances medical education and research by one step (Albert et al., 2024; Canguit et al., 2025).

12.2.2. Storage Solutions

In Picture Archiving and Communication Systems (PACS), best practices in data storage and archiving are crucial to efficiently manage massive amounts of medical imaging data. Tiered storage methodologies are key to delivering balanced performance and cost savings. By organizing data at multiple levels based on accessibility and usage frequency, medical facilities can streamline retrieval while minimizing costs associated with high-performance storage systems. For instance, frequently used images can be stored on fast, expensive storage systems, while less often accessed or aged data can be transferred to slower, less costly systems. This organizational approach not only enhances access speed but also reduces overall storage infrastructure load, thereby addressing the issue posed by exponential growth in medical imaging, as evidenced by the increasing complexity of modern PACS (Nguyen-Chi et al., 2024). Incorporation of advanced compression processes ensures that data are stored more efficiently in PACS. As medical imaging generates a huge amount of data, utilizing practical compression algorithms allows for substantial file size reductions without compromising image quality. Lossless compression methods, in particular, are favored in clinical applications as they ensure diagnostic integrity. And with the advent of sophisticated imaging modalities, the need to deal with larger files drives the evolution of new compression technologies. Such advancements not only help preserve storage space but also increase network data transmission speeds, thereby streamlining the entire process in health facilities. Lastly, solving storage issues with these techniques is essential, as seen by the ongoing rise in imaging procedures in medical diagnosis (Nguyen-Chi et al., 2024).

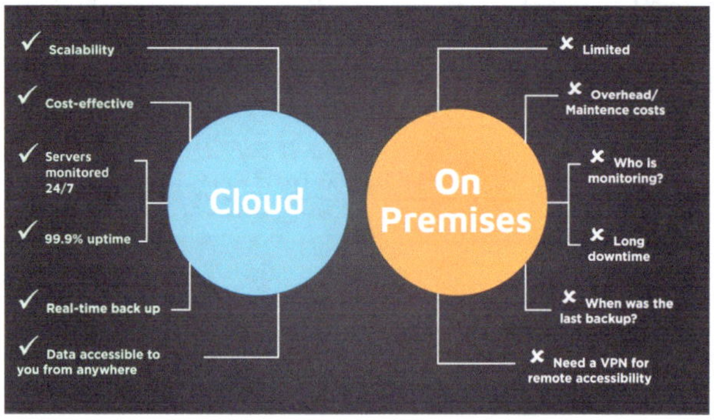

Figure 12.7. Comparison of on-site versus cloud-based PACS storage solutions.

Source: https://cdn.prod.website-files.com/6688504067e38d85fe21517b/668f026419a1a33c43e1aa4c_2_Revamp_Cloud_PACS_vs_On_Prem_b72669ba96.jpeg.

Disaster recovery planning is an essential part of PACS storage solutions, in which the access to and security of critical medical image data must be preserved in the event of unexpected events. Recovery planning not only addresses potential data loss from hardware failures and cyber-attacks, but also data recovery requirements that must be triggered quickly. Some of this involves establishing routine backup processes and tracking redundant storage devices to help protect against single points of failure. At a time when patient treatment increasingly relies on timely access to imaging files, hospitals need to place a high value on disaster recovery processes as part of their broader data management plan. Through robust disaster recovery planning, healthcare entities can reduce risk, uphold patient safety, and maintain continuous operations, thereby improving the reliability of PACS systems (Lebre et al., 2021) (Figure 12.7).

12.2.3. Communication Networks

In the context of Picture Archiving and Communication Systems (PACS), communication networks play a critical role in enabling the free flow of medical image data. They provide a platform for integrating various components of the PACS structure, allowing ready access to images and their associated information. High-latency, high-bandwidth communication networks are needed to handle large file sizes typical of medical imaging, such as CT and MRI scans.

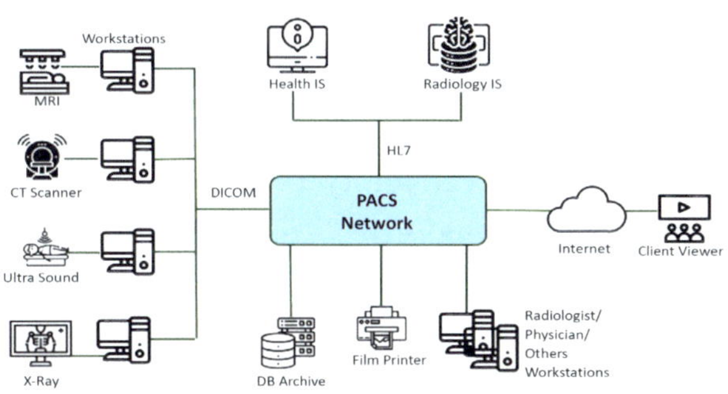

Figure 12.8. Simplified diagram of communication network infrastructure in PACS.

Source: https://www.researchgate.net/publication/358118184/figure/fig1/AS:11431281380133985@1744774813473/Reference-design-for-a-PACS-network-infrastructure.tif.

Such a network is essential because the timely availability of diagnostic images can have a direct impact on clinical decision-making and patient care. In addition, the interconnectivity between imaging centers and hospitals is significantly influenced by the choice of communication protocols and infrastructure, underscoring the need for robust network services that guarantee data integrity and privacy in accordance with healthcare laws. Moreover, the incorporation of web-enabled solutions within PACS greatly enhances communication networks by enabling access to imaging data from remote locations with internet connectivity (Figure 12.8).

By using secure web protocols, radiologists and clinicians can access images and reports on various devices, thereby promoting effective workflow and improved coordination among healthcare professionals. Cloud-native PACS take this potential a notch higher by relying on cloud infrastructure, enabling scalability and flexibility in handling shifting data demands. As hospitals migrate towards these new solutions, it is necessary to consider the impact of communication networks on security and data management. The use of DICOM standards, which govern the exchange of medical data and images, underscores the importance of appropriate network infrastructure to enable smooth interoperability among systems and devices. The connectivity between Health Information Systems (HIS) and Radiology Information Systems (RIS) and communication networks cannot be overstated. The smooth integration of PACS with these systems relies on communication networks that support HL7 interfaces and other messaging standards. These integrations improve order management and reporting processes, enabling a smooth interface between various stakeholders in patient care. An example is the effective implementation of PACS in Malaysian hospitals, which illustrates how communication networks enhance the operational efficiency of medical imaging technology within larger health systems (Nor et al., 2010). The study indicates that these networks influence organizational roles and relationships, thereby affecting the overall performance of healthcare services (Christensen et al., 2010). Consequently, innovation in communication networks is vital for optimizing PACS deployment and enhancing patient outcomes in the dynamic medical imaging environment.

12.3. Benefits of PACS in Medical Imaging

The application of Picture Archiving and Communication Systems (PACS) has transformed medical imaging practice by improving efficiency and the availability of diagnostic information. One of the key benefits of PACS is that it helps to reduce the use of conventional films, which used to cause storage and retrieval problems in medical facilities. With digital image storage, clinicians can quickly retrieve imaging studies in seconds, resulting in quicker diagnosis and enhanced patient care. Its timely availability not only enables communication among healthcare professionals but also enables patients to be given timely, executed treatment plans. Additionally, integrating advanced imaging devices with PACS enables easier collaboration among specialists, improving the overall diagnostic process. Another significant advantage of PACS is its ability to minimize the frequency of redundant imaging exams. Evidence also shows that installing PACS systems can lead to measurable reductions in redundant repeat testing. Research in 10 Ontario hospitals saw modest decreases in duplicate tests ordered within specified time frames post-PACS installation, illustrating its potential in avoiding redundant imaging (Reiner et al., 2008). Although certain imaging modalities, like computed tomography, saw higher rates of duplication after the deployment of PACS, overall, there remains a trend toward the system's contribution to imaging protocol simplification. Such imaging duplication reduction not only optimizes the allocation of resources for the facility but also reduces patient exposure to further radiation, highlighting the safety advantages that come with PACS. In addition, PACS systems also enhance data management and integration with implemented healthcare information systems (HIS) and radiology information systems (RIS). Seamless integration provides an effective order management and reporting process, enabling imaging orders to be processed swiftly and their results reported to the parties involved. Standardized communication protocols, such as HL7, applied atop this integration further support data integrity between platforms. Thus, physicians are better placed to make more effective clinical decisions with integrated, up-to-date patient information. The integration ultimately results in improved patient outcomes and operational effectiveness, signifying the pivotal role of PACS in modern medical imaging practice (Rahman et al., 2020).

12.3.1. Increased Availability of Images

The employment of Picture Archiving and Communication Systems (PACS) has greatly improved the availability of medical images, ensuring that smooth transfer procedures do not hinder diagnostics. By digitizing imaging modality data, PACS eliminates the lead time associated with film-based systems, ensuring that radiologists and referring physicians have real-time access to images. Real-time availability is especially crucial in emergency care, where timely decisions can be a significant factor influencing patient outcomes. Also, PACS integration with Hospital Information Systems (HIS) enables seamless flow of information between departments, and clinicians can access and view images and other medical records later on. Therefore, PACS implementation is a sign of a shift towards a more patient-centered healthcare approach, with increased emphasis on efficiency and better access to essential diagnostic facilities (Canguit et al., 2025). Incorporation of newer technology, such as web-based applications and cloud-native PACS, has provided access to imaging services to more people, particularly those in remote or underserved communities (Figure 12.9).

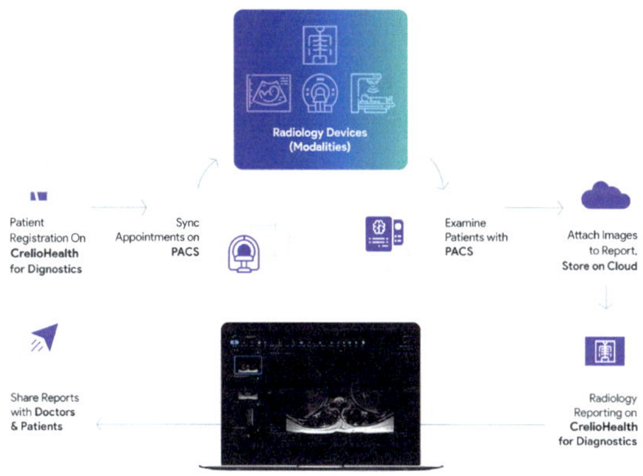

Figure 12.9. Hospital staff accessing patient images remotely via PACS interface.

Source: https://creliohealth.com/assets/img/how-crelio-pacs-radiology-software-works.png.

These infrastructures allow medical care professionals to access imaging data using secure web portals, which is invaluable for those who may not be geographically close to technologically equipped medical facilities. This accessibility enables physicians to collaborate, consult, and share results in real time, regardless of location. Most importantly, remote viewer software enables medical care professionals to view images remotely, enhancing their capability to make accurate decisions promptly. As a result, access to specialist diagnostic services is improved, bridging gaps in healthcare equity and enabling even outlying patients to undergo high-quality imaging and analysis (Joy, 2025). The evolution of PACS technology is also characterized by significant advances in user interfaces and viewing tools, which are crucial for image accessibility. Following the introduction of 2D/3D reconstruction workstations and high-end visualization plug-ins, radiologists now have sophisticated tools that greatly enhance their ability to interpret complex images accurately. Not only do these innovations strengthen the diagnostic process, but they also offer better learning tools for trainee radiologists, as these systems typically form valuable teaching tools. Moreover, performance monitoring and quality control mechanisms built into PACS ensure that radiological equipment is robust and that any accessibility discrepancies are resolved immediately. Therefore, the continuous improvement of PACS, alongside enhancing access to radiological images, also improves the overall quality of radiological services, making the system even more meaningful in modern healthcare (Canguit et al., 2025).

12.3.2. Enhanced Collaboration Among Healthcare Professionals

Better communication between healthcare professionals is one of the key benefits of applying Picture Archiving and Communication Systems (PACS) in medical imaging. Because it possesses a robust infrastructure that facilitates smooth image and report transfer, PACS provides reliable communication among radiologists, referring physicians, and other healthcare providers. This arrangement is significant since it improves clinical decision-making and enhances patient care. For instance, studies have indicated that with effective PACS installation, clinicians expressed high satisfaction with image quality and reliability, which increased team members' confidence and improved the overall patient care experience (Alhur et al., 2024). Also, the availability of digital images reduces consultation time, enabling rapid diagnosis and treatment planning, thereby highlighting the role of collaboration in complex patient cases. Moreover, the introduction of PACS facilitates an innovative impact on workflow efficiency within the healthcare setting. Closer collaboration through computerized interfaces creates enhanced order management and reporting workflows that are critical to delivering timely patient care. As such, clinicians benefit from better communication dynamics, especially in multidisciplinary settings where different specialties must get together to synchronize patient management styles (Figure 12.10).

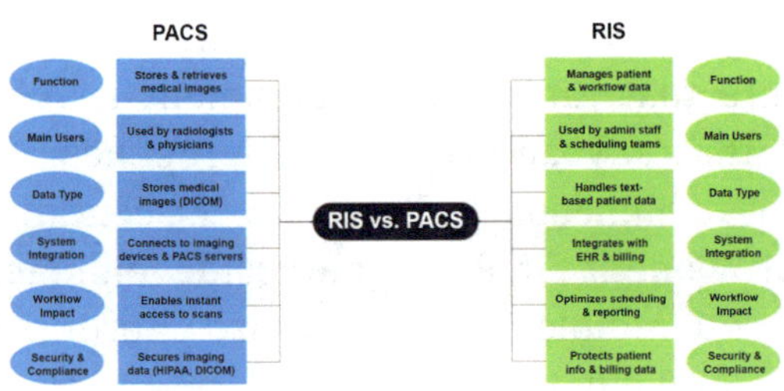

Figure 12.10. Multidisciplinary team using PACS in real-time to discuss patient cases.

Source: https://blog.medicai.io/wp-content/uploads/2025/02/ris-vs-pacs-1024x527.jpg.

The potential to view imaging results through a centralized system facilitates real-time decision-making and discussion, which is imperative in acute scenarios. The innovation heralds a deviation from the standard silos of clinical practice, whose functions become more complementary and collaborative (Nor et al., 2010). PACS endorsement thus not only enhances the functional nature of healthcare delivery but also encourages a professional teamwork culture, which is essential to high-quality patient care. Besides these functional benefits, the PACS-enabled collaboration platform has effects on professional growth for healthcare professionals. When clinicians communicate more through shared imaging facilities, there is potential for mentorship and information sharing among professionals at different levels. Radiologists can exchange ideas with resident doctors or family practitioners, thereby enhancing their diagnostic ability and knowledge of imaging interpretation. Through interaction, there is an environment with ongoing learning and innovation in medical teams. In addition, as new technologies emerge, adaptability in collaborative practice has the potential to enhance healthcare workers' confidence in using these technologies, thereby increasing adoption rates and satisfaction with tools such as PACS (Alhur et al., 2024). Therefore, with more collaboration, not only is the care of the patients enhanced, but also an innovative healthcare workforce that is capable of responding to future challenges.

12.3.3. Increased Efficiency in Workflow

In radiology, the introduction of Picture Archiving and Communication Systems (PACS) has seen revolutionary improvements in workflow efficiency in the healthcare setting. By abandoning traditional film-based modalities for digital modalities, various radiological procedures have been simplified, mainly lowering test acquisition time and image retrieval time. By providing immediate access to high-resolution images, PACS eliminates typical delays in film processing, thereby accelerating diagnosis and treatment planning. As highlighted by ongoing research, implementing digital workflows not only improves operational effectiveness but also promotes greater interaction among healthcare providers, leading to better care coordination. It is imperative in high-volume healthcare facilities, where timely delivery of diagnostic imaging can be decisive for patient treatment and outcome improvement (Canguit et al., 2025). Moreover, PACS integration with hospital information systems (HIS) and radiology information systems (RIS) is a significant advancement in workflow management. Leveraging HL7 interfaces to exchange data smoothly has enabled the establishment of a robust architecture to automate order management and reporting workflows. Automation is not as prone to human errors and facilitates faster processing of radiological orders and reporting results to referring clinicians. Greater interoperability enables imaging data to be queried in real time by clinicians, which improves clinical decision-making in a timely manner (Figure 12.11).

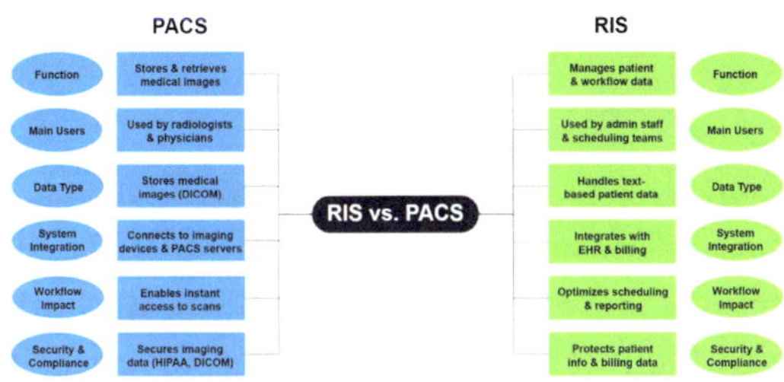

Figure 12.11. Workflow comparison between traditional imaging systems and PACS.

Source: https://blog.medicai.io/wp-content/uploads/2025/02/ris-vs-pacs-1024x527.jpg.

Consequently, the PACS system not only enhances diagnostic accuracy but also facilitates healthcare's broader goal of maximizing quality and efficiency in patient care (Pérez-Sanpablo et al., 2025). Finally, with ongoing advances in PACS technology, artificial intelligence (AI) integration further enhances workflow efficiency by optimizing data analysis and interpretation. Artificial intelligence software embedded in PACS enhances image recognition, thereby facilitating quicker anomaly identification and shorter reporting times.

For instance, studies have indicated that AI-powered software can reduce reporting time by 30-50%, thereby improving overall workflow in radiology departments. Cloud-based PACS offerings support remote access and collaboration, enhancing workflows by allowing healthcare professionals to access images and reports from anywhere, at any time. The result is a new imaging environment that not only assists radiologists but also significantly improves patient care outcomes (Canguit et al., 2025).

12.4. Challenges in Implementing PACS

Implementation of Picture Archiving and Communication Systems (PACS) in healthcare imaging frequently encounters very significant challenges, primarily resulting from organizational and technical complexities. Hospitals vary widely in internal structure, and these differences play a significant role in PACS adoption. As highlighted by recent empirical studies, the external environment —including regulations and policies influenced by health ministries —also plays a role in determining the direction of PACS implementation. For instance, Malaysian hospital observation in the study found that organizational dynamics would impact the success of the technology, and how it is used in real time, as well as long-term impacts on the healthcare infrastructure (Nor et al., 2010). It illustrates that no amount of new technology can make successful PACS integration a reality unless an overall adaptation of existing roles and relationships to the advent of the systems is considered. Other than organizational dynamics, integration of PACS into existing health information systems (HIS) and radiology information systems (RIS) poses significant challenges. Interoperability of many systems is of paramount concern, yet when different platforms and standards are applied, complications arise. The HL7 interfaces intended to facilitate information transfer between systems can often be poorly implemented or misinterpreted, leading to inefficiency and user frustration (Nor et al., 2010). This reality underscores the need for adequate training and ongoing support for medical staff as they adapt to new workflows and technologies. Smooth integration is hindered by unsmooth integration, which can stall productivity, undermine patient care, and ultimately stop the benefits of PACS adoption from being realized. Cost factors remain a barrier to PACS implementation. Excessive initial costs of technology acquisition, installation, and staff training can deter healthcare facilities, particularly in low-resource settings. Even with the technology's capacity for increased efficiency and information management, the investment often ends up translating into budget restraints affecting other vital healthcare services. Thus, hospitals will have difficulty balancing investments in PACS with their overall operational requirements, leading to a piecemeal implementation strategy. To counter such financial limitations, healthcare organizations must explore a tiered storage strategy and disaster recovery planning, which maximizes resources and costs with a guarantee of the sustainability of PACS in their imaging departments.

12.4.1. High Initial Costs

The implementation of Picture Archiving and Communication Systems (PACS) for medical imaging is typically deterred by the cost of the necessary infrastructure and technology, which is often exorbitant. These costs can include hardware and software purchases and installation charges, which can be extremely high financial burdens for health facilities. To many hospitals, especially those in resource-scarce settings, such high upfront costs might lead to resistance to adopting PACS despite its enormous potential to improve efficiency and patient care. As posited in e-health project research, the installation cost of advanced technologies might significantly affect decision-making models in healthcare institutions, considering that administrators must weigh the potential benefits against such high initial costs (Jeyaraj et al., 2011). Also, the start-up costs are further carried over into operational expenses, including training and maintenance. With the integration of the PACS, the hospital also faces the additional challenge of managing the apt system and ongoing staff training. Building an effective user base is key, as staff must be trained to use the system correctly to facilitate integration into existing routines (Figure 12.12).

PACS cost	Cost CXR	Cost CT	Cost MRI	Cost CT contrast	Cost MRI contrast
PACS software	R912 000	R912 000	R912 000	R912 000	R912 000
CR cassettes	R10 000	-	-	-	-
CT	-	R5 000 000	-	R5 000 000	-
MRI	-	-	R9 000 000	-	R9 000 000
Radiologists workstations	R204 027	R204 027	R204 027	R204 027	R204 027
CD publisher	R239 205	R239 205	R239 205	R239 205	R239 205
QC workstation	R121 738	R121 738	R121 738	R121 738	R121 738
Server and hardware	R337 982	R337 982	R337 982	R337 982	R337 982
RIS consoles including software/hardware	R618 736	R618 736	R618 736	R618 736	R618 736
X-ray unit	R991 200	-	-	-	-
Single-slot reader and operator consoles	R212 500	-	-	-	-
Training and labour (radiology)	R154 000	R154 000	R154 000	R154 000	R154 000
Training and labour (hospital)	R42 000	R42 000	R42 000	R42 000	R42 000
Network costs	R21 620	R21 620	R21 620	R21 620	R21 620
Total	**R2 953 010**	**R6 739 310**	**R10 739 310**	**R6 739 310**	**R10 739 310**

PACS, picture archiving and communications systems; CT, computed tomography; MRI, magnetic resonance imaging; CD, compact disc; RIS, radiology information system.

Figure 12.12. Overall costs for chest radiographs and CT and MRI brain scans using the PACS system.

Source: Hospital IT Budget Survey (2024).

In addition, the long-term sustainability of PACS also relies on occasional maintenance and upgrades, which further increase the investment costs for healthcare facilities. This can create inequality in the adoption of technology, with more affluent hospitals purchasing sophisticated systems, further widening disparities in healthcare quality delivery (Nor et al., 2010). Despite the challenges highlighted above, the high cost of initial PACS investment can prompt healthcare organizations to seek innovative financing mechanisms and collaborative models. For example, hospitals may pursue public-private partnerships or leverage government grants to adopt e-health technology. Such financially creative solutions can help ease some of the pressures associated with initial investments and foster more equitable uptake of PACS across diverse healthcare settings. Lastly, while initial investments in PACS can create acute barriers, strategic planning and consensus-building can enable greater integration of innovative medical imaging technologies into healthcare, thereby enhancing the overall quality of patient care (Jeyaraj et al., 2011).

12.4.2. Integration with Existing Systems

The coupling of Picture Archiving and Communication Systems (PACS) with existing health information systems, such as Hospital Information Systems (HIS) and Radiology Information Systems (RIS), is essential in the enhancement of effectiveness in medical image workflows. An unbroken data exchange is enabled by Health Level Seven (HL7) interfaces that facilitate communication among systems. This interoperability allows for streamlined processes to include patient registration, order management, and result delivery. For instance, HL7 standards ensure that imaging orders entered in the HIS are correctly delivered to the PACS, thereby reducing administrative errors and enhancing the overall quality of patient care. Furthermore, this integration goes a long way in supporting the strengthening of integrated medical informatics environments, which in turn enhances decision-making and operational efficiency in healthcare organizations (Pérez-Sanpablo et al., 2025) (Figure 12.13).

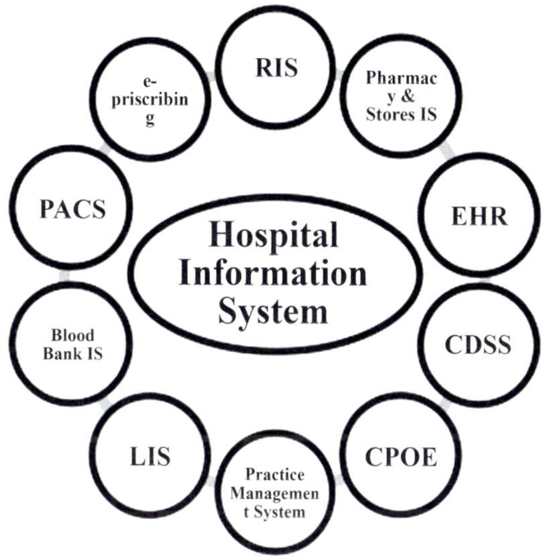

Figure 12.13. Diagram illustrating PACS integration with an existing hospital information system.

Source: https://www.researchgate.net/profile/Kevin-Lee-78/publication/254462532/figure/fig1/AS:297844062867456@1448022966291/Hospital-Information-System.png.

Beyond HL7 interfaces, the second most important aspect of the integration process is the order management functionality embedded within the PACS system. Tight integration of imaging orders and reports with patient records streamlines radiologists' and healthcare providers' workflow. An integrated order management system can help track imaging orders and monitor their completion status, thereby reducing delays in patient care. Moreover, the function of such functionality is better diagnosis accuracy, as physicians have real-time imaging data directly connected to their patients' histories. As evidenced in real-world uses, such integration also encourages a collaborative ecosystem, with better communication among radiologists and the referring professionals, hence better timely intervention and better patient outcomes (Nguyen-Chi et al., 2024). As PACS continues to evolve in the healthcare setting, integrating with reporting procedures is a critical necessity. Efficient reporting processes not only enhance report generation time but also provide consistency and accuracy in diagnostic reports. Adding NLP software to PACS enables automated report generation, resulting in a significant reduction in radiologists' report delivery time. This innovation illustrates how technological improvements are providing value to clinical settings by linking diagnostic imaging data with reporting process workflows. Moreover, by ensuring that reporting processes are HIS and RIS system-compliant, healthcare organizations can achieve a more integrated digital system that, in the long run, promotes service delivery and enforces high-quality standards of patient care (Pérez-Sanpablo et al., 2025).

12.4.3. Data Security and Privacy Concerns

Security and privacy concerns are intrinsic to the use and implementation of Picture Archiving and Communication Systems (PACS) for medical imaging. The transition from traditional film-based imaging to digital platforms increases the vulnerability of confidential patient data. The vulnerability stems from the interconnectedness of systems within healthcare facilities, where intrusions can occur through unauthorized access or inappropriate manipulation of information. The penalties for a breach of data are severe and can lead to unauthorized disclosures of personal health information and the loss of patient trust. Additionally, healthcare organizations must navigate a complex landscape of compliance requirements, such as HIPAA, that set demanding standards for safeguarding patient data. Promoting a culture of compliance and awareness among healthcare staff is essential to mitigate these risks, with an emphasis on ongoing training and system evaluation (D'Assonville et al., 2016). Data Object Definitions and Security Extensions realized via DICOM standards are essential for data integrity and confidentiality in PACS. These standards allow medical images to be securely transmitted, ensuring that data is not only properly formatted but also encrypted to prevent interception during transfer. Security mechanisms, such as user authentication and access control, are necessary to limit access to data by authorized individuals, thereby fortifying the layers of security surrounding sensitive data. Moreover, practices such as anonymizing data can further ensure privacy by removing identifiable information before images are released for review or research collaborative purposes. As healthcare relies increasingly on networked technologies, adherence to DICOM security standards becomes indispensable in safeguarding patient information and creating trust in digital imaging solutions (Rocha et al., 2023) (Figure 12.14).

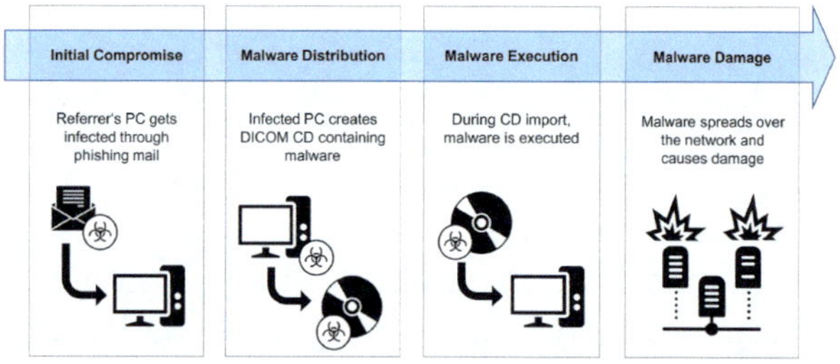

Figure 12.14. Infographic showing common data security threats and countermeasures in PACS.

Source: https://ars.els-cdn.com/content/image/1-s2.0-S1076633220301719-gr1.jpg.

Also, ongoing technological advancements, such as cloud-native PACS solutions, introduce new dimensions to data security and confidentiality concerns. While cloud computing is scalable and easy to use, it also presents potential risks in third-party data handling. Healthcare organizations must ensure that cloud providers have good security procedures and comply with applicable regulatory standards. It is also essential to establish robust disaster recovery planning. This not only prevents data loss but also supports quick recovery in the event of a security breach. Implementing intricate backup procedures and regular vulnerability scanning, institutions can improve their PACS for increasing threats. Prioritizing data protection and addressing privacy issues are ultimately key to the successful implementation and use of PACS for medical imaging, ensuring both operational efficiency and patient safety.

12.5. Future Trends in PACS

The following steps in Picture Archiving and Communication Systems (PACS) will change the world of medical imaging rather fundamentally. The most striking advance would likely be the integration of artificial intelligence (AI) and machine learning technologies. These technologies can enhance image analysis and interpretation by automating routine processes and identifying patterns that are not apparent to the human eye. AI-based algorithms can aid radiologists in diagnosis through decision-support systems that review imaging data for abnormalities. As noted, generative AI can also create user-friendly conversational interfaces to communicate with PACS, thereby improving clinician workflow and patient interaction (Zhang et al., 2023). Furthermore, the continuous evolution of AI will expand its abilities to tackle specific challenges across different medical environments, ultimately leading to quicker and more accurate diagnoses. Along with AI incorporation, cloud-native PACS solutions will likely play an instrumental role in future advancements. While cloud-based applications have adoption disadvantages due to concerns about security as well as latency, innovation within edge computing and federated learning can overcome these restraints (Figure 12.15).

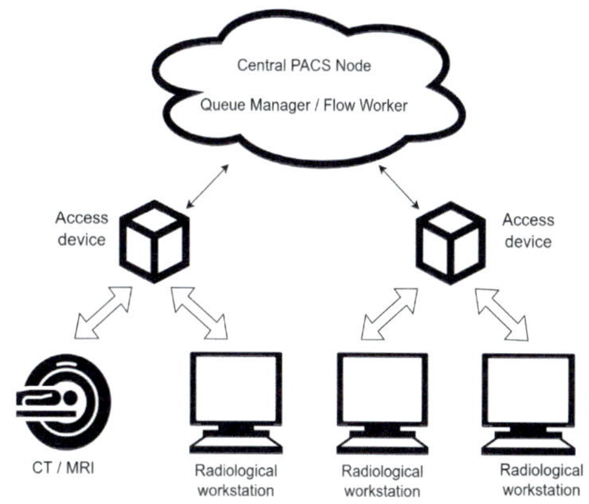

Figure 12.15. Conceptual image of PACS leveraging cloud infrastructure.

Source: https://pub.mdpi-res.com/sensors/sensors-22-08569/article_deploy/html/images/sensors-22-08569-g001.png?1667818698.

Edge computing enables closer-to-source clinical data processing, reducing latency and increasing response times, which is critical for time-critical medical applications. This shift will allow for improved data handling and analysis without compromising patient privacy or data safety. As illustrated by current studies, edge innovative processing has shown promising results superior to those of traditional centralized systems (Qayyum et al., 2022). With advances in technology, PACS deployment in clinical settings will likely change. The incorporation of enhanced visualization capabilities with PACS will also be a future-shaping trend. Improvements in user interfaces, including mobile viewer applications and advanced visualization plugins, will enhance radiologists' access to imaging information. They will accommodate 2D and 3D reconstructions, with the potential for more sophisticated analysis of complex imaging studies. Improved user interfaces will not only enhance the diagnostic opportunities but also aid interdisciplinary collaboration among healthcare providers, which is important for integrated patient care. As healthcare professionals increasingly rely on real-time access to imaging exams from various devices, user-centered design will be the most important factor in encouraging the use of these sophisticated visualization tools. As PACS continues to advance, technological integration among data, analytics, and user interfaces will become the driving force in shaping the future of medical imaging.

12.5.1. Cloud Storage Advancements

Advances in cloud storage technology have radically transformed the Picture Archiving and Communication Systems (PACS) environment in medical imaging.

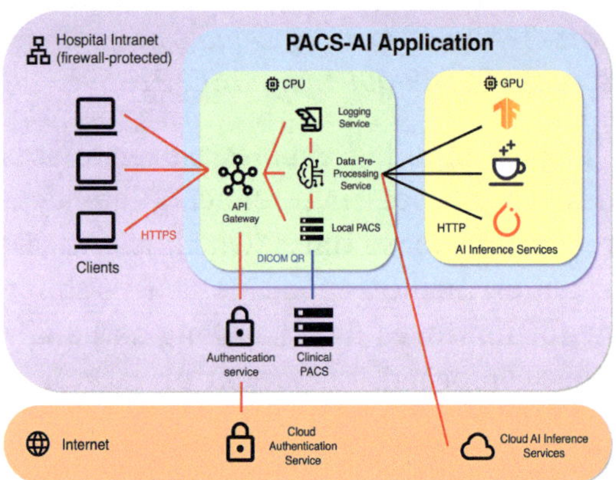

Figure 12.16. AI-driven image analysis dashboard integrated into a PACS workstation.

Source: https://onlinecjc.ca/cms/10.1016/j.cjca.2024.05.025/asset/4a60b20f-de2d-44c8-b9f3-535123f6ddee/main.assets/gr3_lrg.jpg.

Cloud-native PACS technology supports efficient storage, retrieval, and sharing of large volumes of medical images across a distributed platform. This shift towards cloud storage corresponds to the needs of modern healthcare institutions, which increasingly opt for vendor-neutral archives with multi-repository support, as highlighted by recent studies. For example, the implementation of a secure accounting system within open-source repositories demonstrates how cloud-based systems could effectively cater to multi-repository cases without undermining compliance with modern DICOM-Web protocols (Bastião et al., 2020). Moreover, these features facilitate easy horizontal integration with other systems, allowing hospitals to exchange information with various institutions more conveniently than in the past (Figure 12.16).

When health care organizations adopt cloud storage, issues such as data security, privacy, and scalability become important concerns. Cloud PACS may include advanced encryption and security measures that comply with requirements such as HIPAA while providing robust data protection. Inexpensive PACS advances in recent years, using network-attached storage and virtual private networks, illustrate how organizations can leverage cloud capabilities without paying exorbitant costs. These systems not only provide strong data storage and easy installation but also enable remote inspection of data and subsequent cloud-based backup, enhancing the efficiency of operations in smaller and mid-size facilities (Greco et al., 2022). This merger points out the potential of cloud-based storage options to minimize the cost implications of legacy PACS while maximizing availability and dependability. In addition, the ability to deploy tiered storage solutions on cloud servers expands healthcare providers' options to manage their imaging data effectively. These solutions allow sorting data by access frequency, placing high-use images in easily accessible tiers and less frequently used files in costlier, less accessible tiers. Such dynamic archiving methodology is complemented by disaster recovery planning, which uses cloud infrastructure to provide geographically distributed backups to protect against data loss. Therefore, PACS, along with auxiliary cloud storage, not only enables improved operating control but also introduces a new paradigm of scalability and redundancy into radiological imaging areas, commensurate with the expanding needs of the modern health care environment.

12.5.2. Integration with Artificial Intelligence

The integration of artificial intelligence (AI) into Picture Archiving and Communication Systems (PACS) revolutionizes medical imaging, making it much more precise and streamlined. Using machine learning algorithms, PACS can analyze large imaging datasets to assist radiologists in detecting anomalies, thereby accelerating diagnoses.

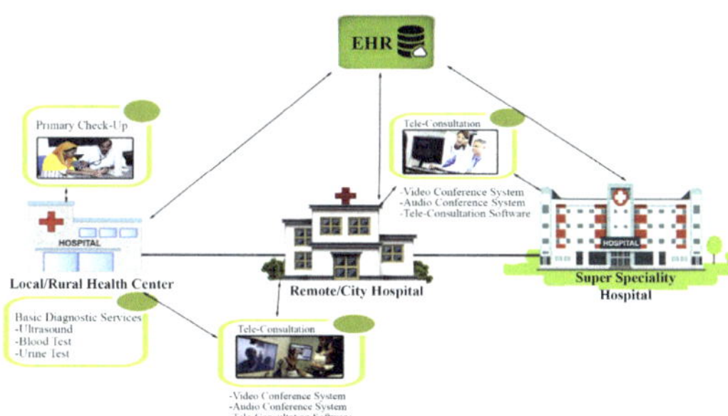

Figure 12.17. PACS enabling remote diagnostics in rural telemedicine programs.

Source: https://ars.els-cdn.com/content/image/3-s2.0-B9780128169483000143-f14-01-9780128169483.jpg.

AI-powered tools also automate report generation and improve communication between health professionals, virtually eliminating workflow bottlenecks. Doctors increasingly regard AI-enhanced PACS as vital to optimized patient outcomes, reflecting a broader healthcare industry trend toward automated systems.

Integration not only increases imaging efficiency but also enhances clinician satisfaction, as evidenced by the association between rising PACS adoption rates and improved healthcare worker experiences (Alhur et al., 2024). Additionally, AI integration into PACS enables higher-level data processing techniques to sustain the system's competency (Figure 12.17).For instance, AI software shines at leveraging historical imaging data to predict future healthcare outcomes and recommend preventive measures based on trends. This forward-thinking approach can be especially helpful in disease prevention, since PACS are no longer storage devices—they have become intelligent platforms facilitating ongoing patient care practices. In addition, the nature of AI technologies enables PACS to remain compliant with evolving DICOM standards and security extensions, addressing both the need for advanced imaging solutions and compliance with healthcare legislation (Abelha et al., 2006). Last but not least, unobtrusively integrating AI facilitates the synergy of technology and healthcare professionals toward improved medical imaging. Also of interest is how AI affects PACS user interfaces and viewing tools. Advanced visualization plugins powered by AI enable radiologists to perform more precise 2D and 3D reconstructions, resulting in clearer images of a patient's health. Such technology makes it easier to improve interaction between clinicians and PACS, allowing for user experiences that arecustomized according to individual requirements and case needs. As a result, healthcare providers have greater satisfaction and improved workflow control. AI-enhanced interfaces also facilitate mobile viewer apps, with remote access to critical imaging information and a smoother approach to patient care. This changing environment further underscores AI's core role in PACS, demonstrating its ability not only to streamline imaging processes but also to support clinicians in their decision-making (Alhur et al., 2024).

12.5.3. Expansion of Telemedicine Applications

The expansion of telemedicine applications presents a significant opportunity to enhance medical image workflows, particularly through the integration of Picture Archiving and

Communication Systems (PACS). Telemedicine enables remote consultations, broadening access for patients in rural or underserved areas. Telemedicine, by enabling radiologists to read medical images at remote locations, not only optimizes the utilization of specialist capacity but also enables timely diagnosis. Such integration also relies on the PACS infrastructure that is readily available to transfer imaging information and support remote viewing applications. When institutions implement telemedicine, they usually find that PACS functionality is well-suited to their need for flexibility and efficiency in the delivery of care. This reflects the fact that expanding the use of telemedicine applications can create strong synergy with PACS capabilities, driving improved patient outcomes and operational efficiencies in healthcare settings. The robust architecture of modern PACS partially mitigates the complexity of telemedicine solutions. Due to breakthroughs in web-based solutions and cloud-native PACS, medical professionals can view and share imaging data without being physically present at specific locations. The technologies are supported by a range of devices, including mobile devices, thereby allowing medical professionals to see essential patient data on the move. This feature is particularly beneficial in the acute care setting, where timely imaging studies are needed to support sound decision-making. Secondly, the DICOM standards used ensure that telemedicine and PACS processes are standardized and can interoperate, adding further value to each system. Through being available and of top quality as regards data integrity, PACS becomes central to effective telemedicine solution implementation, delineating a chief interrelationship that fuels innovation in medical imaging. Though there is clearly an advantage in leveraging telemedicine and PACS, there are definite hurdles to be overcome to optimize their full potential within healthcare systems. Data security, that is, transmission of private medical images, is of the utmost concern. Adherence to security extensions offered in DICOM standards then becomes crucial to safeguarding patient information in telemedicine use. Besides, the high cost of advanced PACS technology may serve as a dampener to adoption in low-resource settings; thus, non-standard solutions like DW-PACS, designed for the developing world, are crucial (Mendel et al., 2015). Transparency into the individual needs of diverse healthcare settings, such as resource-poor environments, will enable more generic telemedicine approaches. Accordingly, careful consideration of security, cost, and flexibility in telemedicine and PACS is vital to the equitable expansion of these technologies across the world's healthcare system.

12.6. Case Studies of PACS Implementation

The implementation of Picture Archiving and Communication Systems (PACS) in healthcare organizations typically reveals the intricate realities of technology adoption in various organizational contexts. A Malaysian hospital case study highlights how outside and inside forces shape the adoption and impact of medical imaging technologies. In particular, the evidence shows that the Ministry of Health role has an apparent effect on implementation strategies, proving that there is a level to which policy frameworks from outside can influence the uptake of innovations. The study also points to the interconnectedness of hospital settings, suggesting that what happens in one institution can affect how another institution approaches PACS. This connectivity is essential, as institutions benefit from collective knowledge and strategic alignment in their technology implementation, validating the need for consideration of local and overall health policies through the implementation process (Nor et al., 2010). Moreover, the experiences of implementers, such as senior managers who must carry out e-health initiatives, are crucial for understanding the determinants that facilitate or hinder PACS normalization. An empirical study grounded in the analytical framework of Normalization Process Theory (NPT) finds that successful PACS integration is underpinned by perceived advantages of professional relationships and goal alignment with organizational objectives. Implementer feedback identifies that if technology enables communication between patients and medical professionals, it establishes a collaborative context in which normalization can occur. Conversely, when things do not go as planned—that is, when misalignment or inefficiency occurs—implementers have lower levels of acceptance and integration, once more highlighting the engagement of stakeholders in the initial stages of implementation. This case-based evidence underscores the need for healthcare organizations to foster a positive organizational culture for technology adoption (Jeyaraj et al., 2011). The case studies also highlight the importance of context-specific implementation strategies that align with the unique needs and circumstances of medical facilities. The contrasted observation of differing implementation experiences is that not all systems reach the same degree of success; some hospitals integrate smoothly, while others do not. The differences may be due to variations in organizational design, staff competence, and prevailing medical imaging practices. Moreover, the interaction between these factors determines the scalability possibility of PACS technologies geographically across locations with varying infrastructural capacities. By depicting these various implementations, the case studies collectively affirm that there cannot be a one-size-fits-all solution. Instead, hospitals must reflect on their practices to inform their strategies, so that PACS not only meets clinical needs but also facilitates seamless workflow integration across the healthcare continuum (Jeyaraj et al., 2011; Nor et al., 2010).

12.6.1. Successful Implementations in Hospitals

Effective implementation of Picture Archiving and Communication Systems (PACS) in hospitals requires a deep understanding of both technical and organizational considerations. Those hospitals that have successfully implemented PACS have tended to do so alongside their current operating processes.

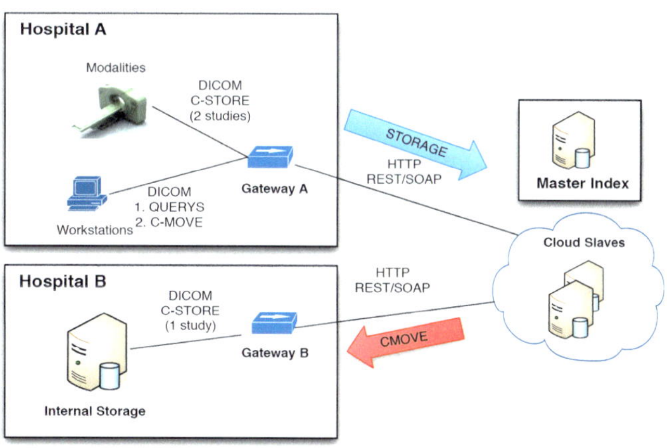

Figure 12.18. Case example of PACS deployment across multiple departments in a large hospital.

Source: https://www.researchgate.net/publication/51223746/figure/fig2/AS:339703791407111@1458003104041/An-illustrative-example-of-the-usage-of-the-PACS-Cloud-across-two-medical-centers.png.

This, in fact, is important because not only does PACS involve enormous financial investments, but it also involves clinical workforce cultural change. By developing a common framework for monitoring and evaluation, for example, the PACS integrated situational alignment (PISA) Framework proposed in the literature, the hospitals get to enhance their responsiveness to emerging technological requirements and, at the same time, optimize patient care. Organizations that prepare for this alignment in planning and implementation stages enhance their chances of achieving effective integration and maximizing PACS technology benefits (Bellika et al., 2006). Selecting an appropriate technological architecture is pivotal to the successful implementation of PACS. Solution choices such as client-server architectures, web-based solutions, and cloud-native platforms each possess distinctive strengths and weaknesses that influence their application in hospital settings (Figure 12.18).

Architectural choices should consider the institution's specific needs and infrastructure capabilities to support both optimized connectivity and system performance. Furthermore, institutions that invest in advanced visualization packages and mobile viewer software typically achieve more stable, user-friendly PACS deployments with enhanced overall usability for clinical users. With these decisions, successful organizations apply architectural agility and integration capability to design environments to facilitate effective data exchange and patient management (Bellika et al., 2006). Quality patient care is ultimately the measure of whether PACS deployments will be successful in hospitals. Quantitative benefits, such as reduced waiting times for imaging reports and improved diagnostic performance, are most essential. Successful deployment, therefore, not only focuses on the technology but also gives user training and supports its due importance during the transitional period. Properly trained personnel for new systems enhance operational effectiveness and user satisfaction. Complete backup and maintenance routines are also crucial to preserve data integrity and availability. By nurturing a culture of continual improvement and responsive feedback, hospitals can customize their PACS solutions to continue addressing clinical requirements over the long term, thereby enhancing overall patient care and institutional reputation (Batenburg et al., 2008).

12.6.2. Lessons Learned From Failed Implementations

The use of Picture Archiving and Communication Systems (PACS) in medical imaging has often been impeded by mistakes gained from unsuccessful projects. The most critical lesson is proper planning that entails not only technical specifications but also user requirements and workflows. The majority of organizations have experienced difficulties due to inadequate assessment of these key factors, resulting in systems that are not aligned with actual requirements. For instance, in digital pathology labs, failure to integrate digital case management appropriately led to inefficient workflows and user dissatisfaction. As has already been found in past experiences, systematic identification of user behavior and operational requirements can significantly enhance the success rate for PACS implementation and increase overall clinical workflow efficiency (Schwen et al., 2023) (Figure 12.19).

Another important lesson is the urgent need for staff training and support before and after PACS installation. Frequently, businesses underestimate the effort required to switch to digital technology, which generates resistance among staff who have no idea how to operate them. For example, hospitals that provided minimal training and support saw high levels of radiologist frustration, leading to under-optimization of the system and decreased diagnostic accuracy. Structured training programs for technical and operational aspects can minimize such challenges, which in turn enhances user confidence and system performance. As a result, ensuring comprehensive training and ongoing support is highly important for overcoming barriers to new technology adoption in health care settings (Qayyum et al., 2022).

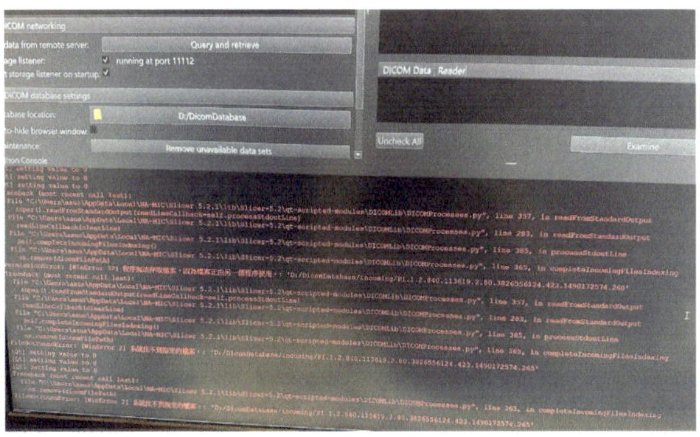

Figure 12.19. Diagram showing Dicom PACS retrieve fail rollout at a regional clinic.

Source: https://us1.discourse-cdn.com/flex002/uploads/slicer/original/3X/c/c/cc8eeef5a95bf0a867f1c0450a6ad13ceeed348c.jpeg.

Last, one of the essential takeaways from failed PACS implementations is an understanding of the evolving context of digital health technology, in particular, data security and system interoperability. With increasingly advanced cyberattacks, failed implementations have also often revealed suboptimal security measures, exposing sensitive patient information in the process. Furthermore, compatibility issues arise when new systems are not compatible with existing healthcare infrastructure, thereby preventing DICOM standards and integration with Radiology Information Systems (RIS) or Health Information Systems (HIS). Firms must conduct rigorous evaluations of their security infrastructure and interoperability challenges, adopting best practices and advanced technologies to ensure seamless integration. Through addressing these interoperability and security needs, hospitals can better plan for efficient PACS installations to meet regulatory as well as operational needs (Qayyum et al., 2022).

12.6.3. Comparative Analysis of Different PACS Solutions

The comparative analysis of different Picture Archiving and Communication Systems (PACS) solutions presents a set of capabilities and issues specific to each architecture. Traditional client-server designs are usually the backbone of most healthcare centers, offering reliability and a centralized model of data access.

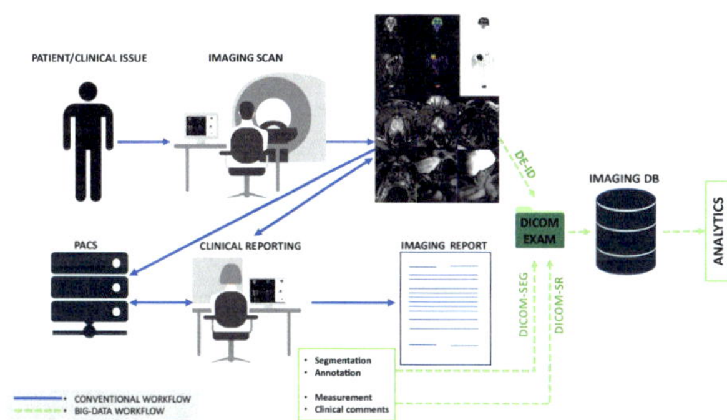

Figure 12.20. DICOM support big data management investigating its use in medical imaging community.

Source: https://media.springernature.com/lw1200/springer-static/image/art%3A10.1186%2Fs13244-021-01081-8/MediaObjects/13244_2021_1081_Fig1_HTML.png.

This will rely on local servers, however, and may increase maintenance costs and limit scalability. Conversely, web-based solutions have emerged as a viable option, enabling remote access to medical images via standard web browsers. This simplicity has facilitated easier use for better collaboration among medical professionals. Differences in network performance, however, can affect the user experience when retrieving data. As the discipline advances, cloud-native PACS solutions leverage the advantages of the cloud for increased scalability, reduced costs, and enhanced disaster recovery, but they also require stringent compliance with data protection standards to protect covered patient information (Figure 12.20).

DICOM standards form the core aspect of PACS functionality, specifying how medical data is structured and conveyed through diverse systems. Under the DICOM standards, data object definitions ensure consistent representation of medical images, enabling interoperability across different vendors' equipment. Network services defined by DICOM also aid in facilitating communication between PACS and imaging modalities, and thus enhancing workflows. But their implementation can vary across PACS solutions, creating compatibility issues that affect clinicians' smooth access to patient records. Therefore, while some systems implement DICOM-compliant services with success, others require additional customization for optimal performance. The challenge is not only in technical compliance with these standards but also in the ongoing need to teach users their correct use to improve patient treatment more effectively through proper data sharing and image archiving. Interfacing the PACS with Hospital Information Systems (HIS) and Radiology Information Systems (RIS) is a key factor in optimizing imaging processes and patient outcomes. Effective HL7 interfaces allow seamless transfer of data, orders, and reports between PACS and these clinical systems. Facilitating synchronized management of orders, PACS solutions accelerate the scheduling of imaging studies and tracking of results, thereby reducing turnaround time for diagnostic reports. Improved reporting workflows are also becoming increasingly popular, enabling radiologists to prepare, review, and release findings more efficiently. However, the degree of integration can vary significantly across PACS solutions, with some offering more robust functionality than others. As healthcare organizations strive to enhance operational effectiveness, the relative assessment of PACS solutions must consider the extent to which the systems are integrated with HIS/RIS, as this directly affects clinical workflow effectiveness and, indirectly, patient satisfaction.

SUMMARY

The evolution of Picture Archiving and Communication Systems (PACS) has dramatically changed the character of medical imaging. PACS facilitate rapid storage, retrieval, and transfer of medical images across healthcare facilities, enhancing patient diagnosis and treatment. With evolving technologies, PACS have integrated advanced features such as cloud-native systems and 3D visualization software, which not only enhance accessibility but also streamline clinical workflows. Moreover, DICOM standards enable numerous imaging modalities and systems to operate harmoniously with one another, ensuring compatibility and interoperability —a key consideration in overall healthcare delivery. The ongoing advancements in user interfaces and data management create many opportunities for PACS, looking forward to ultimately enhancing patient care quality and operational efficiency in medical imaging departments. Despite such progress, the potential of PACS is still underutilized in some areas, significantly reducing its contribution to healthcare. A recent publication indicates the sluggish adoption rate of PACS and Radiological Information Systems (RIS) among Greek public hospitals, with significant operation-related issues. Most hospitals continue to use PACS solely for image storage rather than leveraging its full capabilities. This suggests the necessity for specialized training programs and improved support systems for medical staff, which are critical in facilitating effective PACS integration. Sealing these loopholes not only reinforces image quality management but also delivers an improved experience for patients and healthcare professionals, thereby driving advancements in the field of medical imaging. In the near future, the integration of explainable Artificial Intelligence (AI) into PACS offers opportunities to enhance diagnostic accuracy and efficiency. As deep learning advances in medical imaging, there is a growing need for interpretable decision-making processes, especially in critical healthcare scenarios (Bas et al., 2022). PACS systems need to advance by incorporating AI-driven analytics that provide interpretable insights into image data, thereby assisting radiologists in making more informed decisions. Additionally, incorporating robust feedback mechanisms will enhance system flexibility and user satisfaction, ensuring that PACS will never fall out of step with the constantly evolving needs of medical professionals. The future of PACS, hence, is a matter of not just technology but also of developing a platform for continued learning and system tuning (Konstantinidis et al., 2020).

CLOSER LOOK

THE POWER OF PACS: TECHNOLOGICAL INTEGRATION DRIVING EFFICIENCY AND QUALITY IN MEDICAL IMAGING

With the shift in medical imaging, the impact of Picture Archiving and Communication Systems (PACS) is tremendous and overwhelming. PACS not only streamlines image acquisition, storage, and distribution, but also reengineers workflows within healthcare organizations. Better access to information and greater communication among departments result in smoother interdepartmental collaboration among healthcare professionals, ultimately having a positive impact on patient outcomes. For instance, PACS integration with Radiology Information Systems (RIS) and Health Information Systems (HIS) offers a single platform to handle patient records and imaging orders. Based on research, hospitals that have successfully installed PACS experience a significant reduction in the turnaround time for imaging studies, with direct consequences for treatment decisions and patient satisfaction (Nor et al., 2010). Additionally, PACS use has prompted a reevaluation of professional roles and communication in healthcare facilities. Radiographers and other clinical personnel, as they transition to the new technology, see their roles extend into realms formerly beyond their boundary of authority. The shift produces a promising work environment for increased communication between radiologic technologists and interpreting physicians. Significantly, as these groups coalesce, relationships with non-clinical staff are also altered. As PACS becomes increasingly integrated into hospital operations, it affects the social construction of medical teams, pushing clinicians to be more team-oriented in their practice of patient care (Nor et al., 2010). Not only does this enhance technical efficiency, but it also improves the quality of the medical services being offered. Moreover, as the care structure is further developed, quality assurance and effective training remain essential. Establishing standards for the use of PACS sets best practices for use in various medical specialties. This comprises in-depth training in imaging protocols, archiving requirements, and user interface operations, making all personnel competent and confident in operating the system. Highlighting quality assurance programs puts importance on the need for continuous monitoring of performance, ensuring system reliability and security. With adequate training and resources, healthcare organizations can maximize the benefits of PACS, establish effective workflows, and improve patient care. Finally, successful PACS implementation can convert into improved operational efficiency as well as health outcomes in medical imaging.

REFERENCES

1. Abdul Rahman, M. Q., Ahmad, M. S., Basharie, S. M., Baskaran, R., et al. (2020). Camera stabilizer. https://core.ac.uk/download/12007477.pdf (accessed on 14th July 2025).
2. Abelha, A., Alves, V., Analide, C., Machado, J., et al. (2006). A web-based collaboration approach for teaching in medicine. https://core.ac.uk/download/55607454.pdf (accessed on 14th July 2025).
3. Abo, A., Bailitz, J., Blaivas, M., Chilstrom, M., et al. (2018). Systemwide clinical ultrasound program development: An expert consensus model. https://core.ac.uk/download/213444194.pdf (accessed on 14th July 2025).
4. Alhur, A. (2024). Clinician acceptance and adoption of PACS in radiology services: An exploratory study. https://core.ac.uk/download/617102161.pdf (accessed on 14th July 2025).
5. Bastião, L., Costa, C., & Lebre, R. (2020). A cloud-ready architecture for shared medical imaging repository. http://arxiv.org/abs/1904.05795 (accessed on 14th July 2025).
6. Bonmatí, M. J., Mata Miquel, C., Oliver Malagelada, A., Torrent, M., et al. (2012). MammoApplet: An interactive Java applet tool for manual annotation in medical imaging. https://core.ac.uk/download/81581714.pdf (accessed on 14th July 2025).
7. Breil, B., Dugas, C., Fritz, F., Thiemann, V., et al. (2013). Mapping turnaround times (TAT) to a generic timeline: A systematic review of TAT definitions in clinical domains. https://miami.uni-muenster.de/Record/4acc6511-6fbd-40ac-923d-f29894541e96 (accessed on 14th July 2025).
8. Canguit, J. A., & Sison, M. O. (2025). Diagnostic efficiency, challenges and job satisfaction of radiologic technologists in picture archiving and communication system (PACS). *International Journal of Academic Research in Progressive Education and Development*. https://www.semanticscholar.org/paper/6e8773ca0a4c414bb361eb60203a62a8a09a1723 (accessed on 14th July 2025).
9. Christensen, B., Heaney, D. J., Larsen, F., McFarlane, A., et al. (2010). Transnational comparison: A retrospective study on e-health in sparsely populated areas of the northern periphery. https://core.ac.uk/download/4193249.pdf (accessed on 14th July 2025).
10. Costa, C., Godinho, T. M., Silva, D., Silva, A., et al. (2018). A community-driven validation service for standard medical imaging objects. https://core.ac.uk/download/565356469.pdf (accessed on 14th July 2025).
11. D'Assonville, G. A. (2016). Factors affecting the acceptance and meaningful use of picture archive and communication systems by referring clinicians in private practice. https://core.ac.uk/download/145036514.pdf (accessed on 14th July 2025).
12. Duerinckx, D. (1983). Guest editors' introduction: Digital picture archiving and communication systems in medicine. *IEEE Computer, 16*, 14–16. https://www.semanticscholar.org/paper/3dbbca54d4509f2796cedb1c8ce20ef3cdaa87d9 (accessed on 14th July 2025).
13. Greco, A., Costanza, D., Castiello, E., Meomartino, L., & Coluccia, P. (2022). Description of a low-cost picture archiving and communication system based on network-attached storage. https://core.ac.uk/download/541673461.pdf (accessed on 14th July 2025).

14. Jeyaraj, A., McDonnell, A., Nolan, A., Webster, A., Mackinnon, A. D., Jha, A. K., Yarbrough, A. K., et al. (2011). Why is it difficult to implement e-health initiatives? A qualitative study. https://core.ac.uk/download/10454.pdf (accessed on 14th July 2025).

15. Lebre, R., & Costa, C. (2021). An efficient and reliable architecture for distributing medical imaging data. *2021 International Conference on e-Health and Bioengineering (EHB).* https://www.semanticscholar.org/paper/638aaade10d9f20a3a672ccc40f26d6ffed84d01 (accessed on 14th July 2025).

16. Mendel, J. B., & Schweitzer, A. L. (2015). PACS for the developing world. https://core.ac.uk/download/56528339.pdf (accessed on 14th July 2025).

17. Mohd Nor, R. (2010). The organizational implications of medical imaging in the context of Malaysian hospitals. https://core.ac.uk/download/1588563.pdf (accessed on 14th July 2025).

18. Nguyen-Chi, N., & Nguyen-Thanh, T. (2024). Effective application of patient web portal tool for storage and return of medical records results. *2024 7th International Conference on Green Technology and Sustainable Development (GTSD).* https://www.semanticscholar.org/paper/5a15f4baa859a57dfc540020aac776cd2f7217c8 (accessed on 14th July 2025).

19. Pérez-Sanpablo, J., Quinzaños-Fresnedo, J., Gutiérrez-Martínez, J., Lozano-Rodríguez, I. G., & Roldán-Valadez, E. (2025). Transforming medical imaging: The role of artificial intelligence integration in PACS for enhanced diagnostic accuracy and workflow efficiency. *Current Medical Imaging.* https://www.semanticscholar.org/paper/07234831990987bd706bc40f023eabd193a1d8a2 (accessed on 14th July 2025).

20. Qayyum, A., Ahmad, K., Ahsan, M. A., Al-Fuqaha, A., & Qadir, J. (2022). Collaborative federated learning for healthcare: Multi-modal COVID-19 diagnosis at the edge. *IEEE Open Journal of the Computer Society, 3*, 172–184. https://doi.org/10.1109/ojcs.2022.3206407 (accessed on 14th July 2025).

21. Reiner, B. I., Hayt, D. B., Brenner, D. J., Siegel, E. L., Watkins, J., Tu, J. V., You, J. J., et al. (2008). Impact of picture archiving communication systems on rates of duplicate imaging: A before-after study. https://core.ac.uk/download/pdf/8220407.pdf (accessed on 14th July 2025).

22. Rocha, N. P., & Santos, M. (2023). A big data approach to explore medical imaging repositories based on DICOM. https://core.ac.uk/download/574337620.pdf (accessed on 14th July 2025).

23. Varghese, A. P., Naik, S., Andrabi, S. A. U. H., Luharia, A., Tivaskar, S., John, J., Mishra, G. V., et al. (2024). Emerging applications of picture archiving and communication systems and their impact on research and education: A literature review. *Cureus, 16.* https://www.semanticscholar.org/paper/066cdb62989a87161900f3f3803937092fd37432 (accessed on 14th July 2025).

24. Wong, S. T. C., & Huang, H. K. (1996). A hospital integrated framework for multimodality image base management. *IEEE Transactions on Systems, Man and Cybernetics–Part A, 26*, 455–469. https://www.semanticscholar.org/paper/8f889d163b7fca85752057a4514561e497557abb (accessed on 14th July 2025).

25. Zhang, P., & Boulos, M. N. K. (2023). Generative AI in medicine and healthcare: Promises, opportunities and challenges. *Future Internet, 15*, 286–286. https://doi.org/10.3390/fi15090286 (accessed on 14th July 2025).

INDEX

D

E

F

G

H

I

Q

R

S

T